CLINICAL GASTROENTEROLOGY

Series Editor
George Y. Wu
University of Connecticut Health Center, Farmington, CT, USA

For further volumes:
http://www.springer.com/series/7672

Christophe Faure • Carlo Di Lorenzo
Nikhil Thapar
Editors

Pediatric Neurogastroenterology

Gastrointestinal Motility and Functional Disorders in Children

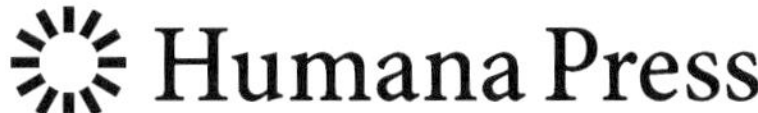

Editors
Christophe Faure
Division of Pediatric Gastroenterology
Sainte-Justine University Health Center
Department of Pediatrics
Université de Montréal
Montréal, QC, Canada

Carlo Di Lorenzo
Division of Pediatric Gastroenterology
Nationwide Children's Hospital
The Ohio State University
Columbus, OH, USA

Nikhil Thapar
Gastroenterology Unit
University College London
Institute of Child Health
Department of Paediatric
Gastroenterology,
Neurogastroenterology, and Motility
Great Ormond Street Hospital
for Children
London, UK

ISBN 978-1-60761-708-2 ISBN 978-1-60761-709-9 (eBook)
DOI 10.1007/978-1-60761-709-9
Springer New York Heidelberg Dordrecht London

Library of Congress Control Number: 2012952724

Printed on acid-free paper

Humana Press is a brand of Springer
Springer is part of Springer Science+Business Media (www.springer.com)

To my parents with love.

Christophe Faure

To my parents for their unconditioned support and love.

Carlo Di Lorenzo

To my beloved father Baldev Sahai Thapar—blessed by your and mum's unending love, forever my guiding light and inspiration.

Nikhil Thapar

To our patients and all the children afflicted by motility and sensory digestive disorders.

Christophe Faure
Carlo Di Lorenzo
Nikhil Thapar

Foreword

Welcome to the first comprehensive textbook of pediatric neurogastroenterology and motility. Thirty years have passed since the first stirrings of interest in this field. A number of factors coalesced to facilitate its evolution from oddity and anecdote to mainstream basic science, epidemiology, and clinical trials. First, there has been an increase in the number of pediatric gastroenterologists, providing a reservoir of intellectual curiosity. Second, medical technology has advanced, so that we measure more, both in the basic science laboratory and in pediatric practice. Third, medical care has improved, so that infants who were dying before diagnosis now live, for example, on parenteral nutrition, so that their pseudo-obstruction can be characterized. Fourth, the 1999 publication of pediatric Rome criteria, symptom-based criteria for the diagnosis of functional gastrointestinal disorders, inspired new investigations into mind–body pediatric medicine. Motility themed advances dominated the first 10 years. During the second 10 years the emphasis shifted to understanding visceral pain and other afferent sensory sensations and reflexes. In the past 10 years the focus has been on brain–gut interactions and the functional gastrointestinal disorders. This text admirably covers all three areas of emphasis. The publication of this volume marks the end of the beginning for pediatric neurogastroenterology and motility.

New Orleans, LA, USA — Paul Hyman

Preface

In the past 20 years, major advances have been achieved in the care of children with pediatric gastrointestinal motility and sensitivity disorders. This is a reflection of the progress that has been made understanding such conditions at the developmental and molecular level as well as the development of novel tools to investigate and treat them. These progresses have led to the birth of a new "Science", namely *Neurogastroenterology*, which is devoted to "study the interface of all aspects of the digestive system with the different branches of the nervous system" and which has now established itself as a major area of clinical practice and research. In the past two decades, there has been an almost exponential increase in publications of scientific papers in the field, a plethora of international fora for the discussion of such conditions and creation of dedicated journals with respectable citation indices. Pediatric neurogastroenterology and motility has not lagged behind and arguably is fast becoming a major and popular subspecialty in its own right.

With this book we aimed to draw upon an extensive international expertise to provide a contemporary state-of-the-art reference textbook for pediatric neurogastroenterology and motility that both specialists and generalists alike will find helpful.

Overview of the Book

The first chapters are dedicated to some of the success stories of the field. Utilizing a range of animal models and studies in the human itself we now have a remarkable understanding of the mechanisms involved in the formation of a functional enteric neuromusculature. It is clear that development is a complex spatiotemporal process involving the coordinated interplay of a number of genes regulating cellular properties and organogenesis. This complexity is reflected in one of the most commonly recognized gut motility disorders, Hirschsprung's disease, a condition caused by a failure of development of the enteric nervous system. The ontogeny of motility patterns within the GI tract is now understood in great detail. Utilizing new technologies, animal models, and some studies in humans, researchers have been able to show that GI motility is regulated by a number of mechanisms that vary in relation to stage of development, maturity, and region within the GI tract. It is very likely that the coming years will see an increasing recognition of the developmental and related functional pathogenic mechanisms underlying a range of disorders involving enteric nerves, muscles and interstitial cells of Cajal. The rich sensory innervation that not only underlies the normal functioning of the GI tract but has increasingly been implicated in a range of functional GI disorders is thoroughly described. This sensory innervation and its processing appear to be plastic and influenced by a number of disease mechanisms and clinical states including infection, inflammation, and psychological stress. How visceral sensation is modulated by the interplay among the CNS, neurogastrointestinal system, inflammation, and gut microbial ecosystem especially in relation to irritable bowel syndrome is addressed in a subsequent chapter. This theme is further developed with the discussion of the bio-psycho-social influences on enteric neuromuscular function and how the social and cultural settings of patients act to modify physiologic responses.

The belly of the book summarizes the practical investigations that are available in the pediatric neurogastroenterologist's armamentarium. In many respects this is where much of the recent strides of the field have taken place, moving it into the realms of a high-tech futuristic specialty. Major highlights have been the advent of impedance and high-resolution manometry technologies, which did not exist when the first textbook on pediatric gastrointestinal motility was published, and are now well accepted and standardized diagnostic techniques. The role of sensitivity tests, namely barostat and satiety drinking tests, in recognizing altered gut sensation as a key pathophysiologic component of functional gastrointestinal disorders, is discussed. The application to clinical investigation of radionucleotide scintigraphy tests which have seen in recent years a wider application given their improved tolerability, cost, and safety profile is described in detail. Older and newer technologies ranging from electrogastrography and transit studies to 3D-ultrasonography and the wireless motility capsule are presented. Finally, there is a discussion of autonomic function testing as indirect measure of gastrointestinal function. The subsequent chapters deal with the practical approach to and description of the pathology of disorders of enteric neuromusculature and the genetic underpinning of motility disorders.

The next section of the book focuses on a journey through the GI tract detailing motility disorders that occur in each region. Feeding and swallowing disorders in a range of GI and systemic diseases are discussed. Pediatric esophageal and gastric motor disorders are summarized, and intestinal pseudo-obstruction syndrome and Hirschsprung's diseases, the most severe forms of GI dysmotility, are discussed in great detail. The book then focuses on secondary (malformative) and postsurgical motor disorders.

The book then transitions from more classic motility disorders to functional GI disorders, arguably one of the most common and challenging group of conditions encountered by primary care providers and subspecialists. The role of the Rome criteria in developing the field of pediatric functional disorders is highlighted. Infant regurgitation and gastroesophageal reflux disease, infantile colic, functional dyspepsia, irritable bowel syndrome, cyclic vomiting syndrome, aerophagia, adolescent rumination syndrome, and functional constipation are discussed.

The final section of the book is dedicated to therapy, including pharmacotherapy, cognitive behavioral therapy, gastric electrical stimulation, intestinal transplantation, and the potential use of stem cells.

Montreal, QC, Canada	Christophe Faure
Columbus, OH, USA	Carlo Di Lorenzo
London, UK	Nikhil Thapar

Acknowledgments

To our wives (Sophie, Daniela, and Catherine) and children (Alexandre, Timothé, Clémentine, Gaspar, Mario, Cristina, Francesca, Valentina, Sachin, Nayan, and Kira) for all their love, support, and patience throughout the preparation of this book.

Montreal, QC, Canada — Christophe Faure
Columbus, OH, USA — Carlo Di Lorenzo
London, UK — Nikhil Thapar

Contents

Contributors

Anthony Alioto, PhD Department of Psychology, Nationwide Children's Hospital, Columbus, OH, USA

Ann Aspirot, MD Department of Surgery, Pediatric Surgery Division, Sainte-Justine University Health Center, University of Montreal, Montreal, QC, Canada

Elizabeth A. Beckett, PhD Discipline of Physiology, School of Medical Sciences, University of Adelaide, Adelaide, SA, Australia

Marc A. Benninga, MD, PhD Department of Pediatric Gastroenterology, Emma Children's Hospital/Academic Medical Centre, Amsterdam, The Netherlands

William Berquist, MD Pediatrics Department, Gastroenterology Division, Lucile Packard Children's Hospital, Stanford University, Stanford, CA, USA

Lorenzo Biassoni, MSc, FRCP Nuclear Medicine, Department of Radiology, Great Ormond Street Hospital for Children, London, UK

Joel C. Bornstein, PhD Department of Physiology, University of Melbourne, Melbourne, VIC, Australia

Osvaldo Borrelli, MD, PhD Division of Neurogastroenterology & Motility, Department of Paediatric Gastroenterology, Great Ormond Street Hospital for Children, London, UK

Roberta Buonavolontà, MD Department of Pediatrics, University of Naples, Naples, Italy

Rosa Burgers, MD Department of Pediatric Gastroenterology, Emma Children's Hospital/Academic Medical Centre, Amsterdam, The Netherlands

Alan J. Burns, PhD Neural Development Unit, UCL Institute of Child Health, London, UK

Julie Castilloux, MD Pediatric Department, Gastroenterology Division, Centre Hospitalier Universitaire Laval, Quebec City, QC, Canada

Gisela Chelimsky, MD Pediatric Gastroenterology Division, Pediatrics Department, Medical College of Wisconsin, Milwaukee, WI, USA

Thomas C. Chelimsky, MD Neurology Department, Medical College of Wisconsin, Milwaukee, WI, USA

Eric Chiou, MD Center for Motility and Functional Gastrointestinal Disorders, Children's Hospital Boston, Boston, MA, USA

Denesh K. Chitkara, MD Pediatric Gastroenterology and Nutrition, Goryeb Children's Hospital, Atlantic Health, Morristown, NJ, USA

Ashish Chogle, MD, MPH Pediatric Gastroenterology, Hepatology and Nutrition Division, Pediatrics Department, Children's Memorial Hospital, Northwestern University, Chicago, IL, USA

Joseph M.B. Croffie, MD, MPH Division of Gastroenterology, Pediatrics Department, James Whitcomb Riley Hospital for Children, Indianapolis, IN, USA

Thierry Devreker, MD Pediatric Gastroenterology Department, Universitair Kinderziekenhuis Brussel, Brussels, Belgium

Carlo Di Lorenzo, MD Division of Pediatric Gastroenterology, Nationwide Children's Hospital, The Ohio State University, Columbus, OH, USA

Christophe Faure, MD Division of Pediatric Gastroenterology, Department of Pediatrics, Sainte-Justine University Health Center, Université de Montréal, Montréal, QC, Canada

David R. Fleisher, MD Pediatric Gastroenterolgy Division, Department of Child Health, University of Missouri School of Medicine, Columbia, MO, USA

Alejandro Flores, MD Pediatric Gastroenterology, Tufts Medical Center, Boston, MA, USA

Sylvie Fortin, PhD Anthropology Department, Université de Montréal, Montréal, QC, Canada

John E. Fortunato, MD Department of Pediatrics, Gastroenterology Division, Wake Forest University, Winston-Salem, NC, USA

Cheryl E. Gariepy, MD Center for Molecular and Human Genetics, The Research Institute at Nationwide Children's Hospital, Columbus, OH, USA

Pediatric Gastroenterology, Hepatology and Nutrition Division, Pediatrics Department, The Ohio State University College of Medicine, Columbus, OH, USA

Jose M. Garza, MD, MS Gastroenterology, Heptaology and Nutrition Division, Pediatrics Department, Cincinnati Children's Hospital Medical Center, Cincinnati, OH, USA

Annie Gauthier, PhD Research Center, Sainte-Justine University Health Center, Montreal, QC, Canada

Valentina Giorgio Division of Neurogastroenterology & Motility, Department of Paediatric Gastroenterology, Great Ormond Street Hospital for Children, London, UK

Jonathan M. Gisser, MD MSc Center for Molecular and Human Genetics, The Research Institute at Nationwide Children's Hospital, Columbus, OH, USA

Division of Pediatric Gastroenterology, Hepatology and Nutrition, Pediatrics Department, The Ohio State University College of Medicine, Columbus, OH, USA

Liliana Gomez, MSc Research Center, Sainte-Justine University Hospital, Montreal, QC, Canada

Roberto Gomez, MD Pediatric Gastroenterology Department, Wake Forest University, Winston-Salem, NC, USA

Olivier Goulet, MD, PhD Pediatrics Department, Hôpital Necker-Enfants Malades at the University of Paris 5 René Descartes, Paris, France

Pediatric Gastroenterology-Hepatology and Nutrition and Reference Center for Rare Digestive Diseases, Intestinal Failure Rehabilitation Center, Paris, France

Ernesto Guiraldes, MD Pontificia Universidad Católica de Chile and Universidad Mayor, Santiago, Chile

Aileen F. Har, MB, BCh Division of Gastroenterology, Pediatrics Department, James Whitcomb Riley Hospital for Children, Indianapolis, IN, USA

Bruno Hauser, MD Paediatric Gastroenterology Hepatology and Nutrition Division, Paediatrics Department, Universitair Kinderziekenhuis Brussel, Brussels, Belgium

Tiffany A. Heanue, PhD Division of Molecular Neurobiology, National Institute for Medical Research, Mill Hill, London, UK

Robert O. Heuckeroth, MD, PhD Pediatric Gastroenterology Division, Pediatrics Department, Washington University School of Medicine in St. Louis, St. Louis, MO, USA

Developmental Biology, St. Louis Children's Hospital, St. Louis, MO, USA

Ryo Hotta, MD, PhD Department of Anatomy and Neuroscience, The University of Melbourne, Melbourne, AustraliaDepartment of Pediatric Surgery, Keio University School of Medicine, Tokyo, Japan

Jeffrey S. Hyams, MD Digestive Diseases, Connecticut Childrens Medical Center, University of Connecticut School of Medicine, Hartford, CT, USA

Paul E. Hyman, MD Gastroenterology Division, Children's Hospital, Louisiana State University, New Orleans, LA, USA

Sabine Irtan, MD Pediatric Surgery, Hôpital Necker-Enfants Malades, University of Paris, Paris, France

Sudarshan R. Jadcherla, MD, FRCPI, DCH, AGAF Department of Pediatrics, Division of Neonatology, Pediatric Gastroenterology and Nutrition, The Ohio State University College of Medicine and Public Health

Section of Neonatology, Nationwide Children's Hospital, Columbus, OH, USA

Ajay Kaul, MD Division of Gastroenterology, Pediatrics Department, Cincinnati Children's Hospital Medical Center, Cincinnati, OH, USA

Oren Koslowe, MD Gastroenterology and Nutrition, Pediatrics Department, Goryeb Children's Hospital/Atlantic Health System, Morristown, NJ, USA

Minou Le-Carlson, MD Pediatric Gastroenterology, Hepatology and Nutrition, Pediatrics Department, Stanford University Medical Center, Lucile Packard Children's Hospital, Palo Alto, CA, USA

Alycia Leiby, MD Pediatric Gastroenterology and Nutrition, Goryeb Children's Hospital, Atlantic Health, Morristown, NJ, USA

B.U.K. Li, MD Division of Gastroenterology, Hepatology and Nutrition, Pediatrics Department, Medical College of Wisconsin, Milwaukee, WI, USA

Keith J. Lindley, MD, PhD Division of Neurogastroenterology & Motility, Department of Paediatric Gastroenterology, Great Ormond Street Hospital for Children, London, UK

Vera Loening-Baucke, MD General Pediatric Division, Pediatrics Department, University of Iowa, Iowa City, IA, USA

Medizinische Klinik und Poliklinik, Gastroenterologie, Hepatologie and Endokrinologie, Charité Universitätsmedizin, Berlin, Germany

H. Nicole Lopez, MD Pediatrics Department, Wake Forest University School of Medicine, Winston-Salem, NC, USA

Massimo Martinelli, MD Pediatric Gastroenterology Division, Pediatrics Department, University of Naples "Federico II", Naples, Italy

Sonia Michail, MD The Children's Medical Center, Gastroenterology, One Children's Plaza, Dayton, OH, USA

Hayat Mousa, MD Pediatric Gastroenterology Hepatology and Nutrition, Department of Pediatrics, Nationwide Children Hospital, Ohio State University, Columbus, OH, USA

Dipa Natarajan, MSc, MPhil, PhD Neural Development Unit, UCL, Institute of Child Health, London, UK

Mun-Wah Ng, MD Pediatrics Department, Pediatrics Department, Gastroenterology & Nutrition Division, Children's, Hospital Los Angeles, Los Angeles, CA, USA

Samuel Nurko, MD, MPH Center for Motility and Functional Gastrointestinal Disorders, Children's Hospital, Boston, MA, USA

Taher Omari, PhD Gastroenterology Unit, Child, Youth and Women's Health Service, School of Paediatrics and Reproductive Health University of Adelaide, Adelaide, SA, Australia

Andrée Rasquin, MD Gastroenterology Division, Pediatrics Department, Hospital Ste Justine, University of Montreal, Montreal, QC, Canada

Brian P. Regan DO Pediatric Gastroenterology, Tufts Medical Center, Boston, MA, USA

Leonel Rodriguez, MD, MS Department of Medicine, Gastroenterology Division, Children's Hospital Boston, Harvard Medical School, Boston, MA, USA

José Luis Roessler, MD Pediatric Gastroenterology Division, Pediatrics Department, Hospital Félix Bulnes, Santiago de, Chile

Nathalie Rommel, MSc, PhD Department Neurosciences, Faculty of Medicine, Experimental Otorhinolaryngology, University of Leuven, Leuven, Belgium

Rachel Rosen, MD, MPH Harvard Medical School, Center for Motility and Functional Gastrointestinal Disorders Children's Hospital Boston, Boston, MA, USA

Marina Russo, MD Department of Pediatrics, University of Naples Federico II, Naples, Italy

Silvia Salvatore, MD Pediatric Department, University of Insubria, Ospedale "F. Del Ponte", Varese, Italy

Miguel Saps, MD Pediatric Gastroenterology, Hepatology and Nutrition Division, Pediatrics Department, Children's Memorial Hospital, Northwestern University, Chicago, IL, USA

Virpi Vanamo Smith, PhD, MRCPath Paediatric Surgery Unit, Institute of Child Head, University College London, London, UK

Manu R. Sood, MD(UK), FRCPCH Pediatric Gastroenterology Division, Medical College of Wisconsin, Children's Hopsital of Wisconsin, Milwaukee, WI, USA

Annamaria Staiano, MD Pediatric Gastoenterology Division, Pediatrics Department, University of Naples "Federico II", Naples, Italy

Bhanu Sunku, MD Mount Kisco Medical Group, Mount Kisco, NY, USA

Alexander Swidsinski, MD, PhD Gastroenterologie, Hepatologie and Endokrinologie, Medizinische Klinik und Poliklinik, Charité Universitätsmedizin, Berlin, Germany

Steven Teich, MD Pediatric Surgery, Nationwide Children's Hospital, Columbus, OH, USA Clinical Surgery, Pediatric Surgery, The Ohio State University, Columbus, OH, USA

Nikhil Thapar, BSc(Hon), BM(Hon), MRCP, MRCPCH, PhD Gastroenterology Unit, University College London, Institute of Child Health, Division of Neurogastroenterology and Motility, London, UK

Department of Paediatric Gastroenterology, Great Ormond Street Hospital for Children, London, UK

Rossella Turco, MD Department of Pediatrics, University of Naples Federico II, Naples, Italy

Miranda A.L. van Tilburg, PhD UNC Center for Functional GI and Motility Disorders, Chapel Hill, NC, USA

Department of Medicine, Division of Gastroenterology and Hepatology, University of North Carolina at Chapel Hill, Chapel Hill, NC, USA

Yvan Vandenplas, MD, PhD Pediatrics, Universitair Ziekenhuis Brussel, Vrye Universiteit Brussel, Brussels, Belgium

Arine M. Vlieger, MD, PhD Department of Pediatrics, St. Antonius Hospital, Nieuwegein, The Netherlands

Heather M. Young, PhD Department of Anatomy & Neuroscience, University of Melbourne, Parkville, VIC, Australia

Nader N. Youssef, MD, FAAP, FACG Adolescent Gastroenterology, Digestive Health Care Center, Hillsborough, NJ, USA

Bella Zeisler, MD Division of Digestive Diseases, Hepatology, and Nutrition, Connecticut Children's Medical Center, Hartford, CT, USA

Part I

Physiology and Development of the Enteric Neuromuscular System and Gastrointestinal Motility

1 Introduction to Gut Motility and Sensitivity

Nikhil Thapar, Christophe Faure, and Carlo Di Lorenzo

The gastrointestinal tract represents one of the most complex and diverse organ of the human body, being capable of a vast array of activities from digestion, absorption and excretion to endocrine and immune functions. Most of these functions are dependent on highly coordinated sensory and effector mechanisms which monitor the GI lumen and wall and respond to specific cues. In conjunction with a drive to maintain homeostasis within the body, the effector mechanisms regulate blood flow, adjust the balance between absorption and secretion, and coordinate mixing and propulsion of luminal contents along the length of the bowel. This latter "motility" activity is executed by region specific peristaltic contractions and emptying mechanisms, which are dependent on highly coordinated interactions among the components of the gut neuromusculature. These components comprise the intrinsic nervous system of the gut (enteric nervous system—ENS), the smooth muscle coats and interstitial cells of Cajal (Fig. 1.1). Each of them is extensive in terms of size and numbers and has an inherent complexity in structure, organization and function. Apart from genetics, further key influences on these elements come from the central and autonomic nervous systems, endocrine system, immune system, intestinal microbiota, and connective tissue. In children, this process is further complicated by ongoing development and growth of the gut and its neuromusculature, changes in environment and diet, and adaptation to postnatal life. It follows, therefore, that there are an enormous range of potential etiopathogenic factors that could result in gut motility disorders.

Sensory functions of the GI tract are similarly important in the understanding of functional disorders. Normally, most of the information originating from the GI tract does not reach the level of conscious perception and is processed in the brainstem. Other sensations such as hunger, fullness, satiety, bloating, and need to defecate that involve adapted behaviors reach the cortex. Extrinsic innervation of the GI tract is composed of vagal, spinal visceral (sympathetic) and sacral nerves. These nerves contain afferent (or sensory) fibers that transmit information from the viscera to the CNS and efferent fibers that transmit information from the CNS to the gut. At the level of

N. Thapar, B.Sc. (Hon), B.M. (Hon), M.R.C.P., M.R.C.P.C.H., Ph.D. (✉)
Division of Neurogastroenterology, and Motility, Department of Gastroenterology, Great Ormond Street Hospital, London WC1N 3JH, UK
e-mail: n.thapar@ucl.ac.uk

C. Faure, M.D.
Division of Pediatric Gastroenterology, Department of Pediatrics, Sainte-Justine University Health Center, Université de Montréal, 3175 Côte Sainte-Catherine, Montréal, H3T1C5, QC, Canada

C. Di Lorenzo, M.D.
Division of Pediatric Gastroenterology, Nationwide Children's Hospital, The Ohio State University, Columbus, OH, USA

C. Faure et al. (eds.), *Pediatric Neurogastroenterology: Gastrointestinal Motility and Functional Disorders in Children*, Clinical Gastroenterology,
DOI 10.1007/978-1-60761-709-9_1, © Springer Science+Business Media New York 2013

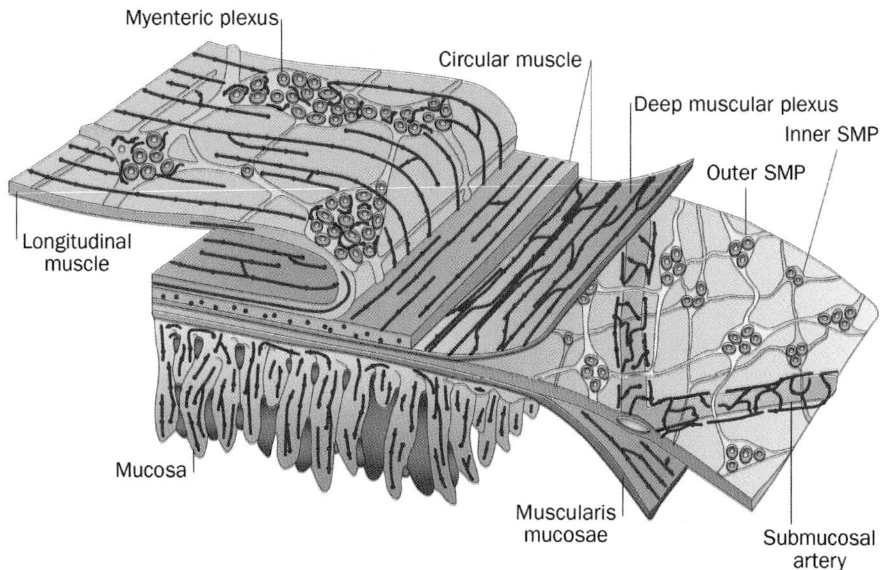

Fig. 1.1 The organization of the ENS of human and medium–large mammals. The ENS has ganglionated plexuses, the myenteric plexus between the longitudinal and circular layers of the external musculature and the SMP that has outer and inner components. Nerve fiber bundles connect the ganglia and also form plexuses that innervate the longitudinal muscle, circular muscle, muscularis mucosae, intrinsic arteries and the mucosa. Innervation of gastroenteropancreatic endocrine cells and gut-associated lymphoid tissue is also present, which is not illustrated here. Abbreviations: *ENS* enteric nervous system, *SMP* submucosal plexus. From Furness JB. The enteric nervous system and neurogastroenterology. Nat Rev Gastroenterol Hepatol. 2012;9(5):286–94. Reprinted with permission from Nature Publishing Group

the gastrointestinal tract, sensory neurons and entero-endocrine cells serve as transducers.

Central processing of visceral sensitivity is complex and involves somatosensory cortex which provides information about intensity and localization of the stimulus, the anterior cingulate cortex which mainly processes pain characteristics and cognitive aspects of the pain experience, insula which integrates internal state of the organism and the prefrontal cortex which is believed to play a key role in the integration of sensory information and in the affective aspect of the sensation. Therefore, it appears that, similar to motor disorders, visceral sensory disorders may result from multiple factors and are prone to be influenced by complex interactions with cognitive and behavioral components.

The Enteric Nervous System

The enteric nervous system (ENS) represents the intrinsic nervous system of the GI tract and is present along its entire length. It is part of the peripheral nervous system and, although it receives inputs from both the CNS and autonomic nervous systems, it is capable of functioning independently from them.

The ENS is one of the largest and more complex components of the peripheral nervous system. It contains as many neurons as the spinal cord and the enteric glial cells share their properties with those in the central nervous system (CNS) [1]. Its complexity in terms of neuronal diversity is similar to that of the CNS [1, 2]. The ENS is organized as plexuses of interconnected

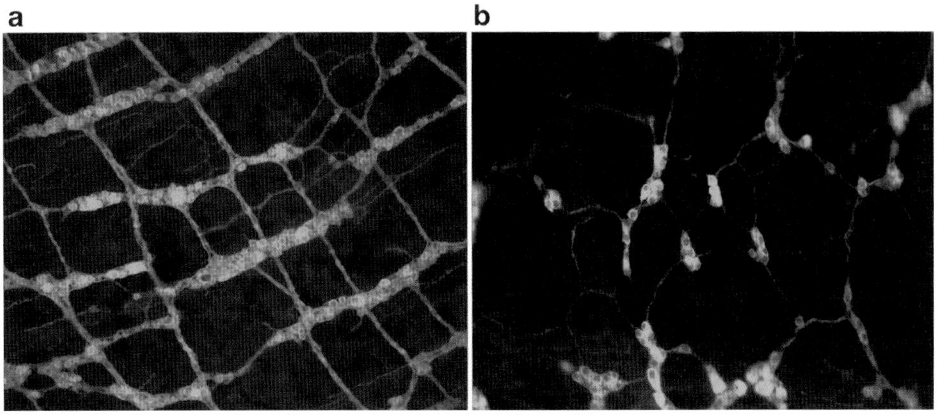

Fig. 1.2 Whole-mount preparation of rat myenteric (**a**) and submucosal (**b**) plexuses (Immunofluorescent staining with an antibody to the neuronal marker PGP9.5). Neuronal cells are grouped together in ganglia that interconnect both within and between the myenteric and submucosal plexuses. The neuronal cells of the plexuses comprise the enteric nervous system, and along with the glial cells, smooth muscle cells and interstitial cells of Cajal are the intrinsic components of the enteric neuromusculature

ganglia that enmesh the GI tract. In the small and large intestine, these plexuses are present in two distinct layers, the outer myenteric plexus that sits between the inner circular and outer longitudinal muscle layers, and the inner submucosal plexus present between the mucosa and the inner circular muscle layer (Fig. 1.2). Recent data has suggested the existence of a third mucosal plexus [3, 4] but little conclusive evidence exists thus far in humans. The ENS comprises neurons and glia organized into aggregates of cell bodies or ganglia. These are interconnected by bundles of nerve fibers that run along the individual plexuses as well as those that run between them. The real complexity of the ENS is revealed at the ultrastructural level where an intricate circuitry is evident. A variety of neuronal subtypes partakes in this and can be classed in terms of functional and structural characteristics. Subclasses include sensory and motor, excitatory and inhibitory. There are other neuronal subtypes and neurotransmitters present within the ENS (Fig. 1.3) akin to and aligned with those present in the CNS befitting the title conferred upon the ENS as the "second brain."

The development of the ENS is similarly complex. The neurons and glia of the ENS all arise from precursor cells derived from the vagal, sacral, and rostral trunk neural crest [5, 6]. These cells migrate into the oral and anal ends of the embryo and enter the foregut and hindgut [7], colonizing the entire gastrointestinal tract. ENS maturity results from an adequate number of correctly differentiated neurons with sufficient axon outgrowth and branching. Several lines of evidence show that enteric neuronal development is not completed at birth. Indeed, in the murine gut, changes in morphology of the plexuses [8] and in the total number of neurons have been reported between in the first 4 weeks of life [9]. Submucosal plexuses appear later than myenteric plexuses, and the number of submucosal neurons also increases during the same time period [10]. New post-mitotic neurons continue to appear until 3 weeks of postnatal life in the rat gut [11]. Although the pan neuronal marker PGP9.5 is present very early in the embryonic gut (E10.5 in the mouse) [12, 13], neurochemical phenotypic differentiation occurs later during embryonic development and even in postnatal life for cholinergic and peptidergic neurons [14, 15]. ENS neurochemical maturation reaches an adult pattern only at 1 month of postnatal life. In infants, data on functional maturation of the ENS are lacking but it has been reported that the number of cell bodies present within ganglia appears to change according to the age of the individual between 1 day of age and 15 years [16].

Type of neuron	Primary transmitter	Secondary transmitters, modulators	Other neurochemical markers	Study
Enteric excitatory muscle motor neuron	ACh	Tachykinin, enkephalin (presynaptic inhibition)	Calretinin, γ-aminobutyric acid	Brookes *et al.* [19]; Holzer & Holzer Petsche [20]; Grider [21]
Enteric inhibitory muscle motor neuron	Nitric oxide	VIP, ATP or ATP-like compound, carbon monoxide	PACAP, opioids	Fahrenkrug *et al.* [22]; Costa *et al.* [23]; Sanders & Ward [24]; Xue *et al.* [25]
Ascending interneuron	ACh	Tachykinin, ATP	Calretinin, enkephalin	Brookes *et al.* [26]
ChAT, NOS descending interneuron	ATP, ACh	ND	Nitric oxide, VIP	Young *et al.* [27]; Brookes [28]
ChAT, 5-HT descending interneuron	ACh	5-HT, ATP	ND	Furness & Costa [29]; Monro *et al.* [30]; Gwynne & Bornstein [31]
ChAT, somatostatin descending interneuron	ACh	ND	Somatostatin	Gwynne & Bornstein [31]; Portbury *et al.* [32]
Intrinsic sensory neuron	ACh, CGRP, tachykinin	ND	Calbindin, calretinin, IB4 binding	Grider [21]; Gwynne & Bornstein [31]; Li & Furness [33]; Johnson & Bornstein [34];
Interneurons supplying secretomotor neurons	ACh	ATP, 5-HT	ND	Suprenant [35]; Monro *et al.* [36]
Noncholinergic secretomotor neuron	VIP	PACAP	NPY (in most species)	Cassuto *et al.* [37]; Banks *et al.* [38]
Cholinergic secretomotor neuron	ACh	ND	Calretinin	Brookes *et al.* [26]; Keast *et al.* [39]
Motor neuron to gastrin cells	GRP, ACh	ND	NPY	Holst *et al.* [40]; Weiget *et al.* [41]
Motor neurons to parietal cells	ACh	Potentially VIP	ND	Nilsson *et al.* [42]; Feldman *et al.* [43]
Sympathetic neurons, motility inhibiting	Noradrenaline	ND	NPY in some species	Finkleman [44]; Macrae *et al.* [45]
Sympathetic neurons, secretion inhibiting	Noradrenaline	Somatostatin (in guinea pig)	ND	Costa & Furness [46]
Sympathetic neurons, vasoconstrictor	Noradrenaline, ATP	Potentially NPY	NPY	Dresel & Wallentin [47]; Furness [48]; Furness *et al.* [49]
Intestinofugal neurons to sympathetic ganglia	ACh	VIP	Opioid peptides, CCK, GRP	Crowcroft *et al.* [50]; Dalsgaard *et al.* [51]; Love & Szurszewski [52]

*This field continues to advance as improved pharmacological and other tools are developed. Some of the information provided here will therefore undoubtedly be superseded in the future. Further details of postsynaptic receptors have been described elsewhere [2, 31]. Abbreviations: 5-HT, 5-hydroxytryptamine; ACh, acetylcholine; CCK, cholecystokinin; ChAT, choline acetyltransferase; CGRP, calcitonin gene-related peptide; GRP, gastrin releasing peptide; ND, not determined; NPY, neuropeptide Y; NOS, nitric oxide synthase; PACAP, pituitary adenylyl-cyclase activating peptide; VIP vasoactive intestinal peptide.

Fig. 1.3 Multiple transmitters of neurons that control digestive function. From Furness JB. The enteric nervous system and Neurogastroenterology. Nat Rev Gastroenterol Hepatol. 2012;9(5):286–94. Reprinted with permission from Nature Publishing Group

Enteric Muscle Coats

The smooth muscle of the gastrointestinal tract, although present within the mucosa and the blood vessels of the submucosa, is primarily organized into three discrete muscle layers. The innermost, muscularis mucosa, sitting between the mucosa and submucosa is the least developed of these layers, being only a few cells in thickness. The other two, grouped within the muscularis propria, are much thicker and comprise the inner circular muscle layer, with its cells arranged concentrically, placed between the submucosa and the myenteric plexus of the ENS, and the outer longitudinal muscle layer, with its cells running along the long axis of the gut, placed between the myenteric plexus and the outermost serosal layer. In the small intestine, the circular muscle appears well developed in sequential segments along its length giving the appearance of concentric rings. In the large intestine, bands of smooth muscle and connective tissue (taenia coli) run on its outside along its length. Their functional role is not completely clear.

The enteric smooth muscle is organized in syncytia of cells that are electrically coupled to elicit upon activation contractile activity of the muscle layers. The circular and longitudinal muscles work in concert by contracting to result in segmentation and shortening to execute peristalsis and aboral propulsion of gastrointestinal luminal contents. Contraction of smooth muscle cells derives from two basic patterns of electrical activity across the membranes of smooth muscle cells: slow waves and spike potentials. The membrane potential of smooth muscle cells fluctuates spontaneously. These fluctuations spread to adjacent cells, resulting in "slow waves" which are waves of partial depolarization. The frequency of slow waves varies according to the localization in the GI tract: in the stomach, they occur at a frequency of 3 per minute, in the duodenum/jejunum 12–15 per minute and in the ileum 8 per minute. Slow wave activity is an intrinsic property of smooth muscle cells independent of intrinsic innervation. "Spike potentials" which result from exposition to excitatory transmitters occur at the crest of the slow waves and provoke muscle contractions at a maximal rhythm dependent upon slow wave frequency.

Interstitial Cells of Cajal

In 1893, a Spanish physician and professor of pathology provided the first description of a distinct group of cells that appeared to reside in the "interstitium" between enteric nerves and smooth muscles. These cells, now termed Interstitial cells of Cajal (ICC), are now established as critical components of the enteric neuromusculature regulating gastrointestinal motility, playing roles as pacemakers and as mediators of enteric motor neurotransmission. They are present in a number of subtypes and morphologies throughout the layers of the GI tract, each of which may relate to distinct physiological functions. One of the key ICC subtypes, ICC-MY, are present in highly branching networks within the myenteric plexus of the small intestine and appear to initiate slow waves that are spread passively to the adjacent electrically coupled smooth muscle cells. Depolarization of neighboring smooth muscle cells leads to activation of the contractile apparatus.

There has been considerable recent interest in the potential role of ICC disorders in the pathogenesis of human gut motility disorders (reviewed by Burns [17]) and loss and reduced ICC numbers have been implicated in Hirschsprung's disease, slow transit constipation, chronic intestinal pseudo-obstruction, and esophageal achalasia. Some debate exists over whether there is true loss of ICCs, de-differentiation or loss of the cell surface receptor that defines ICCs c-kit. ICCs appear capable of transdifferentiation to smooth muscle cells, a cell type with which they share the same mesenchymal progenitor. Regeneration of ICCs also appears possible [18]. Further studies are required to understand the role of ICCs in disease.

Autonomic Nervous System

The autonomic nervous system is also part of the peripheral nervous system and traditionally further subdivided into the parasympathetic and sympathetic nervous systems with craniosacral and thoracolumbar outflows respectively. As previously stated, much of the parasympathetic innervation to the GI tract travels via the vagus nerve and sacral nerves and the sympathetic along mesenteric blood vessels from the prevertebral ganglia. These tracts carry both sensory and motor innervation. Akin to their other functions these two subdivisions schematically function in opposition to each other with the parasympathetic primarily excitatory to gut function by promoting secretion and peristalsis and mainly mediating physiological (nature and composition of the intestinal content and motility and contractile tension of the smooth muscle) rather than harmful sensations, and the sympathetic inhibitory by decreasing peristalsis and reducing perfusion of the GI tract and transmitting information on potentially noxious stimuli. As a consequence, disorders of the autonomic nervous system are related to disturbances in GI motility and sensing.

References

1. Gershon MD, Chalazonitis A, Rothman TP. From neural crest to bowel: development of the enteric nervous system. J Neurobiol. 1993;24:199–214.
2. Furness JB. Types of neurons in the enteric nervous system. J Auton Nerv Syst. 2000;81:87–96.
3. Metzger M, Caldwell C, Barlow AJ, Burns AJ, Thapar N. Enteric nervous system stem cells derived from human gut mucosa for the treatment of aganglionic gut disorders. Gastroenterology. 2009;136:2214–25. e2211–13.
4. Willot S, Gauthier C, Patey N, Faure C. Nerve growth factor content is increased in the rectal mucosa of children with non-constipated irritable bowel syndrome. Neurogastroenterol Motil. 2012;24(8):734–9.

5. Le Douarin NM, Teillet MA. The migration of neural crest cells to the wall of the digestive tract in avian embryo. J Embryol Exp Morphol. 1973;30:31–48.
6. Newgreen D, Young HM. Enteric nervous system: development and developmental disturbances–part 1. Pediatr Dev Pathol. 2002;5:224–47.
7. Chalazonitis A, Rothman TP, Chen J, Vinson EN, MacLennan AJ, Gershon MD. Promotion of the development of enteric neurons and glia by neuropoietic cytokines: interactions with neurotrophin-3. Dev Biol. 1998;198:343–65.
8. Schafer KH, Hansgen A, Mestres P. Morphological changes of the myenteric plexus during early postnatal development of the rat. Anat Rec. 1999;256:20–8.
9. Faussone-Pellegrini MS, Matini P, Stach W. Differentiation of enteric plexuses and interstitial cells of Cajal in the rat gut during pre- and postnatal life. Acta Anat. 1996;155:113–25.
10. McKeown SJ, Chow CW, Young HM. Development of the submucous plexus in the large intestine of the mouse. Cell Tissue Res. 2001;303:301–5.
11. Pham TD, Gershon MD, Rothman TP. Time of origin of neurons in the murine enteric nervous system: sequence in relation to phenotype. J Comp Neurol. 1991;314:789–98.
12. Mori N, Morii H. SCG10-related neuronal growth-associated proteins in neural development, plasticity, degeneration, and aging. J Neurosci Res. 2002;70:264–73.
13. Young HM, Bergner AJ, Muller T. Acquisition of neuronal and glial markers by neural crest-derived cells in the mouse intestine. J Comp Neurol. 2003;456:1–11.
14. Vannucchi MG, Faussone-Pellegrini MS. Differentiation of cholinergic cells in the rat gut during pre- and postnatal life. Neurosci Lett. 1996;206:105–8.
15. Matini P, Mayer B, Faussone-Pellegrini MS. Neurochemical differentiation of rat enteric neurons during pre- and postnatal life. Cell Tissue Res. 1997;288:11–23.
16. Wester T, O'Briain DS, Puri P. Notable postnatal alterations in the myenteric plexus of normal human bowel. Gut. 1999;44:666–74.
17. Burns AJ. Disorders of interstitial cells of Cajal. J Pediatr Gastroenterol Nutr. 2007;45 Suppl 2:S103–6.
18. Faussone-Pellegrini MS, Vannucchi MG, Ledder O, Huang TY, Hanani M. Plasticity of interstitial cells of Cajal: a study of mouse colon. Cell Tissue Res. 2006;352(2):211–17.

Development of the Enteric Neuromuscular System

2

Tiffany A. Heanue and Alan J. Burns

Gut Embryogenesis

The gut begins to from around the fourteenth day after fertilization in the human as an endoderm-derived primitive tube that subsequently becomes surrounded by splanchnic mesoderm. Of the three germ layers, the endoderm gives rise to the epithelial lining and glands, such as the liver and pancreas, of most of the gut, the ectoderm gives rise to the oral cavity (proximal stomatodaeum) and the anus (distal proctodaeum), and the mesoderm-derived splanchnic mesenchyme gives rise to the smooth muscle and connective tissue. As development proceeds and the gut lengthens, it differentiates into three regions; foregut, midgut and hindgut. The foregut subsequently develops into the pharynx, esophagus, stomach, and the proximal portion of the duodenum down to the opening of the bile duct, as well as the liver, biliary system, and pancreas. The midgut gives rise to the remainder of the duodenum, the small intestine and portions of the large intestine including the cecum, appendix, and colon to the distal transverse colon. The hindgut develops into the distal part of the transverse colon, the descending colon, rectum, and proximal part of the anal canal. The blood supply to the foregut, midgut, and hindgut comes from the coeliac artery, the superior mesenteric artery, and the inferior mesenteric artery respectively.

Smooth Muscle Development

Stages of Smooth Muscle Development

The smooth muscle of the gut derives from the splanchic layer of the lateral plate mesoderm, which is recruited to the primitive gut tube by signals derived from the endoderm and is induced to proliferate and undergo gut-specific mesoderm differentiation (reviewed in [1]). Sonic hedgehog (Shh) is a key signaling molecule in early endoderm–mesoderm interactions. Shh is part of the Hedgehog (Hh) family of cell signals known to be involved in crucial developmental processes in both invertebrate and vertebrate species. *Shh* is expressed in the endoderm of the gut and the receptor for Hh, *Patched-1 (Ptc-1)*, is highly expressed in the adjacent mesoderm (reviewed in [2]). *Shh*$^{-/-}$ mice have significant gut defects that include a reduction in smooth muscle [3]. Gli family members (*Gli1*, *Gli2*, *Gli3*), which are all transcription factors mediating the Hh pathway, have also been shown to be involved in gut development. Thus, Hh signaling is essential for GI

T.A. Heanue, Ph.D.
Division of Molecular Neurobiology, National Institute for Medical Research, Mill Hill, London, UK

A.J. Burns, Ph.D. (✉)
Neural Development Unit, UCL Institute of Child Health, 30 Guilford Street, London, WC1N 1EH, UK
e-mail: alan.burns@ucl.ac.uk

C. Faure et al. (eds.), *Pediatric Neurogastroenterology: Gastrointestinal Motility and Functional Disorders in Children*, Clinical Gastroenterology,
DOI 10.1007/978-1-60761-709-9_2,

tract organogenesis and considerable evidence suggests that defects in this pathway are involved in a number of human gut malformations including intestinal transformation of the stomach, duodenal stenosis, reduced smooth muscle, abnormal innervation of the gut, and imperforate anus [3].

Within the embryonic gut, smooth muscle precursors are initially small and round in shape, but as differentiation proceeds, cells become elongated, circumferentially arranged and parallel to one another and will form the circular muscle layer [4]. Cells from the outer portion of the circular layer stretch radially outward, towards the presumptive longitudinal layer, then form bundles and bend perpendicularly to form an L-shape, thus acquiring the correct orientation of the longitudinal muscle layer [4]. The last layer of smooth muscle to form at the base of the mucosal villi, the muscularis mucosa, also forms during embryogenesis [4]. This radial patterning of the gut muscle occurs similarly along the length of the gastrointestinal tract, though exhibiting a rostral to caudal gradient of maturation, and takes place well before birth [5–7]. In the human gut, the longitudinal, circular, and muscluaris mucosae layers of smooth muscle are evident by week 14 of development [7] (Fig. 2.1). The massive (1,000 fold) increase in amount of the smooth muscle of the gut from embryogenesis to adult stages is accomplished by a combination of a three- to fivefold increase in cell size and a 200–300-fold increase in cell number through mitotic division of existing muscle cells [5].

Peristaltic function of the gut requires the development of the contractile apparatus of the smooth muscle cells, which enables the cell to tense and relax, thus generating the contractile motion. The contractile apparatus is composed of bundles of actin and myosin filaments (myofilaments), attached to the cell membrane via actin-rich dense bodies (the functional equivalent of Z lines in skeletal muscle). Upon receipt of contractile stimulus and signal activation, the myosin (thick) filaments slide over the actin (thin) filaments to produce cellular contractions [8]. Myofilaments are oriented in parallel arrays along the long axis of the smooth muscle cells, and cause shortening along this axis. Studies of chick embryonic intestine demonstrate that upon aggregation and elongation of muscle precursors, the first indications of the developing contractile apparatus are evident as thin bundles of actin filaments, which are initially unattached to the cell membrane [5]. Several days later, thick myosin filaments form, which are also unattached to the cell membrane. Soon after birth, however, extensive insertion of the contractile apparatus to the cell membrane is evident, with abundant microtubules oriented parallel to the cell length [5].

Although smooth muscle can undergo spontaneous contractions, coordination of these contractions is regulated through intrinsic innervation by nerves of the ENS (see below). Because smooth muscle cells of the gut are uninuclear, in contrast to multinuclear skeletal muscle cells, neighboring smooth muscle cells communicate via gap junctions to enable passage of electrical impulses between cells and to allow generation of the coordinated progressive wave contractions characteristic of the gut wall. These gap junctions are observed perinatally in intestinal smooth muscle [5] consistent with the neuronally mediated organized peristaltic activity that commences just before feeding begins at birth [9]. However, ENS- and ICC-independent organized spontaneous contractions can also be observed in mouse intestine several days before birth [9]. Because gap junctions are not observed at these earlier time points, the mechanisms enabling such organized smooth muscle contractions are currently unknown.

Smooth Muscle Development Defects in Motility Disorders

Hirschsprung disease (HSCR) is a common developmental disorder characterized by the absence of enteric neurons and glial cells in a variable portion of the distal gut [10–12]. In the aganglionic region of affected gut, the smooth muscle is tonically or spastically contracted, which leads to bowel obstruction. Why an absence of ENS neurons would lead to such muscle contraction is currently unclear. One hypothesis is that this results from the absence of innervation by fibers from relaxant neurons [13, 14], while an alternative model is that over-proliferation of

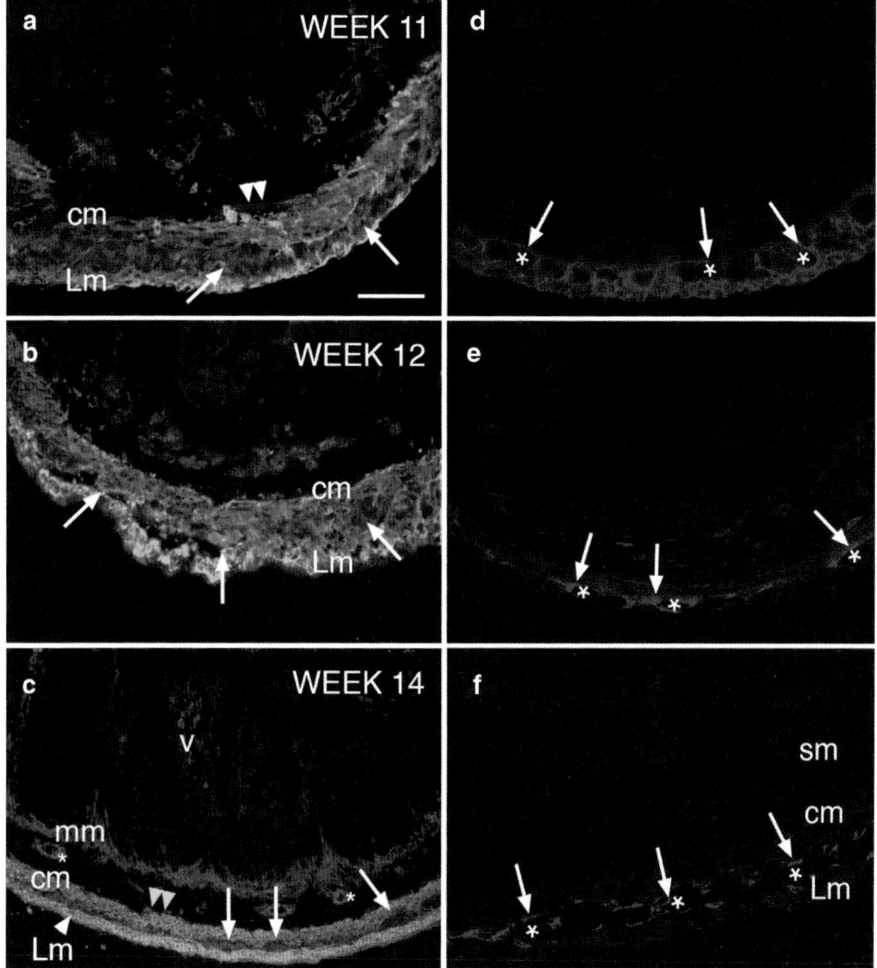

Fig. 2.1 Development of enteric nervous system, smooth muscle, and interstitial cells of cajal within the developing human gut. (**a**) At week 11 of development, α(alpha)SMA-staining (*green*) is apparent in the circular (cm) and longitudinal (Lm) muscle layers, located on either side of the p75^{NTR}-positive (*red*) cells (*arrows*) of the presumptive myenteric plexus. Occasional areas of p75^{NTR} immunoreactivity are also apparent in the region internal to the circular muscle layer, corresponding to the presumptive submucosal plexus (*double arrowheads*). (**b**) At week 12, the circular (cm) and longitudinal (Lm) muscle layers are strongly immunopositive for α(alpha)SMA. Between the muscle layers, p75^{NTR} labeling is present in groups of cells comprising myenteric ganglia (*arrows*). (**c**) At week 14, α(alpha)SMA labeling is strong in the circular (cm) and longitudinal (*arrowhead*, Lm) muscle layers, and weak in the muscularis mucosae (mm), adjacent to the villi (v). The walls of blood vessels within the submucosa are also immunopositive for α(alpha)SMA (*asterisks*). p75^{NTR} staining is present within ganglia of the myenteric plexus (*arrows*) and in nerve fibers within the submucosa (*double arrowheads*). (**d**) At week 11, Kit immunostaining is widespread within the developing smooth muscle layers, particularly surrounding (*arrows*) the presumptive myenteric ganglia (*asterisks*). At week 12 (**e**) and week 14 (**f**), Kit-positive ICC (*arrows*) is restricted to the areas surrounding ganglia (*asterisks*). Scale bar = 50 μm (**a**, **b**); 100 μ(mu)m (**c**). Reproduced with kind permission from Springer Science+Business Media B.V. from original article by Wallace AS, Burns AJ. Development of the enteric nervous system, smooth muscle and interstitial cells of Cajal in the human gastrointestinal tract. Cell Tissue Res. 2009;319:367–82 (modified from Figs. 7 and 8)

extrinsic, stimulatory nerve fibers leads to increased contractility of affected segments [15]. Further experimentation will be necessary to distinguish between these and other models and to shed light on why smooth muscle remains contracted in affected segments in HSCR.

Interestingly, in certain mouse models of HSCR, aganglionic segments exhibit an increased thickness of the circular and longitudinal muscle layers [16] and these thicker muscle regions display an increased contractile force [17, 18]. However, defects in muscle layers are not observed in all models of aganglionosis [19, 20]. Thus, muscle hypertrophy may not provide a generally applicable explanation for tonic contraction of affected segments in HSCR or other motility disorders, although it may provide explanation for disease features in some cases.

Defects in smooth muscle characterize some rare cases of chronic intestinal pseudo-obstruction (CIPO), and these are classified as myopathic CIPO, and like most cases of CIPO, are largely idiopathic [21]. Mouse mutations affecting development of gut smooth muscle have been identified, and include defects in the proliferation of smooth muscle progenitors and radial patterning of the gut [22]. Further studies in mouse or other model organisms are helping to uncover the basic cellular processes required for normal development of smooth muscle, and therefore shed light on the genesis of human gut diseases.

The Enteric Nervous System

The smooth muscle of the gut is innervated by intrinsic neurons of the enteric nervous system (ENS). In addition, extrinsic nerves, comprising vagal and spinal afferent neurons that have their cell bodies outside the gut and communicate to the CNS, make axonal connections to ENS neurons and modify their activity [23–25]. Here we focus on the gut intrinsic ENS, which can function independently of the CNS to maintain local reflex activity to control muscular mixing and peristaltic movements, changes in blood flow, and secretion of water and electrolytes [23].

The ENS consists of interconnected ganglia, containing neurons and glial cells. Ganglia are organized in two plexus layers which span the length the gut, an outer myenteric plexus, situated between the longitudinal and circular muscle layers, and an inner submucosal plexus lying between the circular muscle and the muscularis mucosae [23]. ENS neurons function to make synaptic connections to appropriate target tissues, such as the muscle, the mucosa, and the blood vessels of the gut, and to create interconnections to other ENS neurons and ganglia as well as to extrinsic neurons. Such a wide spectrum of functional requirements is satisfied by vast numbers (millions of neurons in the small intestine [26]) of different neuronal types [27]. Overall the ENS is estimated to contain more neurons than found in the spinal cord [28]. ENS glial cells are even more numerous (fourfold) than neurons and function as support cells for ENS neurons and may also play a role in modulating neuronal activity or in interactions with other gut cell types such as endothelial cells and intestinal epithelial cells [29].

Migration of ENS Precursors

The ENS derives from neural crest cells (NCC) that delaminate from the neural tube and migrate towards the developing gut tube. The primary contribution to the ENS comes from vagal NCC, which begin migration at E9.0–9.5 in the mouse, and by 4 weeks gestation in human, and enter the foregut and move in a rostral to caudal direction to colonize the entire gut tube by E14 in mouse and by 7 weeks gestation in human [7, 30, 31] (see Fig. 2.1). In addition, trunk neural crest from the posterior vagal region makes a small contribution to the foregut ENS [31], whereas the hindgut receives contribution from the sacral neural crest, which begin their migration at a later stage and enter and colonize exclusively the hindgut [32–34]. The myenteric ganglia emerges first during development, whereas the submucosal plexus originates later when cells from the myenteric plexus migrate through the circular muscle towards the submucosa [35] and are clearly seen in the submucosal region of the human intestine at 11 weeks of gestation [7] (see Fig. 2.1).

A variety of studies have examined the behavior and pattern of migratory enteric neural crest-derived cells (ENCCs) as they move into and along the developing gut. Time-lapse movies of fluorescently labeled ENCCs, which are rendered fluorescent through dye-labeling of cells or use of transgenic mice possessing fluorescent ENCCs, have enabled their migratory behaviors to be monitored. ENCCs are found to advance through the gut steadily as multicellular strands, with a few isolated cells preceding the migratory wavefront [36–38]. The pattern of advance changes as ENCCs reach the cecum, when the advancing strand pauses and cells separate and adopt a solitary meandering behavior [37]. After several hours, the cells leave the cecum and continue movement through the hindgut as a network of interconnected cells to complete gut colonization [36]. Interestingly, immature neurons that are being generated even as ENCCs are migrating through the gut (see below) also exhibit rostral to caudal migration, albeit more slowly than their ENCC precursors [39]. Approximately half of the immature neurons migrate by caudal movement of cell bodies along long leading processes [39].

Among the signals involved in directing migration of NCC along the gut, perhaps the best understood are the components of the RET pathway [40]. Loss of RET signaling results in gut aganglionosis in mice [41] and the *RET* gene is the main gene implicated in HSCR in humans [10, 42, 43]. Within the gut, the RET receptor and the glycosylphosphatidylinositol (GPI)-linked GDNF family receptor α(alpha)1 (GFRα(alpha)1) co-receptor are expressed on NCC, and the ligand, glial cell line-derived neurotrophic factor (GDNF), is expressed within the gut mesenchyme (Fig. 2.2), and has been shown, in vitro, to be a chemoattractant for NCC [44]. Consistent with this in vitro finding, GDNF is expressed in the stomach when the ENCC wavefront is in the esophagus, and is elevated in the cecum as ENCC migrate towards this distal part of the gut. Thus, it appears that NCC move towards centers of GDNF expression that are upregulated progressively further along the gut. More extensive information concerning the molecular mechanisms involved in ENS development can be found in the following reviews [11, 45, 46].

Proliferation in the ENS

The colonization of the entire gut takes place over many days (E9.0–E14 in the mouse), and from week 4 to 7 in human gestation [7], and during this period the gut is growing considerably in length, and continues to grow during further embryonic and postnatal stages. In order to continue expansion into caudal gut regions as well as to keep pace with the expanding length of the already colonized gut regions, the relatively small number of ENCCs must therefore increase greatly in number throughout the gut. For that reason, it is not surprising that proliferation of ENCCs is observed and is essentially equivalent at all rostral–caudal positions [47]. Nevertheless, the size of the starting pool of ENS progenitors has a significant impact on the capacity of ENCCs to completely colonize the gut. In a number of experimental conditions in which the initial pool of ENCCs is reduced, there is a failure of ENCC to colonize the distal gut [19, 33, 48], or to appropriately populate the entire gut with ENS neurons [49]. Moreover, mathematical models which suggest that ENCC proliferation is a key driver of colonization have been substantiated by experimental data [50].

Regarding molecular mechanisms influencing ENCC proliferation, the RET ligand, GDNF, has been shown to to increase the proliferation rate and numbers of enteric neural precursors in vitro and in vivo [49, 51, 52]. An additional level of control of GDNF/RET signaling is mediated by factors such as those within the endothelin receptor-B (EDNRB) pathway. Activation of EDNRB specifically enhances the effect of RET signaling on the proliferation of uncommitted ENS progenitors [53] and the EDNRB ligand, endothelin-3 (ET-3) which directly regulates ENCC proliferation and differentiation [54], modulates the action of GDNF by inhibiting neuronal differentiation [52]. Another mediator of GDNF/RET signaling is Prokineticin-1 (Prok-1) which has been shown to maintain proliferation and differentiation of ENCCs [55]. Another factor shown to be involved in ENCC proliferation is retinoic acid (RA), which enhances proliferation of subsets of ENS precursors and increases neuronal differentiation [56].

Differentiation in the ENS

The mature ENS contains a large variety of neuronal cell types and glial cells, with neuronal

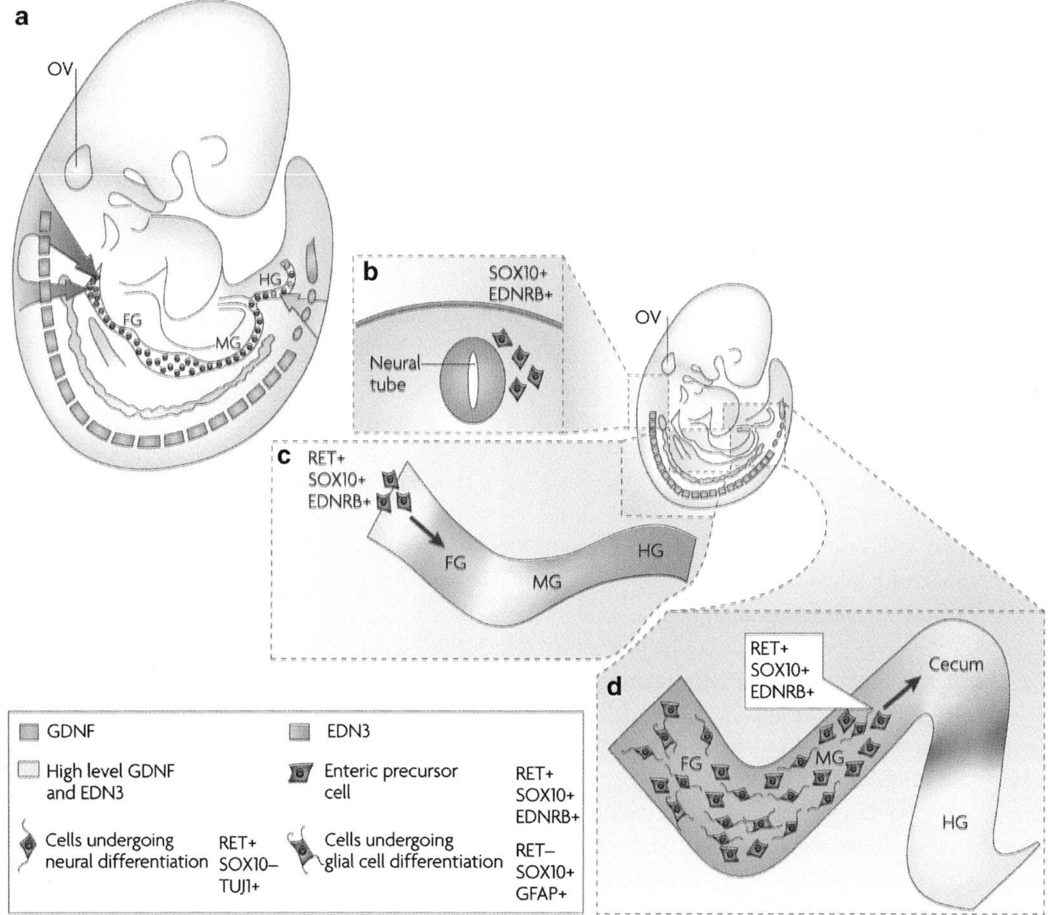

Fig. 2.2 Sources, migratory routes and gene expression in neural crest cells contributing to the ENS. (**a**) At approximately embryonic day (E) 8.5–9 in the mouse, vagal neural crest cells (*red arrow*) invade the anterior foregut and migrate in a rostral to caudal direction to colonize the entire foregut (FG), midgut (MG), cecum, and hindgut (HG) and give rise to the majority of the enteric nervous system (ENS, *red dots*). Colonization is complete by E15.5. The most caudal vagal neural crest cells, emanating from a region overlapping with the most anterior trunk neural crest cells (*blue arrow*), make a small contribution to the ENS of the esophagus and the anterior stomach (*blue dots*). Finally, sacral neural crest cells (*yellow arrow*) also make a small contribution, beginning their migration at approximately E13.5 and migrating in a caudal to rostral direction to colonize the colon (*yellow dots*). (**b**) As vagal neural crest cells (*red*) emigrate from the neural tube, they express SRY-box 10 (SOX10) and endothelin receptor B (EDNRB). (**c**) Upon entering the foregut at E9–9.5, enteric neural crest-derived cells (ENCCs) begin to express RET. Within the gut mesenchyme, the RET ligand glial cell-line-derived neurotrophic factor (GDNF) is expressed at high levels in the stomach (*green*) and the EDNRB ligand endothelin 3 (EDN3) is expressed in the midgut and hindgut (pink). (**d**) As ENCCs migrate caudally at approximately E11, they encounter high levels of GDNF and EDN3 expression in the cecum (*yellow*). Cells behind the wavefront begin progressive differentiation towards neural and glial cell fates. Beginning at E11.5, GDNF and EDN3 are expressed in the distal hindgut (not shown). Reproduced from Heanue and Pachnis (2007) Enteric nervous system development and Hirschsprung's disease: advances in genetic and stem cell studies. Nat Rev Neurosci 8(6): 466–79. Panel (**a**) modified, with permission from The Company of Biologists Ltd, from Durbec et al. (1996) Development 122(1): 349–58

types distinguishable on the basis of their morphologies, immunohistochemical profiles, and electrophysiological properties [27, 57–59]. Even as ENCCs are migrating through rostral gut regions, some of these ENCCs are undergoing neuronal differentiation [38, 60, 61], thus beginning the process of generating the wide range of neuronal cell types present in the mature ENS. Nevertheless, ENS progenitor cells persist amongst the pool of ENCCs and differentiation of distinct neuronal types continues throughout embryonic and postnatal development [59, 62]. Differentiation of glial cells begins in the late embryonic period, around E15, and continues during the postnatal period [59, 63]. Interestingly, cells expressing early neural differentiation markers can continue to proliferate [47, 60], thus providing an additional mechanism to expand ENS cell number to populate the continuously growing gut.

In order to generate the distinct classes of ENS neurons and glial cells, there is a progression during ENCC development from bipotential ENS progenitor cells, capable of giving rise to both neurons and glial cells, to separate neural and glial progenitor cells (see Fig. 2.2), and the further subdivision of neural progenitors into precursors of the distinct neuronal types. While the advancement of cells through the stages of this progressive lineage restriction can be identified using molecular markers [59] (Fig. 2.2), the factors influencing the changes in cell state are largely unknown. Indeed, in only a few instances have transcription factors, such as *Mash1*, which generates some serotonergic neurons [30], or *Hand2*, which is involved in the development of vasoactive intestinal polypeptide (VIP) neurons [64] and in terminal differentiation [65], been identified. In most cases, genes affecting development of the ENS affect all lineages due to defects in the survival or proliferation of early progenitor cells (reviewed in [45]). The capacity for ENS progenitor cells to be propagated in culture has the potential in future to complement gene deletion studies in elucidation of the factors controlling progressive ENS lineage restriction.

It has been postulated that defects in the development of specific subtypes of enteric neurons may underline certain motility disorders [27]. Although some ENS neurons of the human myenteric plexus have been characterized [66–68], the cataloging of ENS subtypes may still be too preliminary to enable motility disorders to be analyzed on this basis.

Ganglia Formation and Connectivity in the ENS

Ganglia are the functional units of the ENS. To perform their tasks, they must contain the appropriate number of neuronal subtypes and innervate appropriate targets that is, the muscle layers, the mucosa, and the blood vessels [23]. Unfortunately, the mechanisms controlling the formation of ganglia, the generation of neuronal diversity, and the processes of establishing appropriate axonal connections are not well understood. Nevertheless, some insights concerning ganglia formation can be obtained from various gut motility disorders. In contrast to HSCR patients that have hindgut aganglionosis and megacolon, gut dysmotility has also been reported in patients where enteric ganglia are abnormally large in size and/or number of neurons "hyperganglionosis," or reduced in size "hypoganglionosis." Hyperganglionosis occurs either as ganglioneuromas associated with multiple endocrine neoplasia type 2B (MEN2B), a heritable disorder due to M918T missense mutation in the RET gene [69], or as intestinal neuronal dysplasia (IND), a controversial, inconsistently described entity, characterized by features that include increased density of submucosal ganglia, increased numbers of ganglion cells per submucosal ganglion, and/or ectopic placement of ganglia [70]. Mice with mutations in the homeobox gene *Enx* (*Hox11L1*) have been suggested as a model for IND since these animals have megacolon and increased numbers of large intestinal myenteric ganglion cells [71]. In contrast to hyperganglionosis, hypoganglionosis, another condition that is difficult to diagnose by suction biopsy, has been associated with intestinal pseudo-obstruction (reviewed in [72]). Although the molecular mechanisms causing hypoganglionosis are unclear, the smaller ganglia may result from failure of development of neuronal subclasses [73], or from gene dosage effects since *Gdnf*$^{+/-}$ and *Ret*$^{+/-}$ mice have hypoganglionosis [74, 75].

Regarding establishment of neuronal projections within the ENS, limited data reveal that early-generated neurons that transiently exhibit tyrosine hydroxylase (TH) immunoreactivity have long leading processes that project caudally, and will eventually give rise to caudally projecting neurons that innervate the circular muscle or other myenteric neurons [76]. This observation led to the suggestion that the same factors that guide migration of ENCCs in a rostral to caudal direction, or the migrating ENCCs themselves, are influencing the direction of axonal outgrowth of this neuronal population. In the zebrafish, a correlation has been made between the orientation of smooth muscle cells and the direction of axonal projections; as circular muscle cells begin to differentiate and elongate around the circumferential axis, ENS neurons begin to extend axons circumferentially around the gut [77]. Whether such a putative organizer role for smooth muscle cell exists similarly in other vertebrate species is currently unknown. Finally, although neurons are known to make axonal connections to target tissues and express synaptic proteins even at embryonic stages [78–80], it is unknown at what time point neurons are making functionally active synaptic connections, as the relevant electrophysiological analysis has yet to be performed.

Development of Interstitial Cells of Cajal

ICC—Different Forms, Different Functions

Interstitial cells of Cajal (ICC) are small network-forming cells located within the gut muscle layers that were first described by the Spanish neuroanatomist Ramon Santiago y Cajal in the late 1800s. However, it has only been in the last two decades that great progress has been made in our understanding of the morphology and physiological roles of ICC. These advances have been primarily due to the discovery that ICC express *c-kit*, the proto-oncogene that encodes the receptor tyrosine kinase Kit, the ligand for which is stem cell factor (SCF), and that anti-Kit antibody specifically labels ICC [81]. Consequently, studies using anti-Kit antibody in gut from humans and laboratory animals have revealed a range of different ICC morphologies in different gut regions ([82]; for reviews see [83, 84]).

To investigate the physiological role(s) of ICC, their development was disrupted using either injection of anti-Kit antibody into mice to block ICC formation, or genetically, using *W* mutant mice that have loss-of-function mutations in the *c-kit* gene, or *steel* mutant mice that are deficient in the SCF ligand for Kit. Morphological analysis of anti-kit injected mice, or *W* or *steel* mutants, revealed a lack of ICC within the myenteric plexus of the small intestine, and physiological studies demonstrated a lack of intestinal pacemaker activity in the same gut region [81, 85–87]. Thus, these studies demonstrated that ICC associated with the myenteric plexus are necessary for pacing electrical slow wave activity and contractions within GI muscles.

In addition to the pacemaker role for ICC, a role for ICC in the mediation of neurotransmission, as originally proposed by Cajal, has seemed likely since long, thin intramuscular ICC are closely apposed to varicose nerve terminals, and electrically coupled via gap junctions to neighboring smooth muscle cells [88]. Analysis of stomach tissues from *W* mutant mice that are deficient in intramuscular ICC, but have normal patterns of enteric nerve fibers and smooth muscle cells, demonstrated a lack of nitric oxide-mediated neuroregulation of smooth muscle [88]. These, and more recent findings for other neurotransmitters confirm that intramuscular ICC play a fundamental role in the reception and transduction of both inhibitory and excitatory enteric motor neurotransmission [89].

Embryological Origin of ICC

ICC are derived from the mesoderm. Lecoin et al. [20], using quail-chick interspecies grafting to genetically label the vagal neural crest cell-derived precursors of the ENS, demonstrated that in chimeric embryos, the ENS cells were of quail (donor) origin whereas ICC were of chick (host) origin and therefore belonged to the gut mesenchyme lineage and were not neural crest-derived. These authors also cultured aneural chick gut on the chick chorioallantoic membrane and found that ICC developed in the absence of enteric neurons, thus concluding that ICC are of mesodermal origin and develop independently from the enteric neurons with which they subsequently form anatomical and functional relations. The same year, Young et al. [90], also using gut explants, but in this case from the mouse, demonstrated that when aganglionic segments of large intestine were explanted under the renal capsule of adult mice, ICC but not neurons developed in these explants, again indicating that ICC do not arise from the neural crest.

In the human gut, Kit-positive ICC have been identified as early as week 9 of development, after the colonization of the gut by NCC and following the differentiation of the circular muscle layer. Unlike these other cell types, ICC do not appear to mature in a rostrocaudal wave, as Kit immunoreactivity is more defined in the hindgut than in the midgut at week 9. ICC rapidly mature and, by week 11, Kit immunoreactivity is restricted to cells surrounding the myenteric ganglia [7] (see Fig. 2.1), in a pattern that is more organized in the midgut than in the hindgut. Similar reports of ICC surrounding myenteric ganglia have been described in the human fetal small bowel [91, 92]. ICC development in the human therefore appears to lag behind that of the ENS by at least 3 weeks and slightly behind that of smooth muscle differentiation, as evidenced by αSMA immunoreactivity. A similar developmental lag for ICC has also been reported in the mouse embryo [93], as ICC form after the gut has been colonized by neural precursors and after the development of αSMA immunopositive muscle.

ICC in Human Gastrointestinal Motility Disorders

Loss of ICC, or disruption of ICC networks, has been reported in a wide range of GI diseases, including achalasia, CIPO, HSCR, inflammatory bowel diseases, slow transit constipation, and others (for reviews see [83, 94, 95]). However, in many cases it is difficult to determine whether defects in ICC networks are the cause of motility disorders, or whether disrupted ICC networks are a consequence of gut dysfunction. For example, in disease states, a lack of Kit-labeling could either indicate an actual loss of ICC from the gut tissues, or a loss of Kit expression from ICC which are still present within the gut but that may have a different phenotype. Experimental findings support the idea that ICC can change phenotype (or loose Kit expression) under certain conditions or insult. For example, in studies where Kit receptors were blocked during development, ICC almost entirely disappeared from the small intestine. However, closer examination revealed that ICC had not undergone apoptosis, but had developed ultrastructural features similar to smooth muscle cells. These findings highlight plasticity between ICC and smooth muscle cells that is regulated by Kit signaling [96, 97]. In addition to transdifferentiation, ICC appear to have some capacity for regeneration. In experiments where the mouse intestine was exposed to a chemical insult which induced loss of the myenteric plexus associated ICC, a few weeks later, cells with ICC-like features began to reappear [98, 99]. A further example of the difficulty in interpreting potential loss/reduction of ICC is in human HSCR. Some studies of HSCR tissues have reported a reduction in the cellular density of ICC or "disrupted" ICC networks within the aganglionic region [100, 101], whereas others have observed normal ICC networks in aganglionic gut [102, 103]. The latter findings, together with the data outlined above from chick and mouse gut showing the ICC develop in gut deprived of neural crest-derived ENS precursors [20, 90, 104], suggest that ICC can develop in the absence of enteric neurons.

ENS/Smooth Muscle/ICC Developmental Interactions

Here we have outlined some key developmental aspects of gastrointestinal smooth muscle, the enteric nervous system, and ICC, which together comprise the gut neuromusculature. The neurons and glia of the ENS are derived from the neural crest, whereas the smooth muscle and ICC originate from mesoderm-derived mesenchyme. In order to colonize the entire length of the gut, and become orientated into myenteric and submucosal ganglia, NCC receive essential signaling cues expressed by the developing smooth muscle. ICC, which are closely related to smooth muscle cells but critically differ in their requirement for Kit signaling, appear to be able to develop in the absence of enteric neurons, but whether they form normal, functional networks in these circumstances is still open to debate. Smooth muscle also develops in the absence of ENS cells but in some mouse models of aganglionosis, gut muscle appears to be abnormal. Thus, developmental interrelationships between the these three cell types are crucial for formation of a functioning gastrointestinal tract, and a better understanding of how ENS cells, smooth muscle, and ICC develop and interact will help shed light on the pathophysiology of gut neuromuscular diseases.

References

1. Roberts DJ. Molecular mechanisms of development of the gastrointestinal tract. Dev Dyn. 2000;219:109–20.
2. van den Brink GR. Hedgehog signaling in development and homeostasis of the gastrointestinal tract. Physiol Rev. 2007;87:1343–75.
3. Ramalho-Santos M, Melton DA, McMahon AP. Hedgehog signals regulate multiple aspects of gastrointestinal development. Development. 2000;127:2763–72.
4. Masumoto K, Nada O, Suita S, Taguchi T, Guo R. The formation of the chick ileal muscle layers as revealed by alpha-smooth muscle actin immunohistochemistry. Anat Embryol. 2000;201:121–9.
5. Gabella G. Development of visceral smooth muscle. Results Probl Cell Differ. 2002;38:1–37.
6. McHugh KM. Molecular analysis of smooth muscle development in the mouse. Dev Dyn. 1995;204:278–90.
7. Wallace AS, Burns AJ. Development of the enteric nervous system, smooth muscle and interstitial cells of Cajal in the human gastrointestinal tract. Cell Tissue Res. 2005;319:367–82.
8. Gunst SJ, Zhang W. Actin cytoskeletal dynamics in smooth muscle: a new paradigm for the regulation of smooth muscle contraction. Am J Physiol Cell Physiol. 2008;295:C576–87.
9. Burns AJ, Roberts RR, Bornstein JC, Young HM. Development of the enteric nervous system and its role in intestinal motility during fetal and early postnatal stages. Semin Pediatr Surg. 2009;18:196–205.
10. Amiel J, Sproat-Emison E, Garcia-Barcelo M, et al. Hirschsprung disease, associated syndromes and genetics: a review. J Med Genet. 2008;45:1–14.
11. Young HM, Newgreen D, Burns AJ. The Development of the enteric nervous system in relation to Hirschsprung's disease. In: Ferretti P, Copp AJ, Tickle C, Moore G, editors. Embryos, genes and birth defects. 2nd ed. Chichester: John Wiley and Sons; 2006. p. 263–300.
12. Kenny SE, Tam PK, Garcia-Barcelo M. Hirschsprung's disease. Semin Pediatr Surg. 2010;19:194–200.
13. Bealer JF, Natuzzi ES, Buscher C, et al. Nitric oxide synthase is deficient in the aganglionic colon of patients with Hirschsprung's disease. Pediatrics. 1994;93:647–51.
14. Larsson LT, Shen Z, Ekblad E, Sundler F, Alm P, Andersson KE. Lack of neuronal nitric oxide synthase in nerve fibers of aganglionic intestine: a clue to Hirschsprung's disease. J Pediatr Gastroenterol Nutr. 1995;20:49–53.
15. Yamataka A, Miyano T, Okazaki T, Nishiye H. Correlation between extrinsic nerve fibers and synapses in the muscle layers of bowels affected by Hirschsprung's disease. J Pediatric Surg. 1992;27:1213–6.
16. Tennyson VM, Pham TD, Rothman TP, Gershon MD. Abnormalities of smooth muscle, basal laminae, and nerves in the aganglionic segments of the bowel of lethal spotted mutant mice. Anat Rec. 1986;215:267–81.
17. Hillemeier C, Biancani P. Mechanical properties of obstructed colon in a Hirschsprung's model. Gastroenterology. 1990;99:995–1000.
18. Won KJ, Torihashi S, Mitsui-Saito M, et al. Increased smooth muscle contractility of intestine in the genetic null of the endothelin ETB receptor: a rat model for long segment Hirschsprung's disease. Gut. 2002;50:355–60.
19. Barlow AJ, Wallace AS, Thapar N, Burns AJ. Critical numbers of neural crest cells are required in the pathways from the neural tube to the foregut to ensure complete enteric nervous system formation. Development. 2008;135:1681–91.
20. Lecoin L, Gabella G, Le Douarin N. Origin of the c-kit-positive interstitial cells in the avian bowel. Development. 1996;122:725–33.
21. Antonucci A, Fronzoni L, Cogliandro L, et al. Chronic intestinal pseudo-obstruction. World J Gastroenterol. 2008;14:2953–61.
22. Mao J, Kim BM, Rajurkar M, Shivdasani RA, McMahon AP. Hedgehog signaling controls mesenchymal growth in the developing mammalian digestive tract. Development. 2010;137:1721–9.
23. Furness JB. The enteric nervous system. Oxford: Blackwell Publishing; 2006.
24. Furness JB, Jones C, Nurgali K, Clerc N. Intrinsic primary afferent neurons and nerve circuits within the intestine. Prog Neurobiol. 2004;72:143–64.

25. Powley TL. Vagal input to the enteric nervous system. Gut. 2000;47 Suppl 4:iv30–2. discussion iv36.
26. Gabella G. The number of neurons in the small intestine of mice, guinea-pigs and sheep. Neuroscience. 1987;22:737–52.
27. Hao MM, Young HM. Development of enteric neuron diversity. J Cell Mol Med. 2009;13:1193–210.
28. Gershon MD, Chalazonitis A, Rothman TP. From neural crest to bowel: development of the enteric nervous system. J Neurobiol. 1993;24:199–214.
29. Ruhl A. Glial cells in the gut. Neurogastroenterol Motil. 2005;17:777–90.
30. Blaugrund E, Pham TD, Tennyson VM, et al. Distinct subpopulations of enteric neuronal progenitors defined by time of development, sympathoadrenal lineage markers and Mash-1-dependence. Development. 1996;122:309–20.
31. Durbec PL, Larsson-Blomberg LB, Schuchardt A, Costantini F, Pachnis V. Common origin and developmental dependence on c-ret of subsets of enteric and sympathetic neuroblasts. Development. 1996;122:349–58.
32. Anderson RB, Stewart AL, Young HM. Phenotypes of neural-crest-derived cells in vagal and sacral pathways. Cell Tissue Res. 2006;323:11–25.
33. Burns AJ, Champeval D, Le Douarin NM. Sacral neural crest cells colonise aganglionic hindgut in vivo but fail to compensate for lack of enteric ganglia. Dev Biol. 2000;219:30–43.
34. Burns AJ, Le Douarin NM. The sacral neural crest contributes neurons and glia to the post-umbilical gut: spatiotemporal analysis of the development of the enteric nervous system. Development. 1998;125:4335–47.
35. McKeown SJ, Chow CW, Young HM. Development of the submucous plexus in the large intestine of the mouse. Cell Tissue Res. 2001;303:301–5.
36. Druckenbrod NR, Epstein ML. The pattern of neural crest advance in the cecum and colon. Dev Biol. 2005;287:125–33.
37. Druckenbrod NR, Epstein ML. Behavior of enteric neural crest-derived cells varies with respect to the migratory wavefront. Dev Dyn. 2007;236:84–92.
38. Young HM, Bergner AJ, Anderson RB, et al. Dynamics of neural crest-derived cell migration in the embryonic mouse gut. Dev Biol. 2004;270:455–73.
39. Hao MM, Anderson RB, Kobayashi K, Whitington PM, Young HM. The migratory behavior of immature enteric neurons. Dev Neurobiol. 2009;69:22–35.
40. Manie S, Santoro M, Fusco A, Billaud M. The RET receptor: function in development and dysfunction in congenital malformation. Trends Genet. 2001;17:580–9.
41. Schuchardt A, D'Agati V, Larsson-Blomberg L, Costantini F, Pachnis V. Defects in the kidney and enteric nervous system of mice lacking the tyrosine kinase receptor Ret. Nature. 1994;367:380–3.
42. Tam PK, Garcia-Barcelo M. Genetic basis of Hirschsprung's disease. Pediatr Surg Int. 2009;25:543–58.
43. Lantieri F, Griseri P, Ceccherini I. Molecular mechanisms of RET-induced Hirschsprung pathogenesis. Ann Med. 2006;38:11–9.
44. Young HM, Hearn CJ, Farlie PG, Canty AJ, Thomas PQ, Newgreen DF. GDNF is a chemoattractant for enteric neural cells. Dev Biol. 2001;229:503–16.
45. Heanue TA, Pachnis V. Enteric nervous system development and Hirschsprung's disease: advances in genetic and stem cell studies. Nat Rev. 2007;8:466–79.
46. Gershon MD. Developmental determinants of the independence and complexity of the enteric nervous system. Trends Neurosci. 2010;33:446–56.
47. Young HM, Turner KN, Bergner AJ. The location and phenotype of proliferating neural-crest-derived cells in the developing mouse gut. Cell Tissue Res. 2005;320:1–9.
48. Stanchina L, Baral V, Robert F, et al. Interactions between Sox10, Edn3 and Ednrb during enteric nervous system and melanocyte development. Dev Biol. 2006;295:232–49.
49. Gianino S, Grider JR, Cresswell J, Enomoto H, Heuckeroth RO. GDNF availability determines enteric neuron number by controlling precursor proliferation. Development. 2003;130:2187–98.
50. Simpson MJ, Zhang DC, Mariani M, Landman KA, Newgreen DF. Cell proliferation drives neural crest cell invasion of the intestine. Dev Biol. 2007;302:553–68.
51. Heuckeroth RO, Lampe PA, Johnson EM, Milbrandt J. Neurturin and GDNF promote proliferation and survival of enteric neuron and glial progenitors in vitro. Dev Biol. 1998;200:116–29.
52. Hearn CJ, Murphy M, Newgreen D. GDNF and ET-3 differentially modulate the numbers of avian enteric neural crest cells and enteric neurons in vitro. Dev Biol. 1998;197:93–105.
53. Barlow A, de Graaff E, Pachnis V. Enteric nervous system progenitors are coordinately controlled by the G protein-coupled receptor EDNRB and the receptor tyrosine kinase RET. Neuron. 2003;40:905–16.
54. Nagy N, Goldstein AM. Endothelin-3 regulates neural crest cell proliferation and differentiation in the hindgut enteric nervous system. Dev Biol. 2006;293(1):203–17.
55. Ngan ES, Shum CK, Poon HC, et al. Prokineticin-1 (Prok-1) works coordinately with glial cell line-derived neurotrophic factor (GDNF) to mediate proliferation and differentiation of enteric neural crest cells. Biochim Biophys Acta. 2008;1783:467–78.
56. Sato Y, Heuckeroth RO. Retinoic acid regulates murine enteric nervous system precursor proliferation, enhances neuronal precursor differentiation, and reduces neurite growth in vitro. Dev Biol. 2008;320:185–98.
57. Rothman TP, Sherman D, Cochard P, Gershon MD. Development of the monoaminergic innervation of the avian gut: transient and permanent expression of phenotypic markers. Dev Biol. 1986;116:357–80.

58. Sang Q, Young HM. The identification and chemical coding of cholinergic neurons in the small and large intestine of the mouse. Anat Rec. 1998;251:185–99.
59. Young HM, Bergner AJ, Muller T. Acquisition of neuronal and glial markers by neural crest-derived cells in the mouse intestine. J Comp Neurol. 2003;456:1–11.
60. Baetge G, Gershon MD. Transient catecholaminergic (TC) cells in the vagus nerves and bowel of fetal mice: relationship to the development of enteric neurons. Dev Biol. 1989;132:189–211.
61. Young HM, Ciampoli D, Hsuan J, Canty AJ. Expression of Ret-, p75(NTR)-, Phox2a-, Phox2b-, and tyrosine hydroxylase-immunoreactivity by undifferentiated neural crest-derived cells and different classes of enteric neurons in the embryonic mouse gut. Dev Dyn. 1999;216:137–52.
62. Pham TD, Gershon MD, Rothman TP. Time of origin of neurons in the murine enteric nervous system: sequence in relation to phenotype. J Comp Neurol. 1991;314:789–98.
63. Rothman TP, Tennyson VM, Gershon MD. Colonization of the bowel by the precursors of enteric glia: studies of normal and congenitally aganglionic mutant mice. J Comp Neurol. 1986;252:493–506.
64. Hendershot TJ, Liu H, Sarkar AA, et al. Expression of Hand2 is sufficient for neurogenesis and cell type-specific gene expression in the enteric nervous system. Dev Dyn. 2007;236:93–105.
65. D'Autreaux F, Morikawa Y, Cserjesi P, Gershon MD. Hand2 is necessary for terminal differentiation of enteric neurons from crest-derived precursors but not for their migration into the gut or for formation of glia. Development. 2007;134:2237–49.
66. Hens J, Vanderwinden JM, De Laet MH, Scheuermann DW, Timmermans JP. Morphological and neurochemical identification of enteric neurones with mucosal projections in the human small intestine. J Neurochem. 2001;76:464–71.
67. Porter AJ, Wattchow DA, Brookes SJ, Costa M. The neurochemical coding and projections of circular muscle motor neurons in the human colon. Gastroenterology. 1997;113:1916–23.
68. Wattchow DA, Porter AJ, Brookes SJ, Costa M. The polarity of neurochemically defined myenteric neurons in the human colon. Gastroenterology. 1997;113:497–506.
69. Hofstra RM, Landsvater RM, Ceccherini I, et al. A mutation in the RET proto-oncogene associated with multiple endocrine neoplasia type 2B and sporadic medullary thyroid carcinoma. Nature. 1994;367:375–6.
70. Meier-Ruge WA, Bruder E, Kapur RP. Intestinal neuronal dysplasia type B: one giant ganglion is not good enough. Pediatr Dev Pathol. 2006;9:444–52.
71. Shirasawa S, Yunker AM, Roth KA, Brown GA, Horning S, Korsmeyer SJ. Enx (Hox11L1)-deficient mice develop myenteric neuronal hyperplasia and megacolon. Nature Med. 1997;3:646–50.
72. Dingemann J, Puri P. Isolated hypoganglionosis: systematic review of a rare intestinal innervation defect. Pediatr Surg Int. 2010;26:1111–5.
73. Gershon MD. The enteric nervous system: a second brain. Hosp Pract (Off Ed). 1999;34:31–2. 35–38, 41–32 passim.
74. Shen L, Pichel JG, Mayeli T, Sariola H, Lu B, Westphal H. Gdnf haploinsufficiency causes Hirschsprung-like intestinal obstruction and early-onset lethality in mice. Am J Hum Genet. 2002;70:435–47.
75. Carniti C, Belluco S, Riccardi E, et al. The Ret(C620R) mutation affects renal and enteric development in a mouse model of Hirschsprung's disease. Am J Pathol. 2006;168:1262–75.
76. Young HM, Jones BR, McKeown SJ. The projections of early enteric neurons are influenced by the direction of neural crest cell migration. J Neurosci. 2002;22:6005–18.
77. Olden T, Akhtar T, Beckman SA, Wallace KN. Differentiation of the zebrafish enteric nervous system and intestinal smooth muscle. Genesis. 2008;46:484–98.
78. Heanue TA, Pachnis V. Expression profiling the developing mammalian enteric nervous system identifies marker and candidate Hirschsprung disease genes. PNAS 2006;103:6919–24.
79. Vannucchi MG, Faussone-Pellegrini MS. Synapse formation during neuron differentiation: an in situ study of the myenteric plexus during murine embryonic life. J Comp Neurol. 2000;425:369–81.
80. Vohra BP, Tsuji K, Nagashimada M, et al. Differential gene expression and functional analysis implicate novel mechanisms in enteric nervous system precursor migration and neuritogenesis. Dev Biol. 2006;298:259–71.
81. Maeda H, Yamagata A, Nishikawa S, et al. Requirement of c-kit for development of intestinal pacemaker system. Development. 1992;116:369–75.
82. Burns AJ, Herbert TM, Ward SM, Sanders KM. Interstitial cells of Cajal in the guinea-pig gastrointestinal tract as revealed by c-Kit immunohistochemistry. Cell Tissue Res. 1997;290:11–20.
83. Vanderwinden JM, Rumessen JJ. Interstitial cells of Cajal in human gut and gastrointestinal disease. Microsc Res Tech. 1999;47:344–60.
84. Rumessen JJ, Vanderwinden JM. Interstitial cells in the musculature of the gastrointestinal tract: Cajal and beyond. Int Rev Cytol. 2003;229:115–208.
85. Torihashi S, Ward SM, Nishikawa S, Nishi K, Kobayashi S, Sanders KM. c-kit-dependent development of interstitial cells and electrical activity in the murine gastrointestinal tract. Cell Tissue Res. 1995;280:97–111.
86. Ward SM, Burns AJ, Torihashi S, Sanders KM. Mutation of the proto-oncogene c-kit blocks development of interstitial cells and electrical rhythmicity in murine intestine. J Physiol. 1994;480:91–7.
87. Huizinga JD, Thuneberg L, Kluppel M, Malysz J, Mikkelsen HB, Bernstein A. W/kit gene required for interstitial cells of Cajal and for intestinal pacemaker activity. Nature. 1995;373:347–9.

88. Burns AJ, Lomax AE, Torihashi S, Sanders KM, Ward SM. Interstitial cells of Cajal mediate inhibitory neurotransmission in the stomach. PNAS 1996;93:12008–13.
89. Ward SM, McLaren GJ, Sanders KM. Interstitial cells of Cajal in the deep muscular plexus mediate enteric motor neurotransmission in the mouse small intestine. J Physiol. 2006;573:147–59.
90. Young HM, Ciampoli D, Southwell BR, Newgreen DF. Origin of interstitial cells of Cajal in the mouse intestine. Dev Biol. 1996;180:97–107.
91. Kenny SE, Connell G, Woodward MN, et al. Ontogeny of interstitial cells of Cajal in the human intestine. J Pediatr Surg. 1999;34:1241–7.
92. Wester T, Eriksson L, Olsson Y, Olsen L. Interstitial cells of Cajal in the human fetal small bowel as shown by c-kit immunohistochemistry. Gut. 1999;44:65–71.
93. Wu JJ, Rothman TP, Gershon MD. Development of the interstitial cell of Cajal: origin, kit dependence and neuronal and nonneuronal sources of kit ligand. J Neurosci Res. 2000;59:384–401.
94. Sanders KM, Ordog T, Ward SM. Physiology and pathophysiology of the interstitial cells of Cajal: from bench to bedside. IV. Genetic and animal models of GI motility disorders caused by loss of interstitial cells of Cajal. Am J Physiol Gastrointest Liver Physiol. 2002;282:G747–56.
95. Burns AJ. Disorders of interstitial cells of Cajal. J Pediatr Gastroenterol Nutr. 2007;45 Suppl 2:S103–6.
96. Torihashi S, Nishi K, Tokutomi Y, Nishi T, Ward S, Sanders KM. Blockade of kit signaling induces transdifferentiation of interstitial cells of cajal to a smooth muscle phenotype. Gastroenterology. 1999;117:140–8.
97. Sanders KM, Ordog T, Koh SD, Torihashi S, Ward SM. Development and plasticity of interstitial cells of Cajal. Neurogastroenterol Motil. 1999;11:311–38.
98. Faussone-Pellegrini MS, Vannucchi MG, Ledder O, Huang TY, Hanani M. Plasticity of interstitial cells of Cajal: a study of mouse colon. Cell Tissue Res. 2006;325(2):211–7.
99. Huizinga JD, Zarate N, Farrugia G. Physiology, injury, and recovery of interstitial cells of Cajal: basic and clinical science. Gastroenterology. 2009;137:1548–56.
100. Yamataka A, Kato Y, Tibboel D, et al. A lack of intestinal pacemaker (c-kit) in aganglionic bowel of patients with Hirschsprung's disease. J Pediatric Surg. 1995;30:441–4.
101. Vanderwinden JM, Rumessen JJ, Liu H, Descamps D, De Laet MH, Vanderhaeghen JJ. Interstitial cells of Cajal in human colon and in Hirschsprung's disease. Gastroenterology. 1996;111:901–10.
102. Horisawa M, Watanabe Y, Torihashi S. Distribution of c-Kit immunopositive cells in normal human colon and in Hirschsprung's disease. J Pediatric Surg. 1998;33:1209–14.
103. Newman CJ, Laurini RN, Lesbros Y, Reinberg O, Meyrat BJ. Interstitial cells of Cajal are normally distributed in both ganglionated and aganglionic bowel in Hirschsprung's disease. Pediatric Surg Int. 2003;19:662–8.
104. Ward SM, Ordog T, Bayguinov JR, et al. Development of interstitial cells of Cajal and pacemaking in mice lacking enteric nerves. Gastroenterology. 1999;117:584–94.

Development of Gut Motility

3

Heather M. Young, Elizabeth A. Beckett,
Joel C. Bornstein, and Sudarshan R. Jadcherla

Introduction

Coordinated movements of the gastrointestinal tract are crucial for the primary functions of this organ: digestion of food, absorption of nutrients and removal of waste products. Several complex motor patterns involving coordinated contractions and relaxations of the external muscle layers of the gut have distinct roles in gut motility (see section below). These motility patterns have been intensively studied and characterized in adults, but there is far less known about gut motility during development. Here we review the types of motor patterns that are present in the gut of developing laboratory animals and humans. We also discuss the mechanisms that regulate intestinal movements during development.

H.M. Young, Ph.D. (✉)
Department of Anatomy & Neuroscience, University of Melbourne, 3010, Parkville, VIC, Australia
e-mail: h.young@unimelb.edu.au

E.A. Beckett, Ph.D.
Discipline of Physiology, School of Medical Sciences, University of Adelaide, Adelaide, SA, Australia

J.C. Bornstein, Ph.D.
Department of Physiology, University of Melbourne, Melbourne, VIC, Australia

S.R. Jadcherla, M.D., F.R.C.P.I., D.C.H., A.G.A.F.
Department of Pediatrics, Division of Neonatology, Pediatric Gastroenterology and Nutrition, The Ohio State University College of Medicine and Public Health; Section of Neonatology, Nationwide Children's Hospital, Columbus, OH, USA

Motility Patterns and Their Control Mechanisms in the Mature Gut

Coordinated movements of the gastrointestinal tract include mixing, propagating motor activities and receptive relaxation. These movements are regulated by multiple control systems including extrinsic neurons, intrinsic neurons (the enteric nervous system, ENS), interstitial cells of Cajal (ICC) and myogenic mechanisms, which can all operate simultaneously [1, 2]. The relative contribution of each control system to a particular activity varies between different regions of the gastrointestinal tract [3]. Furthermore, as discussed later in this article, recent studies in animal models also show that the relative contribution of different control systems to contractile activity in the intestine also varies with developmental age [4]. Thus, the control of gut motility is very complex [2].

The primary function of the esophagus is to act as a conduit between the pharynx and the stomach, and the only motor pattern is peristalsis. During the pharyngeal phase of swallowing, the upper esophageal sphincter (UES) relaxes, and there is then a sequential contraction of esophageal muscle from the proximal to the distal end, followed by lower esophageal sphincter (LES) relaxation, so as to allow the bolus to enter the

C. Faure et al. (eds.), *Pediatric Neurogastroenterology: Gastrointestinal Motility and Functional Disorders in Children*, Clinical Gastroenterology,
DOI 10.1007/978-1-60761-709-9_3,

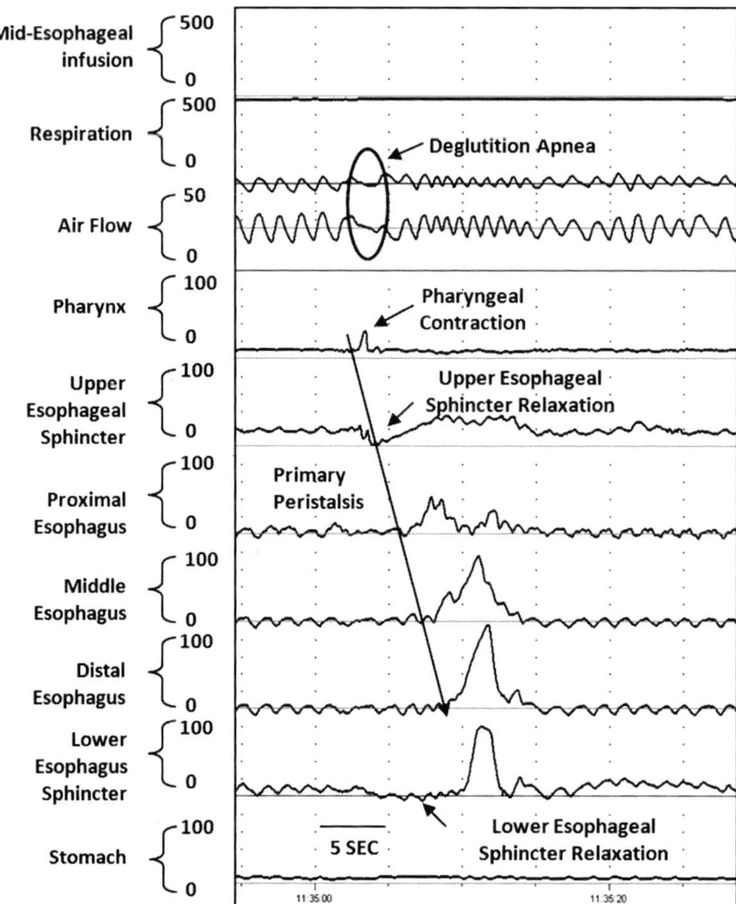

Fig. 3.1 An example of spontaneous primary esophageal peristalsis in a premature infant evoked upon pharyngeal contraction. Such sequences facilitate swallowing and esophageal clearance. Note the brief respiratory modification and deglutition apnea during pharyngeal waveform suggesting cross-communications between the pharynx and airway

stomach. This integrated sequence of reflexes induced by swallowing constitutes *primary peristalsis* (Fig. 3.1). Peristalsis is also induced by esophageal distension, which is termed *secondary peristalsis*. In humans, the upper third of the esophagus, which is striated muscle, is controlled entirely by neurons in the brainstem via the vagus nerves. The lower, smooth muscle regions of the esophagus are controlled by the vagus nerve, intrinsic neurons and myogenic mechanisms [3].

Different motor patterns occur in the proximal and distal stomach [3]. In the proximal stomach, receptive relaxation and accommodation occur, which are both mediated by neurons in the brainstem via vago-vagal reflexes. The distal stomach exhibits different motor patterns in the fed and fasted states. In the fed state, the distal stomach grinds and mixes. Extrinsic neurons are not essential for this contractile activity, but it can be modulated by vagal pathways. Migrating motor complexes (MMCs) are waves of strong contractions that sweep slowly along the gastrointestinal tract in the fasted state to clear indigestible food, mucous and epithelial debris. In humans, MMCs occur around once every 2–4 h, and most originate in the distal stomach and propagate along the small intestine [3]. The initiation of MMCs is modulated by vagal input and motilin released from the duodenum, while the propagation of MMCs is coordinated by enteric neurons.

Multiple motor patterns occur in the small and large intestines. Segmentation, alternating stationary waves of contraction and relaxation, mixes intestinal contents with digestive enzymes and exposes nutrients to the absorptive epithelium (small intestine) or facilitates water extraction (colon). Peristalsis, contraction waves that migrate in an anal direction, moves intestinal contents to new gut regions and is essential for elimination of undigested material. MMCs, which are initiated in the stomach or proximal duodenum, propagate along significant lengths of the intestine. In humans, MMCs occur only in the fasted state and only in the small intestine [3]. In other species, however, MMCs can occur in both the fed and fasted states and also occur in the colon. Haustration, the mixing of feces to absorb water, occurs in sac-like structures called haustrations of the large intestine of some species including humans.

Studies in animal models have shown that the ENS is essential for segmentation in the small intestine [5]. Peristalsis in the small and large intestines is controlled by an interplay between the ENS, ICC, and myogenic mechanisms [2]. However, the ENS is essential for intestinal peristalsis as revealed by the bowel obstruction caused by the aganglionic region of infants with Hirschsprung's disease. The ENS is also essential for the initiation and propagation of the MMC in the small intestine, although the CNS and hormones can modulate MMCs [3]. Studies in the rabbit colon have shown that haustral formation and propagation is neurally mediated [6]. Furthermore, water and electrolyte secretion is regulated by the ENS, as is the integration between motility and secretion [7].

Development of Motility Patterns and Their Control Mechanisms—Studies of Laboratory Animals

Unlike humans, the mechanisms controlling motility patterns during development can be examined in intact segments of gut of laboratory animals in vitro or in vivo. Most studies of mammals have been performed using segments of fetal or postnatal mouse intestine in vitro. However, because larval zebrafish are transparent, propagating contractile activity and transit studies using fluorescent food have been performed in zebrafish in vivo [8–13]. In this section we focus by necessity on the small and large intestines as there are relatively few studies on the development of motility patterns and their control mechanisms in the esophagus and stomach of laboratory animals.

Motility Patterns Present in the Developing Gut

Although fetal mammals receive nutrition solely via the placenta, contractile activity in the gut commences well before birth. The esophagus of preterm piglets (delivered by caesarean section at 91% of full gestation) exhibits esophageal contractions in response to oral feeding, but compared to term piglets, the frequency of contractions is lower and the contractions propagate at a lower velocity [14]. In fetal mice, shallow contractions that propagate both orally and anally are first observed in preparations of small intestine in vitro at embryonic day (E) 13.5 (the gestation period for a mouse is around 19 days) [4]. Moreover, propagating contractions are observed in zebrafish larvae before the yolk sac is fully absorbed [8–11]. The physiological role of prenatal (or pre-yolk sac absorption) gastrointestinal contractile activity is unclear. Fetal mammals swallow amniotic fluid, which advances along the gut [15–17], and this meconium progresses towards the distal regions of bowel during late fetal stages [18]. Although it is highly likely that the propagating contractile activity that occurs prior to birth contributes to the propulsion of meconium anally prior to birth, this has yet to be conclusively demonstrated.

Development of Enteric Neurons and Their Role in Motility During Development

The ENS arises from neural crest-derived cells that emigrate primarily from the caudal hindbrain

[19, 20], although sacral level neural crest cells also give rise to some enteric neurons, mainly in the colon and rectum [21, 22]. Neuronal differentiation commences early as pan-neuronal markers are first expressed by a subpopulation of neural crest-derived cells as they are migrating along the gut in fetal mice and rats [23, 24].

In the mature ENS, there are many different subtypes of enteric neurons [25]. In the developing mouse gut, cells expressing markers for some enteric neuron subtypes are present shortly after the first expression of pan-neuronal proteins [26], but different enteric neuron subtypes develop at different ages [27]. Expression of neuronal nitric oxide synthase (nNOS—the synthetic enzyme for nitric oxide), and choline acetyltransferase (ChAT, the synthetic enzyme for acetylcholine) by developing enteric neurons have been the most extensively studied. nNOS neurons in the mature ENS include interneurons and inhibitory motor neurons to the external muscle layers [28]. ChAT neurons include excitatory interneurons and excitatory motor neurons to the external muscle layers [29]. In both zebrafish and mice, nNOS neurons are one of the first enteric neuron subtypes to appear during development [10, 26, 30, 31]. In guinea-pigs, although the total number of myenteric neurons in the small intestine increases between neonatal and adult stages, the total number of nNOS neurons in the neonatal guinea-pig is the same as in adults and so the percentage of myenteric neurons expressing nNOS declines during postnatal development [32]. In zebrafish, the proportion of enteric neurons expressing nNOS does not change between 72 and 120 hpf (hours post-fertilization) [31]. In the rat, however, the proportion of myenteric neurons expressing NOS increases postnatally [33]. ChAT immunoreactivity is not detected until late in embryonic development in the mouse [34] although uptake of ^{3}[H]-choline is detected considerably earlier [35]. Similarly, although ChAT immunoreactivity is detectable in the zebrafish brain during embryonic development and in the ENS of adult zebrafish, ChAT immunoreactivity is not detectable in the ENS during zebrafish embryonic development [31]. In rats, the percentage of ChAT-immunoreactive myenteric neurons increases during postnatal development [33]. Changes in the proportions of some subtypes of enteric neurons have also been reported between weaning and adulthood in rats and guinea-pig, suggesting that the ENS is not fully mature at weaning [36–38].

The development of the innervation of the muscle layers has been examined in a number of species. In the dog, the plexuses of nerve fibers in the small intestine and colon are immature at birth [39]. In the guinea-pig ileum, the density of cholinergic nerve fibers in myenteric ganglia and in the tertiary plexus is higher at neonatal stages than in adults [32], whereas in the mouse colon the density of cholinergic nerve fibers in the circular muscle layer increases during early postnatal stages [40]. These differences might reflect the fact that mice are born at a developmentally earlier age than guinea-pigs.

Although enteric neuron differentiation commences prior to the presence of propagating contractile activity, studies in mice and zebrafish using pharmacological inhibitors of neural activity or mutants lacking enteric neurons have shown that the first motility patterns are not neurally mediated [4, 11]. There is therefore a significant delay between when enteric neurons first develop and when neurally mediated motility patterns are observed. This very likely reflects the fact that the neural circuitry mediating motility patterns involves at least three different types of neurons [41], which must develop and then form the appropriate synaptic connections with each other and with target cells. In mice, neurally mediated motility patterns are not observed until shortly before birth in the duodenum [4], and a week after birth in the colon [40]. In longitudinal muscle strips from postnatal rats, electrical field stimulation-induced contractions are reduced by a muscarinic acetylcholine receptor antagonist starting at postnatal day (P) 14, whereas inhibition of nNOS caused a significant increase in the contractile response only from P36 [33]. Thus, cholinergic neuromuscular transmission to the longitudinal muscle in the rat colon does not develop until postnatal stages and precedes the development of nitric oxide-mediated transmission. In the mouse small intestine, cholinergic neuromuscular transmission commences at late fetal stages [42]. In contrast, cholinergic neuromuscular transmission in the guinea-pig taenia and in the frog gut commences after inhibitory or nitric oxide-mediated transmission [43, 44]. In the longitudinal muscle of human and guinea-pig intestine, nitric oxide-mediated transmission is relatively more prominent at postnatal stages than in adults [32, 45].

In summary, although enteric neurons develop early, the first gastrointestinal motility patterns are not neurally mediated. However, neurally mediated contractile activity is prominent by birth, and is essential for propulsive activity as shown by the bowel obstruction that occurs proximal to the aganglionic region in infants with Hirschsprung's disease. The first subtype of enteric neuron to develop is the nNOS neurons, and although there are some exceptions, nitric oxide-mediated transmission develops earlier and/or is more prominent during pre- and postnatal development than in adults. As the relative importance of different neurotransmitters to gastrointestinal contractile activity changes significantly during development, drugs that successfully treat motility disorders in adults will not necessarily have similar effects in infants and children.

Development of Interstitial Cells of Cajal (ICC) and Their Role in Motility During Development

In the adult gut, there are several different subpopulations of ICC, most of which are in close association with enteric neurons [46]. Different subpopulations of ICC play different roles. For example, ICC at the level of the myenteric plexus (ICC-MY) mediate slow waves, the electrical events that time the occurrence of phasic contractions [47–50], and ICC within the circular muscle act as intermediaries in neuromuscular transmission [51, 52].

Unlike enteric neurons and glia, ICC do not arise from the neural crest during embryological development as ICC develop in explants of avian and mammalian embryonic gut which have been removed prior to the arrival of neural crest cells in that region [53, 54]. Furthermore, ICC are distributed normally and slow wave activity is generated in the bowel of mutant mice lacking enteric neurons [55, 56]. Hence ICC development and maintenance is independent of crest-derived cells in mice. In an infant with intestinal aganglionosis extending into the jejunum, abundant ICC were present in the myenteric region, but degenerating ICC were observed in the circular muscle of the aganglionic region [57]. Thus, in humans, ICC also arise independently of neurons, although some subpopulations of ICC may directly or indirectly require neurons for their long term survival.

Developmental studies in mice suggest that smooth muscle cells and ICC arise from a common mesenchymal precursor [58, 59] and that differentiation to the ICC phenotype during embryogenesis is dependent upon cellular signaling via the tyrosine kinase receptor, Kit [42, 59–61]. The natural ligand for the Kit receptor is stem cell factor (SCF or *steel*), which is expressed in both enteric neurons and smooth muscle cells [55, 56, 62]. Mutations leading to deficiency of Kit in W/W^v mice or membrane bound SCF in Sl/Sl^d mice result in disruptions of particular ICC populations and aberrant gastrointestinal motility [47–49]. Both migrating motor complexes and higher frequency phasic contractions can be recorded from the small intestine of W/W^v mice, which lack intestinal ICC-MY [63], but the phasic contractions are characteristically abrupt and uncoordinated [64]. Treatment of embryonic jejunal explants with Kit-neutralizing antibodies prior to the emergence of cells with the ultrastructural characteristics of ICC prevents the development of ICC and slow wave activity [42]. The postnatal maintenance of ICC also appears dependent upon Kit-signaling as injection of Kit neutralizing antibodies resulted in loss of ICC and lethal paralytic ileus in neonatal mice [61]. Loss of ICC due to Kit blockade is accompanied by a loss of electrical slow wave activity in the small intestine and reduced neural responses in the small bowel and colon [65]. In the absence of Kit-signaling, ICC appear to differentiate to a smooth muscle phenotype, but appear to retain, at least in the short term, the ability to regenerate the ICC phenotype if Kit signaling is restored [60].

During embryogenesis there is a rostral-to-caudal development of ICC along the gastrointestinal tract. In embryonic mice, the circular muscle layer differentiates prior to the longitudinal muscle layer. Nearly all of the mesenchymal cells between the serosa and the newly formed circular muscle layer, consisting of precursors of both longitudinal muscle and ICC, initially express Kit [42, 65]. As embryonic development progresses a subpopulation of these mesenchymal precursors lose expression of Kit and differentiate into longitudinal smooth muscle [59]. The Kit-positive cells on the circular muscle side of this newly formed longitudinal muscle layer develop into the anastomosing network termed ICC-MY.

Motility patterns of the stomach during development have not been extensively researched using laboratory animals. In mouse, 2 days prior to birth, ICC-MY and slow wave activity are present in the gastric antrum whilst spindle shaped intramuscular ICC (ICC-IM) are evident and neurally mediated responses can be recorded from the gastric fundus [66].

Intramuscular ICC (ICC-IM) are closely associated with the varicose terminals of both excitatory and inhibitory motor nerves and without ICC-IM neural transmission from enteric motor neurons is significantly compromised [51, 52].

Despite this close anatomical arrangement between nerves and ICC-IM, the outgrowth of motor nerve processes does not appear to be dependent upon the presence of ICC as the distribution of both excitatory and inhibitory nerve processes is normal in *W/W^v* fundus muscles devoid of ICC-IM. In contrast, the terminal processes of vagal intramuscular arrays do not ramify within the circular muscle layer of the stomach in the absence of ICC-IM [67, 68].

Electrical rhythmicity can be recorded from segments of mouse small intestine 3 days prior to birth [42, 60]. However, the first propagating contractions in mouse intestine are evident in the mid stages of embryonic development (embryonic day 13), prior to the emergence of a Kit positive ICC network and slow wave activity at embryonic day 18 [4]. The frequency of these initial contractions is similar in wildtype mice and in mutant (*W/W^v*) mice lacking ICC-MY, providing further evidence that these contractile patterns are myogenic[1] rather than ICC-mediated. Closer to the time of birth, after anastomosing networks of ICC-MY have established, slow waves and phasic contractions occur at a similar frequency suggesting that myogenic contractions become entrained by ICC-MY [4]. Around 5 days after birth, a second layer of Kit-positive cells, termed ICC-DMP, are evident in the region of the deep muscular plexus of the rodent small intestine [59, 65, 69, 70]. Development of neuromuscular responses to stimulation is concomitant with the development of ICC-DMP and blockade of ICC-DMP development with Kit neutralizing antibodies has been shown to lead to a severe attenuation of postjunctional responses to nerve stimulation [71] suggesting their role as mediators of neurotransmission in the intestine.

Role of Myogenic Mechanisms in Intestinal Motility During Development

Studies in embryonic mice and zebrafish have shown that the first intestinal motility patterns to appear during development, spontaneous contractions that propagate anally and orally, are not mediated by neurons or ICC [4, 11]. Hence the contractions must be myogenic, that is, generated by the smooth muscle cells themselves. Motility patterns that are not mediated by either neurons or ICC are present in the intestine of mature animals, but under normal conditions are not very prominent [72, 73]. However, propagating contractions in other organs of mature animals, including the upper urinary tract, vas deferens and uterus are entirely myogenic in origin [74]. In the duodenum and colon of fetal mice, the myogenic contractions require the entry of extracellular calcium [4], but it is unknown how they are initiated or propagated.

[1] In the field of gastrointestinal motility, the term "myogenic" has been used to describe contractile activity generated by ICC as well as muscle cells, but here we use the term myogenic to refer to contractions specifically originating from the muscle cells themselves.

Environmental Influences on Motility Patterns During Development

The composition of gut contents changes dramatically immediately after birth and then at weaning. There is evidence from piglets that the introduction of solid food at weaning induces changes in some of the properties of MMCs [75], but it is unknown whether changes in luminal contents immediately following birth also induce changes in motility patterns. Dietary components have recently been shown to affect motility and gene expression in the ENS of mature rats; in particular, long term exposure to resistant starch diet enhanced colonic propulsive motility and increased the number of ChAT immunoreactive myenteric neurons [76]. Furthermore, piglets treated with a probiotic showed increases in the expression of some neurotransmitters in submucosal, but not myenteric, neurons [77]. Additional studies are required to determine whether the changes in motility patterns that occur during postnatal development are induced by, or coincident with, dietary changes.

Motility is likely to be altered during fetal hypoxic stress as the transit of fluoescein-labeled luminal contents along the small intestine in fetal rabbits is decreased after a 1-h hypoxic episode [17].

Motility in Human Neonates and Children

In human infants, gastrointestinal motility is very complex, and as in laboratory animals, is almost certainly influenced by maturational changes in the CNS and ENS, gut muscle and ICC, as well as diet and changing anatomical postures during infancy. Furthermore, in the vulnerable high risk infant in intensive care units, hypoxia, inflammation, sepsis and other comorbidity conditions can complicate the feeding process and gastrointestinal transit.

Immunohistochemical studies of human fetuses have shown that neurons, muscle and ICC differentiate from proximal-to-distal and that the longitudinal and circular muscle layers and myenteric and submucosal plexuses have a mature appearance by week 14 [78, 79]. As in laboratory mammals, many subtypes of enteric neurons develop prior to birth [27]. Kit-expressing ICC-MY first appear around weeks 7–9 [78, 79]. In the stomach, ICC-MY, ICC-IM (intramuscular), and ICC-SEP (ICC located within connective tissue septa separating muscle bundles) are all present by the end of the fourth month of development [80].

The simple physiological functions of the neonatal foregut, midgut, and hindgut, respectively, are to facilitate (1) safe feeding by steering ingested material away from the airway, (2) gastrointestinal transit and mixing of luminal contents to permit absorption and propulsion, and (3) evacuation of excreta to modify the intestinal milieu. In this section on human neonates, we review the developmental aspects of (1) pharyngo-esophageal motility, (2) gastric motility, (3) small intestinal motility, and (4) colonic motility.

Developmental Pharyngo-Esophageal Motility in Human Neonates

Swallowing Prior to Birth

Numerous studies have shown that the human fetus swallows amniotic fluid [15, 81]. By 11 weeks gestation, the ability to swallow has developed and by 18–20 weeks sucking movements appear. There is an increase in the volume swallowed with gestational age, and by near term, the human fetus swallows around 500 ml of amniotic fluid per day [81]. Studies using a sheep model have shown that, as in adults, swallowing in near-term fetuses involves central cholinergic mechanisms [82].

Upper and Lower Esophageal Sphincter Functions and Esophageal Peristalsis in Human Neonates

Using micromanometry methods, upper esophageal sphincter (UES), esophageal body and lower esophageal sphincter (LES) functions have been characterized in neonates [83–85]. The resting UES tone increases with maturation from around

18 mmHg in 33 week preterm infants, to 26 mmHg in full term born neonates compared to 53 mmHg in adults. In contrast, the motor events associated with LES relaxation in healthy preterm infants 33 weeks and older have similar characteristics to adults [86].

In 33 weeks preterm infants, primary esophageal peristalsis occurs, but considerable maturation occurs pre- and postnatally [83, 85]. For example, evaluation of consecutive spontaneous solitary swallows in preterm infants at 33 weeks, preterm infants at 36 weeks, full term infants and adults showed significant age-dependent changes in the amplitude and velocity of the peristaltic contractions [84].

During anterograde movement of a bolus following swallowing or during retrograde movement of a bolus during gastroesophageal reflux events, the bolus comes in close proximity to the airway. Peristalsis is the single most important function that ensures clearance of luminal contents away from the airway. During primary esophageal peristalsis, there is a respiratory pause called deglutition apnea that occurs during the pharyngeal phase of swallow (see Fig. 3.1). This brief inhibition in respiration is due to a break in respiratory cycle (inspiratory or expiratory) and is a normal reflex. On the other hand, during esophageal provocation events (for example, infusion via a manometry catheter, or gastroesophageal reflux) proximal esophageal contraction and distal esophageal relaxation result in secondary peristalsis, which occurs independent of central swallowing mechanisms (Fig. 3.2) [87–89]. These reflexes prevent the ascending spread of the bolus and promote descending propulsion to ensure esophageal clearance.

Secondary esophageal and UES contractile reflexes have been compared in 33 weeks and 36 weeks mean post menstrual age premature infants [90]. The occurrence of secondary peristalsis was volume dependent, and the characteristics matured with age. Furthermore, as the premature infant grew older, the occurrence of secondary peristalsis increased significantly with increment in dose volumes of air or liquids. Thus, it appears that vago-vagal protective reflex mechanisms that facilitate esophageal clearance are present in healthy premature neonates, but these mechanisms mature with age.

Esophageal provocation can also result in an increase in UES pressure [87, 88]. This reflex is the *esophago-UES-contractile reflex,* and is mediated by the vagus. The UES contractile reflex has been studied in premature infants, and like secondary peristalsis, the occurrence of UES contractile reflex is volume dependent, and the reflex matures during prenatal stages. This reflex may provide protection to the airways by limiting the proximal extent of the refluxate during spontaneous gastroesophageal reflux events.

Gastric Motility in Human Neonates

Scant information is available about receptive relaxation in the fundus in human neonates. Ultrasound studies of the fetal stomach detected gastric emptying as early as 13 weeks of gestation [91], and the length of gastric emptying cycles in fetuses increases just prior to birth [92]. The rate of gastric emptying is not influenced by nonnutritive sucking, but is influenced by calorific value and stress: Calorically denser formula accelerates gastric emptying and extreme stress, such as the presence of systemic illness, delays gastric emptying [93].

Small Intestinal Motility in Human Neonates

In 28–37 weeks of gestation preterm infants, the majority of the contractile activity in the small intestine consists of clusters of low amplitude contractions that propagate for a short distance or not at all [94]. Propagating, cyclical MMCs with clearly defined phases develop between 37 weeks and term [95].

In adults, motilin, which is released from mucosal cells in the duodenum, is an important regulator of MMCs, and initiation of phase III of the MMC (intense rhythmic contractions) in the

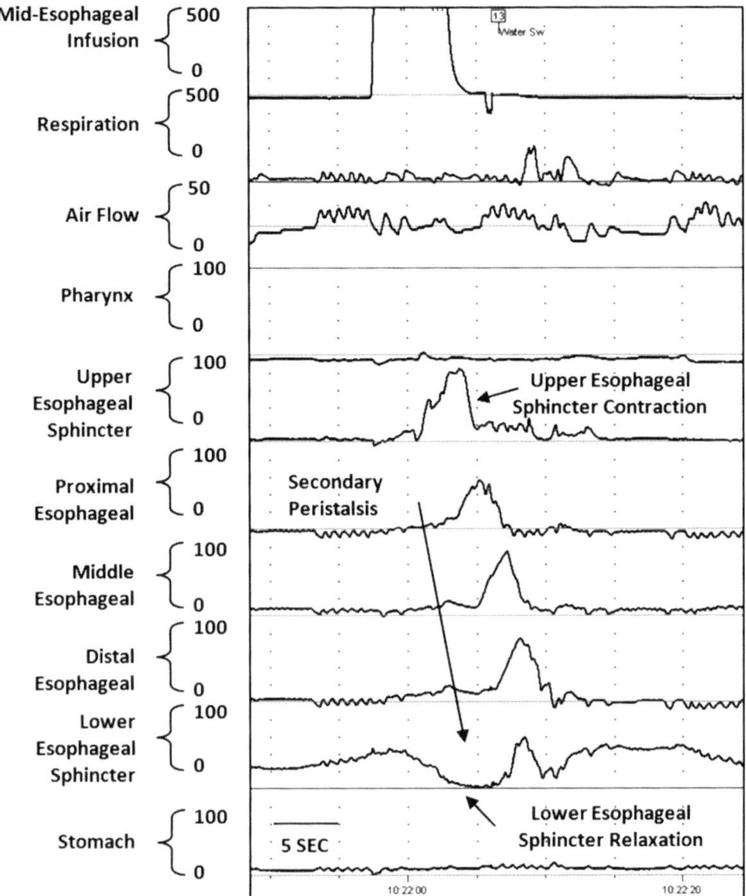

Fig. 3.2 Swallow independent secondary esophageal peristalsis in a premature infant in response to a mid-esophageal infusion. Such sequences are evoked during esophageal provocations and contribute to esophageal and airway protection by facilitating clearance

antrum is correlated with an increase in plasma concentrations of motilin [3]. In human neonates, the fasting plasma concentrations of motilin are similar to those in adults, but there are no detectable increases in motilin levels coincident with the initiation of MMCs [96]. The antibiotic, erythromycin, is also a motilin receptor agonist and accelerates gastric emptying in adults [97]. Erythromycin triggers initiation of the MMC in preterm infants whose gestational ages exceed 32 weeks [98]. Administration of erythromycin fails to trigger MMCs in infants younger than 32 weeks, suggesting immaturity of the neuronal circuitry mediating MMCs or that the motilin receptor cannot be activated by erythromycin at these ages.

Developmental Colonic Motility in Human Neonates

There is a marked lack of data on colonic motility in neonatal humans owing to technical limitations and ethical concerns.

Mechanisms Controlling Motility in Human Infants and Children

As in laboratory animals, enteric neurons and ICC appear to be essential for normal motility in human infants and children. An essential role for enteric neurons in gut motility after birth is best demonstrated by Hirschsprung's disease, where the segment lacking enteric neurons is unable to propel gut contents. Genetic alterations of Kit, and reduced ICC density, have recently been directly linked to a severe case of idiopathic constipation and megacolon in a 14 year old child [99], demonstrating the critical relationship between Kit function, ICC development and functional gastrointestinal motility patterns in the human intestine. Other studies have reported alterations in ICC networks in Hirschsprung's disease, chronic idiopathic intestinal pseudoobstruction, and pediatric constipation [100–106], but these defects may be an indirect consequence, rather than the cause, of the gut dysfunction. However, it is important to remember that motility disorders in children are not necessarily due to defects in neurons or ICC. For example, studies in mice have shown that defects in the gut muscle can also result in motility defects [107].

References

1. Sanders KM. Regulation of smooth muscle excitation and contraction. Neurogastroenterol Motil. 2008;20 Suppl 1:39–53.
2. Huizinga JD, Lammers WJ. Gut peristalsis is governed by a multitude of cooperating mechanisms. Am J Physiol Gastrointest Liver Physiol. 2009;296(1):G1–8.
3. Hasler WL. Motility of the small intestine and colon. In: Yamada T, editor. Textbook of gastroenterology, vol. 1. 5th ed. Philadelphia: Wiley-Blackwell; 2009. p. 231–63.
4. Roberts RR, Ellis M, Gwynne RM, et al. The first intestinal motility patterns in fetal mice are not mediated by neurons or interstitial cells of Cajal. J Physiol. 2010;588(Pt 7):1153–69.
5. Gwynne RM, Thomas EA, Goh SM, Sjovall H, Bornstein JC. Segmentation induced by intraluminal fatty acid in isolated guinea-pig duodenum and jejunum. J Physiol. 2004;556(Pt 2):557–69.
6. Lentle RG, Janssen PW, Asvarujanon P, Chambers P, Stafford KJ, Hemar Y. High-definition spatiotemporal mapping of contractile activity in the isolated proximal colon of the rabbit. J Comp Physiol B. 2008;178(3):257–68.
7. Wood JD. Enteric nervous system: sensory physiology, diarrhea and constipation. Curr Opin Gastroenterol. 2010;26(2):102–8.
8. Holmberg A, Schwerte T, Fritsche R, Pelster B, Holmgren S. Ontogeny of intestinal motility in correlation to neuronal development in zebrafish embryos and larvae. J Fish Biol. 2003;63:318–31.
9. Holmberg A, Schwerte T, Pelster B, Holmgren S. Ontogeny of the gut motility control system in zebrafish Danio rerio embryos and larvae. J Exp Biol. 2004;207(Pt 23):4085–94.
10. Holmberg A, Olsson C, Holmgren S. The effects of endogenous and exogenous nitric oxide on gut motility in zebrafish Danio rerio embryos and larvae. J Exp Biol. 2006;209(Pt 13):2472–9.
11. Holmberg A, Olsson C, Hennig GW. TTX-sensitive and TTX-insensitive control of spontaneous gut motility in the developing zebrafish (Danio rerio) larvae. J Exp Biol. 2007;210(Pt 6):1084–91.
12. Kuhlman J, Eisen JS. Genetic screen for mutations affecting development and function of the enteric nervous system. Dev Dyn. 2007;236(1): 118–27.
13. Field HA, Kelley KA, Martell L, Goldstein AM, Serluca FC. Analysis of gastrointestinal phys-iology using a novel intestinal transit assayin zebrafish. Neurogastroenterol Motil. 2009;21(3):304–12.
14. Rasch S, Sangild PT, Gregersen H, Schmidt M, Omari T, Lau C. The preterm piglet—a model in the study of oesophageal development in preterm neonates. Acta Paediatr. 2010;99(2):201–8.
15. McLain Jr CR. Amniography studies of the gastrointestinal motility of the human fetus. Am J Obstet Gynecol. 1963;86:1079–87.
16. Sase M, Lee JJ, Park JY, Thakur A, Ross MG, Buchmiller-Crair TL. Ontogeny of fetal rabbit upper gastrointestinal motility. J Surg Res. 2001;101(1): 68–72.
17. Sase M, Lee JJ, Ross MG, Buchmiller-Crair TL. Effect of hypoxia on fetal rabbit gastrointestinal motility. J Surg Res. 2001;99(2):347–51.
18. Anderson RB, Enomoto H, Bornstein JC, Young HM. The enteric nervous system is not essential for the propulsion of gut contents in fetal mice. Gut. 2004;53(10):1546–7.
19. Yntema CL, Hammond WS. The origin of intrinsic ganglia of trunk viscera from vagal neural crest in the chick embryo. J Comp Neurol. 1954;101:515–41.
20. Le Douarin NM, Teillet MA. The migration of neural crest cells to the wall of the digestive tract in avian embryo. J Embryol Exp Morphol. 1973;30(1):31–48.
21. Burns AJ, Le Douarin NM. The sacral neural crest contributes neurons and glia to the post- umbilical gut: spatiotemporal analysis of the development of the enteric nervous system. Development. 1998;125(21):4335–47.
22. Kapur RP. Colonization of the murine hindgut by sacral crest-derived neural precursors: experimental support for an evolutionarily conserved model. Dev Biol. 2000;227(1):146–55.
23. Baetge G, Pintar JE, Gershon MD. Transiently catecholaminergic (TC) cells in the bowel of the fetal rat: precursors of noncatecholaminergic enteric neurons. Dev Biol. 1990;141(2):353–80.
24. Baetge G, Schneider KA, Gershon MD. Development and persistence of catecholaminergic neurons in

cultured explants of fetal murine vagus nerves and bowel. Development. 1990;110(3):689–701.
25. Furness JB. Types of neurons in the enteric nervous system. J Auton Nerv Syst. 2000;81(1–3):87–96.
26. Hao MM, Moore RE, Roberts RR, et al. The role of neural activity in the migration and differentiation of enteric neuron precursors. Neurogastroenterol Motil. 2010;22(5):e127–37.
27. Hao MM, Young HM. Development of enteric neuron diversity. J Cell Mol Med. 2009;13(7):1193–210.
28. Brookes SJ. Neuronal nitric oxide in the gut. J Gastroenterol Hepatol. 1993;8(6):590–603.
29. Brookes SJ. Classes of enteric nerve cells in the guinea-pig small intestine. Anat Rec. 2001;262(1):58–70.
30. Branchek TA, Gershon MD. Time course of expression of neuropeptide Y, calcitonin gene-related peptide, and NADPH diaphorase activity in neurons of the developing murine bowel and the appearance of 5-hydroxytryptamine in mucosal enterochromaffin cells. J Comp Neurol. 1989;285(2):262–73.
31. Uyttebroek L, Shepherd IT, Harrisson F, et al. Neurochemical coding of enteric neurons in adult and embryonic zebrafish (Danio rerio). J Comp Neurol. 2010;518(21):4419–38.
32. Patel BA, Dai X, Burda JE, et al. Inhibitory neuromuscular transmission to ileal longitudinal muscle predominates in neonatal guinea pigs. Neurogastroenterol Motil. 2010;22(8):909–18. e236–907.
33. de Vries P, Soret R, Suply E, Heloury Y, Neunlist M. Postnatal development of myenteric neurochemical phenotype and impact on neuromuscular transmission in the rat colon. Am J Physiol Gastrointest Liver Physiol. 2010;299(2):G539–47.
34. Hao MM, Boesmans W, Van den Abbeel C, Bornstein JC, Young HM, Vanden Berghe P. Neuronal activity in developing enteric neurons. Australian Neuroscience Society Abstracts. 2010
35. Rothman TP, Gershon MD. Phenotypic expression in the developing murine enteric nervous system. J Neurosci. 1982;2(3):381–93.
36. Vannucchi MG, Faussone-Pellegrini MS. Differentiation of cholinergic cells in the rat gut during pre- and postnatal life. Neurosci Lett. 1996;206(2–3):105–8.
37. Matini P, Mayer B, Faussone-Pellegrini MS. Neurochemical differentiation of rat enteric neurons during pre- and postnatal life. Cell Tissue Res. 1997;288(1):11–23.
38. Abalo R, Vera G, Rivera AJ, Moro-Rodriguez E, Martin-Fontelles MI. Postnatal maturation of the gastrointestinal tract: a functional and immunohistochemical study in the guinea-pig ileum at weaning. Neurosci Lett. 2009;467(2):105–10.
39. Daniel EE, Wang YF. Control systems of gastrointestinal motility are immature at birth in dogs. Neurogastroenterol Motil. 1999;11(5):375–92.
40. Roberts RR, Murphy JF, Young HM, Bornstein JC. Development of colonic motility in the neonatal mouse-studies using spatiotemporal maps. Am J Physiol Gastrointest Liver Physiol. 2007;292(3):G930–8.
41. Bornstein JC, Costa M, Grider JR. Enteric motor and interneuronal circuits controlling motility. Neurogastroenterol Motil. 2004;16 Suppl 1:34–8.
42. Ward SM, Harney SC, Bayguinov JR, McLaren GJ, Sanders KM. Development of electrical rhythmicity in the murine gastrointestinal tract is specifically encoded in the tunica muscularis. J Physiol (Lond). 1997;505(Pt 1):241–58.
43. Zagorodnyuk VP, Hoyle CH, Burnstock G. An electrophysiological study of developmental changes in the innervation of the guinea-pig taenia coli. Pflugers Arch. 1993;423(5–6):427–33.
44. Sundqvist M, Holmgren S. Ontogeny of excitatory and inhibitory control of gastrointestinal motility in the African clawed frog, Xenopus laevis. Am J Physiol Regul Integr Comp Physiol. 2006;291(4):R1138–44.
45. Wittmeyer V, Merrot T, Mazet B. Tonic inhibition of human small intestinal motility by nitric oxide in children but not in adults. Neurogastroenterol Motil. 2010;22:e1078–282.
46. Burns AJ, Herbert TM, Ward SM, Sanders KM. Interstitial cells of Cajal in the guinea-pig gastrointestinal tract as revealed by c-Kit immunohistochemistry. Cell Tissue Res. 1997;290(1):11–20.
47. Ward SM, Burns AJ, Torihashi S, Sanders KM. Mutation of the proto-oncogene c-kit blocks development of interstitial cells and electrical rhythmicity in murine intestine. J Physiol. 1994;480(Pt 1):91–7.
48. Huizinga JD, Thuneberg L, Kluppel M, Malysz J, Mikkelsen HB, Bernstein A. W/kit gene required for interstitial cells of Cajal and for intestinal pacemaker activity. Nature. 1995;373(6512):347–9.
49. Ward SM, Burns AJ, Torihashi S, Harney SC, Sanders KM. Impaired development of interstitial cells and intestinal electrical rhythmicity in steel mutants. Am J Physiol. 1995;269(6 Pt 1):C1577–85.
50. Hirst GD, Edwards FR. Generation of slow waves in the antral region of guinea-pig stomach–a stochastic process. J Physiol. 2001;535(Pt 1):165–80.
51. Burns AJ, Lomax AE, Torihashi S, Sanders KM, Ward SM. Interstitial cells of Cajal mediate inhibitory neurotransmission in the stomach. Proc Natl Acad Sci U S A. 1996;93(21):12008–13.
52. Ward SM, Beckett EA, Wang X, Baker F, Khoyi M, Sanders KM. Interstitial cells of Cajal mediate cholinergic neurotransmission from enteric motor neurons. J Neurosci. 2000;20(4):1393–403.
53. Lecoin L, Gabella G, Le Douarin N. Origin of the c-kit-positive interstitial cells in the avian bowel. Development. 1996;122(3):725–33.
54. Young HM, Ciampoli D, Southwell BR, Newgreen DF. Origin of interstitial cells of Cajal in the mouse intestine. Dev Biol. 1996;180(1):97–107.
55. Ward SM, Ordog T, Bayguinov JR, et al. Development of interstitial cells of Cajal and pacemaking in mice

lacking enteric nerves. Gastroenterology. 1999;117(3):584–94.
56. Wu JJ, Rothman TP, Gershon MD. Development of the interstitial cell of cajal: origin, kit dependence and neuronal and nonneuronal sources of kit ligand. J Neurosci Res. 2000;59(3):384–401.
57. Huizinga JD, Berezin I, Sircar K, et al. Development of interstitial cells of Cajal in a full-term infant without an enteric nervous system. Gastroenterology. 2001;120(2):561–7.
58. Kluppel M, Huizinga JD, Malysz J, Bernstein A. Developmental origin and Kit-dependent development of the interstitial cells of cajal in the mammalian small intestine. Dev Dyn. 1998;211(1):60–71.
59. Torihashi S, Ward SM, Sanders KM. Development of c-Kit-positive cells and the onset of electrical rhythmicity in murine small intestine. Gastroenterology. 1997;112(1):144–55.
60. Beckett EA, Ro S, Bayguinov Y, Sanders KM, Ward SM. Kit signaling is essential for development and maintenance of interstitial cells of Cajal and electrical rhythmicity in the embryonic gastrointestinal tract. Dev Dyn. 2007;236(1):60–72.
61. Maeda H, Yamagata A, Nishikawa S, Yoshinaga K, Kobayashi S, Nishi K. Requirement of c-kit for development of intestinal pacemaker system. Development. 1992;116(2):369–75.
62. Young HM, Torihashi S, Ciampoli D, Sanders KM. Identification of neurons that express stem cell factor in the mouse small intestine. Gastroenterology. 1998;115(4):898–908.
63. Spencer NJ, Sanders KM, Smith TK. Migrating motor complexes do not require electrical slow waves in the mouse small intestine. J Physiol. 2003;553(Pt 3):881–93.
64. Hennig GW, Spencer NJ, Jokela-Willis S, et al. ICC-MY coordinate smooth muscle electrical and mechanical activity in the murine small intestine. Neurogastroenterol Motil. 2010;22(5):e138–51.
65. Torihashi S, Ward SM, Nishikawa S, Nishi K, Kobayashi S, Sanders KM. c-kit-dependent development of interstitial cells and electrical activity in the murine gastrointestinal tract. Cell Tissue Res. 1995;280(1):97–111.
66. Ward SM, Sanders KM. Physiology and pathophysiology of the interstitial cell of Cajal: from bench to bedside. I. Functional development and plasticity of interstitial cells of Cajal networks. Am J Physiol Gastrointest Liver Physiol. 2001;281(3):G602–11.
67. Fox EA, Phillips RJ, Martinson FA, Baronowsky EA, Powley TL. C-Kit mutant mice have a selective loss of vagal intramuscular mechanoreceptors in the forestomach. Anat Embryol (Berl). 2001;204(1):11–26.
68. Fox EA, Phillips RJ, Byerly MS, Baronowsky EA, Chi MM, Powley TL. Selective loss of vagal intramuscular mechanoreceptors in mice mutant for steel factor, the c-Kit receptor ligand. Anat Embryol (Berl). 2002;205(4):325–42.
69. Faussone-Pellegrini MS. Cytodifferentiation of the interstitial cells of Cajal related to the myenteric plexus of mouse intestinal muscle coat. An E.M. study from foetal to adult life. Anat Embryol (Berl). 1985;171(2):163–9.
70. Faussone-Pellegrini MS, Matini P, Stach W. Differentiation of enteric plexuses and interstitial cells of Cajal in the rat gut during pre- and postnatal life. Acta Anat (Basel). 1996;155(2):113–25.
71. Ward SM, McLaren GJ, Sanders KM. Interstitial cells of Cajal in the deep muscular plexus mediate enteric motor neurotransmission in the mouse small intestine. J Physiol. 2006;573(Pt 1):147–59.
72. Roberts RR, Bornstein JC, Bergner AJ, Young HM. Disturbances of colonic motility in mouse models of Hirschsprung's disease. Am J Physiol Gastrointest Liver Physiol. 2008;294(4):G996–1008.
73. Hennig GW, Gregory S, Brookes SJ, Costa M. Non-peristaltic patterns of motor activity in the guinea-pig proximal colon. Neurogastroenterol Motil. 2010;22(6):e207–17.
74. Lang RJ, Takano H, Davidson ME, Suzuki H, Klemm MF. Characterization of the spontaneous electrical and contractile activity of smooth muscle cells in the rat upper urinary tract. J Urol. 2001;166(1):329–34.
75. Lesniewska V, Laerke HN, Hedemann MS, Hojsgaard S, Pierzynowski SG, Jensen BB. The effect of change of the diet and feeding regimen at weaning on duodenal myoelectrical activity in piglets. Animal Sci. 2000;71:443–51.
76. Soret R, Chevalier J, De Coppet P, et al. Short-chain fatty acids regulate the enteric neurons and control gastrointestinal motility in rats. Gastroenterology. 2010;138(5):1772–82.
77. di Giancamillo A, Vitari F, Bosi G, Savoini G, Domeneghini C. The chemical code of porcine enteric neurons and the number of enteric glial cells are altered by dietary probiotics. Neurogastroenterol Motil. 2010;22(9):e271–8.
78. Fu M, Tam PK, Sham MH, Lui VC. Embryonic development of the ganglion plexuses and the concentric layer structure of human gut: a topographical study. Anat Embryol. 2004;208(1):33–41.
79. Wallace AS, Burns AJ. Development of the enteric nervous system, smooth muscle and interstitial cells of Cajal in the human gastrointestinal tract. Cell Tissue Res. 2005;319(3):367–82.
80. Radenkovic G, Ilic I, Zivanovic D, Vlajkovic S, Petrovic V, Mitrovic O. C-kit-immunopositive interstitial cells of Cajal in human embryonal and fetal oesophagus. Cell Tissue Res. 2010;340(3):427–36.
81. Ross MG, Nijland MJ. Development of ingestive behavior. Am J Physiol. 1998;274(4 Pt 2):R879–93.
82. Shi L, Mao C, Zeng F, Zhu L, Xu Z. Central cholinergic mechanisms mediate swallowing, renal excretion, and c-fos expression in the ovine fetus near term. Am J Physiol Regul Integr Comp Physiol. 2009;296(2):R318–25.

83. Omari TI, Miki K, Fraser R, et al. Esophageal body and lower esophageal sphincter function in healthy premature infants. Gastroenterology. 1995;109(6):1757–64.
84. Jadcherla SR, Duong HQ, Hofmann C, Hoffmann R, Shaker R. Characteristics of upper oesophageal sphincter and oesophageal body during maturation in healthy human neonates compared with adults. Neurogastroenterol Motil. 2005;17(5):663–70.
85. Staiano A, Boccia G, Salvia G, Zappulli D, Clouse RE. Development of esophageal peristalsis in preterm and term neonates. Gastroenterology. 2007;132(5):1718–25.
86. Omari TI, Miki K, Davidson G, et al. Characterisation of relaxation of the lower oesophageal sphincter in healthy premature infants. Gut. 1997;40(3):370–5.
87. Jadcherla SR. Manometric evaluation of esophageal-protective reflexes in infants and children. Am J Med. 2003;115(Suppl 3A):157S–60.
88. Jadcherla SR. Upstream effect of esophageal distention: effect on airway. Curr Gastroenterol Rep. 2006;8(3):190–4.
89. Gupta A, Gulati P, Kim W, Fernandez S, Shaker R, Jadcherla SR. Effect of postnatal maturation on the mechanisms of esophageal propulsion in preterm human neonates: primary and secondary peristalsis. Am J Gastroenterol. 2009;104(2):411–9.
90. Jadcherla SR, Duong HQ, Hoffmann RG, Shaker R. Esophageal body and upper esophageal sphincter motor responses to esophageal provocation during maturation in preterm newborns. J Pediatr. 2003;143(1):31–8.
91. Sase M, Miwa I, Sumie M, Nakata M, Sugino N, Ross MG. Ontogeny of gastric emptying patterns in the human fetus. J Matern Fetal Neonatal Med. 2005;17(3):213–7.
92. Sase M, Miwa I, Sumie M, et al. Gastric emptying cycles in the human fetus. Am J Obstet Gynecol. 2005;193(3 Pt 2):1000–4.
93. Berseth CL. Motor function in the stomach and small intestine in the neonate. NeoReviews. 2006;7:e28–33.
94. Berseth CL. Gestational evolution of small intestine motility in preterm and term infants. J Pediatr. 1989;115(4):646–51.
95. Bisset WM, Watt JB, Rivers RP, Milla PJ. Ontogeny of fasting small intestinal motor activity in the human infant. Gut. 1988;29(4):483–8.
96. Jadcherla SR, Klee G, Berseth CL. Regulation of migrating motor complexes by motilin and pancreatic polypeptide in human infants. Pediatr Res. 1997;42(3):365–9.
97. Janssens J, Peeters TL, Vantrappen G, et al. Improvement of gastric emptying in diabetic gastroparesis by erythromycin. Preliminary studies. N Engl J Med. 1990;322(15):1028–31.
98. Jadcherla SR, Berseth CL. Effect of erythromycin on gastroduodenal contractile activity in developing neonates. J Pediatr Gastroenterol Nutr. 2002;34(1):16–22.
99. Breuer C, Oh J, Molderings GJ, et al. Therapy-refractory gastrointestinal motility disorder in a child with c-kit mutations. World J Gastroenterol. 2010;16(34):4363–6.
100. Isozaki K, Hirota S, Miyagawa J, Taniguchi M, Shinomura Y, Matsuzawa Y. Deficiency of c-kit+ cells in patients with a myopathic form of chronic idiopathic intestinal pseudo-obstruction. Am J Gastroenterol. 1997;92(2):332–4.
101. Kenny SE, Connell MG, Rintala RJ, Vaillant C, Edgar DH, Lloyd DA. Abnormal colonic interstitial cells of Cajal in children with anorectal malformations. J Pediatr Surg. 1998;33(1):130–2.
102. Yamataka A, Ohshiro K, Kobayashi H, et al. Abnormal distribution of intestinal pacemaker (C-KIT-positive) cells in an infant with chronic idiopathic intestinal pseudoobstruction. J Pediatr Surg. 1998;33(6):859–62.
103. Wedel T, Spiegler J, Soellner S, et al. Enteric nerves and interstitial cells of Cajal are altered in patients with slow-transit constipation and megacolon. Gastroenterology. 2002;123(5):1459–67.
104. Taguchi T, Suita S, Masumoto K, Nagasaki A. An abnormal distribution of C-kit positive cells in the normoganglionic segment can predict a poor clinical outcome in patients with Hirschsprung's disease. Eur J Pediatr Surg. 2005;15(3):153–8.
105. Burns AJ. Disorders of interstitial cells of Cajal. J Pediatr Gastroenterol Nutr. 2007;45 Suppl 2:S103–6.
106. Bettolli M, De Carli C, Jolin-Dahel K, et al. Colonic dysmotility in postsurgical patients with Hirschsprung's disease. Potential significance of abnormalities in the interstitial cells of Cajal and the enteric nervous system. J Pediatr Surg. 2008;43(8):1433–8.
107. Angstenberger M, Wegener JW, Pichler BJ, et al. Severe intestinal obstruction on induced smooth muscle-specific ablation of the transcription factor SRF in adult mice. Gastroenterology. 2007;133(6):1948–59.

Visceral Sensitivity

4

Christophe Faure

The central nervous system (CNS) continuously receives information from the gastrointestinal (GI) tract related to the state of the organs and to the content of the gut. The CNS must integrate this information with inputs from other organs or from the environment in order to initiate suitable responses. Most of the information originating from the GI tract does not reach the level of conscious perception and is processed in the brainstem, below cortical level. Other sensations such as hunger, fullness, satiety, gas, focal gut distension, and need to defecate (as well as their physiological correlates, i.e., gastric and rectal distension) that involve adapted behaviors reach the cortex.

Abnormally heightened visceral sensitivity may lead to abdominal pain and functional GI disorders (FGID). Indeed, visceral hypersensitivity is considered a central pathophysiological mechanism of FGID [1]. Gastrointestinal pain is reported as dull, vague, and diffusely localized. Cutting, crushing (e.g., mucosal biopsy sampling) of the GI tract are not perceived when applied to conscious subjects. Stimuli for visceral pain include distension or traction on the mesentery as well as ischemia and inflammation, events that stimulate afferent nerve terminals.

C. Faure, M.D. (✉)
Division of Pediatric Gastroenterology, Department of Pediatrics, Sainte-Justine University Health Center, Université de Montréal, 3175 Côte Sainte-Catherine, Montréal, H3T1C5, QC, Canada
e-mail: christophe.faure@umontreal.ca

Neuroanatomy and Processing of Gastrointestinal Tract Sensitivity

Visceral Innervation (Fig. 4.1)

Similar to somatic sensitivity, gut afferent signals reach conscious perception through a three-neuron chain. Extrinsic innervation of the GI tract is composed of vagal afferents, spinal visceral afferents, and sacral afferents [2]. These nerves contain efferent fibers that transmit information from the CNS to the gut and afferent (or sensory) fibers that transmit information from the viscera to the CNS. Visceral afferent fibers are composed of sensory neurons that, arising from the cell body, project two neurites, one as peripheral fiber and one as central fiber. Visceral afferents participate to visceral sensation and in local reflexes controlling GI functions. Somatic and spinal visceral afferents converging on dorsal horn neurons result in viscerosomatic projection or referred pain.

Vagal Innervation

Vagal innervation is provided by the vagus nerve which innervates esophagus, stomach, small intestine, caecum, and proximal colon. Sensory afferent neurons predominate numerically in the vagus nerve. Cell bodies are located in nodose ganglia and the central processes terminate in the nucleus of the solitary tract (NTS).

C. Faure et al. (eds.), *Pediatric Neurogastroenterology: Gastrointestinal Motility and Functional Disorders in Children*, Clinical Gastroenterology,
DOI 10.1007/978-1-60761-709-9_4, © Springer Science+Business Media New York 2013

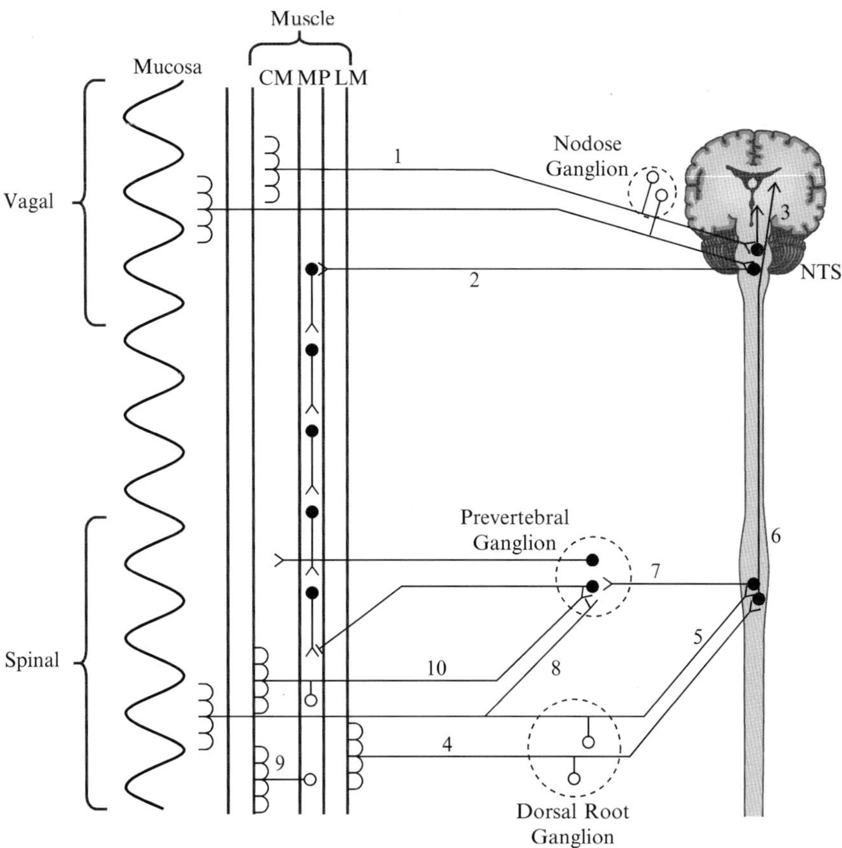

Fig. 4.1 Spinal and vagal innervation of the gastrointestinal tract. **Upper portion**: sensory information from vagal receptors is carried by vagal afferent nerves **(1)** with nerve cell bodies in the nodose ganglion to the sensory nucleus of the solitary tract (NTS). Second order neurons transmit the information either to higher centers in the CNS **(3)** or via efferent vagal fibers **(2)** in the form of vagovagal reflexes back to the ENS. **Lower portion**: sensory information from spinal receptors located in the mucosa, muscle or serosa is carried by spinal afferent fibers **(4)** with nerve cell bodies in the dorsal root ganglion to second-order neurons in the spinal cord. Second-order neurons transmit the information either to the CNS **(6)** or via sympathetic nerves **(7)** to prevertebral ganglia, to the ENS, and to the gastrointestinal muscle (spinal reflex). Collaterals of spinal afferents also form short reflex loops with postganglionic sympathetic nerves in the prevertebral ganglion **(8)**. In addition to spinal afferents, sensory structures with nerve cell bodies are also located within the intestinal wall **(9,10)**. *CM* circular muscle layer, *MP* myenteric plexus, *LM* longitudinal muscle layer. From: Mayer EA, Raybould HE. Role of visceral afferent mechanisms in functional bowel disorders. Gastroenterology 1990;99:1688–704, copyright Elsevier. Adapted with kind permission of Elsevier

Vagal afferents are believed to be mainly mediating physiological rather than harmful sensations, transmitting information on nature and composition of the intestinal content and motility and contractile tension of the smooth muscle.

Spinal Innervation

Visceral afferents running in the spinal cord are referred as "spinal afferents" when the term "sympathetic innervation" is restricted to spinal efferent innervation [2]. Spinal innervation is provided by the greater splanchnic nerve which forms three main ganglia from which they distribute to the viscera: the celiac ganglion distributes nerves to the esophagus, stomach, and duodenum; the superior mesenteric ganglion distributes nerves to the intestines down to the ascending colon and the inferior mesenteric ganglion to the colon from the hepatic flexure to the rectum. Sensory afferent neurons account for 10–20% of fibers in spinal afferents and cell bodies are located in dorsal root ganglia (DRG) at the cervical, thoracic, and upper lumbar spine [2].

Their central processes terminate in the dorsal horn of the spinal cord. Spinal afferents transmit information on potentially noxious mechanical or chemical stimuli and are involved in sensation of visceral pain. However, it should be kept in mind that, in the CNS, vagal inputs likely integrate with the inputs from the spinal pathways and therefore perception of pain is the result of modulation of vagal and spinal afferences [3]. Vagal and spinal afferents are predominantly unmyelinated C-fibers or thinly myelinated A-delta fibers with low conduction velocity.

Sacral Innervation

The distal third of the colon is innervated by the pelvic nerve and the pudendal nerve. This part of the GI tract receives dual spinal innervation from splanchnic and pelvic afferents [3]. Pelvic spinal afferents innervate the pelvic organs through parasympathetic nerves. Cell bodies are located in the DRG.

Sensory Terminals

At the level of the gastrointestinal tract, sensory neurons and enteroendocrine cells serve as transducers. Vagal mechanoreceptors are located in the mucosa or muscle layer and spinal receptors are located in the mucosa, muscle, or serosa [4]. Gut sensory terminals and receptors include mechanoreceptors, chemoreceptors, thermoreceptors, and nociceptors [5]. Recently, most evidence points toward polymodality of the visceral receptors.

Vagal Terminals

Vagal sensory endings terminate in the intestinal wall in three different ways [4]. "Intramuscular arrays" are located within the circular or longitudinal muscle layers and appear to be stretch receptors. "Intraganglionic endings" (IGLE) are situated at the surface of myenteric ganglia and are activated by tension of the gut wall. They are supposed to transmit signals that are perceived as nonpainful sensation of fullness. Mucosal projections extend into the lamina propria and correspond to mucosal receptors [6].

Spinal Terminals

Spinal terminals are less well characterized and are anatomically not clearly identifiable. Studies have shown that mechanonociceptors mediating transduction of pain evoked after high amplitude distension are spinal afferents [4]. Fine "varicose branching axons" that appear as specialized endings can be demonstrated in the serosa and mesenteries around blood vessels [6]. The mechanisms of mechanotransduction are currently unknown.

Enteroendocrine Cells

Enteroendocrine cells are contained within the intestinal mucosa throughout the GI tract distal to the esophagogastric junction and provide an interface between external milieu and terminal endings of afferents. They resemble the sensory cells in the lingual epithelium taste buds. They have an apical tuft of microvilli exposed to the luminal content and release bioactive molecules (serotonin—synthetized by enterochromaffin (EC) cells—and hormones such as CCK, leptin, orexin, ghrelin) that stimulate afferent terminal in the lamina propria in response to appropriate stimuli. Enteroendocrine cells are involved in chemosensitivity and respond to nutrients playing a key role in the glucose homeostasis [7]. It has also been recently shown that gut is able to "taste" odorants, spices and bitter taste via enteroendocrine cells [8]. EC cells contain serotonin which is known to be released in response to chemical stimuli [9] and plays a key role in the gut mechanosensitivity in response to mucosal deformation. When acting on 5-HT_3 receptors, serotonin release is involved in the peristaltic reflex by activating intrinsic neurons (IPAN) and in visceral sensations by activating mucosal endings of sensory afferents.

Receptors on Visceral Afferents Involved in Visceral Pain

A large number of bioactive substances and chemical mediators have been implicated in the sensory signal transduction of visceral pain [10]. These substances produce their effects by three distinct processes: (1) direct activation of a receptor, which generally involves the opening of ion channels; (2) sensitization which results

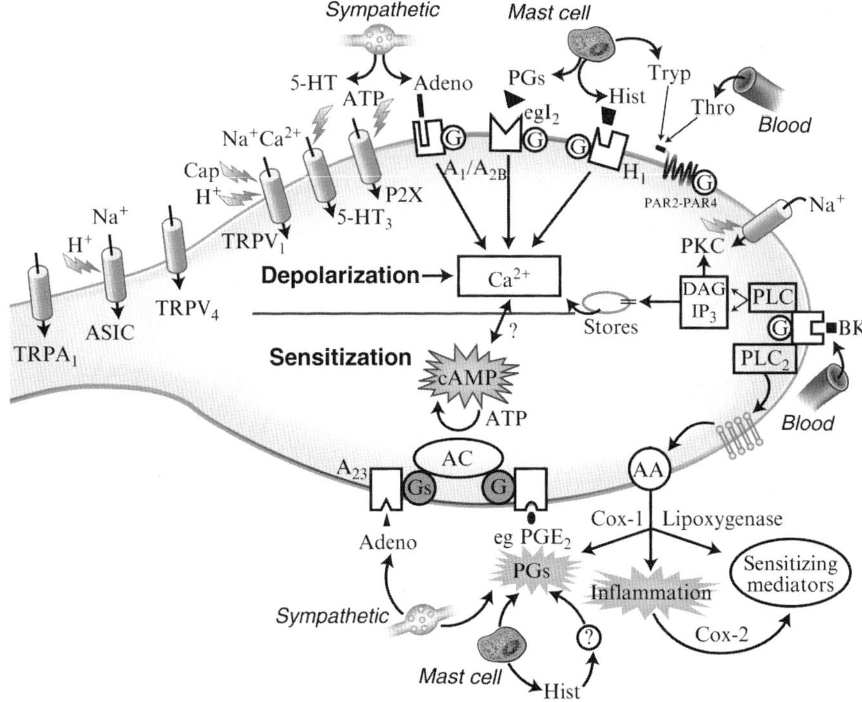

Fig. 4.2 Some of the potential receptor mechanisms underlying activation (depolarization) and sensitization at the terminal of a gastrointestinal sensory afferent [11, 12]. Separate mechanisms underlie activation and sensitization. Some mediators such as serotonin (5-HT) cause activation via 5-HT3 receptors, whereas others like PGE2 acting at EP2 receptors sensitize visceral afferent responses to other stimuli. Still others, for example, adenosine (Adeno), cause both stimulation and sensitization, possibly through distinct receptor mechanisms. Bradykinin (BK) has a self-sensitizing action, stimulating discharge through activation of phospholipase C (PLC) and enhancing excitability via prostaglandins (PGs) after activation of phospholipase A2 (PLA2). Inflammatory mediators can be released from different cell types (e.g., sympathetic varicosities, mast cells, lymphocytes, and blood vessels) present in or around the afferent nerve terminal. 5-HT, ATP, H+and capsaicin (Cap) can directly activate cation channels (NSCCs) such as TRPA1 [13], TRPV1 [13–15], P2X [16], TRPV4 [17, 18], and ASIC [14, 15]. Adenosine, histamine, prostaglandins (not PGE2), and proteases such as mast cell tryptase (Tryp) and thrombin (Thro) act on G protein-coupled receptors (PAR2 [19] and PAR4 [20]) leading to a calcium-dependent modulation of ion channel activity. Sensitization, however, may be mediated by increased intracellular cAMP. Adenosine and PGE2 can generate cAMP directly through G protein-coupled stimulation of adenylate cyclase (AC). In contrast, histamine (Hist) may act indirectly through the generation of prostaglandins. The actions of cAMP downstream are currently unknown but may involve modulation of ion channels, interaction with other second messengers (e.g., calcium), or even changes in receptor expression. AA, arachidonic acid; ASIC, Acid-sensing ion channels; COX-1, COX-2, cyclooxygenase-1 and –2; DAG, diacylglycerol; IP3, inositol 1,4,5-trisphosphate; PARs, protease activated receptors; TRPA1, Transient receptor potential cation channel A1; TRPV1 and TRPV4, transient receptor potential cation channel subfamily V member 1 and 4. From Kirkup AJ, Brunsden AM, Grundy D. Receptors and transmission in the brain-gut axis: potential for novel therapies. I. Receptors on visceral afferents. Am J Physiol Gastrointest Liver Physiol 2001;280:G787-94. Modified with permission from The American Physiological Society

in afferent hyperexcitability; and (3) through genetic change that alters the phenotype of the afferent nerve (alterations in the expression or activity of channels and receptors). Figure 4.2 depicts the complexity of receptors and bioactive substances involved in visceral sensitivity in terminal afferents.

Central Pathways of Visceral Sensitivity

Vagal Central Pathway

Vagal afferents project in the brainstem to the NTS which displays a viscerotopic organization [21]. The NTS acts as a relay for the enormous amount of data originating from the abdominal viscera and, in turn, it sends out a network to the motor nucleus (nucleus ambiguus [NA] and dorsal motor nucleus [DMN]) providing the circuits for basic reflex of the GI tract. The NTS also projects fibers to higher centers: (1) information is relayed to parabrachial nuclei (PBN), which in turn are connected to higher brain centers (amygdala system) and (2) long projections terminate in the thalamus, hypothalamus, and anterior cingulate cortex (ACC) and insular cortical regions regulating arousal, emotional, autonomic, and behavioral responses [2, 3].

Spinal Central Pathway

After entering the spinal cord, first-order neurons make synapse in the dorsal horn and second-order neurones project to the brain through a number of different tracts: spinoreticular, spinomesencephalic, spinohypothalamic, and spinothalamic [22]. The spinothalamic tract is classically subdivided into lateral spinothalamic tract that mediates the sensory-discriminative aspects of pain (localization, intensity), and medial spinothalamic tract mediating the motivational-affective aspects of pain (suffering, unpleasantness). The lateral spinothalamic tract projects to the ventral posterior lateral nucleus of the sensory thalamus, from which information is relayed to the somatosensory cortex (S1 and S2), and the insula cortex. The medial spinothalamic tract projects to medial dorsal and ventral medial posterior nuclei of the thalamus and mainly projects, with spinoreticular, spinomesencephalic, and spinohypothalamic tracts, onto brainstem and midbrain structures such as reticular formation, NTS, periaqueductal gray (PAG) and PBN. From these structures, third-order neurons project to areas involved in emotional functioning, like the anterior cingulated cortex ACC and the orbitomedial prefrontal cortex (PFC).

Central Processing of Visceral Sensitivity

The main function of somatosensory cortex (S1 and S2) is to provide information about intensity and localization of the stimulus (sensory-discriminative). The ACC mainly processes pain affects (unpleasantness, pain-related anxiety) and cognitive aspects of the pain experience (attention, anticipation). However, important interactions between these two systems are certainly present. The insula integrates internal state of the organism and encodes sensory and emotional information related to pain. The prefrontal cortex is believed to play a key role in the integration of sensory information and in the affective aspect of the sensation. Furthermore, this region is also involved in the generation of and the choice between autonomic and behavioral response patterns, and has been shown to be a putative biological substrate of cognitive influences (including placebo effect) on emotions and the affective dimension of pain.

Quantitative meta-analysis techniques have recently permitted to pool the results of 18 studies conducted between 2000 and 2010 using PET or fMRI in controls and IBS subjects undergoing supraliminal rectal distension (painful or not). Data from the healthy control subjects confirm that regions activated in response to supraliminal rectal distension include zones associated with visceral sensation (bilateral anterior insula, bilateral midcingulate cortex, and right thalamus), emotional arousal (right perigenual ACC), and regions associated with attention and modulation of arousal (left inferior parietal, left lateral, and right medial prefrontal cortex) [23].

Descending Modulatory Pathways

Pain afferent stimuli reaching brain structures induce projections able to modulate ongoing transmission of those inputs at the level of the dorsal horn thus achieving a descending modulatory control. Descending modulation can be inhibitory, facilitatory, or both [2, 22].

At the cortical level, the ACC is the key region involved in this control through projections toward the amygdala and the PAG. Thus, cognitive and affective factors may exert influence on pain transmission through the ACC. The amygdala and the PAG project in turn to the locus coeruleus, the raphe nuclei, and the rostrolateral ventral medulla, which then send projections to the dorsal horn and modulate the synaptic transmission of sensory information at this level.

Visceral Hypersensitivity

Definitions applied in visceral sensitivity have been borrowed from the somatic pain field. *Hypersensitivity* is defined as an increased sensation of stimuli (appraised by measurement of threshold volumes or pressure for first sensation or pain). *Hyperalgesia* is an increased pain sensation to a certain painful stimulus and *allodynia* a stimulus previously not perceived as being painful that becomes painful. *Visceral hypersensitivity* is defined as an exaggerated perceptual response (hyperalgesia, allodynia, abnormal somatic referral) in response to peripheral events. Theoretically, visceral hypersensitivity could be the result of changes in visceral afferent signal processing (reflecting increased visceral afferent input to the brain from the gut such as peripheral sensitization at the level of the gastrointestinal tract) or a consequence of alterations in pain modulation mechanisms (i.e., central sensitization or pain inhibition process at the level of the central nervous system), or due to a variable combinations of these pathways.

In pediatrics, several independent groups have reported that 75–100% of children affected by IBS have a low rectal sensory threshold for pain (i.e., visceral hypersensitivity) as compared to control children [24–28]. In adults, the prevalence of visceral hypersensitivity varies from 20% [29] to 94% [30] across studies suggesting that visceral hypersensitivity is a more reliable diagnostic marker in children than in adults.

Aberrant viscerosomatic projections have also been reported in children with IBS and FAP who, in response to rectal distension, refer their sensation to aberrant sites compared to the controls, i.e., with abdominal projections on dermatomes T8 to L1 wherein controls referred their sensation to the S3 dermatome. In adults and in children, visceral hypersensitivity has been shown to be "organ-specific" with a low rectal sensitivity threshold in IBS patients [30–37], a low gastric sensitivity threshold in FD [38–41] and "diffuse" hypersensitivity in mixed IBS+FD patients [42].

Data from studies on visceral hypersensitivity in FGID and specifically in IBS favor the presence of heterogeneous causes and mechanisms in a population of patients. Animal models have permitted investigations to uncover cellular and molecular abnormalities in the gastrointestinal tract as well as in the CNS (spinal cord and brain) [43, 44]. In humans, studies have similarly found several changes in the rectal and colonic mucosa (inflammation, mast cell infiltration, serotonin pathway anomalies…) in IBS patients. Functional brain imaging techniques have permitted to demonstrate, in adults, the importance of a role for CNS dysregulation of pain processing in IBS. Recently, preliminary data on visceral afferents have been obtained in humans predicting significant progress in this field [45, 46].

Peripheral Mechanisms

Inflammation

It is accepted that IBS onset may be triggered by enteric bacterial infection that may have consequences on local inflammation, EC cell and mast cell counts [47, 48]. Low-grade inflammation has been reported in the enteric ganglia [49] and the mucosa [49, 50] of patients with IBS. The mucosal inflammation has been reported to correlate with fatigue and depression in adults with IBS [51]. Proinflammatory cytokine (IL-1, IL-6, and TNF-α(alpha)) production by peripheral blood mononuclear cells is upregulated in patients with IBS [52]. The major role of inflammation in IBS has been confirmed by microarray studies on colonic specimens that have emphasized the key role of inflammatory cells in FGID [53].

Mast Cell Hyperplasia and Mucosal Innervation

Abnormal mast cell numbers (increase [54–56] or decrease [57]) and close proximity to mucosal enteric neurites has been reported in stressed rats [54, 55] and noted in the descending colon of adult patients with IBS [56, 57]. Mast cell activation might be a means whereby psychological factors perpetuate mucosal inflammation; in animal studies, stress increases mast cell numbers and activation [54, 55]. In humans, cold stress induces mast cell degranulation in the gut [58], and in IBS, both fatigue and depression scores correlate significantly with the mast cell counts of the lamina propria [51]. It has been shown that the mucosa releases mediators that activate afferent nerves and might therefore mediate visceral hypersensitivity [59]. Tryptase [19, 59] and nerve growth factor (NGF) [60, 61], secreted by activated mast cells, have been reported as involved in visceral hypersensitivity.

Serotonin (5HT) Pathway

Serotonin is secreted by enterochromaffin (EC) cells and plays a critical role in the regulation of GI motility, secretion, and sensation through specific receptors [62–66]. The 5HT transporter (SERT) terminates the actions of 5HT by removing it from the interstitial space [67–69]. Changes in EC cell numbers and 5HT content, release, and uptake have been demonstrated in an animal model of post-infectious visceral hypersensitivity [70]. Coates et al. [71] reported also that mucosal 5HT, tryptophan hydroxylase-1 messenger RNA (TpH1, the rate-limiting enzyme in the biosynthesis of 5HT) and SERT mRNA were all significantly reduced in colonic mucosa of adult patients with IBS. Camilleri et al. [72] did not confirm results on SERT mRNA. In children 5HT content was found significantly higher in the rectal mucosa of pediatric subjects with IBS as compared to controls and SERT mRNA was significantly lower in patients than in controls [73]. Park et al. [74] have shown a correlation between EC cells and rectal hypersensitivity in adults suggesting that these cells play a role in visceral sensitivity.

PAR2 and PAR4

Protease-activated receptors (PAR) are G-protein-coupled receptors that are activated after cleavage by proteases of their N-terminal domain, which releases a tethered ligand that binds and activates the receptor. In the GI tract, PARs can be activated by mast cell tryptase, pancreatic trypsin, and exogenous proteinases [80]. PAR-1, PAR-2, and PAR-4 are distributed throughout the GI tract. PAR-1 and PAR-2 are involved in modulation of intestinal inflammation [81, 82] and PAR-2 [83] and PAR-4 are key players in visceral pain and hypersensitivity. Activation of PAR-2 is pronociceptive [19, 84] and PAR-4 is conversely an inhibitor of visceral hypersensitivity [20, 85]. It is conceivable that visceral hypersensitivity may result from disequilibrium between the pronociceptive effect of PAR-2 activation (or overexpression) incorrectly counterbalanced by the antinociceptive effect of PAR-4 activation (or low expression).

TRPV1 and TRPV4

A role of TRPV1 in visceral hypersensitivity is supported by several studies in rodents showing that TRPV1 mediates visceral nociception behavior [14, 15, 75]. In adult humans, a potential role of TRPV1 is supported by a higher density of TRPV1 fibers in the colonic mucosa of patients with IBS as compared to controls [76]. Interestingly, Sugiuar et al. [77] have shown that TRPV1 function is enhanced by 5HT in colonic sensory neurons and Gatti et al. [78] have reported that PAR-2 activation exaggerates TRPV1-induced cough. TRPV4 mediates somatic mechanosensation. Recent studies have also emphasized the role of TRPV4 expression and function in visceral nociception [17, 18, 79]. TRPV4 is expressed in visceral afferent neurons [18] and epithelial colonic cells [17]. Interestingly, TRPV4 is thought to be the mediator of PAR-2 induced colonic sensitization [17, 79]. Whether TRPV4 expression at the colonic level participates in the transmission of the nociceptive message is unknown. No human studies on TRPV4 are currently available.

Other Potential Mechanisms

Voltage gated sodium channels and cannabinoid receptors have been reported as involved in visceral sensitivity in animal studies but data in humans are lacking [86].

Central Mechanisms

When measured by using rectal distensions in humans, the perceptual response expressed by the subject and measured as the rectal sensory threshold can be separated into two components according to the signal detection theory [87–89]: the *perceptual sensitivity* (the physiological capacity of the neurosensory apparatus of the rectum to detect intraluminal distension, i.e., the ability to detect intraluminal distension) and the *response bias* (how the sensation is reported). The *perceptual sensitivity* reflects the ability of the organ to detect and transduce the stimulus to the central nervous system. The *response bias* is the reporting behavior (intensity, painfulness) which is a cognitive process influenced by past experience and psychological state. Though perceptual sensitivity can be related to peripheral mechanisms, response bias results from central modulation of the stimuli and processing of the sensation.

Central Sensitization

Central sensitization is a phenomenon that has been described in chronic somatic pain [90, 91]: that is a peripheral injury triggers a long-lasting increase in the excitability of spinal cord neurons inducing an increase in the afferent activity secondary to profound changes in the gain of the somatosensory system. This central facilitation results in allodynia, hyperalgesia, and a receptive field expansion that enables input from non-injured tissue to produce pain (secondary hyperalgesia). In an animal model of stress-induced visceral hyperalgesia, spinal microglia activation has been shown to play a key role in facilitation of pain stimuli [92]. In humans, using RIII reflex, evidence of an alteration (facilitation) of spinal modulation of nociceptive processing has been shown in IBS [93]. Alterations of pain inhibition processes in IBS have also been reported [94].

Dysregulation of Pain Processing

Functional cerebral imaging techniques have brought significant progress in the understanding of cortical and subcortical processing of pain in IBS. The results of the previously cited quantitative meta-analysis of 18 studies conducted in adult controls and IBS subjects undergoing supraliminal rectal distension (painful or not) support a role for CNS dysregulation of pain processing in IBS [23]. IBS subjects show a greater extent of brain activity than controls, in regions associated with visceral afferent processing and emotional arousal. Since similar differences are observed in sham distension and during anticipation of the actual rectal stimulus, they cannot be completely related to increased afferent input from the GI tract suggesting that, at least in some patients, the visceral hypersensitivity can be related to anomalies of central processing of visceral sensations.

The association of visceral hypersensitivity with somatic thermal hyperalgesia has been reported by some authors at least in a subset of IBS adult patients [35, 94, 95] suggesting that abnormal pain processing may be present in these patients. One pediatric study did not found such somatic thermal or mechanical hyperalgesia but showed a decreased sensitivity at the thenar [96].

Increased response bias (i.e., a tendency to report as painful visceral sensations) with a similar perceptual sensitivity than controls (i.e., same ability as controls to discriminate rectal distensions) which favors the hypothesis of a central abnormal processing of visceral sensations has been reported by one group [97] but was not confirmed by others [98].

References

1. Drossman D, Camilleri M, Mayer E, Whitehead W. AGA technical review on irritable bowel syndrome. Gastroenterology. 2002;123:2108–31.
2. Aziz Q, Thompson DG. Brain-gut axis in health and disease. Gastroenterology. 1998;114:559–78.
3. Bielefeldt K, Christianson JA, Davis BM. Basic and clinical aspects of visceral sensation: transmission in the CNS. Neurogastroenterol Motil. 2005;17:488–99.
4. Berthoud HR, Blackshaw LA, Brookes SJ, Grundy D. Neuroanatomy of extrinsic afferents supplying the gastrointestinal tract. Neurogastroenterol Motil. 2004;16 Suppl 1:28–33.
5. Brierley SM. Molecular basis of mechanosensitivity. Auton Neurosci. 2010;153:58–68.
6. Blackshaw LA, Brookes SJ, Grundy D, Schemann M. Sensory transmission in the gastrointestinal tract. Neurogastroenterol Motil. 2007;19:1–19.
7. Raybould HE. Gut chemosensing: Interactions between gut endocrine cells and visceral afferents. Auton Neurosci. 2010;153:41–6.
8. Braun T, Voland P, Kunz L, Prinz C, Gratzl M. Enterochromaffin cells of the human gut: sensors for spices and odorants. Gastroenterology. 2007;132:1890–901.
9. Bertrand PP, Kunze WA, Bornstein JC, Furness JB, Smith ML. Analysis of the responses of myenteric neurons in the small intestine to chemical stimulation of the mucosa. Am J Physiol. 1997;273:G422–35.
10. Beyak MJ. Visceral afferents—determinants and modulation of excitability. Auton Neurosci. 2010;153:69–78.
11. Kirkup AJ, Brunsden AM, Grundy D. Receptors and transmission in the brain-gut axis: potential for novel

therapies. I. Receptors on visceral afferents. Am J Physiol Gastrointest Liver Physiol. 2001;280:G787–94.
12. Christianson JA, Bielefeldt K, Altier C, Cenac N, Davis BM, Gebhart GF, High KW, Kollarik M, Randich A, Undem B, Vergnolle N. Development, plasticity and modulation of visceral afferents. Brain Res Rev. 2009;60:171–86.
13. Brierley SM, Hughes PA, Page AJ, Kwan KY, Martin CM, O'Donnell TA, Cooper NJ, Harrington AM, Adam B, Liebregts T, Holtmann G, Corey DP, Rychkov GY, Blackshaw LA. The ion channel TRPA1 is required for normal mechanosensation and is modulated by algesic stimuli. Gastroenterology. 2009;137:2084–2095 e3.
14. Jones 3rd RC, Xu L, Gebhart GF. The mechanosensitivity of mouse colon afferent fibers and their sensitization by inflammatory mediators require transient receptor potential vanilloid 1 and acid-sensing ion channel 3. J Neurosci. 2005;25:10981–9.
15. Jones 3rd RC, Otsuka E, Wagstrom E, Jensen CS, Price MP, Gebhart GF. Short-term sensitization of colon mechanoreceptors is associated with long-term hypersensitivity to colon distention in the mouse. Gastroenterology. 2007;133:184–94.
16. Masamichi S, Bin F, Gebhart GF. Peripheral and central P2X3 receptor contributions to colon mechanosensitivity and hypersensitivity in the mouse. Gastroenterology. 2009;13(6):2096–104.
17. Cenac N, Altier C, Chapman K, Liedtke W, Zamponi G, Vergnolle N. Transient receptor potential vanilloid-4 has a major role in visceral hypersensitivity symptoms. Gastroenterology. 2008;135:937–46. 946 e1–2.
18. Brierley SM, Page AJ, Hughes PA, Adam B, Liebregts T, Cooper NJ, Holtmann G, Liedtke W, Blackshaw LA. Selective role for TRPV4 ion channels in visceral sensory pathways. Gastroenterology. 2008;134:2059–69.
19. Cenac N, Andrews CN, Holzhausen M, Chapman K, Cottrell G, Andrade-Gordon P, Steinhoff M, Barbara G, Beck P, Bunnett NW, Sharkey KA, Ferraz JG, Shaffer E, Vergnolle N. Role for protease activity in visceral pain in irritable bowel syndrome. J Clin Invest. 2007;117:636–47.
20. Auge C, Balz-Hara D, Steinhoff M, Vergnolle N, Cenac N. Protease-activated receptor-4 (PAR(4)): a role as inhibitor of visceral pain and hypersensitivity. Neurogastroenterol Motil. 2009;21(11):1189–e107.
21. Altschuler SM, Bao XM, Bieger D, Hopkins DA, Miselis RR. Viscerotopic representation of the upper alimentary tract in the rat: sensory ganglia and nuclei of the solitary and spinal trigeminal tracts. J Comp Neurol. 1989;283:248–68.
22. Van Oudenhove L, Demyttenaere K, Tack J, Aziz Q. Central nervous system involvement in functional gastrointestinal disorders. Best Pract Res Clin Gastroenterol. 2004;18:663–80.
23. Tillisch A, Mayer E, Labus J. Quantitative meta-analysis identifies brain regions activated during rectal distension in irritable bowel syndrome. Gastroenterology. 2011;140:91–100.
24. Faure C, Wieckowska A. Somatic referral of visceral sensations and rectal sensory threshold for pain in children with functional gastrointestinal disorders. J Pediatr. 2007;150:66–71.
25. Van Ginkel R, Voskuijl WP, Benninga MA, Taminiau JA, Boeckxstaens GE. Alterations in rectal sensitivity and motility in childhood irritable bowel syndrome. Gastroenterology. 2001;120:31–8.
26. Iovino P, Tremolaterra F, Boccia G, Miele E, Ruju FM, Staiano A. Irritable bowel syndrome in childhood: visceral hypersensitivity and psychosocial aspects. Neurogastroenterol Motil. 2009;21:940–e74.
27. Di Lorenzo C, Youssef NN, Sigurdsson L, Scharff L, Griffiths J, Wald A. Visceral hyperalgesia in children with functional abdominal pain. J Pediatr. 2001;139:838–43.
28. Halac U, Noble A, Faure C. Rectal sensory threshold for pain is a diagnostic marker of irritable bowel syndrome and functional abdominal pain in children. J Pediatr. 2010;156:60–65 e1.
29. Camilleri M, McKinzie S, Busciglio I, Low PA, Sweetser S, Burton D, Baxter K, Ryks M, Zinsmeister AR. Prospective study of motor, sensory, psychologic, and autonomic functions in patients with irritable bowel syndrome. Clin Gastroenterol Hepatol. 2008;6:772–81.
30. Mertz H, Naliboff B, Munakata J, Niazi N, Mayer E. Altered rectal perception is a biological marker of patients with irritable bowel syndrome. Gastroenterology. 1995;109:40–52.
31. Whitehead WE, Holtkotter B, Enck P, Hoelzl R, Holmes KD, Anthony J, Shabsin HS, Schuster MM. Tolerance for rectosigmoid distention in irritable bowel syndrome. Gastroenterology. 1990;98:1187–92.
32. Bouin M, Plourde V, Boivin M, Riberdy M, Lupien F, Laganiere M, Verrier P, Poitras P. Rectal distention testing in patients with irritable bowel syndrome: sensitivity, specificity, and predictive values of pain sensory thresholds. Gastroenterology. 2002;122:1771–7.
33. Schmulson M, Chang L, Naliboff B, Lee OY, Mayer EA. Correlation of symptom criteria with perception thresholds during rectosigmoid distension in irritable bowel syndrome patients. Am J Gastroenterol. 2000;95:152–6.
34. Bradette M, Delvaux M, Staumont G, Fioramonti J, Bueno L, Frexinos J. Evaluation of colonic sensory thresholds in IBS patients using a barostat. Definition of optimal conditions and comparison with healthy subjects. Dig Dis Sci. 1994;39:449–57.
35. Bouin M, Meunier P, Riberdy-Poitras M, Poitras P. Pain hypersensitivity in patients with functional gastrointestinal disorders: a gastrointestinal-specific defect or a general systemic condition? Dig Dis Sci. 2001;46:2542–8.
36. Naliboff BD, Munakata J, Fullerton S, Gracely RH, Kodner A, Harraf F, Mayer EA. Evidence for two distinct perceptual alterations in irritable bowel syndrome. Gut. 1997;41:505–12.

37. Spetalen S, Jacobsen MB, Vatn MH, Blomhoff S, Sandvik L. Visceral sensitivity in irritable bowel syndrome and healthy volunteers: reproducibility of the rectal barostat. Dig Dis Sci. 2004;49:1259–64.
38. Coffin B, Azpiroz F, Guarner F, Malagelada JR. Selective gastric hypersensitivity and reflex hyporeactivity in functional dyspepsia. Gastroenterology. 1994;107:1345–51.
39. Tack J, Caenepeel P, Fischler B, Piessevaux H, Janssens J. Symptoms associated with hypersensitivity to gastric distention in functional dyspepsia. Gastroenterology. 2001;121:526–35.
40. Tack J, Caenepeel P, Corsetti M, Janssens J. Role of tension receptors in dyspeptic patients with hypersensitivity to gastric distention. Gastroenterology. 2004;127:1058–66.
41. Mertz H, Fullerton S, Naliboff B, Mayer EA. Symptoms and visceral perception in severe functional and organic dyspepsia. Gut. 1998;42:814–22.
42. Bouin M, Lupien F, Riberdy M, Boivin M, Plourde V, Poitras P. Intolerance to visceral distension in functional dyspepsia or irritable bowel syndrome: an organ specific defect or a pan intestinal dysregulation? Neurogastroenterol Motil. 2004;16:311–4.
43. Mayer EA, Collins SM. Evolving pathophysiologic models of functional gastrointestinal disorders. Gastroenterology. 2002;122:2032–48.
44. Mayer EA, Bradesi S, Chang L, Spiegel BM, Bueller JA, Naliboff BD. Functional GI disorders: from animal models to drug development. Gut. 2008;57:384–404.
45. Peiris M, Bulmer DC, Baker MD, Boundouki G, Sinha S, Hobson A, Lee K, Aziz Q, Knowles CH. Human visceral afferent recordings: preliminary report. Gut. 2011;60:204–8.
46. Jiang W, Adam IJ, Kitsanta P, Tiernan J, Hill C, Shorthouse A, Grundy D. 'First-in-man': characterising the mechanosensitivity of human colonic afferents. Gut. 2011;60:281–2.
47. Saps M, Pensabene L, Di Martino L, Staiano A, Wechsler J, Zheng X, Di Lorenzo C. Post-infectious functional gastrointestinal disorders in children. J Pediatr. 2008;152:812–6. 816 e1.
48. Spiller R, Garsed K. Postinfectious irritable bowel syndrome. Gastroenterology. 2009;136:1979–88.
49. Tornblom H, Lindberg G, Nyberg B, Veress B. Full-thickness biopsy of the jejunum reveals inflammation and enteric neuropathy in irritable bowel syndrome. Gastroenterology. 2002;123:1972–9.
50. Chadwick VS, Chen W, Shu D, Paulus B, Bethwaite P, Tie A, Wilson I. Activation of the mucosal immune system in irritable bowel syndrome. Gastroenterology. 2002;122:1778–83.
51. Piche T, Saint-Paul MC, Dainese R, Marine-Barjoan E, Iannelli A, Montoya ML, Peyron JF, Czerucka D, Cherikh F, Filippi J, Tran A, Hebuterne X. Mast cells and cellularity of the colonic mucosa correlated with fatigue and depression in irritable bowel syndrome. Gut. 2008;57:468–73.
52. Liebregts T, Adam B, Bredack C, Roth A, Heinzel S, Lester S, Downie-Doyle S, Smith E, Drew P, Talley NJ, Holtmann G. Immune activation in patients with irritable bowel syndrome. Gastroenterology. 2007;132:913–20.
53. Aerssens J, Camilleri M, Talloen W, Thielemans L, Gohlmann HW, Van Den Wyngaert I, Thielemans T, De Hoogt R, Andrews CN, Bharucha AE, Carlson PJ, Busciglio I, Burton DD, Smyrk T, Urrutia R, Coulie B. Alterations in mucosal immunity identified in the colon of patients with irritable bowel syndrome. Clin Gastroenterol Hepatol. 2008;6:194–205.
54. Gue M, Del Rio-Lacheze C, Eutamene H, Theodorou V, Fioramonti J, Bueno L. Stress-induced visceral hypersensitivity to rectal distension in rats: role of CRF and mast cells. Neurogastroenterol Motil. 1997;9:271–9.
55. Eutamene H, Theodorou V, Fioramonti J, Bueno L. Acute stress modulates the histamine content of mast cells in the gastrointestinal tract through interleukin-1 and corticotropin-releasing factor release in rats. J Physiol. 2003;553:959–66.
56. Barbara G, Stanghellini V, De Giorgio R, Cremon C, Cottrell GS, Santini D, Pasquinelli G, Morselli-Labate AM, Grady EF, Bunnett NW, Collins SM, Corinaldesi R. Activated mast cells in proximity to colonic nerves correlate with abdominal pain in irritable bowel syndrome. Gastroenterology. 2004;126:693–702.
57. Klooker TK, Braak B, Koopman KE, Welting O, Wouters MM, van der Heide S, Schemann M, Bischoff SC, van den Wijngaard RM, Boeckxstaens GE. The mast cell stabiliser ketotifen decreases visceral hypersensitivity and improves intestinal symptoms in patients with irritable bowel syndrome. Gut. 2010;59:1213–21.
58. Santos J, Saperas E, Nogueiras C, Mourelle M, Antolin M, Cadahia A, Malagelada JR. Release of mast cell mediators into the jejunum by cold pain stress in humans. Gastroenterology. 1998;114:640–8.
59. Barbara G, Wang B, Stanghellini V, de Giorgio R, Cremon C, Di Nardo G, Trevisani M, Campi B, Geppetti P, Tonini M, Bunnett NW, Grundy D, Corinaldesi R. Mast cell-dependent excitation of visceral-nociceptive sensory neurons in irritable bowel syndrome. Gastroenterology. 2007;132:26–37.
60. van den Wijngaard RM, Klooker TK, Welting O, Stanisor OI, Wouters MM, van der Coelen D, Bulmer DC, Peeters PJ, Aerssens J, de Hoogt R, Lee K, de Jonge WJ, Boeckxstaens GE. Essential role for TRPV1 in stress-induced (mast cell-dependent) colonic hypersensitivity in maternally separated rats. Neurogastroenterol Motil. 2009;21(10):1107–e94.
61. Barreau F, Salvador-Cartier C, Houdeau E, Bueno L, Fioramonti J. Long-term alterations of colonic nerve-mast cell interactions induced by neonatal maternal deprivation in rats. Gut. 2008;57:582–90.
62. Gershon MD. Review article: roles played by 5-hydroxytryptamine in the physiology of the bowel. Aliment Pharmacol Ther. 1999;13 Suppl 2:15–30.

63. Gershon MD. Nerves, reflexes, and the enteric nervous system: pathogenesis of the irritable bowel syndrome. J Clin Gastroenterol. 2005;39:S184–93.
64. Tack J, Sarnelli G. Serotonergic modulation of visceral sensation: upper gastrointestinal tract. Gut. 2002;51:77i–80.
65. Camilleri M. Serotonergic modulation of visceral sensation: lower gut. Gut. 2002;51:81i–6.
66. Mawe GM, Coates MD, Moses PL. Review article: intestinal serotonin signalling in irritable bowel syndrome. Aliment Pharmacol Ther. 2006;23:1067–76.
67. Chen JX, Pan H, Rothman TP, Wade PR, Gershon MD. Guinea pig 5-HT transporter: cloning, expression, distribution, and function in intestinal sensory reception. Am J Physiol. 1998;275:G433–48.
68. Chen JJ, Li Z, Pan H, Murphy DL, Tamir H, Koepsell H, Gershon MD. Maintenance of serotonin in the intestinal mucosa and ganglia of mice that lack the high-affinity serotonin transporter: Abnormal intestinal motility and the expression of cation transporters. J Neurosci. 2001;21:6348–61.
69. Wade PR, Chen J, Jaffe B, Kassem IS, Blakely RD, Gershon MD. Localization and function of a 5-HT transporter in crypt epithelia of the gastrointestinal tract. J Neurosci. 1996;16:2352–64.
70. Spiller RC, Jenkins D, Thornley JP, Hebden JM, Wright T, Skinner M, Neal KR. Increased rectal mucosal enteroendocrine cells, T lymphocytes, and increased gut permeability following acute Campylobacter enteritis and in post-dysenteric irritable bowel syndrome. Gut. 2000;47:804–11.
71. Coates MD, Mahoney CR, Linden DR, Sampson JE, Chen J, Blaszyk H, Crowell MD, Sharkey KA, Gershon MD, Mawe GM, Moses PL. Molecular defects in mucosal serotonin content and decreased serotonin reuptake transporter in ulcerative colitis and irritable bowel syndrome. Gastroenterology. 2004;126:1657–64.
72. Camilleri M, Andrews CN, Bharucha AE, Carlson PJ, Ferber I, Stephens D, Smyrk TC, Urrutia R, Aerssens J, Thielemans L, Gohlmann H, van den Wyngaert I, Coulie B. Alterations in expression of p11 and SERT in mucosal biopsy specimens of patients with irritable bowel syndrome. Gastroenterology. 2007;132:17–25.
73. Faure C, Patey N, Gauthier C, Brooks EM, Mawe GM. Serotonin signaling is altered in irritable bowel syndrome with diarrhea but not in functional dyspepsia in pediatric age patients. Gastroenterology. 2010;139:249–58.
74. Park JH, Rhee PL, Kim G, Lee JH, Kim YH, Kim JJ, Rhee JC, Song SY. Enteroendocrine cell counts correlate with visceral hypersensitivity in patients with diarrhoea-predominant irritable bowel syndrome. Neurogastroenterol Motil. 2006;18:539–46.
75. Winston J, Shenoy M, Medley D, Naniwadekar A, Pasricha PJ. The vanilloid receptor initiates and maintains colonic hypersensitivity induced by neonatal colon irritation in rats. Gastroenterology. 2007;132:615–27.
76. Akbar A, Yiangou Y, Facer P, Walters JR, Anand P, Ghosh S. Increased capsaicin receptor TRPV1 expressing sensory fibres in irritable bowel syndrome and their correlation with abdominal pain. Gut. 2008;57:923–9.
77. Sugiuar T, Bielefeldt K, Gebhart GF. TRPV1 function in mouse colon sensory neurons is enhanced by metabotropic 5-hydroxytryptamine receptor activation. J Neurosci. 2004;24:9521–30.
78. Gatti R, Andre E, Amadesi S, Dinh TQ, Fischer A, Bunnett NW, Harrison S, Geppetti P, Trevisani M. Protease-activated receptor-2 activation exaggerates TRPV1-mediated cough in guinea pigs. J Appl Physiol. 2006;101:506–11.
79. Sipe WE, Brierley SM, Martin CM, Phillis BD, Cruz FB, Grady EF, Liedtke W, Cohen DM, Vanner S, Blackshaw LA, Bunnett NW. Transient receptor potential vanilloid 4 mediates protease activated receptor 2-induced sensitization of colonic afferent nerves and visceral hyperalgesia. Am J Physiol Gastrointest Liver Physiol. 2008;294:G1288–98.
80. Kawabata A, Matsunami M, Sekiguchi F. Gastrointestinal roles for proteinase-activated receptors in health and disease. Br J Pharmacol. 2008;153 Suppl 1:S230–40.
81. Steinhoff M, Vergnolle N, Young SH, Tognetto M, Amadesi S, Ennes HS, Trevisani M, Hollenberg MD, Wallace JL, Caughey GH, Mitchell SE, Williams LM, Geppetti P, Mayer EA, Bunnett NW. Agonists of proteinase-activated receptor 2 induce inflammation by a neurogenic mechanism. Nat Med. 2000;6:151–8.
82. Hyun E, Andrade-Gordon P, Steinhoff M, Vergnolle N. Protease-activated receptor-2 activation: a major actor in intestinal inflammation. Gut. 2008;57:1222–9.
83. Coelho AM, Vergnolle N, Guiard B, Fioramonti J, Bueno L. Proteinases and proteinase-activated receptor 2: a possible role to promote visceral hyperalgesia in rats. Gastroenterology. 2002;122:1035–47.
84. Kayssi A, Amadesi S, Bautista F, Bunnett NW, Vanner S. Mechanisms of protease-activated receptor 2-evoked hyperexcitability of nociceptive neurons innervating the mouse colon. J Physiol. 2007;580:977–91.
85. Annahazi A, Gecse K, Dabek M, Ait-Belgnaoui A, Rosztoczy A, Roka R, Molnar T, Theodorou V, Wittmann T, Bueno L, Eutamene H. Fecal proteases from diarrheic-IBS and ulcerative colitis patients exert opposite effect on visceral sensitivity in mice. Pain. 2009;144:209–17.
86. Akbar A, Walters JR, Ghosh S. Review article: visceral hypersensitivity in irritable bowel syndrome: molecular mechanisms and therapeutic agents. Aliment Pharmacol Ther. 2009;30:423–35.
87. Mcmillan NA, Creelman CD. Detection theory: a user's guide. New York: Laurence Elbaum Associates Inc.; 2005.
88. Clark WC. Pain sensitivity and the report of pain: an introduction to sensory decision theory. Anesthesiology. 1974;40:272–87.

89. Harvey LOJ. Detection sensitivity and response bias. In: http://psych.colorado.edu/~lharvey/p4165/p4165_2003_spring/2003_Spring_pdf/P4165_SDT.pdf, ed, 2003.
90. Woolf CJ. Central sensitization: implications for the diagnosis and treatment of pain. Pain. 2011;152:S2–15.
91. Zhang J, Shi XQ, Echeverry S, Mogil JS, De Koninck Y, Rivest S. Expression of CCR2 in both resident and bone marrow-derived microglia plays a critical role in neuropathic pain. J Neurosci. 2007;27:12396–406.
92. Bradesi S, Svensson CI, Steinauer J, Pothoulakis C, Yaksh TL, Mayer EA. Role of spinal microglia in visceral hyperalgesia and NK1R up-regulation in a rat model of chronic stress. Gastroenterology. 2009;136(1339–48):e1–2.
93. Coffin B, Bouhassira D, Sabate JM, Barbe L, Jian R. Alteration of the spinal modulation of nociceptive processing in patients with irritable bowel syndrome. Gut. 2004;53:1465–70.
94. Piche M, Arsenault M, Poitras P, Rainville P, Bouin M. Widespread hypersensitivity is related to altered pain inhibition processes in irritable bowel syndrome. Pain. 2010;148:49–58.
95. Zhou Q, Fillingim RB, Riley 3rd JL, Malarkey WB, Verne GN. Central and peripheral hypersensitivity in the irritable bowel syndrome. Pain. 2010;148:454–61.
96. Zohsel K, Hohmeister J, Flor H, Hermann C. Somatic pain sensitivity in children with recurrent abdominal pain. Am J Gastroenterol. 2008;103:1517–23.
97. Dorn SD, Palsson OS, Thiwan SI, Kanazawa M, Clark WC, van Tilburg MA, Drossman DA, Scarlett Y, Levy RL, Ringel Y, Crowell MD, Olden KW, Whitehead WE. Increased colonic pain sensitivity in irritable bowel syndrome is the result of an increased tendency to report pain rather than increased neurosensory sensitivity. Gut. 2007;56:1202–9.
98. Corsetti M, Ogliari C, Marino B, Basilisco G. Perceptual sensitivity and response bias during rectal distension in patients with irritable bowel syndrome. Neurogastroenterol Motil. 2005;17:541–7.

Inflammation, Microflora, Motility, and Visceral Sensitivity

5

Sonia Michail and Mun-Wah Ng

Introduction

This chapter addresses the relationship between the gut microflora and the neurogastrointestinal system. It is divided into several sections that further dissect the contribution of the bacterial content of the gut towards the development of motility disorders, with a main focus on the most common functional and visceral hypersensitivity disorder—irritable bowel syndrome (IBS).

The Effect of the Brain on Gut Environment

Communication between the brain and the gut (see Fig. 5.1) is modulated by the autonomic nervous system, both sympathetic and parasympathetic. This gut–brain axis controls gut functions ranging from gastrointestinal secretions to motility and immune response. In turn, the vitality of the gut microbiome, at least in part, is determined by the gastrointestinal transit and motility which, when impaired, can affect the delivery of nutrients to the microbiota. For example, impaired intestinal transit caused by disarray of the migrating motor complexes (MMC) can result in the development of small bowel bacterial overgrowth [1]. Disordered MMC contractions are common in IBS where decreased MMC contractions in the small bowel are seen in constipation-predominant IBS, and accelerated intestinal transit in diarrhea-predominant IBS [2]. In addition, the autonomic nervous system modulates gastrointestinal mucus secretion which forms the biofilm, home to the many of the enteric microbiota [3]. It also influences immune activation of the gut, directly, through modulation of the response of the gut immune cells to luminal bacteria, or indirectly, through modification of the ability of luminal bacteria to reach the gut immunocytes. Interestingly, stress and stressful stimuli can enhance the permeability of the intestinal epithelium, which allows bacterial antigens to cross the intestinal epithelium triggering an immune response in the intestinal mucosa [4–9] and causing a significant reduction in the tight junction proteins which leads to a compromise in the epithelial barrier function and the development of leaky gut [10]. Therefore, the brain and its axis can greatly influence the gut milieu.

Mucosal-Gut Microbial Interaction

Stress can also play an important role in mucosal-microbiome interaction and host protection. For example, secretion of mucosal

S. Michail, M.D. (✉)
The Children's Medical Center, Gastroenterology, One Children's Plaza, Dayton, OH 45404, USA
e-mail: sonia.michail@hotmail.com

M.-W, Ng, M.D.
Pediatrics Department, Gastroenterology & Nutrition Division, Children's Hospital Los Angeles, Los Angeles, CA, USA

C. Faure et al. (eds.), *Pediatric Neurogastroenterology: Gastrointestinal Motility and Functional Disorders in Children*, Clinical Gastroenterology,
DOI 10.1007/978-1-60761-709-9_5, © Springer Science+Business Media New York 2013

defensins, which are antimicrobial peptides, can play an important role in host defense mechanisms against inflammatory and infectious diseases of the gastrointestinal tract [11]. The secretion of such defensins by Paneth cells is enhanced by stress [12]. Stress can also impact the secretion of neuroendocrine signaling molecules such as catecholamines, serotonin, and cytokines, which are secreted by neurons, immune cells, and enterochromaffin cells, into the gut lumen in response to different stress stimuli [13–15]. Furthermore, norepinephrine release in the intestine during stress and trauma induces expression of virulence factors in *Pseudomonas aeruginosa* which contributes to gut-derived sepsis [16], stimulates the growth of several other strains of enteric pathogens, and intensify the virulence of *Campylobacter jejuni* [17]. These reports can help us appreciate the association of stressful events with the development of gastrointestinal disease such gastroenteritis and subsequent development of post infectious IBS [18].

Bidirectional Signaling

The gut microbiome, much like the enteric nervous system, can affect the intestinal motility. For example, *Lactobacillus acidophilus* and *Bifidobacterium bifidum* are capable of promoting motility, while other members of the gut microbiome such as Escherichia species can inhibit or slow down the intestinal transit [19]. Gut bacteria can also modulate gut transit indirectly through the production of microbial metabolites such as short-chain fatty acids or peptides such as *N*-formylmethionyl–leucine–phenylalanine [20–22]. Disturbance in the intricate balance between different enteric microbial populations might, therefore, predispose the host to altered gut motility and secretion, which results in diarrhea or constipation. These changes are, in turn, likely to influence the balance of enteric microbiota. Therefore, the gut microbiome can directly influence gut homeostasis by the regulation of bowel motility and modulation of visceral pain and immune responses [23–26] (Fig. 5.1).

Irritable Bowel Syndrome

IBS is a common disorder afflicting millions of adults and children around the world. From the pediatric perspective, it is estimated that IBS affects up to 25% of school-age children and adolescents, accounts for a significant number (2–4%) of office visits to primary care doctors, and represents about 25–50% of all patients who visit a gastroenterologist's clinic [27]. The past several years have witnessed an emergence of new concepts related to the pathophysiology of IBS, which include alterations in gut motility, small-bowel bacterial overgrowth, microscopic inflammation, visceral hypersensitivity, and changes related to the brain–gut microbial axis.

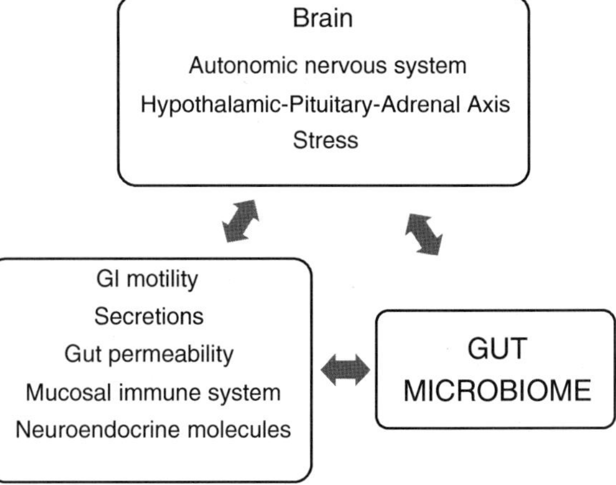

Fig. 5.1 Bidirectional relationship of the brain–gut–enteric microbiota axis

Altered Gut Motility

In IBS, disordered gut motility has been observed along the length of the gastrointestinal tract [28–31]. The major migrating complex (MMC), which consists of periodic, contractions that sweep the luminal contents from the stomach to the colon, becomes disorganized. Several studies have shown that patients with IBS tend to have abnormalities in these contractions. For example, Vassallo et al. measured colonic electronic barostat and perfusion manometry in 16 subjects and demonstrated a greater frequency of prolonged, high amplitude and greater preprandial colonic motility, which may explain the increased perception of pain in these patients. Other studies assessing colonic transit times in IBS, showed a shorter colonic transit in patients with diarrhea-predominant IBS [32, 33] consistent with the presenting symptomatololgy. More importantly, the dysmotility seen in these patients can predispose them to develop small-bowel bacterial overgrowth, which is another proposed etiology for the development of IBS symptoms.

The Contribution of the Gut Microbiome Towards IBS

Small-Bowel Bacterial Overgrowth

Small-bowel bacterial overgrowth has emerged as a possible cause of IBS since Vantrappen and colleagues' work which suggested that it may occur in specific motility disorder such as a reduction in the major migrating complex [1]. Further studies have confirmed this finding in this patient population [34–36]. A large study of 202 patients with IBS found that 78% of these patients had evidence of bacterial overgrowth demonstrated by abnormal lactulose-methane-hydrogen breath testing. In the study, 25 of 47 patients experienced eradication of bacterial overgrowth on follow-up after treatment with antibiotics. Analysis of this subset of patients revealed that those who had successful eradication of bacterial overgrowth reported improvement in their IBS symptoms [37]. Another study by Pimentel showed that 84% of 111 patients with IBS had abnormal breath testing. These patients were then randomized to receive neomycin or placebo for 1 week. A follow-up questionnaire revealed that patients in the neomycin group reported a 35% reduction in symptomatology as compared to 11.4% in the placebo group [38]. More recently, Peralta and colleagues assessed 97 patients who met Rome II criteria and found that 56% of these patients had positive lactulose breath tests [39].

Although the exact mechanisms by which altered fecal flora induce disease are poorly understood, it has been shown that fecal short chain fatty acids produced by microbiota, which are critical for maintenance of the colonic epithelium, are significantly reduced in children with diarrhea-predominant IBS [40]. Symptoms especially related to gas production are reduced by an exclusion diet, suggesting an alteration in the activity of hydrogen-consuming bacteria and further emphasizing the importance of fermentation in the pathogenesis of IBS [41]. Lactulose breath testing in IBS subjects does not seem to reflect malabsorption but the pattern of hydrogen excretion is suggestive of bacterial overgrowth [42] and suggests that IBS might be associated with rapid excretion of gaseous products of fermentation [43]. On the other hand, increased bacterial methane production was seen with constipation-predominant IBS [44]. Postprandial serotonin release was also blunted [45], suggesting a possible neurochemical basis for impaired motor function. The discovery that specific changes in gut microbiota contribute to IBS pathophysiology could aid in the development of new therapeutic strategies [46, 47].

The Gut Microbiome in IBS

The gut microbiome is the array of microorganisms that dwell along the human gastrointestinal tract. The human microbiota is estimated to contain as many as 10^{14} bacterial cells-a number that is 10 times greater than the number of human cells present in our bodies [48–50]. The microbiota colonizes every surface in contact with the external environment but the colon is the most heavily colonized and is estimated to contain over 70% of all the organisms in the human body.

The human gut has a large surface area [51] and is rich in nutrients, making it a preferred site for bacterial colonization. The architecture of this population is dynamic and evolves from birth to adulthood. It is influenced by the diet, state of health, external environment and other similar factors. The microbiome is closely associated with many aspects of human health, from nutritional status to immune and stress response. The intricate balance in the make-up of the gut microbial population, as well as the presence or absence of key microbial elements is crucial in ensuring health of the host. Although it is embraced as largely beneficial, it has been postulated that altered bacterial populations or products of bacterial metabolism may contribute to the development of disease in the gastrointestinal tract as well as remote areas of the body. The mechanisms through which microbiota exerts its beneficial or negative influences on the host include the production of signaling pathways and recognition of bacterial proteins by intestinal epithelial and mucosal host immune cells.

Recent data propose a role for the gut microbiota in the development of both central and peripheral neural processes. These interactions, termed the "brain–gut–enteric microbiota axis" [52], as discussed, can be bidirectional, with potential ramifications for disruption of this axis leading to abnormal neurogenic stimulation of the enteric system and the development of disorders such as IBS. The activation of any of the central nervous system and the gut–brain axis has potential in influencing enteric microbiota both directly through interaction between the gut microbiome and the host, and indirectly via changes in their environment [3].

In animal studies, the impact of stress on the composition of the enteric microbiota has become evident [53, 54]. Stress was characterized by transient reductions in the levels of the enteric microbiota in rhesus monkeys. In postnatal, maternal separation-induced stress, reduction in *Lactobacilli* was associated with the appearance of stress-indicative behaviors.

So is there a quantitative difference in the gut bacteria in IBS? Several studies are beginning to address this question. Osipov and colleagues demonstrate that the concentration of *Streptomycetes*, *Rhodococci*, and other members of the *Actinomycetales* order become dozen folds higher in quantity [55]. In another study by Malinen, a reduction of *Lactobacilli*, *Clostridium coccoides*, and *Bifidobacterium catenulatem* counts were seen in diarrhea-predominant IBS compared with healthy individuals [56]. Si and colleagues noted a reduction of fecal *Bifidobacteria* and an increase in *Enterobacteriaceae, as well as lowered resistance to* microbial colonization of the bowel in patients with IBS [57]. Taken together, these studies show encouraging associations between the gut microbiome and IBS.

Intestinal Inflammation

Considerable attention has been recently directed towards the possibility of microscopic inflammation as a contributor to the development of IBS [58, 59]. Low-grade inflammation found in biopsies of different parts of the intestine in subjects with IBS has fueled this concept [47, 58, 60, 61]. The release of certain inflammatory mediators such as cytokines, interleukins, and histamine, may affect nearby enteric nerves, causing alteration in gut function and sensory perception leading to IBS symptomatology [60, 62]. The study by Chadwick et al. led the way to the new concept of IBS as an inflammatory condition. In their study of 77 IBS subjects, 55% were diarrhea predominant; and none had a confirmed infectious origin for IBS [58]. While 38 subjects had normal histology, 31 demonstrated microscopic inflammation and 8 fulfilled histologic criteria for lymphocytic colitis. Interestingly, even in the group with normal histology, immunohistology demonstrated inflammation with increased intraepithelial lymphocytes as well as an increase in CD3+ and CD25+ cells in the lamina propria. Therefore, all subjects had mucosal immune activation.

Additional studies further support the role of inflammation in IBS. Gonsalkorale and colleagues demonstrated that subjects with IBS have a reduction in interleukin-10 (IL-10), which has an anti-inflammatory effect [63]. Barbara and colleagues' work demonstrate an increase in colonic mast cell degranulation with direct correlation between the proximity of mast cells in the mucosa and clinical pain severity [62]. Furthermore, Tornblom and colleagues examined full-thickness jejunal biopsies in 10 subjects obtained during laparoscopy [64] and noted low-grade infiltration of lymphocytes in the myenteric plexus in all patients and many had evidence of neuronal degeneration, longitudinal muscle hypertrophy and abnormalities in the number and size of interstitial cells of Cajal. There is also evidence to support an alteration in the ratio between the cytokines IL-10 and IL-12 favoring a Th1 response similar to what is seen in peripheral blood mononuclear cells [65]. Spiller further proposed that the inflammatory changes could represent an immune response to an initial enteric infection in individuals who become susceptible by a relative deficiency of anti-inflammatory cytokines [66].

Although embracing this theory broadens therapeutic options, yet efforts to treat the inflammation in an attempt to improve symptoms have been largely unsuccessful. Subjects with post-infectious IBS randomized to either prednisolone 30 mg daily versus placebo showed no improvement in their symptoms even though T lymphocytes decreased by 22% as compared to 11.5% in the placebo group [67]. Therefore, the clinical significance and application of this important concept of IBS being an inflammatory condition are yet to be defined.

Modulation of Visceral Hypersensitivity

Visceral hypersensitivity is becoming more recognized as a potential contributor to the development of pain in IBS. Studies are now beginning to utilize the concept of the gut microbiome and probiotics to modulate this visceral hypersensitivity. Animal studies using the probiotic *Lactobacillus farciminis* demonstrate significant attenuation of stress-induced proteins during colorectal distension in rats and suggest a link to the epithelial cell cytoskeletal contraction [25, 26]. A study by Verdu showed that administration of *Lactobacillus paracasei* attenuates the antibiotic induced visceral hypersensitivity in mice [68]. Perhaps the most interesting link between gut bacteria and visceral sensitivity is highlighted by Rousseaux et al. [69] establishing that oral administration of *L. acidophilus* induced the expression of mu-opioid and cannabinoid receptors in epithelial cells, and mediated analgesic functions in the intestine in a manner similar to that induced by morphine.

Potential Therapeutic Applications

The modification of the enteric microbiota to treat subjects with IBS and visceral hypersensitivity is attractive due to its ease, relative safety, and current lack of other effective therapeutic alternatives. Such modifications can be achieved by the administration of antibiotics, probiotics, or prebiotics. Clinical studies have produced variable responses to such treatments and vary depending on age, predominant symptoms, and bowel habits. Our current understanding of IBS pathophysiology remains incomplete, and although the complexity of the network of interactions within the enteric microbiota and visceral hypersensitivity is emerging, some studies have provided evidence for a beneficiary role for enhancement or manipulation of the gut bacteria. The use of nonabsorbable antimicrobial therapies such as Rifaximin has shown some promise and probiotics and prebiotics are also emerging as potential therapies. A recent study by Pimentel [70] validated that rifaximin therapy for 2 weeks provided significant relief of IBS symptoms, bloating, abdominal pain, and diarrhea. In another study, 54 patients with positive lactulose breath tests were treated with a 7-day course of rifaximin. Follow-up after 3 weeks revealed that half of their subjects had a subsequent negative lactulose breath test and a statistically significant improvement in symptoms. These results were similar to those found in another recent study by Majewski and associates, in which a 4-week course of rifaximin led to improvement in IBS-related symptoms and a negative breath test in patients who previously had positive tests [71]. Although these results are encouraging, other researchers have failed to confirm these findings and further research is needed in this area [72].

An important study by O'Mahony et al. [65] showed that *Bifidobacterium infantis* not only resulted in symptom reduction in IBS, but also correlated with normalization of proinflammatory cytokines, suggesting an immune modulating effect of probiotics. The study by Bazzocchi et al. [73] is the first observation showing a clinical improvement related to changes in the composition of the fecal bacterial flora, fecal biochemistry and colonic motility pattern, all of which was induced by administration of probiotics, in patients with functional diarrhea. In constipation-predominant IBS, Agrawal and colleagues [74] show improvements in abdominal girth and gastrointestinal transit, as well as reduced symptomatology after 4 weeks of *Bifidobacerterium lactis* consumption.

Pediatric studies addressing the role of probiotics in IBS have recently emerged (Table 5.1). A study published by Bausserman and Michail [75] designed to determine whether oral administration of the probiotic *Lactobacillus GG* under randomized, placebo-controlled, double-blinded conditions would improve symptoms of IBS in children, showed a lower incidence of perceived abdominal distension but did not alter any of the other parameters. Another double-blinded, randomized controlled trial by Gawronska et al. [76] designed to determine the efficacy of a 4-week therapy with *Lactobacillus rhamnosus GG* (LGG) in treating functional abdominal pain disorders (FAPD) in children showed a higher incidence of treatment success (i.e., no pain) in children with IBS receiving the probiotic. A more recent study by Guandalini and colleagues [77] suggests a beneficial role for VSL#3 (Sigma-Tau Pharmaceuticals, Inc.) in children with IBS. Finally, reports of amelioration of symptoms of bloating and flatulence in patients with IBS when treated with a poorly absorbed antibiotic, Rifaximin [77, 78], and the poorly absorbed antibiotic Neomycin has been effective in reducing symptoms and decreasing hydrogen and methane production in IBS [38, 79], suggesting major role for intestinal bacteria as a contributor to symptoms of IBS.

Conclusions

Strong evidence suggests that the gut microbiome plays an important role in functional gastrointestinal disorders and interactions between the gut and the nervous system influence intestinal motility and inflammation. Although several reports suggest a disruption in the balance of the enteric microbiota in patients with IBS, considerably more data are needed to establish whether these changes are merely seen due to the dysmotility or indeed there is a causative role for these findings. While most of the studies addressing the role of the enteric bacteria rely on traditional culture techniques to identify the microbiome, studies utilizing molecular technology in identifying the microbiota would prove useful in further investigating the role of these bacteria in gastrointestinal symptomatology and disease. Results from a small number of well-designed, randomized, controlled, clinical trials suggest that, not only does regular intake of certain probiotic bacteria help to treat the symptoms of IBS, but their effects go beyond symptoms and are associated with modulation of biological parameters, such as intestinal transit, abdominal girth and inflammatory markers that in turn influence the gut–brain axis.

Further understanding of the gut microbiota will improve our knowledge of their role in health and disease, and allow for improved future therapeutic and prophylactic modalities. Although significant strides have been made in our journey of deciphering the codes of the gut microbiome, our ability to delve deep into this fascinating organ has been hampered by the complexities of its inhabitants. The introduction of non-culture-based molecular techniques that enable quantitative assessment of the entire enteric microbiota coupled with encouraging results from probiotic research continue to improve our understanding in this area.

Table 5.1 Summary of published pediatric reports of probiotic role in irritable bowel syndrome

Author	Year	Type of probiotic	Duration in weeks	Population	Type of trial	Outcome of study
Bausserman and Michail [75]	2005	LGG (10^{10} CFU given BID)	6	Age: 6–20 ($n=50$)	R, DB, PC	Lower incidence of perceived abdominal distention in LGG group, but no difference in other parameters
Gawronska [76]	2007	LGG (3×10^{9} CFU given BID)	4	Age : 6–16 ($n=104$)	R, DB, PC	LGG group more likely to have no pain, reduced frequency of pain, but not pain severity than controls
Guandalini [77]	2010	VSL#3 (4–11 y/o: 1 sachet daily; 12–18 y/o: 1 sachet BID)	6	Age : 4–18 ($n=59$)	R, DB, PC	Relief of symptoms, lowered abdominal pain/discomfort, bloating/gassiness, and life disruption in VSL#3 group

R randomized, *PC* placebo controlled, *DB* double-blinded, *LGG Lactobacillus GG*, *VSL#3* proprietary mixture of *Bifidobacterium breve, Bifidobacterium longum, Bifidobacterium infantis, Lactobacillus acidophilus, Lactobacillus plantarum, Lactobacillus paracasei, Lactobacillus bulgaricus,* and *Streptococcus thermophilus* (Sigma-Tau Pharmaceuticals, Inc.)

References

1. Vantrappen G, et al. The interdigestive motor complex of normal subjects and patients with bacterial overgrowth of the small intestine. J Clin Invest. 1977;59(6):1158–66.
2. Wang SH, et al. A research of migrating motor complex in patients with irritable bowel syndrome. Zhonghua Nei Ke Za Zhi. 2009;48(2):106–10.
3. Macfarlane S, Dillon JF. Microbial biofilms in the human gastrointestinal tract. J Appl Microbiol. 2007;102(5):1187–96.
4. Kiliaan AJ, et al. Stress stimulates transepithelial macromolecular uptake in rat jejunum. Am J Physiol. 1998;275(5 Pt 1):G1037–44.
5. Groot J, et al. Stress-induced decrease of the intestinal barrier function. The role of muscarinic receptor activation. Ann N Y Acad Sci. 2000;915:237–46.
6. Yates DA, et al. Adaptation of stress-induced mucosal pathophysiology in rat colon involves opioid pathways. Am J Physiol Gastrointest Liver Physiol. 2001;281(1):G124–8.
7. Soderholm JD, et al. Neonatal maternal separation predisposes adult rats to colonic barrier dysfunction in response to mild stress. Am J Physiol Gastrointest Liver Physiol. 2002;283(6):G1257–63.
8. Soderholm JD, et al. Chronic stress induces mast cell-dependent bacterial adherence and initiates mucosal inflammation in rat intestine. Gastroenterology. 2002;123(4):1099–108.
9. Jacob C, et al. Mast cell tryptase controls paracellular permeability of the intestine. Role of protease-activated receptor 2 and beta-arrestins. J Biol Chem. 2005;280(36):31936–48.
10. Demaude J, et al. Phenotypic changes in colonocytes following acute stress or activation of mast cells in mice: implications for delayed epithelial barrier dysfunction. Gut. 2006;55(5):655–61.
11. Salzman NH, et al. Enteric defensins are essential regulators of intestinal microbial ecology. Nat Immunol. 2010;11(1):76–83.
12. Alonso C, et al. Maladaptive intestinal epithelial responses to life stress may predispose healthy women to gut mucosal inflammation. Gastroenterology. 2008;135(1):163–172 e1.
13. Stephens RL, Tache Y. Intracisternal injection of a TRH analogue stimulates gastric luminal serotonin release in rats. Am J Physiol. 1989;256(2 Pt 1):G377–83.
14. Santos J, et al. Release of mast cell mediators into the jejunum by cold pain stress in humans. Gastroenterology. 1998;114(4):640–8.
15. Hughes DT, Sperandio V. Inter-kingdom signalling: communication between bacteria and their hosts. Nat Rev Microbiol. 2008;6(2):111–20.
16. Alverdy J, et al. Gut-derived sepsis occurs when the right pathogen with the right virulence genes meets the right host: evidence for in vivo virulence expression in *Pseudomonas aeruginosa*. Ann Surg. 2000;232(4):480–9.
17. Cogan TA, et al. Norepinephrine increases the pathogenic potential of *Campylobacter jejuni*. Gut. 2007;56(8):1060–5.
18. Dunlop SP, et al. Relative importance of enterochromaffin cell hyperplasia, anxiety, and depression in postinfectious IBS. Gastroenterology. 2003;125(6):1651–9.
19. Mazmanian SK, Round JL, Kasper DL. A microbial symbiosis factor prevents intestinal inflammatory disease. Nature. 2008;453(7195):620–5.
20. Barbara G, et al. Interactions between commensal bacteria and gut sensorimotor function in health and disease. Am J Gastroenterol. 2005;100(11):2560–8.
21. Malbert CH. The ileocolonic sphincter. Neurogastroenterol Motil. 2005;17 Suppl 1:41–9.
22. Dass NB, et al. The relationship between the effects of short-chain fatty acids on intestinal motility in vitro and GPR43 receptor activation. Neurogastroenterol Motil. 2007;19(1):66–74.
23. Husebye E, et al. Influence of microbial species on small intestinal myoelectric activity and transit in germ-free rats. Am J Physiol Gastrointest Liver Physiol. 2001;280(3):G368–80.
24. Rhee SH, et al. Pathophysiological role of Toll-like receptor 5 engagement by bacterial flagellin in colonic inflammation. Proc Natl Acad Sci USA. 2005;102(38):13610–5.
25. Ait-Belgnaoui A, et al. *Lactobacillus farciminis* treatment attenuates stress-induced overexpression of Fos protein in spinal and supraspinal sites after colorectal distension in rats. Neurogastroenterol Motil. 2009;21(5):567–73. e18–9.
26. Ait-Belgnaoui A, et al. *Lactobacillus farciminis* treatment suppresses stress induced visceral hypersensitivity: a possible action through interaction with epithelial cell cytoskeleton contraction. Gut. 2006;55(8):1090–4.
27. Everhart JE, Renault PF. Irritable bowel syndrome in office-based practice in the United States. Gastroenterology. 1991;100(4):998–1005.
28. Di Lorenzo C, et al. Antroduodenal manometry in children and adults with severe non-ulcer dyspepsia. Scand J Gastroenterol. 1994;29(9):799–806.
29. Fenton TR, Harries JT, Milla PJ. Disordered small intestinal motility: a rational basis for toddlers' diarrhoea. Gut. 1983;24(10):897–903.
30. Vassallo MJ, et al. Colonic tone and motility in patients with irritable bowel syndrome. Mayo Clin Proc. 1992;67(8):725–31.
31. Cann PA, et al. Irritable bowel syndrome: relationship of disorders in the transit of a single solid meal to symptom patterns. Gut. 1983;24(5):405–11.
32. Manabe N, et al. Lower functional gastrointestinal disorders: evidence of abnormal colonic transit in a 287 patient cohort. Neurogastroenterol Motil. 2010;22(3):293-e82.
33. Horikawa Y, et al. Gastrointestinal motility in patients with irritable bowel syndrome studied by using radiopaque markers. Scand J Gastroenterol. 1999;34(12):1190–5.

34. de Boissieu D, et al. Small-bowel bacterial overgrowth in children with chronic diarrhea, abdominal pain, or both. J Pediatr. 1996;128(2):203–7.
35. Pimentel M, et al. Methane, a gas produced by enteric bacteria, slows intestinal transit and augments small intestinal contractile activity. Am J Physiol Gastrointest Liver Physiol. 2006;290(6):G1089–95.
36. Pimentel M, et al. Lower frequency of MMC is found in IBS subjects with abnormal lactulose breath test, suggesting bacterial overgrowth. Dig Dis Sci. 2002;47(12):2639–43.
37. Pimentel M, Chow EJ, Lin HC. Eradication of small intestinal bacterial overgrowth reduces symptoms of irritable bowel syndrome. Am J Gastroenterol. 2000;95(12):3503–6.
38. Pimentel M, Chow EJ, Lin HC. Normalization of lactulose breath testing correlates with symptom improvement in irritable bowel syndrome. a double-blind, randomized, placebo-controlled study. Am J Gastroenterol. 2003;98(2):412–9.
39. Peralta S, et al. Small intestine bacterial overgrowth and irritable bowel syndrome-related symptoms: experience with Rifaximin. World J Gastroenterol. 2009;15(21):2628–31.
40. Treem WR, et al. Fecal short-chain fatty acids in patients with diarrhea-predominant irritable bowel syndrome: in vitro studies of carbohydrate fermentation. J Pediatr Gastroenterol Nutr. 1996;23(3):280–6.
41. King TS, Elia M, Hunter JO. Abnormal colonic fermentation in irritable bowel syndrome. Lancet. 1998;352(9135):1187–9.
42. Pimentel M, Kong Y, Park S. Breath testing to evaluate lactose intolerance in irritable bowel syndrome correlates with lactulose testing and may not reflect true lactose malabsorption. Am J Gastroenterol. 2003;98(12):2700–4.
43. Dear KL, Elia M, Hunter JO. Do interventions which reduce colonic bacterial fermentation improve symptoms of irritable bowel syndrome? Dig Dis Sci. 2005;50(4):758–66.
44. Pimentel M, et al. Methane production during lactulose breath test is associated with gastrointestinal disease presentation. Dig Dis Sci. 2003;48(1):86–92.
45. Pimentel M, Kong Y, Park S. IBS subjects with methane on lactulose breath test have lower postprandial serotonin levels than subjects with hydrogen. Dig Dis Sci. 2004;49(1):84–7.
46. Quigley EM. Bacterial flora in irritable bowel syndrome: role in pathophysiology, implications for management. J Dig Dis. 2007;8(1):2–7.
47. Barbara G, et al. New pathophysiological mechanisms in irritable bowel syndrome. Aliment Pharmacol Ther. 2004;20 Suppl 2:1–9.
48. Ley RE, Peterson DA, Gordon JI. Ecological and evolutionary forces shaping microbial diversity in the human intestine. Cell. 2006;124(4):837–48.
49. Savage DC. Microbial ecology of the gastrointestinal tract. Annu Rev Microbiol. 1977;31:107–33.
50. Whitman WB, Coleman DC, Wiebe WJ. Prokaryotes: the unseen majority. Proc Natl Acad Sci USA. 1998;95(12):6578–83.
51. Gebbers JO, Laissue JA. Immunologic structures and functions of the gut. Schweiz Arch Tierheilkd. 1989;131(5):221–38.
52. Rhee SH, Pothoulakis C, Mayer EA. Principles and clinical implications of the brain-gut-enteric microbiota axis. Nat Rev Gastroenterol Hepatol. 2009;6(5):306–14.
53. Schaedler RW, Dubos RJ. The fecal flora of various strains of mice. Its bearing on their susceptibility to endotoxin. J Exp Med. 1962;115:1149–60.
54. Bailey MT, Coe CL. Maternal separation disrupts the integrity of the intestinal microflora in infant rhesus monkeys. Dev Psychobiol. 1999;35(2):146–55.
55. Osipov GA, et al. [Clinical significance of studies of microorganisms of the intestinal mucosa by culture biochemical methods and mass fragmentography]. Eksp Klin Gastroenterol. 2003;(4):59–67, 115
56. Malinen E, et al. Analysis of the fecal microbiota of irritable bowel syndrome patients and healthy controls with real-time PCR. Am J Gastroenterol. 2005;100(2):373–82.
57. Si JM, et al. Intestinal microecology and quality of life in irritable bowel syndrome patients. World J Gastroenterol. 2004;10(12):1802–5.
58. Chadwick VS, et al. Activation of the mucosal immune system in irritable bowel syndrome. Gastroenterology. 2002;122(7):1778–83.
59. Gwee KA, et al. Increased rectal mucosal expression of interleukin 1beta in recently acquired post-infectious irritable bowel syndrome. Gut. 2003;52(4):523–6.
60. Weston AP, et al. Terminal ileal mucosal mast cells in irritable bowel syndrome. Dig Dis Sci. 1993;38(9):1590–5.
61. Faure C, et al. Serotonin signaling is altered in irritable bowel syndrome with diarrhea but not in functional dyspepsia in pediatric age patients. Gastroenterology. 2010;139(1):249–58.
62. Barbara G, et al. Activated mast cells in proximity to colonic nerves correlate with abdominal pain in irritable bowel syndrome. Gastroenterology. 2004;126(3):693–702.
63. Cremonini F, et al. Effect of CCK-1 antagonist, dexloxiglumide, in female patients with irritable bowel syndrome: a pharmacodynamic and pharmacogenomic study. Am J Gastroenterol. 2005;100(3):652–63.
64. Tornblom H, et al. Full-thickness biopsy of the jejunum reveals inflammation and enteric neuropathy in irritable bowel syndrome. Gastroenterology. 2002;123(6):1972–9.
65. O'Mahony L, et al. Lactobacillus and bifidobacterium in irritable bowel syndrome: symptom responses and relationship to cytokine profiles. Gastroenterology. 2005;128(3):541–51.
66. Spiller RC. Role of nerves in enteric infection. Gut. 2002;51(6):759–62.
67. Dunlop SP, et al. Randomized, double-blind, placebo-controlled trial of prednisolone in post-infectious irritable bowel syndrome. Aliment Pharmacol Ther. 2003;18(1):77–84.

68. Verdu EF, et al. Specific probiotic therapy attenuates antibiotic induced visceral hypersensitivity in mice. Gut. 2006;55(2):182–90.
69. Rousseaux C, et al. *Lactobacillus acidophilus* modulates intestinal pain and induces opioid and cannabinoid receptors. Nat Med. 2007;13(1):35–7.
70. Pimentel M, et al. Rifaximin therapy for patients with irritable bowel syndrome without constipation. N Engl J Med. 2011;364(1):22–32.
71. Majewski M, McCallum RW. Results of small intestinal bacterial overgrowth testing in irritable bowel syndrome patients: clinical profiles and effects of antibiotic trial. Adv Med Sci. 2007;52:139–42.
72. Yamini D, Pimentel M. Irritable bowel syndrome and small intestinal bacterial overgrowth. J Clin Gastroenterol. 2010;44(10):672–5.
73. Bazzocchi G, et al. Intestinal microflora and oral bacteriotherapy in irritable bowel syndrome. Dig Liver Dis. 2002;34 Suppl 2:S48–53.
74. Agrawal A, et al. Clinical trial: the effects of a fermented milk product containing *Bifidobacterium lactis* DN-173-010 on abdominal distension and gastrointestinal transit in irritable bowel syndrome with constipation. Aliment Pharmacol Ther. 2008;29(1):104–14.
75. Bausserman M, Michail S. The use of Lactobacillus GG in irritable bowel syndrome in children: a double-blind randomized control trial. J Pediatr. 2005;147(2):197–201.
76. Gawronska A, et al. A randomized double-blind placebo-controlled trial of Lactobacillus GG for abdominal pain disorders in children. Aliment Pharmacol Ther. 2007;25(2):177–84.
77. Guandalini S, et al. VSL#3 improves symptoms in children with irritable bowel syndrome: a multicenter, randomized, placebo-controlled, double-blind, crossover study. J Pediatr Gastroenterol Nutr. 2010;51(1):24–30.
78. Sharara AI, et al. A randomized double-blind placebo-controlled trial of rifaximin in patients with abdominal bloating and flatulence. Am J Gastroenterol. 2006;101(2):326–33.
79. Frissora CL, Cash BD. Review article: the role of antibiotics vs. conventional pharmacotherapy in treating symptoms of irritable bowel syndrome. Aliment Pharmacol Ther. 2007;25(11):1271–81.

Integration of Biomedical and Psychosocial Issues in Pediatric Functional Gastrointestinal and Motility Disorders

6

Miranda A.L. van Tilburg

Introduction

Treating gastrointestinal symptoms in children is often more difficult than it may seem. Consider the following case. *Johnny is a 6 year old child who presents with nausea and abdominal pain. Upon history taking the child appears to experience early satiety and some minor weight loss. You notice pallor and irritability. After thorough diagnostic work-up John is diagnosed with delayed gastric emptying. The family is sent home with a prescription for Metoclopramide and referral to a dietician. Several months later Johnny returns to you and appears to be doing well. Pallor has disappeared and weight loss has been stopped. Nevertheless problems continue at home around feeding. Johnny still refuses food and continues to complain of nausea and abdominal pain. You suspect psychological factors may be playing a role. The symptoms started around the time Johnny's parents got a divorce. Mother seems anxious and Johnny is out of school regularly around fear of symptoms.*

This scenario is recognizable for many clinicians working with children who suffer from functional gastrointestinal and motility disorders. Psychosocial factors often play a role in these disorders and no clinician working with this group of patients will deny its influence. But the interpretation of how psychological symptoms affect the etiology and maintenance of these disorders varies considerably among clinicians. Are psychological issues primary causes of some disorders? Can psychological disturbances affect digestive processes? In the case of Johnny: Were the continuation of his symptoms after successful treatment of the gastric emptying, primarily due to: (1) anxiety of his family, who may too easily over-interpret normal symptoms as signaling disease; or (2) was there a behavioral component to his symptoms in the first place, that was not addressed with medication therapy thereby leading to ineffective treatment? Answers to some of these questions can affect the course of suggested treatment for Johnny and other children like him. In this chapter, first the theoretical models explaining the role of psychosocial issues in health and disease will be discussed. These are implicit working models guiding clinical care and scientific research and are important to explore. Then, the current scientific evidence for the role of psychosocial factors on physiological functioning will be presented.

M.A.L. van Tilburg, Ph.D. (✉)
UNC Center for Functional GI and Motility Disorders, 130 Mason Farm Rd. #4105. CB 7080, Chapel Hill, NC 27599-7080, USA

Department of Medicine, Division of Gastroenterology and Hepatology, University of North Carolina at Chapel Hill, Chapel Hill, NC, USA
e-mail: tilburg@med.unc.edu

C. Faure et al. (eds.), *Pediatric Neurogastroenterology: Gastrointestinal Motility and Functional Disorders in Children*, Clinical Gastroenterology,
DOI 10.1007/978-1-60761-709-9_6, © Springer Science+Business Media New York 2013

Psychological Issues in Health and Disease

Biomedical Model: A Symptom Has Either a Physiological or Psychological Origin

Under guidance of the biomedical model, medicine has seen one of the greatest advances in its existence over the past centuries. It has been responsible for some of the most impressive discoveries of modern Medicine such as the development of penicillin, vaccines, etc. It is still widely popular today among many clinicians and patients. The biomedical model envisions a direct relation between disease and symptom: Cause A will lead to symptoms B. The more disease causing A is present the more symptoms will be observed. If A is eradicated the symptoms will disappear. This straightforward model of health and disease focuses primarily on biological origins; but argues that in lieu of a disease or structural abnormality, psychological factors can cause symptoms. For example, if no biomedical reason can be found for stomachaches (such as lactose intolerance) then these symptoms can be attributed to psychosocial distress, i.e., anxiety or school avoidance. The biomedical model is simple and elegant but completely ignores contextual influences on health and disease: Symptoms are either caused by biological or psychological causes. This straight-forward and appealing approach has led to the notion that if symptoms are not in "the body" it must be "all in the head." It also explains our fascination with drugs as a "quick fix" for *real* symptoms worthy of a clinician's time while behavioral or supportive therapy have become synonym to treating symptoms that are either feigned or a result from being "crazy" and not belonging in a physician's office.

Biopsychosocial Model: Symptoms Can Be Altered by Psychosocial Processes

By the mid 70s of the last century the powerful biomedical model started to show little cracks. It became clear that there was no perfect association between biomedical processes and symptoms. For example, under the biomedical model the frequency and amount of gastric acid refluxing into the esophagus should explain the intensity of heartburn complaints. However, there are patients with very severe acid reflux for years, who are not symptomatic until developing Barrett's esophagus. On the other hand, there are others with minimal acid reflux whose life is severely affected by their symptoms. The only way to explain these findings with the biomedical model is to see the first person as a "tough" or stoic child, silently suffering while continuing with his/her life, while the second is a "wimp" complaining at the tiniest bit of discomfort. The first elicits admiration and the second contempt. However, imperfect associations between biomedical processes and symptoms are so ubiquitous that they seem to be the rule rather than the exemption. The biopsychosocial model, first proposed by Dr. Engel [1], posits that biochemical alterations do not directly translate into illness. The appearance of symptoms is an interplay between many factors including biomedical, psychological, and social factors, e.g., bacteria A leads to more symptoms under stressful circumstances.

The biopsychosocial model has been widely adopted by researchers and clinicians to explain health and disease and is particularly useful for understanding and studying functional gastrointestinal disorders. There is a robust literature describing the influence of both physiological and psychological factors on the illness presentation of functional gastrointestinal disorders in particular irritable bowel syndrome (IBS). These studies will be discussed later in this chapter.

System Theory: Physiological and Psychological Processes Are Constantly Interacting to Cause Symptoms

Although the biopsychosocial model was presented by Dr. Engel as a system theory it is nowadays often presented in a reductionist way. Some authors reduce mental and social phenomena to basic biological phenomena such as activation of the autonomous or central nervous system (CNS) and

Hypothalamic-Pituitary-Adrenal (HPA) axis [2]. Johnny from our case at the beginning of the chapter may be anxious which leads to CNS and HPA axis activation, interacting through the brain–gut axis with the enteric nervous system culminating in gastrointestinal symptoms. Systems theory acknowledges that psychosocial processes undoubtedly have biological correlates. However, it argues that the different systems—biological, psychological, and social—interact with each other but cannot be reduced to the lowest—molecular—level. The reasoning behind this is simple: we cannot understand the meaning of psychosocial processes by purely studying its biological correlates; subjective phenomena are equally important.

The biopsychosocial model is also sometimes reduced to a hierarchy of unidirectional cause and effects relationships which includes causes, precipitants, modulators, or sustaining forces [3]. In Johnny's case anxiety and delayed gastric emptying can be thought to independently cause or sustain his symptoms and it is up to the physician to decide which one is most important and thus should be treated first. Viewing psychosocial and biomedical factors as somewhat independent processes largely denies the reality of the situation in which there are feedback loops between all parts of the system. Johnny's delayed gastric emptying caused pain and fullness, which made him anxious around food. His fears of having pain after a meal in turn may have led to hypervigilance and increased the sensitivity of his nerves to normal digestive processes thereby worsening his symptoms. Thus, anxiety is both cause and effect in this circular loop.

Systems theory is an attempt to understand these complex feedback loops over time and discovering the interrelated causes that sustain specific symptom over time. Unfortunately such nice integrated models of proximal causes and effects over time are difficult to study. The need for complex study designs and statistical methods has seriously hampered the testing of systems theory in functional gastrointestinal and motility disorders. Recent developments of system theory methodology in other fields show promise for application in functional gastrointestinal and motility disorders.

The Brain–Gut Axis

Nowadays the role of psychosocial variables in functional gastrointestinal and motility disorders is widely recognized and the biopsychosocial approach is commonly endorsed in explaining these disorders. The biopsychosocial model postulates that psychosocial factors can interact with the gut through the brain–gut axis: the bidirectional communication between enteric nervous system in the gut and the brain. This means that emotions and thoughts have the capability to affect gastrointestinal sensation, motility, and inflammation. Reciprocally, gastrointestinal processes are able to affect perception, mood, and behavior. Dysregulation of the brain–gut axis is thought to be at the core of many functional gastrointestinal disorders.

With regularity the question is asked whether psychological issues are a cause or consequence of the brain–gut axis dysregulation. Some authors have found increased anxiety before a diagnosis of functional gastrointestinal and motility disorders [4] while others have argued that increased psychosocial distress may be a consequence of having to deal with a chronic, unpredictable condition [5]. A large community based study found that both positions may be right: Psychosocial comorbidity was as likely to be present *before* as *after* seeking care for abdominal pain [6]. The question is if it really helps to know which one came first. If we conceive of our body as a system in which psychosocial and biomedical factors interact continually, then the question of what came first is not relevant. Both factors will interact to cause symptoms and understanding the disorder is exploring this interaction. For example, in the case of fecal incontinence we do not ask if the child was constipated first and then became anxious about evacuation of large bowel movements; or anxious about potty training and then experienced large stools due to withholding. Both may be true and will lead to the same symptom: fecal incontinence. Both factors need to be addressed to ensure successful resolution of symptoms. Thus, rather than trying to solve the "Chicken-and-egg" dilemma we should focus on understanding how the different components of the system interact to create these symptoms. In the following section we summarize the literature on psychosocial influences on functional gastrointestinal and motility disorders.

Psychosocial Influences on Functional Gastrointestinal and Motility Disorders

There are many psychosocial aspects relevant to functional gastrointestinal and motility disorders such as personality [7], self-esteem [8, 9], early childhood experiences [10, 11], to name only a few. Out of all the possibly relevant psychosocial factors the most often studied is the concept of stress. We all know what stress is and what it feels like. However, defining stress is more elusive than it seems. First there are the events that may be stressful: being stopped by a policeman for speeding, giving a speech in front of several colleagues, taking your child to the Emergency Room. These are called stressors. Second, there are individual reactions to stress: feelings of anger/fear, trouble concentrating, and physical reactions such as accelerated heartbeat, tensed muscles and increased perspiration. It is important to realize that not all potential stressors lead to stress reactions and that stress can be both positive and negative. What is stressful for one person may be pleasurable to another or have little impact whatsoever to a third person. A parachute jump or deep sea dive may elicit enormous fear and anxiety in some while others find it highly pleasurable and for very experienced professionals it may just a simple routine. Therefore, stress is a subjective experience created by the appraisal of an environmental demand as harmful, threatening or challenging and appraisal of our ability to meet this demand [12]. If a person has adequate resources to deal with a difficult situation he or she may not experience stress; but if the demand (almost) exceeds one's resources a person will be under a great deal of stress. When the term "stress" is used it may refer to the following: (1) the stressors, which are usually major life events such as trauma, abuse or divorce but can also be the cumulative effect of small daily hassles; (2) the subjective experience of stress which is usually measured by self-reports of perceived stress; and (3) stress reactions which includes behavioral (e.g., withdrawal or confrontation), emotional (e.g., anger, fear, anxiety, depression), and physiological reactions (e.g., skin conductivity, blood pressure, cortisol, and catecholamines). Thus, stress in addition to being itself, is also causing itself and resulting in itself. It is important to realize which aspect of stress is being referred to when reading and interpreting the scientific literature on stress.

Stress can be felt in the gut. We are all familiar with the typical butterflies associated with young love, feeling squeamish when being forced to deliver bad news and the run to the bathroom before the start of an important race or game. Stress has been found to alter gut functioning. It has effects on GI sensory, motor, and immune functioning; which are also etiological pathways for many functional gastrointestinal and motility disorders.

Stress and Gastrointestinal Motor Functioning

Motility disturbances are a hallmark symptom of many functional gastrointestinal and motility disorders which may result in symptoms such as altered stool consistency, nausea, or bloating. There is evidence to suggest that stress induces changes in motility. For example, under stressful conditions gastric emptying decreases and colonic transit accelerates [13, 14]. These stress-induced motility changes are caused by increases in corticotrophin-releasing factor (CRF). CRF is best known as the principal instigator of the physiological response to stress through the Hypothalamic-Pituitary-Adrenal (HPA) axis and CRF 1 receptors have been found to regulate behavioral reactions to stress [15–18]. But the effects of stress on motility seem to operate outside of this system. It has been reported that activation of CRF receptors in the brain induces propulsive motor function and diarrhea without involving the HPA axis, but rather through stimulation of autonomic nervous system [19, 20]. Central CRF stimulates the vagal nerves innervating to the proximal colon which results in release of colonic serotonin [19, 21]. Serotonin is involved in various gastrointestinal motility processes such as the gastric accommodation reflex, small bowel transit, and the colonic response to feeding [22]. Therefore serotonin abnormalities in the gut can lead to motility disturbances in functional gastrointestinal and motility disorders [22]. This is supported by the fact that medications aimed at altering gut serotonin have been found to be effective in treating several functional gastrointestinal and motility disorders including IBS, constipation, functional dyspepsia, and gastroparesis [22].

In addition to motility, CRF receptors have also been implicated in visceral hypersensitivity and immune functioning (for an over view see Tache et al. [23]), the two topics which are discussed next.

Stress and Gastrointestinal Sensory Functioning

One of the most consistent findings in painful functional gastrointestinal and motility disorders is visceral hypersensitivity. Hypersensitivity to gut distension—the reporting of first sensation of pain at lower levels of pressure than normal—has been found in more than half of adult patients who suffer from IBS and functional dyspepsia [24]. Visceral sensitivity is usually measured by using the barostat technique. The barostat inflates a balloon to different pressure levels in the stomach, colon, or rectum while the patient is asked to report level of discomfort and pain (for guidelines on using the barostat in children see van den Berg et al. [25]). As the barostat technique is invasive there are few studies in children. The results of these studies show that visceral hypersensitivity is a common phenomenon in children with painful gastrointestinal disorders [25–27]. In addition, visceral *hypo*sensitivity in the rectum has been reported in children with constipation [28, 29]. Reduced sensation in the rectum corroborates the fact that these children do not easily feel an urge to defecate.

The role of stress on visceral sensitivity has only been examined in abdominal pain related functional gastrointestinal disorders. Many studies have found reduced pain thresholds in reaction to stress—which is equivalent to more easily reporting pain under stress. Studies in rats have shown that early-life stress is associated with colonic hypersensitivity in adulthood [30–34]. In humans, acute stress, induced by cold water hand immersion (physical stressor) or dichotomous listening (mental stressor), seems to reduce pain thresholds as well [35, 36]. But other types of stressor have yielded mixed effects. Past stressful experiences (e.g., abuse history) and psychological distress (e.g., anxiety or depression) have been associated with decreased pain thresholds in some studies [26, 37–40] while others have reported no effects of stress at all [26, 39, 41–43]. Thus, most studies report increased sensitivity with stress but some did not find any effects and one study actually found decreased sensitivity [44]. The reason for the inconclusive evidence may be related to the way visceral sensitivity is measured.

In most barostat protocols increasing levels of pressure are presented to the patient who is asked to indicate first perception of discomfort. This experimental design is believed to be vulnerable to psychological response biases in particular fear of pain [45]. Naliboff and colleagues found that when offering unpredictable changes in volume, differences in pain thresholds between IBS patients and controls disappeared [46]. Dorn and colleagues added to these findings by showing that rather than increased neurosensory sensitivity (the ability to discriminate between pressure levels), lower pain thresholds in IBS are explained primarily by an increased psychological tendency to report pain [47]. One of the non-sensory cues that influence pain threshold ratings is hypervigilance to symptoms. IBS patients have a higher tendency to label visceral sensations as unpleasant during barostat testing [46]. Thus, visceral hypersensitivity can either be caused by hypervigilance or perceptual sensitivity and both may have associations with stress. Dorn found some indication that increased psychological distress is associated with hypervigilance but others have not been able to replicate this [46–48].

If we assume that under certain circumstances stress can affect visceral sensitivity, an important question becomes at what level in the neural system these effects are most dominant. Sensations from the gastrointestinal tract are relayed to spinal dorsal horn. Visceral sensory information is then conveyed to supraspinal sites and finally to cortical areas where they are perceived [49]. Descending emotional pathways via the periaqueductal gray to the dorsal horn can amplify or suppress new afferent signals from the gut. Amplification of these signals can occur at any level in this neural pathway. Evidence is building that the Central Nervous System is an important site of modulating the pain response. Brain responses to visceral stimuli are increased in IBS patients compared to controls in areas related to conscious experience of visceral sensations (specifically the Insular Cortex) as well as areas related to emotion modulation and emotional response to threat including the Anterior Cingulate Cortex, hypothalamus, and the amygdala. Thus, IBS patients tend to responds with more affective and attentional responses to visceral stimuli. In addition, decreased activation in the periaqueductal gray shows decreased efferent inhibition of pain signals [49].

Though the brain is the most likely level for psychological input to interface with visceral input, very few studies have investigated the role of psychological factors in modulating the Central Nervous System response to visceral sensations Berman and colleagues studied anticipation of visceral pain [50]. They found that negative affect reduces anticipatory brain stem inhibition. Reduced anticipatory brain stem inhibition in turn was associated with increased brain responsiveness to actual distention [50]. Ringel and colleagues observed that during rectal distension, patients with IBS and abuse history show greater posterior/middle dorsal and anterior cingulate cortex activation, as well as reduced activity of the supragenual anterior cingulate (a region implicated in pain inhibition and arousal) [51, 52]. In a case report of a patient with of severe IBS and posttraumatic stress disorder, resolution of emotional distress was associated with reduction in activation of the midcingulate cortex, prefrontal area 6/44, and the somatosensory cortex, areas associated with pain intensity encoding [53]. Thus, there is evidence that psychological factors can influence brain reactions to visceral pain, specifically areas related to emotion modulation, but the exact mechanism still needs to be determined.

Stress and Gastrointestinal Immune Functioning

The role of the immune system in functional gastrointestinal and motility disorders, specifically IBS, has received a lot of attention in the past decade. This line of research initially focused on patients who developed IBS following an infectious gastroenteritis. Later, low grade inflammation within the gut wall as well as altered immunological function and alterations in gut flora were found in functional gastrointestinal disorders of noninfectious origin including IBS, functional dyspepsia, and noncardiac chest pain [54–56]. Many innate and adaptive immune parameters have been studied but among the most robust findings are increased levels of mast cells, monocytes, and T-cells as well as increased intestinal permeability (for a review see Ohman and Simren [57]). Although most studies have been done in adults, increased gut inflammation has also been shown in children who suffer from functional abdominal pain [58–61]. Outside the field of gastroenterology, there are many studies which suggest that psychological distress affects the immune system in healthy adults (for a meta-analysis see Denson et al. [62]). For example stress reduces antigens production following vaccinations [63, 64], increases susceptibility to colds [65] and meditation decreases IL-6 responses to a laboratory psychosocial stressor [66]. The role of stress on the immune system in functional gastrointestinal and motility disorders has received little attention. In rats and rodents stress increased low-grade inflammation in the gut postinfection [67] as well as esophageal and intestinal permeability [68]. Studies in humans also suggest that stress is associated with low grade inflammation in functional gastrointestinal disorders. Piche et al. [69] and Schurman et al. [61] observed that depression and anxiety scores in IBS patients are correlated with increased mast cell counts. Dinan and colleagues [70] found that increased stress response in IBS patients (measured by plasma adrenocorticotropic hormone levels after CRF administration) is associated with increased IL-6 levels. Anxiety has been reported to be associated with increases in cytokine levels in IBS but only after exposure to Escherichia coli lipopolysaccharides [71]. These are early indicators that stress and the immune system interact in functional gastrointestinal and motility disorders.

Psychological distress may affect immunological response and reducing stress could be helpful. But there is also data to suggest that immune activation may *drive* psychological distress and brain related changes. Activation of the immune system either by viral infection or by administration of cytokines or lypopolysaccharide (found on the outer membrane of gram-negative bacteria) induces cytokine secretion and trigger depression and anxiety in healthy volunteers [72, 73]. In addition, immune-targeted therapies such as interferon-alpha treatment for Hepatitis C or cancer have been known to induce anxiety and depression in a significant percentage of patients [74–76]. Those who develop major depression during treatment have increased pretreatment IL6 and IL-10 concentrations [77]. These findings suggest that that increased immune activation is a causal risk for the development of major depression. Based on these observations Goehler et al. [78] have suggested that "*Some of the negative affective experiences associated with gastrointestinal disorders may not be under the voluntary control of the patient.*"

Although it yet has to be determined how infections in the gut influence the brain and mood, it has been suggested that the brain may react directly to the bacterial composition of the GI tract [78, 79]. The gut contains different species of microbiota, many of which still need to be characterized by culture. Imbalances in gastrointestinal microbiota, or "dysbiosis," have been found in many chronic gastrointestinal disorders such as IBD [80], antibiotic-induced diarrhea [81, 82] and IBS [83–85]. Inducing dysbiosis, either with the use of oral antibiotics or by replacing the microbiota, leads to low grade inflammation, visceral hyperalgesia, and behavioral changes in mice; symptoms changes that are also characteristic of many functional gastrointestinal disorders [86–88]. Dysbiosis may stimulate the vagal nerve. The vagal nerve has been implicated both in neurological control of the immune system particularly cytokine control [89] as well as in dysregulation of the brain–gut interactions in functional gastrointestinal disorders [90]. Vagal sensory neurons react to potentially dangerous bacteria in the GI tract independently of an immunological reaction to their presence: It has been reported that the vagal nerve is stimulated hours before bacteria are able to colonize [91, 92]. In fact mice with dysbiosis show anxiety-like behavior in the absence of circulating pro-inflammatory cytokines and classic sickness behaviors [93]. In addition, administration of a probiotic reduced anxiety-like behavior in mice with colitis, but only if they had an intact vagus nerve [94]. Thus, the vagal nerve can provide signal to the brain on dysbiosis before inflammatory responses reach the brain through the systemic circulation. Goehler argues that the adaptive value of enhanced anxiety during gut infection may lay in threat avoidance [78]. Behavioral responses to an infection such as psychomotor retardation may leave an animal vulnerable to predators. Avoidance of dangerous situations such as open spaces is essential and accomplished by early inducement of anxiety to stimulate threat avoidance. This will put the animal in less danger once sickness behaviors are full-blown. Given that even low grade inflammation can induce alterations in mood, this may be partially responsible for increased anxiety and depression in functional gastrointestinal disorders.

Conclusion

There is clear evidence that psychosocial factors can alter gut physiology. Stress-induced changes in CRF leads to motility disturbances such as decreased gastric emptying and increased colonic transit. In addition, patients who are distressed usually display increased visceral hypersensitivity which is under the control of emotion-regulation areas of the central nervous system. Although not studied extensively in functional gastrointestinal and motility disorders there is a large body of literature suggesting that stress alters immune functioning. The reverse—that alterations in physiology can affect stress levels—has not been studied widely. There is some evidence that immune activation may induce psychological distress. This process may be driven by changes in gut microbiota which are relayed to the brain through the vagus nerve.

One caveat to the above line of research is the almost exclusive focus on a single disease entity: IBS. More research is needed in other functional gastrointestinal disorders to determine if the effects of stress on gut physiology are general to a larger group of patients. In addition, pediatric studies are largely lacking. Childhood offers a unique psychosocial environment embedded within different stages of psychosocial and physiological development. Studying these factors would add an extra dimension to the current literature. For example, we know very little about the psychosocial influences on our youngest patients: those with infant regurgitation or toddler's diarrhea. We also have not studied the role of other typical childhood psychosocial factors such as parental stress on gut physiology. More research is needed to guide our understanding of psychosocial factors in childhood functional gastrointestinal and motility disorders.

In summary, in order to thoroughly understand functional gastrointestinal and motility disorders it is important to look beyond the biomedical causes of these disorders and also consider personal and social factors that influence the symptom report of patients. Clearly psychosocial factors play a role in symptom perception and illness behaviors as well. Recent studies have shown that children with similar symptoms may show very differential outcomes depending on their psychosocial profile [95, 96]. The child with good coping skills and low anxiety will likely improve quickly, while the child who is anxious, has poor coping skills, experiences a lot of stressful life events, and has feelings of low self-worth is more likely to continue to suffer from pain and impairment. Johnny—our case from the beginning of this chapter—was not helped by exclusively treating the biological factors that were driving his symptoms. He needed an integrated treatment approach that consisted of improving delayed gastric emptying (physiological factor) as well as helping him overcome his fear of eating (personal factor) and his mother's anxiety (social factor). Symptoms in children with functional gastrointestinal disorders result from an interplay among biomedical causes and many possible psychosocial factors such as anxiety, depression, hypervigilance to symptoms, inadequate coping, the way parents respond to their pain, bullying, unsanitary toilets at school and many more.

References

1. Engel GL. The need for a new medical model: a challenge for biomedicine. Science. 1977;196:129–36.
2. Wilhelmsen I. Brain-gut axis as an example of the bio-psycho-social model. Gut. 2000;47 Suppl 4:iv5–7.
3. Borrell-Carrio F, Suchman AL, Epstein RM. The biopsychosocial model 25 years later: principles, practice, and scientific inquiry. Ann Fam Med. 2004;2:576–82.
4. Campo JV, Bridge J, Ehmann M, Altman S, Lucas A, Birmaher B, Di LC, Iyengar S, Brent DA. Recurrent abdominal pain, anxiety, and depression in primary care. Pediatrics. 2004;113:817–24.
5. Walker LS, Garber J, Greene JW. Psychosocial correlates of recurrent childhood pain: a comparison of pediatric patients with recurrent abdominal pain, organic illness, and psychiatric disorders. J Abnorm Psychol. 1993;102:248–58.
6. Chitkara DK, Talley NJ, Weaver AL, van Tilburg MAL, Katusic S, Locke GR, Rucker MJ, Whitehead WE. Abdominal pain and co-morbid complaints from childhood to adulthood in a population based birth cohort. Gastroenterology. 2006;130:A502.
7. Merlijn VP, Hunfeld JA, van der Wouden JC, Hazebroek-Kampschreur AA, Koes BW, Passchier J. Psychosocial factors associated with chronic pain in adolescents. Pain. 2003;101:33–43.
8. Walker LS, Claar RL, Garber J. Social consequences of children's pain: when do they encourage symptom maintenance? J Pediatr Psychol. 2002;27:689–98.
9. Claar RL, Walker LS, Smith CA. Functional disability in adolescents and young adults with symptoms of irritable bowel syndrome: the role of academic, social, and athletic competence. J Pediatr Psychol. 1999;24:271–80.
10. Chitkara DK, van Tilburg MA, Blois-Martin N, Whitehead WE. Early life risk factors that contribute

to irritable bowel syndrome in adults: a systematic review. Am J Gastroenterol. 2008;103:765–74.
11. van Tilburg MA, Runyan DK, Zolotor AJ, Graham JC, Dubowitz H, Litrownik AJ, Flaherty E, Chitkara DK, Whitehead WE. Unexplained gastrointestinal symptoms after abuse in a prospective study of children at risk for abuse and neglect. Ann Fam Med. 2010;8:134–40.
12. Lazarus RS, Folkman S. Stress, appraisal, and coping. New York: Springer; 1984.
13. Lenz HJ, Raedler A, Greten H, Vale WW, Rivier JE. Stress-induced gastrointestinal secretory and motor responses in rats are mediated by endogenous corticotropin-releasing factor. Gastroenterology. 1988;95:1510–7.
14. Tache Y, Martinez V, Million M, Rivier J. Corticotropin-releasing factor and the brain-gut motor response to stress. Can J Gastroenterol. 1999;13(Suppl A):18A–25A.
15. Smith GW, Aubry JM, Dellu F, Contarino A, Bilezikjian LM, Gold LH, Chen R, Marchuk Y, Hauser C, Bentley CA, Sawchenko PE, Koob GF, Vale W, Lee KF. Corticotropin releasing factor receptor 1-deficient mice display decreased anxiety, impaired stress response, and aberrant neuroendocrine development. Neuron. 1998;20:1093–102.
16. Stenzel-Poore MP, Heinrichs SC, Rivest S, Koob GF, Vale WW. Overproduction of corticotropin-releasing factor in transgenic mice: a genetic model of anxiogenic behavior. J Neurosci. 1994;14:2579–84.
17. Sutton RE, Koob GF, Le MM, Rivier J, Vale W. Corticotropin releasing factor produces behavioural activation in rats. Nature. 1982;297:331–3.
18. Timpl P, Spanagel R, Sillaber I, Kresse A, Reul JM, Stalla GK, Blanquet V, Steckler T, Holsboer F, Wurst W. Impaired stress response and reduced anxiety in mice lacking a functional corticotropin-releasing hormone receptor 1. Nat Genet. 1998;19:162–6.
19. Stengel A, Tache Y. Neuroendocrine control of the gut during stress: corticotropin-releasing factor signaling pathways in the spotlight. Annu Rev Physiol. 2009;71:219–39.
20. Larauche M, Kiank C, Tache Y. Corticotropin releasing factor signaling in colon and ileum: regulation by stress and pathophysiological implications. J Physiol Pharmacol. 2009;60 Suppl 7:33–46.
21. Nakade Y, Fukuda H, Iwa M, Tsukamoto K, Yanagi H, Yamamura T, Mantyh C, Pappas TN, Takahashi T. Restraint stress stimulates colonic motility via central corticotropin-releasing factor and peripheral 5-HT3 receptors in conscious rats. Am J Physiol Gastrointest Liver Physiol. 2007;292:G1037–44.
22. Gershon MD, Tack J. The serotonin signaling system: from basic understanding to drug development for functional GI disorders. Gastroenterology. 2007;132:397–414.
23. Tache Y, Kiank C, Stengel A. A role for corticotropin-releasing factor in functional gastrointestinal disorders. Curr Gastroenterol Rep. 2009;11:270–7.
24. Kellow JE, Azpiroz F, Delvaux M, Gebhart GF, Mertz HR, Quigley EM, Smout AJ. Applied principles of neurogastroenterology: physiology/motility sensation. Gastroenterology. 2006;130:1412–20.
25. van den Berg MM, Di LC, van Ginkel R, Mousa HM, Benninga MA. Barostat testing in children with functional gastrointestinal disorders. Curr Gastroenterol Rep. 2006;8:224–9.
26. Di Lorenzo C, Youssef NN, Sigurdsson L, Scharff L, Griffiths J, Wald A. Visceral hyperalgesia in children with functional abdominal pain. J Pediatr. 2001;139:838–43.
27. Halac U, Noble A, Faure C. Rectal sensory threshold for pain is a diagnostic marker of irritable bowel syndrome and functional abdominal pain in children. J Pediatr. 2010;156:60–5.
28. Voskuijl WP, van Ginkel R, Benninga MA, Hart GA, Taminiau JA, Boeckxstaens GE. New insight into rectal function in pediatric defecation disorders: disturbed rectal compliance is an essential mechanism in pediatric constipation. J Pediatr. 2006;148:62–7.
29. van den Berg MM, Voskuijl WP, Boeckxstaens GE, Benninga MA. Rectal compliance and rectal sensation in constipated adolescents, recovered adolescents and healthy volunteers. Gut. 2008;57:599–603.
30. Tyler K, Moriceau S, Sullivan RM, Greenwood-van MB. Long-term colonic hypersensitivity in adult rats induced by neonatal unpredictable vs predictable shock. Neurogastroenterol Motil. 2007;19:761–8.
31. Ren TH, Wu J, Yew D, Ziea E, Lao L, Leung WK, Berman B, Hu PJ, Sung JJ. Effects of neonatal maternal separation on neurochemical and sensory response to colonic distension in a rat model of irritable bowel syndrome. Am J Physiol Gastrointest Liver Physiol. 2007;292:G849–56.
32. Schwetz I, McRoberts JA, Coutinho SV, Bradesi S, Gale G, Fanselow M, Million M, Ohning G, Tache Y, Plotsky PM, Mayer EA. Corticotropin-releasing factor receptor 1 mediates acute and delayed stress-induced visceral hyperalgesia in maternally separated Long-Evans rats. Am J Physiol Gastrointest Liver Physiol. 2005;289:G704–12.
33. Bradesi S, Eutamene H, Garcia-Villar R, Fioramonti J, Bueno L. Acute and chronic stress differently affect visceral sensitivity to rectal distension in female rats. Neurogastroenterol Motil. 2002;14:75–82.
34. Ait-Belgnaoui A, Bradesi S, Fioramonti J, Theodorou V, Bueno L. Acute stress-induced hypersensitivity to colonic distension depends upon increase in paracellular permeability: role of myosin light chain kinase. Pain. 2005;113:141–7.
35. Murray CD, Flynn J, Ratcliffe L, Jacyna MR, Kamm MA, Emmanuel AV. Effect of acute physical and psychological stress on gut autonomic innervation in irritable bowel syndrome. Gastroenterology. 2004;127:1695–703.
36. Thoua NM, Murray CD, Winchester WJ, Roy AJ, Pitcher MC, Kamm MA, Emmanuel AV. Amitriptyline modifies the visceral hypersensitivity response to acute stress in the irritable bowel syndrome. Aliment Pharmacol Ther. 2009;29:552–60.
37. Geeraerts B, Van OL, Fischler B, Vandenberghe J, Caenepeel P, Janssens J, Tack J. Influence of abuse his-

tory on gastric sensorimotor function in functional dyspepsia. Neurogastroenterol Motil. 2009;21:33–41.
38. Van OL, Vandenberghe J, Geeraerts B, Vos R, Persoons P, Demyttenaere K, Fischler B, Tack J. Relationship between anxiety and gastric sensorimotor function in functional dyspepsia. Psychosom Med. 2007;69:455–63.
39. Whitehead WE, Crowell MD, Davidoff AL, Palsson OS, Schuster MM. Pain from rectal distension in women with irritable bowel syndrome: relationship to sexual abuse. Dig Dis Sci. 1997;42:796–804.
40. de Medeiros MT, Carvalho AF, de Oliveira Lima JW, Dos Santos AA, de Oliveira RB, Nobre E, Souza MA. Impact of depressive symptoms on visceral sensitivity among patients with different subtypes of irritable bowel syndrome. J Nerv Ment Dis. 2008;196:711–4.
41. Van OL, Vandenberghe J, Dupont P, Geeraerts B, Vos R, Dirix S, Van LK, Bormans G, Vanderghinste D, Demyttenaere K, Fischler B, Tack J. Regional brain activity in functional dyspepsia: a H(2)(15)O PET study on the role of gastric sensitivity and abuse history. Gastroenterol. 2010;139:36–47.
42. van der Veek PP, Van Rood YR, Masclee AA. Symptom severity but not psychopathology predicts visceral hypersensitivity in irritable bowel syndrome. Clin Gastroenterol Hepatol. 2008;6:321–8.
43. Anderson JL, Acra S, Bruehl S, Walker LS. Relation between clinical symptoms and experimental visceral hypersensitivity in pediatric patients with functional abdominal pain. J Pediatr Gastroenterol Nutr. 2008;47:309–15.
44. Ringel Y, Whitehead WE, Toner BB, Diamant NE, Hu Y, Jia H, Bangdiwala SI, Drossman DA. Sexual and physical abuse are not associated with rectal hypersensitivity in patients with irritable bowel syndrome. Gut. 2004;53:838–42.
45. Whitehead WE, Delvaux M, Azpiroz F, Barlow J, Bradley L, Camilleri M, Crowell MD, Enck P, Fioramonti J, Track J, Mayer EA, Morteau O, Phillips SF, Thompson DG, Wingate DL. Standardization of barostat procedures for testing smooth muscle tone and sensory thresholds in the gastrointestinal tract. Dig Dis Sci. 1997;42:223–41.
46. Naliboff BD, Munakata J, Fullerton S, Gracely RH, Kodner A, Harraf F, Mayer EA. Evidence for two distinct perceptual alterations in irritable bowel syndrome. Gut. 1997;41:505–12.
47. Dorn SD, Palsson OS, Thiwan SI, Kanazawa M, Clark WC, van Tilburg MA, Drossman DA, Scarlett Y, Levy RL, Ringel Y, Crowell MD, Olden KW, Whitehead WE. Increased colonic pain sensitivity in irritable bowel syndrome is the result of an increased tendency to report pain rather than increased neurosensory sensitivity. Gut. 2007;56:1202–9.
48. Gomborone JE, Dewsnap PA, Libby GW, Farthing MJ. Selective affective biasing in recognition memory in the irritable bowel syndrome. Gut. 1993;34:1230–3.
49. Mayer EA, Aziz Q, Coen S, Kern M, Labus JS, Lane R, Kuo B, Naliboff B, Tracey I. Brain imaging approaches to the study of functional GI disorders: a Rome working team report. Neurogastroenterol Motil. 2009;21:579–96.
50. Berman SM, Naliboff BD, Suyenobu B, Labus JS, Stains J, Ohning G, Kilpatrick L, Bueller JA, Ruby K, Jarcho J, Mayer EA. Reduced brainstem inhibition during anticipated pelvic visceral pain correlates with enhanced brain response to the visceral stimulus in women with irritable bowel syndrome. J Neurosci. 2008;28:349–59.
51. Ringel Y, Drossman DA, Turkington TG, Bradshaw B, Hawk TC, Bangdiwala S, Coleman RE, Whitehead WE. Regional brain activation in response to rectal distension in patients with irritable bowel syndrome and the effect of a history of abuse. Dig Dis Sci. 2003;48:1774–81.
52. Ringel Y, Drossman DA, Leserman JL, Suyenobu BY, Wilber K, Lin W, Whitehead WE, Naliboff BD, Berman S, Mayer EA. Effect of abuse history on pain reports and brain responses to aversive visceral stimulation: an FMRI study. Gastroenterology. 2008;134:396–404.
53. Drossman DA, Ringel Y, Vogt BA, Leserman J, Lin W, Smith JK, Whitehead W. Alterations of brain activity associated with resolution of emotional distress and pain in a case of severe irritable bowel syndrome. Gastroenterology. 2003;124:754–61.
54. Spiller RC. Role of infection in irritable bowel syndrome. J Gastroenterol. 2007;42 Suppl 17:41–7.
55. Kindt S, Van OL, Broekaert D, Kasran A, Ceuppens JL, Bossuyt X, Fischler B, Tack J. Immune dysfunction in patients with functional gastrointestinal disorders. Neurogastroenterol Motil. 2009;21:389–98.
56. Collins SM, Denou E, Verdu EF, Bercik P. The putative role of the intestinal microbiota in the irritable bowel syndrome. Dig Liver Dis. 2009;41:850–3.
57. Ohman L, Simren M. Pathogenesis of IBS: role of inflammation, immunity and neuroimmune interactions. Nat Rev Gastroenterol Hepatol. 2010;7:163–73.
58. Shulman RJ, Eakin MN, Czyzewski DI, Jarrett M, Ou CN. Increased gastrointestinal permeability and gut inflammation in children with functional abdominal pain and irritable bowel syndrome. J Pediatr. 2008;153:646–50.
59. Taylor TJ, Youssef NN, Shankar R, Kleiner DE, Henderson WA. The association of mast cells and serotonin in children with chronic abdominal pain of unknown etiology. BMC Res Notes. 2010;3:265.
60. Faure C, Patey N, Gauthier C, Brooks EM, Mawe GM. Serotonin signaling is altered in irritable bowel syndrome with diarrhea but not in functional dyspepsia in pediatric age patients. Gastroenterology. 2010;139:249–58.
61. Schurman JV, Singh M, Singh V, Neilan N, Friesen CA. Symptoms and subtypes in pediatric functional dyspepsia: relation to mucosal inflammation and psychological functioning. J Pediatr Gastroenterol Nutr. 2010;51:298–303.
62. Denson TF, Spanovic M, Miller N. Cognitive appraisals and emotions predict cortisol and immune

responses: a meta-analysis of acute laboratory social stressors and emotion inductions. Psychol Bull. 2009;135:823–53.
63. Glaser R, Sheridan J, Malarkey WB, MacCallum RC, Kiecolt-Glaser JK. Chronic stress modulates the immune response to a pneumococcal pneumonia vaccine. Psychosom Med. 2000;62:804–7.
64. Kiecolt-Glaser JK, Glaser R, Gravenstein S, Malarkey WB, Sheridan J. Chronic stress alters the immune response to influenza virus vaccine in older adults. Proc Natl Acad Sci U S A. 1996;93:3043–7.
65. Cohen S, Tyrrell DA, Smith AP. Psychological stress and susceptibility to the common cold. N Engl J Med. 1991;325:606–12.
66. Pace TW, Negi LT, Adame DD, Cole SP, Sivilli TI, Brown TD, Issa MJ, Raison CL. Effect of compassion meditation on neuroendocrine, innate immune and behavioral responses to psychosocial stress. Psychoneuroendocrinology. 2009;34:87–98.
67. Leng YX, Wei YY, Chen H, Zhou SP, Yang YL, Duan LP. Alteration of cholinergic and peptidergic neurotransmitters in rat ileum induced by acute stress following transient intestinal infection is mast cell dependent. Chin Med J (Engl). 2010;123:227–33.
68. Caso JR, Leza JC, Menchen L. The effects of physical and psychological stress on the gastro-intestinal tract: lessons from animal models. Curr Mol Med. 2008;8:299–312.
69. Piche T, Saint-Paul MC, Dainese R, Marine-Barjoan E, Iannelli A, Montoya ML, Peyron JF, Czerucka D, Cherikh F, Filippi J, Tran A, Hebuterne X. Mast cells and cellularity of the colonic mucosa correlated with fatigue and depression in irritable bowel syndrome. Gut. 2008;57:468–73.
70. Dinan TG, Quigley EM, Ahmed SM, Scully P, O'Brien S, O'Mahony L, O'Mahony S, Shanahan F, Keeling PW. Hypothalamic-pituitary-gut axis dysregulation in irritable bowel syndrome: plasma cytokines as a potential biomarker? Gastroenterol. 2006;130:304–11.
71. Liebregts T, Adam B, Bredack C, Roth A, Heinzel S, Lester S, Downie-Doyle S, Smith E, Drew P, Talley NJ, Holtmann G. Immune activation in patients with irritable bowel syndrome. Gastroenterol. 2007;132:913–20.
72. Miller AH, Maletic V, Raison CL. Inflammation and its discontents: the role of cytokines in the pathophysiology of major depression. Biol Psychiatry. 2009;65:732–41.
73. Yirmiya R, Pollak Y, Morag M, Reichenberg A, Barak O, Avitsur R, Shavit Y, Ovadia H, Weidenfeld J, Morag A, Newman ME, Pollmacher T. Illness, cytokines, and depression. Ann N Y Acad Sci. 2000;917:478–87.
74. Capuron L, Gumnick JF, Musselman DL, Lawson DH, Reemsnyder A, Nemeroff CB, Miller AH. Neurobehavioral effects of interferon-alpha in cancer patients: phenomenology and paroxetine responsiveness of symptom dimensions. Neuropsychopharmacology. 2002;26:643–52.
75. Reichenberg A, Yirmiya R, Schuld A, Kraus T, Haack M, Morag A, Pollmacher T. Cytokine-associated emotional and cognitive disturbances in humans. Arch Gen Psychiatry. 2001;58:445–52.
76. Constant A, Castera L, Dantzer R, Couzigou P, de Ledinghen V, Demotes-Mainard J, Henry C. Mood alterations during interferon-alfa therapy in patients with chronic hepatitis C: evidence for an overlap between manic/hypomanic and depressive symptoms. J Clin Psychiatry. 2005;66:1050–7.
77. Wichers MC, Kenis G, Leue C, Koek G, Robaeys G, Maes M. Baseline immune activation as a risk factor for the onset of depression during interferon-alpha treatment. Biol Psychiatry. 2006;60:77–9.
78. Goehler LE, Lyte M, Gaykema RP. Infection-induced viscerosensory signals from the gut enhance anxiety: implications for psychoneuroimmunology. Brain Behav Immun. 2007;21:721–6.
79. Collins SM, Bercik P. The relationship between intestinal microbiota and the central nervous system in normal gastrointestinal function and disease. Gastroenterology. 2009;136:2003–14.
80. Lepage P, Colombet J, Marteau P, Sime-Ngando T, Dore J, Leclerc M. Dysbiosis in inflammatory bowel disease: a role for bacteriophages? Gut. 2008;57:424–5.
81. Jacobs Jr NF. Antibiotic-induced diarrhea and pseudomembranous colitis. Postgrad Med. 1994;95:111–20.
82. McFarland LV. Epidemiology, risk factors and treatments for antibiotic-associated diarrhea. Dig Dis. 1998;16:292–307.
83. Codling C, O'Mahony L, Shanahan F, Quigley EM, Marchesi JR. A molecular analysis of fecal and mucosal bacterial communities in irritable bowel syndrome. Dig Dis Sci. 2010;55:392–7.
84. Kassinen A, Krogius-Kurikka L, Makivuokko H, Rinttila T, Paulin L, Corander J, Malinen E, Apajalahti J, Palva A. The fecal microbiota of irritable bowel syndrome patients differs significantly from that of healthy subjects. Gastroenterology. 2007;133:24–33.
85. Malinen E, Rinttila T, Kajander K, Matto J, Kassinen A, Krogius L, Saarela M, Korpela R, Palva A. Analysis of the fecal microbiota of irritable bowel syndrome patients and healthy controls with real-time PCR. Am J Gastroenterol. 2005;100:373–82.
86. Verdu EF, Bercik P, Verma-Gandhu M, Huang XX, Blennerhassett P, Jackson W, Mao Y, Wang L, Rochat F, Collins SM. Specific probiotic therapy attenuates antibiotic induced visceral hypersensitivity in mice. Gut. 2006;55:182–90.
87. Burton MB, Gebhart GF. Effects of intracolonic acetic acid on responses to colorectal distension in the rat. Brain Res. 1995;672:77–82.
88. Bercik P, Denou E, Collins J, Jackson W, Lu J, Jury J, Deng Y, Blennerhassett P, Macri J, McCoy KD, Verdu EF, Collins SM. The intestinal microbiota affect central levels of brain-derived neurotropic factor and behavior in mice. Gastroenterology. 2011;141:599–609.
89. Rosas-Ballina M, Tracey KJ. Cholinergic control of inflammation. J Intern Med. 2009;265:663–79.
90. Goehler LE, Gaykema RP, Hansen MK, Anderson K, Maier SF, Watkins LR. Vagal immune-to-brain com-

munication: a visceral chemosensory pathway. Auton Neurosci. 2000;85:49–59.
91. Lyte M, Li W, Opitz N, Gaykema RP, Goehler LE. Induction of anxiety-like behavior in mice during the initial stages of infection with the agent of murine colonic hyperplasia Citrobacter rodentium. Physiol Behav. 2006;89:350–7.
92. Goehler LE, Gaykema RP, Opitz N, Reddaway R, Badr N, Lyte M. Activation in vagal afferents and central autonomic pathways: early responses to intestinal infection with *Campylobacter jejuni*. Brain Behav Immun. 2005;19:334–44.
93. Lyte M, Varcoe JJ, Bailey MT. Anxiogenic effect of subclinical bacterial infection in mice in the absence of overt immune activation. Physiol Behav. 1998;65:63–8.
94. Bercik P, Park AJ, Sinclair D, Khoshdel A, Lu J, Huang X, Deng Y, Blennerhassett PA, Fahnestock M, Moine D, Berger B, Huizinga JD, Kunze W, McLean PG, Bergonzelli GE, Collins SM, Verdu EF. The anxiolytic effect of *Bifidobacterium longum* NCC3001 involves vagal pathways for gut-brain communication. Neurogastroenterol Motil. 2011;23(12):1132–9.
95. Mulvaney S, Lambert EW, Garber J, Walker LS. Trajectories of symptoms and impairment for pediatric patients with functional abdominal pain: a 5-year longitudinal study. J Am Acad Child Adolesc Psychiatry. 2006;45:737–44.
96. Walker LS, Baber KF, Garber J, Smith CA. A typology of pain coping strategies in pediatric patients with chronic abdominal pain. Pain. 2008;137:266–75.

Functional Gastrointestinal Disorders: An Anthropological Perspective

7

Sylvie Fortin, Liliana Gomez, and Annie Gauthier

Introduction

In the biomedical and social sciences, the strong tendency towards specialization of knowledge and practices often leads to a separation of the biopsychosocial and cultural aspects of the experience of illness. In this chapter, our objective is to highlight the main contributions of anthropology to the field of medicine, and especially the specialty of functional gastrointestinal disorders (FGIDs). First, we present the most recent epidemiological data, along with an overview of the current state of research into these disorders. Second, we briefly explain the anthropological approach and method, underscoring its main contributions to the understanding of FGIDs. Then we look at the contributions of anthropology to studies on patient–clinician relations with respect to FGIDs. We wind up with some concluding remarks and proposals for avenues of research and thought.

S. Fortin, Ph.D. (✉)
Anthropology Department, Université de Montréal, C.P. 6128, Succ. Centre-ville, Montréal, Québec, Canada, H3C3J7
e-mail: sylvie.fortin@umontreal.ca

L. Gomez, M.Sc.
Research Center, Sainte-Justine University Hospital, Montreal, Quebec, Canada

A. Gauthier, Ph.D.
Research Center, Sainte-Justine University Health Center, Montreal, Quebec, Canada

Epidemiology

Functional gastrointestinal disorders (FGIDs) may be defined as gastrointestinal dysfunction in the absence of apparent physiological lesions. The prevalence rates of FGIDs are 13–20% in the general Canadian population, 10–15% in the global population [1], and approximately 10% in the pediatric population [2].

In some of the first prevalence studies of FGIDs, it was suggested that non-Western countries were less affected than Western countries [3, 4]. Yet in South Africa, an increase in consultations for this type of disorder was observed with recent industrialization and the advent of extensive lifestyle changes. Also, studies in Nigeria [5, 6], Kenya [7], and Ivory Coast [8] found prevalence rates similar to those in North America. Last, some studies report a tendency towards an evening out of prevalence rates of these disorders in various countries: United States 10–15%, Sweden 13.5%, China 15.9%, Singapore 8.6%, Pakistan 14%, Taiwan 22.1%, and Nigeria 26.1% [9]. Although different instruments used to measure prevalence make international data comparisons difficult, variations in rates have been attributed to food, hygiene, and psychosocial factors [10, 11].

Also, population studies in a number of countries suggest significant similarities in the perception of symptoms and decisions to seek medical help for FGIDs [7, 12–16]. Sex differences have

C. Faure et al. (eds.), *Pediatric Neurogastroenterology: Gastrointestinal Motility and Functional Disorders in Children*, Clinical Gastroenterology,
DOI 10.1007/978-1-60761-709-9_7, © Springer Science+Business Media New York 2013

been pointed out, however: in cases of FGIDs, women, regardless of national origin, are more likely than men to express their pain and seek medical help [7, 17–19]. While knowledge in the field is constantly advancing, much is still unknown about the factors involved in the onset and evolution of FGIDs [20, 21]. Nevertheless there seems to be consensus that FGIDs are caused and maintained by a combination of biological, psychological, and social factors.[1]

In the three-pronged bio–psycho–social model, genetic factors, along with environmental factors in the early years of life, family upbringing with respect to food and digestion, specific family dynamics, exposure to infections, types of somatization, and various ways of expressing and developing narratives of suffering [22, 23], are considered to form the basis of physiological processes (abnormal motility or visceral hypersensitivity) and psychosociological processes (susceptibility to stresses of everyday life, psychological condition, coping skills, development of social support). In each person with an FGID, these interactive processes lead to an individual constellation of symptoms and behaviors that influence the person's reactions to the disorder. Given this complexity, multidisciplinary research would seem to be essential and of great benefit in supporting clinicians who work with children, adults, and families affected by FGIDs. Pooling biomedical and social science expertise makes it possible to build on acquired epidemiological and clinical knowledge to better grasp the protective and vulnerability factors associated with the onset and evolution of FGIDs, and gain a better understanding of the intricate relationship between the biological, social, and cultural dimensions of the human body.

[1] The generally accepted hypothesis to explain the pain is that there is a combination of sensory and motor activity along the brain–gut axis. It appears that the information we receive from the outside through our senses and perceptions (emotions, thoughts, smells, sights), by the nature of the neural connections in the higher centers, can affect gastrointestinal sensations, motility, hormone secretion, and inflammation [8]. This physiological action seems to have a variable influence on the endocrine system, immune function, and human behavior.

Contributions of Anthropological Approach and Method to Understanding of FGIDs

Medical anthropology is keenly interested in the interaction between the body and its social and cultural setting that is so fundamental to FGIDs. Classically, it distinguishes between three related concepts:

1. *Disease*—Medically identified pathology (organic dysfunction, psychological deficit, etc.).
2. *Illness*—Patient's subjective experience (disease as experienced).
3. *Sickness*—Disease as a social phenomenon: representations of the disease and the patient, but also health problems such as maltreatment and substance abuse. From this standpoint, anthropology approaches the body as both a physical and symbolic entity, a cultural and organic construct, rooted in a specific time and place [24].

The question of FGIDs therefore cannot be confined to merely the abdominal region; it must be broadened and deepened to include personal experience, life trajectory, and relationships with others and the social setting. To anthropologists, the body is also a mediator that lets a person give form to a discomfort or distress that cannot otherwise be expressed. FGIDs are seen as indicative of restrictive social, political, and economic living conditions, or painful events or situations that leave their marks on the body.

Together, these different levels of understanding of the body constitute "the personal experience of disease," which involves the social world, subjectivity, and psychophysiological processes [25]: a reciprocal relationship between the patient's social world and body/self or, in other words, between the patient's outer and inner environments [23].

Anthropological methods (whether taking a phenomenological, ethnographic, or grounded-theory approach) can lead to a better understanding of the experiences of children with FGIDs, in a number of ways. Observing family situations and conducting in-depth interviews with families and children, often at home, can reveal dimensions missed in clinical encounters or by standardized instruments, which often use closed questions, or that provide further illumination of existing data. For example, children and their mothers sometimes have trouble stating exactly how often abdominal pain has occurred within a given time frame, so their answers do not always correspond to the options offered by the Rome III criteria. The same is true of the location of the pain and other accompanying symptoms [26]. Through the use of anthropological methods, the intensity and description of the pain are better understood in a context that makes sense to the children and their families, in keeping with the concept of illness [23, 27] described above.

The anthropological approach to FGIDs thus follows interview guidelines that focus on the narratives of children and their parents, requiring careful listening to what they have to say and close attention to the practices in their living environments that shape their experiences. From this perspective, verbal and nonverbal communication, as well as the dynamics and practices observed intertwine, thus enriching the data to be analyzed. The accounts recorded in the clinical setting can then be compared with the narratives and observations collected through anthropological study and placed in perspective so that they shed light on each other, with a view to gaining a deeper understanding of the various processes involved.

Analytical models vary according to the specific research questions being examined. For example, in a recent multidisciplinary (anthropological and pediatric gastroenterological) exploratory study of children with FGIDs and their families (users and nonusers of health-care services) [28], we used the "signs, meanings, actions" model [29]. This model made it possible to articulate the children's and parents' point of view as it pertained to (1) signs, that is, the perception of symptoms related to FGIDs; (2) meanings and explanations attributed to them; and (3) actions undertaken to ease the pain and chosen therapeutic paths. Thematic analyses by migrant versus nonmigrant respondents, as well as gastroenterological clinic patients versus nonpatients, provided answers to our initial research questions related to the underrepresentation of migrant children in the overall pediatric FGID patient population. While this kind of method is particularly well suited to qualitative data analysis, it does not ensure statistical accuracy. The interest of this approach lies in its capacity to bring out the quality of the sample and the depth of the information gathered. The ultimate goal is to better understand the phenomenon at hand, focusing on its internal logic, rather than its generalization [30, 31].

The Patient–Physician Relationship

One of anthropology's contributions to medicine is the fact that it situates each patient and his or her family in their own specific life situation. This approach is even more appropriate for a pediatric population, since children seek support and help from their parents when they are in pain, of course, but also because it is the parents who, on the child's behalf, seek a cure, turning to medical and health institutions to varying degrees. In-depth knowledge of the family's life and internal dynamics helps us better define the roles each family member may play in mobilizing various formal and informal resources, both individual and community, to relieve FGIDs. In addition to a better grasp of the wealth, variability and limitations of the resources used, in-depth knowledge of the family's life fosters a better appreciation of the interaction between family climate and the search for solutions, or even the origin of the problem. All this information is invaluable to clinicians and in designing treatment plans that are sensitive to the patient's life situation.

Beyond the family's curative strategies and practices, the anthropological approach explores and delves more deeply into the children's and families' explanations and interpretations of gastrointestinal symptoms. These explanatory models are a way of addressing the etiology of problems based on the experiences and words of the people concerned. They offer explanations of episodes of illness and influence how patients and clinicians alike behave with regard to health problems.

Similarly, these explanations are one of the most important dimensions in establishing good communications and developing a solid therapeutic alliance between children, their parents, and the gastroenterologist [32]. Yet the different parties concerned do not always agree on the same explanatory model. In fact, a series of studies on professional and lay etiological models of diseases have highlighted the potential differences between the frameworks that determine the actions and approaches of experts and those of the people consulting the experts [33, 34]. It is important to examine these differences for several reasons:

1. In clinical practice, doctors often have trouble sharing their knowledge of FGIDs, due to the patient's or family's reluctance or refusal to accept an outside expert's explanation of the symptoms.
2. Divergent perceptions and practices associated with strongly contrasting sociocultural points of reference in a pluralistic setting can lead to communication problems.
3. The perceptions and conceptions of FGID symptoms are often not associated with plain or objective facts, but much more with personal interpretations.

Furthermore, for children and their parents, categories of explanations may be approached from different angles and take on a variety of connotations. Here, once again, the study mentioned earlier involving 43 Montreal families of diverse origins [28, 35] found that food, stress, and heredity were the main lay explanations of abdominal pain. However, these explanations are invested with different meanings from one cultural group to another and from one family to another, or even within the same household. For example, respondents express different relationships to the category "food," depending on whether they are talking about its instrumental, nutritional, social, or emotional dimensions. These different connotations affect the way families respond to abdominal pain. As Cook [32] points out, better knowledge of the different meanings attributed to food, as well as of the eating habits of children and their families, is essential to a successful partnership between health professionals and the children, adults, and families who consult them.

A number of studies have documented problems in clinical encounters concerning FGIDs. Researchers talk about unsatisfactory therapeutic relationships, repeated consultations, and often superfluous and sometimes even harmful interventions [36–39]. To a certain extent, these problems reflect the limitations of our conception of FGIDs. In this context, an anthropological approach makes it possible to nurture the caregiver–patient–family relationship and explore its many issues, such as how the gastroenterologist, the child, and the family members negotiate meanings and roles; areas of agreement and disagreement among these different parties; or even the impact of the diagnosis and medical recommendations on the child's life. An anthropological approach can document what it is that patients and their families take away from the clinical encounter, advice offered, and practices suggested; their impressions of how well they have been heard and of whether the child is on the road to better health. As in other research settings [26, 40–42], it is very much a matter of enriching the encounter with different types of expert and lay knowledge and negotiating about them, in a spirit of disciplinary complementarity (anthropology, medicine) and possible contribution to new analytical paradigms and new clinical approaches.

Finally, given that many children and adults who suffer from FGIDs do not seek medical help [43–46], anthropological research on families who did not consult a doctor (or were not recruited through a health-care institution) may reveal invaluable information about FGIDs. We are thinking here more particularly of sociocultural protective and vulnerability factors related to the onset and evolution of FGIDs, the updating of which requires methods that can continually be adjusted to suit people's specific life situations. Family relationships, for example, and more specifically those between parents and children, may channel and soothe stomach pains, just as they may, in another context, exacerbate tensions that may trigger them. Depending on the context, these relationships may support or hinder the mobilization of care resources both within the family and in the broader sphere of health-care services. This means that the same factors may both protect children's health in some cases and increase their vulnerability in others. By putting the different factors into context, anthropology provides a framework for thinking about FGIDs from a pluralistic perspective, as they are experienced by different groups of human beings, in settings that can be unique or quite similar.

Conclusion

Anthropology has made many valuable contributions to the gastroenterology of FGIDs. Qualitative data supplement epidemiological statistics by providing depth and informative details on the social and symbolic world of children and their families. This information helps identify the protective and vulnerability factors associated with these disorders, provides clues about the necessary conditions of a better therapeutic alliance, and aids in understanding the dynamics at work when people seek health services. Last, by combining the social and biological dimensions, anthropology reminds us that we need to consider culture differently, taking as a starting point the people who embody it; to be open to potential medical pluralism; and to work with a view to developing fruitful interdisciplinary partnerships that will advance science and help children and their families.

References

1. Birtwhistle R. Irritable bowel syndrome: are complementary and alternative medicine treatments useful? Can Fam Physician. 2009;55:126–7.
2. Ramchandani P, Stein A, Wiles N, et al. The impact of recurrent abdominal pain: predictors of outcome in a large population cohort. Acta Paediatr. 2007;96:697–701.
3. Danivat D, Tankeyoon M, Sriratanaban A. Prevalence of irritable bowel syndrome in a non-Western population. BMJ. 1988;296:263–7.
4. Walker A, Segal I. Epidemiology of noninfective intestinal diseases in various ethnic groups in South Africa. Isr J Med Sci. 1979;154:309–33.
5. Okeke EN, Agaba EI, Gwamzhi L, Achinge GI, Angbazo D, Malu AO. Prevalence of irritable bowel syndrome in a Nigerian student population. Afr J Med Sci. 2005;34:33–6.
6. Olubuyide IO, Olawuyi F, Fasanmade AA. A study of irritable bowel syndrome diagnosed by Manning criteria in an African population. Dig Dis Sci. 1995;40:983–5.
7. Lule GN, Amayo E. Irritable bowel syndrome in Kenyans. East Afr Med J. 2002;79:360–3.
8. Soubeyrand J, Condat JM, Leleu JP, Ticolat R, Niamkey E, Beda BY. Functional colonic pathology in the Ivory Coast. Sem Hop. 1983;59:247–51.
9. Quigley E, Gwee KA, Olano C, et al. Irritable bowel syndrome: a global perspective. Global guideline. Munich: World Gastroenterology Organisation; 2009, p. 20
10. Heizer WD, McGovern S. The role of diet in symptoms of irritable bowel syndrome in adults: a narrative review. J Am Diet Assoc. 2009;109:1204–14.
11. Zuckerman MJ, Drossman DA, Foland JA, et al. Comparison of bowel patterns in Hispanics and non-Hispanic whites. Dig Dis Sci. 1995;40:1763–9.
12. Barakzai MD, Fraser D. The effect of culture on symptom reporting: Hispanics and irritable bowel syndrome. J Am Acad Nurse Pract. 2007;19:261–7.
13. Gwee KA, Ghoshal UC. Epidemiology of irritable bowel syndrome in Asia: something old, something new, something borrowed. J Gastroenterol Hepatol. 2009;24:1601–7.
14. Landau DA, Levy Y, Bar-Dayan Y. The prevalence of gastrointestinal diseases in Israeli adolescents and its association with body mass index, gender and Jewish ethnicity. J Clin Gastroenterol. 2008;42:903–9.
15. Lu CL, Chen CY, Luo JC, et al. Significance of Rome II-defined functional constipation in Taiwan and comparison with constipation-predominant irritable bowel syndrome. Aliment Pharmacol Ther. 2006;24:429–38.
16. Wigington WC, Johnson WD, Minocha A. Epidemiology of irritable bowel syndrome among African Americans as compared with whites: a population-based study. Clin Gastroenterol Hepatol. 2005;3:647–53.
17. Baretic M, Jurcic D, Mihanovic M, et al. Epidemiology of irritable bowel syndrome in Croatia. Coll Antropol. 2002;26(Suppl):85–91.
18. Heitkemper M. Irritable bowel syndrome: does gender matter? J Psychosom Res. 2008;64:583–7.
19. Shen Y, Nahas R. Complementary and alternative medicine for treatment of irritable bowel syndrome. Can Fam Physician. 2009;55:143–8.
20. Howell S, Talley N, Quine S, et al. The irritable bowel syndrome has origins in the childhood socioeconomic environment. Am J Gastroenterol. 2004;99:1572–8.
21. Rosh J. Recurrent abdominal pain and the pediatric gastroenterologist: how are we functioning? J Pediatr Gastroenterol Nutr. 2010;50:6–7.
22. Kirmayer L, Young A, Robbins J. Symptom attribution in cultural perspective. Can J Psychiatry. 1994;39:584–95.
23. Kleinman A. The illness narratives: suffering, healing and the human condition. New York: Basic; 1988.

24. Scheper-Hughes N, Lock M. The mindful body: a prolegomenon to future work in medical anthropology. Med Anthropol Q. 1987;1:6–41.
25. Kleinman A, Seeman D, Albrecht G, Fitzpatrick, Ray, editors. Handbook of social studies in health and medicine. Thousand Oaks, CA: Sage; 2000. p. xxvii.
26. Gomez L. Les maux de ventre des enfants haïtiens de Montréal: entre la recomposition culturelle et la souffrance familiale. Université de Montréal; 2010.
27. Fassin D. Entre politiques du vivant et politiques de la vie. Anthropol Soc. 2000;24:95–116.
28. Fortin S, Faure C, Bibeau G, Rasquin, A. Facteurs socioculturels de protection et de vulnérabilité dans l'apparition et l'évolution des troubles fonctionnels de l'intestin: les perspectives des enfants et de leur famille et leurs recours aux services. Fonds de recherche en santé du Québec; 2009–2011.
29. Corin E, Bibeau G. Articulation et variation des systèmes de signes, de sens et d'action. Psychopathol Afr. 1992;24:183–204.
30. Glaser B, Strauss A. The discovery of grounded theory: strategies for qualitative research. Chicago: Aldine; 1967.
31. Melia K. Recognizing quality in qualitative research. In: Bourgeault I, Dingwall R, De Vries R, editors. Sage handbook of qualitative methods in health research. Los Angeles: Sage; 2010. p. 559–74.
32. Waissman R. Book review. Cook J, Dommergues J-P. L'enfant malade et le monde médical: dialogue entre familles et soignants. Sci Soc Santé. 1993;13:137–9.
33. Crushell E, Doherty M, Gormally S, et al. Importance of parental conceptual model of illness in severe recurrent abdominal pain. Pediatrics. 2003;112:1368–72.
34. Kleinman A. Patients and healers in the context of culture: an exploration of culture. Berkeley, CA: University of California Press; 1980.
35. Gauthier A, Fortin S, Gomez L, Bibeau G, Rasquin A, Faure C, et al. Pathways to care in FGIDs: the issues, diversity and equality in health and care. (under review).
36. Longstreth GF, Yao JF. Irritable bowel syndrome and surgery: a multivariable analysis. Gastroenterology. 2004;126:1665–73.
37. Masters K. Recurrent abdominal pain, medical intervention, and biofeedback: what happened to the biopsychosocial model? Appl Psychophysiol Biofeedback. 2006;31:155–65.
38. Talley N. Unnecessary abdominal and back surgery in irritable bowel syndrome: time to stem the flood now? Gastroenterology. 2004;126:1899–903.
39. Wilson S, Roberts L, Roalfe A, Bridge P. Prevalence of irritable bowel syndrome: a community survey. Br J Gen Pract. 2004;54:495–502.
40. Fortin S. The paediatric clinic as negotiated social space. Anthropol Med. 2008;15:175–87.
41. Gauthier A, Bibeau G, Alvarez F. Créer des espaces de négociation entre famille et équipe soignante lors de traitements de pointe en pédiatrie: illustrations et réflexions. Intervention. 2008;129:58–68.
42. Gauthier A, Corin E, Rousseau C. À la croisée des récits: explorer la rencontre clinique en début de psychose. L'Évol Psychiat. 2008;73:639–54.
43. Drossman DA, Sandler RS, McKee DC, Lovitz AJ. Bowel patterns among subjects not seeking health care: use of a questionnaire to identify a population with bowel dysfunction. Gastroenterology. 1982;83:529–34.
44. Hungin A, Whorwell PJ, Tack J, Mearin F. The prevalence, patterns and impact of irritable bowel syndrome: an international survey of 40,000 subjects. Aliment Pharmacol Ther. 2003;17:643–50.
45. Nurko S. The tip of the iceberg: the prevalence of functional gastrointestinal diseases in children. J Pediatr. 2009;154:313–5.
46. Thompson W, Heaton KW. Functional bowel disorders in apparently healthy people. Gastroenterology. 1980;79:283–8.

Part II

Motility and Sensory Testing

Esophageal Manometry

8

Roberta Buonavolontà, Marina Russo,
Rossella Turco, and Annamaria Staiano

Introduction

The esophagus acts as a conduit for the aboral transport of food from the mouth to the stomach. The three structural components of the esophagus are the upper esophageal sphincter (UES), the esophageal body, and the lower esophageal sphincter (LES) [1]. The UES is a physiologically defined as a zone of high intraluminal pressure between the pharynx and the cervical esophagus which comprises the functional activity of three adjacent muscles together with cartilage and connective tissue. The main functions of the UES are to provide the most proximal physical barrier of the gastrointestinal (GI) tract against pharyngeal and laryngeal reflux during esophageal peristalsis, and to avoid the entry of air into the digestive tract during negative intrathoracic pressure events, such as inspiration. The UES relaxes both transiently during swallowing, in order to allow the entry of a bolus into the esophagus, and during belching and vomiting, in order to allow the egress of gastric contents from the esophageal lumen. The UES is present by at least 32 weeks gestation and is functional at birth [2]. However, swallowing coordination may be poor in the first week of life and in premature infants <1,500 g [3, 4]. Structurally, the UES is ~0.5–1 cm long at birth and increases in length to ~3 cm in the adult [1].

The LES is the high pressure zone localized at the esophago-gastric junction, which regulates the flow of contents between the esophagus and the stomach. The main function of the LES is to create a high-pressure zone to prevent retrograde movement of gastric content into the esophagus. During swallowing and belching, the LES promptly relaxes in order to allow the passage of ingested food or air in appropriate directions. At the time of swallowing, the LES relaxes promptly in response to the initial neural discharge from the swallowing center in order to minimize resistance to flow across the esophago-gastric junction. This relaxation starts within 2 seconds after the peristaltic contraction has begun in the proximal esophagus and lasts 5–10 s until the peristaltic wave reaches the distal esophagus. During relaxation, LES pressure falls to the level of gastric pressure. As the LES relaxes (an active process), it is passively opened by the bolus propelled by the peristaltic wave. The LES relaxation is followed by an after-contraction of the upper part of sphincter, which likely represents the end of contraction wave as it reaches the distal esophagus. Swallow-induced LES relaxation is part of

R. Buonavolontà, M.D.
Department of Pediatrics, University of Naples, Naples, Italy

M. Russo, M.D. • R. Turco, M.D.
Department of Pediatrics, University of Naples Federico II, Naples, Italy

A. Staiano, M.D. (✉)
Pediatric Gastoenterology Division, Pediatrics Department, University of Naples "Federico II", via Pansini 5, Naples 80131, Italy
e-mail: staiano@unina.it

C. Faure et al. (eds.), *Pediatric Neurogastroenterology: Gastrointestinal Motility and Functional Disorders in Children*, Clinical Gastroenterology,
DOI 10.1007/978-1-60761-709-9_8, © Springer Science+Business Media New York 2013

primary peristalsis [5]. Like the UES, LES length increases with age, from 1 cm in the newborn to 2–4 cm in the adult [6, 7]. LES pressure also varies with age, going from 7 mmHg in a premature infant of 27 weeks gestation to 18 mmHg at term and from 10 to 45 mmHg in adults [8, 9].

Esophageal manometry has been considered the "gold standard" test for the evaluation of esophageal motor function. Esophageal manometry allows the physician to assess peristalsis by measuring the shape, amplitude and duration of the esophageal contractions [10]. The clinical use of esophageal manometry is in defining the contractile characteristics of the esophagus in an attempt to identify pathological conditions. Esophageal manometry is performed differently in children than in adults because of the differences in size of the esophagus, cooperation by the patient, and neurologic and developmental maturation. These differences require special equipment as well as technical expertise to perform the study, handle the patient, and properly interpret the findings [11].

Equipment

A manometric apparatus consists of a pressure sensors and transducers combination, which detects the intraluminal pressure and changes it into an electrical signal, and a recording device to amplify, record, and store that electrical signal. Although each component can potentially affect recording fidelity, most attention is rightfully focused on the pressure sensor and transducer combination. Recorders (whether they are ink writing polygraphs, thermal writing polygraphs, or computers with analogue to digital converters) all possess response characteristics far in excess of that required for recording esophageal pressure complexes. Specific recorders are most easily distinguished by the number of pressure signals (channels) that can be recorded simultaneously, ease of use, convenience of data storage, accessibility of stored data, and price. The pressure sensor and transducer components of a manometric assembly function as a matched pair and are available in two general designs: water-perfused catheters with volume displacement transducers or strain gauge transducers with solid-state circuitry. Each design has distinct advantages and disadvantages. With water-perfused systems, a pneumohydraulic pump perfuses distilled water through the lumens of the multilumen manometric catheter. Each lumen is connected to an external volume displacement pressure transducer and terminates at a side-hole or sleeve channel within the esophagus, sensing the intraluminal pressure at that position by the relative obstruction to the flow of the perfusate. In addition to having well defined, time-tested response characteristics, other advantages of the perfused manometric system are (1) relatively inexpensive, (2) easy availability of 8-lumen extruded polyvinyl tubes that can be made into manometric assemblies of varied sensor configuration, (3) compatibility with sleeve devices for assessing sphincter function, and (4) temperature stability. Disadvantages of perfused manometric systems are as follows: (1) proper equipment maintenance, which is essential for the system to achieve published response characteristics, requires relatively skilled personnel; and (2) recording characteristics are unsuitable for accurate pharyngeal studies [8].

The main alternative to the water-perfused manometric system is a manometric assembly incorporating strain gauge sensors and solid-state electronic elements. In these manometric systems, the manometric probe contains the transducers at fixed locations along its length. The probe plugs into a small box containing the electronic elements, connected to the recorder. The advantages of intraluminal strain gauge systems are (1) their vastly expanded frequency response, making them suitable for recording any intraluminal pressure activity and (2) their less cumbersome nature compared with perfusion pumps, requiring less skilled personnel to perform clinical studies and less equipment maintenance. The main disadvantages are as follows: (1) the manometric probes are expensive, sometimes fragile, and unmodifiable; (2) manometric probes are subject to several physical constraints with respect to the number of sensing elements and the proximity of the elements to each other; and

(3) there is no equivalent of a sleeve device compatible with this system [8].

With either system, the spacing of the sensing ports depends on the size of the patient. The interval between perfusion ports or transducers may need to be as close as 1–3 cm apart to accommodate the shorter esophagus in infants. During perfusion in infants and small children, the perfusion rate may need to be lower because of the size of the esophagus, the fluid tolerance of infants, and the potential for aspiration. Care must be exercised to compensate for the slower flow rate by decreasing the system compliance [11].

Performing the Test

Esophageal manometry is best performed without sedation. In many children, however, sedation is necessary. Midazolam and chloral hydrate have been shown to be effective with minimal or no influence on pressure measurements [12, 13]. A natural reflex swallow may be induced in young infants and neurologically abnormal children by gently blowing in the child's face (Santmyer swallow) [14].

The single most difficult technical aspect of esophageal manometry in children is cooperation. Physicians performing manometry in children must have great patience. The patient's cooperation can, however, be improved by the use of age-appropriate relaxation techniques. For example, infants relax with swaddling and use of a pacifier. Toddlers are comforted by having a favorite blanket or toy. School-age children benefit from being allowed to handle and examine equipment before the procedure. Adolescents benefit from a thorough review of what to expect before the procedure. Recording artifacts are common in the pediatric patient and occur more commonly than in adults. Specific behaviors (e.g., crying or squirming) should be noted on the tracing itself to allow proper interpretation upon completion of the study [11].

Despite the technical advances, considerable time and expertise are required to obtain a technically adequate and maximally informative study of esophageal function by this technique. At present, abnormal motor activity as measured by "conventional manometry" is defined in terms of a few basic patterns: incomplete sphincter relaxation, esophageal spasm, hypertensive contractions, and loss of tone and motility [15–17]. This classification is simple; however, even for experienced physiologists in specialist centers, interobserver agreement in the interpretation of manometric measurements is poor [18]. Only achalasia and severe diffuse esophageal spasm are specific disorders with manometric abnormalities that are absent in healthy subjects. Other esophageal motility disorders are poorly defined, often include "abnormalities" that can be found in symptom-free individuals as well [19, 20] and are inconsistent over time [21].

High Resolution Manometry

High-resolution manometry (HRM) was developed to increase interpretative consistency and diagnostic accuracy of esophageal manometry [22, 23]. Addition of the dimension of spatial relationship to conventional recording methods has two minimum requirements: recording sites that are positioned closely enough (usually at 1-cm intervals) to allow accurate interpolation of data between sites and an appropriate computer system for acquisition of the data and creation and display of the desired three-dimensional plots [22]. Axial interpolation has already proved useful in understanding the correct relationship of pressure data when unusual wave forms occur, for example, multi-peaked waves [23]. Three-dimensional topographical plots are convenient methods of visually representing the large amount of data provided by the increased number of recording sites.

Both perfused (Medical Measurement Systems, Enschede, The Netherlands) and solid-state systems (Manoscan and Manoview, Sierra Scientific, Los Angeles, USA) to perform HRM are now available. The water-perfused catheters for HRM with 21–32 channels and, more recently, up to 36 pressure sensors, contain smaller lumina, which are perfused at very low rates. In children, at least 80% of the esophageal body and one sphincter could be sampled with the catheter with 21 lumens in either a proximal or distal recording position. With this design, a 20 cm segment is sampled simultaneously. Data acquired by HRM can be analyzed and presented either as multiple line plots or as a spatiotemporal plot.

Three types of data display can be generated and are available for review immediately after completion of the recording sessions, each taking into consideration both time and space relationships of manometric data. Surface plots are three-dimensional representations examined from different elevations or perspectives; contour plots represent three-dimensional data in a single "overhead" perspective as is commonly used to display geographic or weather data; and axial transformations represent data at a single time across all of the recording channels, the dimension of time being represented by an animation of the data frames. In all cases, the initial step involves alignment of the manometric data on a planar surface [22].

The *surface plots* are created by exporting three dimensional data sets to a program specifically designed for geographic mapping. The developed system creates x, y, z data sets for specified time intervals following designated event markers inserted during analysis. For these data sets, x represents the recording site position on the catheter in cm, y the time after the event marker in seconds, and z the pressure amplitude at that time and location in mmHg. In creating surface plots, a grid of data is first established, the gridline interval being determined by the investigator for both the x and y directions. For the purposes of esophageal plotting, gridlines are usually positioned at 0.2 cm and 0.2-s intervals. The z value (pressure amplitude) is interpolated at each grid intersection using available neighboring data for establishing the most appropriate value. Resultant plots can be tilted forward or rotated as required to best visualize the three-dimensional data [22]. *Contour plots* represent an overhead perspective of surface plots, each contour ring encircling amplitudes of equal or greater value than that specified on the color legend. A series of concentric rings indicates a regional pressure peak on the plot. In the developed system the plot baseline can be shifted as required for zero adjustment (e.g., to match intragastric pressure). Likewise, the first contour level as well as the pressure interval for subsequent rings can be modified as required. The *axial transformations* of manometric data are available only on the developed system. Individual frames are created by splining data across all recording sites at a specified time following an inserted or adjusted event marker. All frames are then viewed as an animated movie, the animation speed adjusted by the investigator (Figs. 8.1 and 8.2) [22].

On a theoretical level, HRM provides advantages over conventional techniques for the assessment of esophageal function. One of the most important advantages of HRM is that it makes diagnostic esophageal manometry easier and quicker to perform. It takes away the need for a pull-through and precise positioning of the manometric catheter with respect to the LES. Manometry can thus simply be performed by a lab technician or nurse, and only limited experience in esophageal manometry is required. The pattern of esophageal peristalsis and sphincter activity defines whether esophageal motor activity is normal or abnormal. The intra-bolus pressure and esophago-gastric pressure gradient define whether or not this activity is consistent with effective function. On a practical level, HRM makes it easy to acquire good quality pressure measurements from the esophagus, facilitates positioning of the catheter and removes the need for a pull-through procedure. Moreover spatiotemporal plots of pressure information make it easy to identify normal and abnormal patterns of esophageal motility [15].

Clinical Use of High Resolution Manometry

The advantages of HRM have been described in a series of recent publications [24]. Closely spaced pressure channels provide detailed pressure information that reveals the segmental nature of esophageal peristalsis. This is important because motor abnormalities can be limited to a short segment of the esophagus and will be missed by pressure sensors spaced too far apart

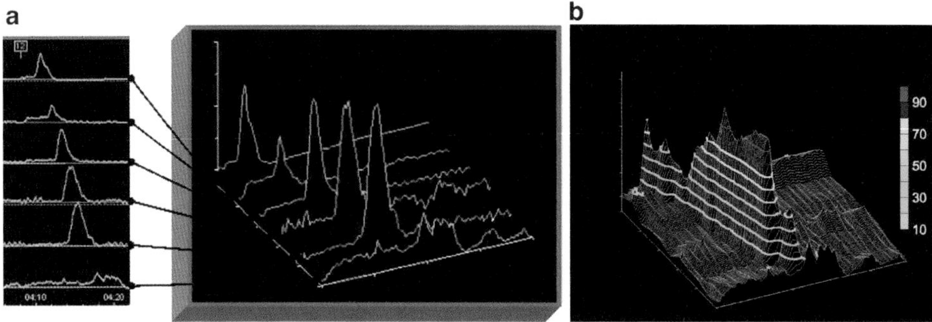

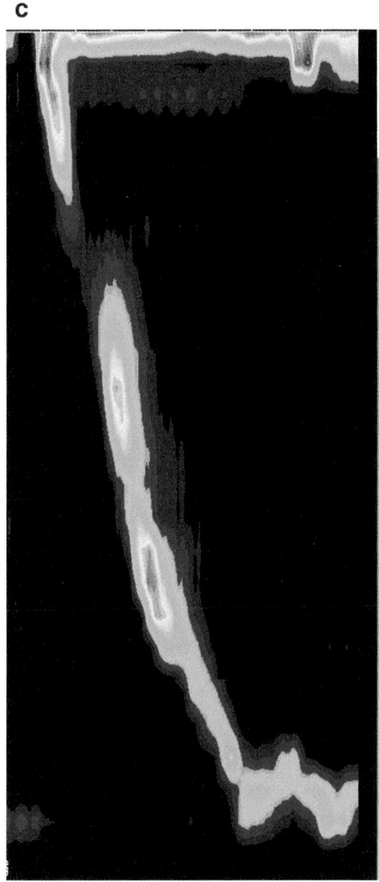

Fig. 8.1 High resolution manometry. (**a**) Tracings are aligned on a planar surface so that spatial relationships of pressure data between recording sensors can be established. (**b**) Interpolation of pressure data between sensors is performed, and colors are applied to pressure levels according to a scale. (**c**) Overhead "contour maps" reveal the segmental nature of esophageal peristalsis

[25, 26]. HRM increases the accuracy by which bolus transport can be predicted from manometry [25]. This is significant because abnormal bolus transport is a more important cause of esophageal symptoms than manometric abnormalities per se [27]. HRM identifies patients with poor coordination between the proximal and mid-esophagus (wide "transition zone"), focal hypotensive contractions or focal spasm that would be missed by conventional manometry.

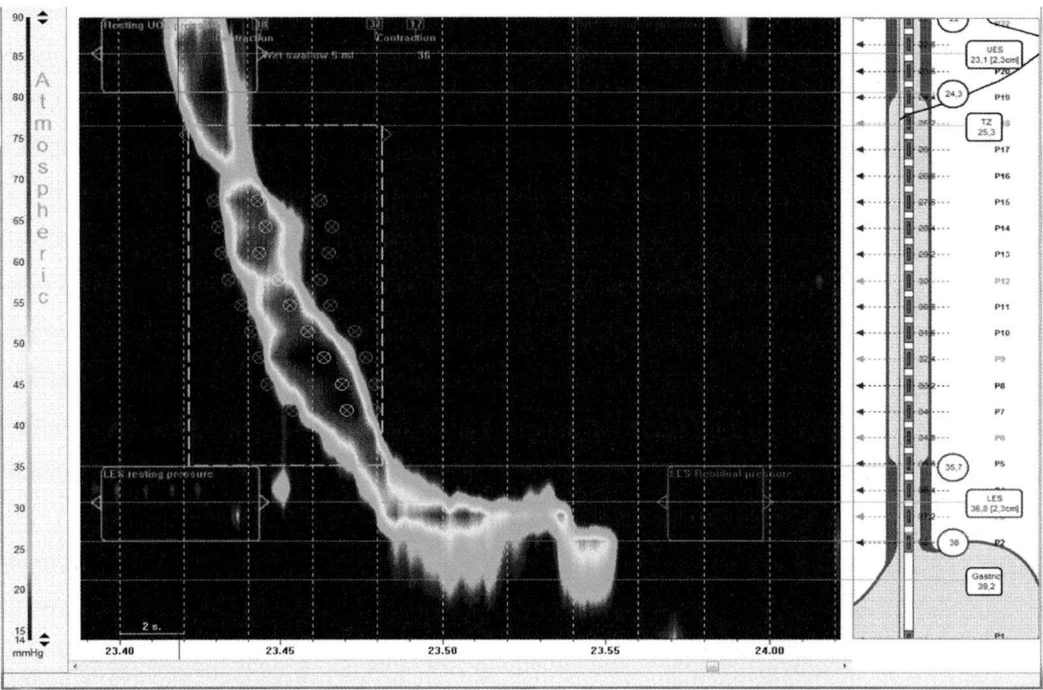

Fig. 8.2 A complete peristaltic chain is seen in this image. The segmental pressure architecture resembles what is seen in the healthy adult. The three intersegmental troughs are indicated on the figure, and the pressure amplitudes represented by the isobaric contour regions are shown in the color legend (in mmHg above gastric baseline pressure; pressures below the first isobaric contour are shown in *dark blue*)

Crucially, HRM can distinguish between abnormalities that disturb bolus transport from abnormalities that have no effect on function (i.e., improves sensitivity *and* specificity of manometric investigation) [25]. The measurement of pressure gradients within the esophageal body and across the gastro-esophageal junction (GEJ) provides an objective assessment of the forces that direct bolus transport [28]. The clinical importance of this is illustrated by the finding that the pressure gradient across the GEJ has higher accuracy for the diagnosis of achalasia than conventional measurements of sphincter relaxation (Figure 8.3) [29]. HRM has been shown to increase diagnostic accuracy. In a group of 212 unselected adult patients, Clouse et al. reported manometric disagreement in 12% between HRM and conventional manometry. Compared against "final diagnosis" six months after the investigation, conventional manometry failed to identify several patients with achalasia and other causes of hypotensive and aperistaltic motility disorders, while the topographical method correctly identified all patients with achalasia within the group with aperistalsis. They concluded that the topographical methods are more accurate than traditional techniques in diagnosing the type of severe motor dysfunction and provide additional information important in the clinical practice of esophageal manometry [30].

Published case series supply vivid examples of clinically important pathology detected by HRM that was not provided (or not properly appreciated) by conventional investigation:

1. The loss of coordination (wide "transition zone") between the proximal (striated) and mid-distal (smooth muscle) esophagus.
2. Focal esophageal spasm limited to the mid-esophagus.
3. Detection of an abnormal pressure gradient (i.e., resistance to flow) localizes pathology within the pharynx and UES (e.g., cricopharyngeal bar) [31].

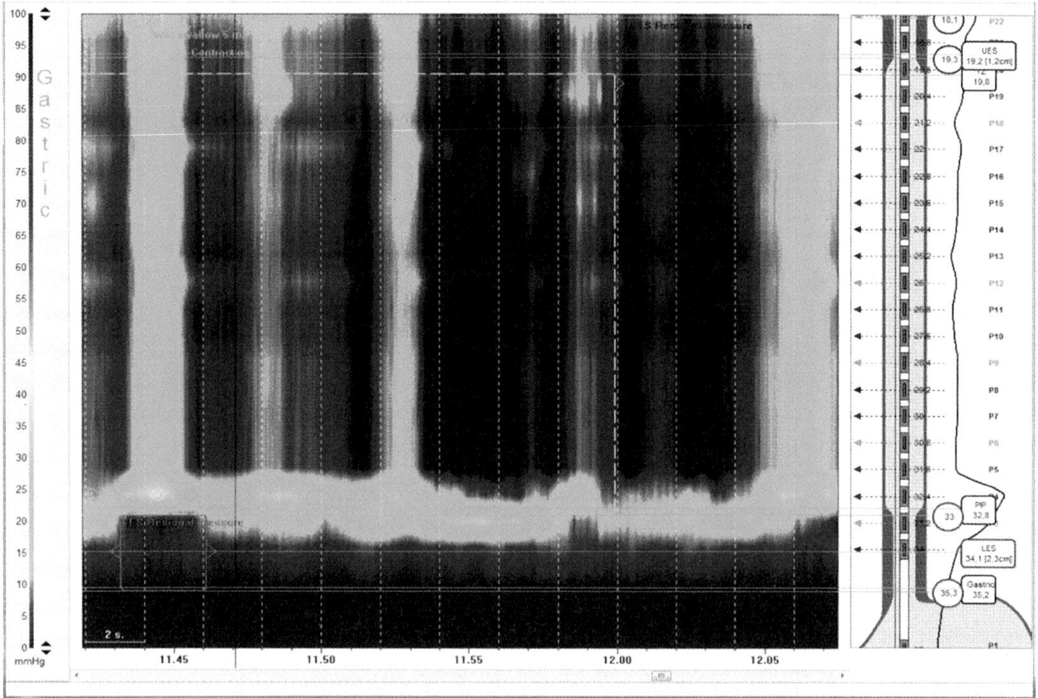

Fig. 8.3 Peristaltic segments are absent in this child with achalasia. The peristaltic chain is replaced by isobaric contour stripes spanning the esophageal body

4. Functional (e.g., achalasia) resistance to bolus transport across the GEJ can be measured and pseudo-relaxation of the LES in vigorous achalasia is clearly seen.
5. Structural resistance to bolus transport caused by peptic stricture, extrinsic compression can be identified on HRM. This ability to differentiate the functional and structural anatomy of the GEJ greatly improves the ability to identify problems post-fundoplication [25].

One important observation made in adults that accentuates the value of HRM is that esophageal peristalsis is comprised a specific chain of sequential pressure segments. These segments, one in the striated-muscle region and two in the smooth-muscle region, appear as concentrated pressure loci separated from each other by lower amplitude pressure troughs on the three-dimensional maps [26, 32–35].

Staiano et al. reported that the same chain of pressure segments identified previously in adults was recognized in every child with the exception of seven with aperistalsis, six of whom were ultimately diagnosed as having achalasia [32]. The first and second pressure troughs were similarly distributed across esophageal length in each age group, but the third trough was located proportionately less closely to the upper margin of the resting LES in the neonates compared with infants/toddlers or children [32]. The first pressure segment was more consistently present in children than in the other two age groups, and the percentage of swallows with the third pressure trough was decreased in neonates compared with children. Consequently, completely formed peristaltic chains were less commonly observed in the neonates, but the number of subjects was too small to confirm that this was a clinically meaningful finding [32]. No differences were found in the presence or distribution of the pressure segments within the esophageal body in subjects who had symptoms ultimately attributed to esophageal disease or who had other explanations for the presenting complaints.

Staiano et al. have recently demonstrated in an HRM study of healthy preterm and term neonates that maturation of the peristaltic chain continues to occur through late gestation and beyond term birth. The same segmental architecture of peristalsis was observed in term and preterm neonates as reported previously in children and adults, and no additional pressure segments or troughs were identified by subjective review of the maps. It was suggested that maturation may continue through the infant/toddler period such that presence of the complete peristaltic chain at rates matching the adult pattern only becomes most evident during childhood years [36].

Although the three contraction segments could be identified in each age subgroup (neonates, infants/toddlers, children), the percentage of complete peristaltic chains appeared reduced in the very small number of neonates studied. The segmental architecture was distinctive for each infant such that identifying peristaltic sequences was simple using high-resolution manometric techniques. The second and third segments overlapped in the distal esophagus as they do in adults [23] such that part of the segment would extend into the neighboring region, yet a set of concentric isobaric contour lines focused on the region (the defining characteristics of a segment) was absent. The first and third segments were present in ≥50% of swallows in very few of the preterm neonates and in a significantly larger proportion of full-term neonates. In contrast, the second segment was well developed in ≥50% of swallows in all preterm and full-term neonates, even in the youngest of studied subjects [36]. These findings indicate that the second segment develops early and is most consistently present, even in preterm neonates. This segment may have particular value in esophageal clearance [37], its early development, thus, being of teleologic importance [36]. In addition, the authors demonstrated that although all the segments can be identified in infants as young as 27 weeks of gestational age at the time of examination, the consistency of their presence continues to increase through the normal gestational period. At full term, only 55% of swallows have a complete segmental chain, indicating that further development occurs in early infancy. These results support a potential role of inadequate esophageal body motor function in the presentation or manifestations of GERD in infants [36].

Recently, Goldani et al. have illustrated the use of HRM in a pediatric age group while using a standardized protocol and analytical method. Despite the inherent limitations of the pediatric population, the authors introduced a new protocol in unsedated children in the context of a clinical setting, moving from research into clinical application. The ability to analyze data using spatiotemporal plots normalized to gastric baseline pressure eliminates a great deal of motion artifacts, which previously required many children to be sedated for the procedure [38]. The additional use of solid swallow has been described in adults to diagnose esophageal spasm in patients with dysphagia who underwent normal conventional manometry [39]. Goldani et al. were the first to describe the usefulness of solid swallows in pediatric patients. Further studies are needed to determine normal patterns of esophageal solid bolus transit in children, given the finding that healthy adults may need more than one swallow to clear solid boluses from the esophagus, and that subjects have poor perception of whether such boluses cleared the esophagus on any given swallow [40].

Goldani et al. introduced the new parameter DCIa, which may be useful for the assessment of hypotensive peristalsis in patients with peristaltic dysfunction. On the basis of all the evidence presented above, we advocate that children should ideally not be sedated for HRM and should adhere to the following protocol: (1) identify LES using standard manometry tracing if necessary; (2) run a baseline recording of LES pressure, allowing for an initial 3 min " settling down " period. Once all relevant structures are identified; (3) administer (a) wet swallows—ten swallows at a minimum of 20 s intervals of 0.5–5.0 ml, aiming for the maximal tolerated volume, 5 ml for those older than 5 years of age, 2 ml for those under 5 years, 0.5–1 ml for infants, and consider wet swallows unsafe in patients with oropharyngeal dysphagia, (b) check MRS offering about 100 ml of liquid by means of a straw or a bottle (increases sensitivity to LES dysfunction, e.g., intrabolus pressure is high in achalasia), (c) consider solid swallows if the patient has symptoms triggered by the consumption of solid food (increases diagnostic sensitivity and clinical significance of manometric findings), preferably test the triggering solid food or at least one slice of toast in subsequent amounts of 2×3 cm in size. This protocol is adapted from what is recommended in adults [15] and is expected to fit into the pediatric age. Conventional analytical methods and the new DCIa variable may be useful to further clarify paradigms regarding the pathophysiology of motility abnormalities and consequently improve the diagnosis of pediatric esophageal motility disorders [40].

Esophageal dysmotility is frequent in children suffering from esophageal atresia (EA) and tracheo-esophageal fistula and frequently is associated with gastroesophageal reflux (GER). The incidence of GER varies from 41% based on symptoms only [17] to 68% measured by pH monitor, 72% by barium swallow, and 65% by scintiscan [41]. The dysmotility may be congenital. Cheng et al. reported a Chinese boy with achalasia, identified by the esophageal conventional manometry, associated with EA [42]. In adults, Dutta et al. reported that the pressure and contractility profile of the esophagus was abnormal in the majority of patients, even in the absence of symptoms [43]. In children, no data exist yet regarding the use of HRM in children treated for EA.

Gastroesophageal reflux, often severe and with respiratory complications, occurs with increased frequency among children with psychomotor retardation. It has been reported that GER occurs in up to 70–75% of children with cerebral palsy [44]; however, the mechanisms underlying its occurrence in neurologically impaired children (NIC) are poorly understood. In neurologically normal adults and children, simultaneous esophageal manometry and pH monitoring have shown that GER is usually due to a transient LES relaxation; whereas other mechanisms, including reduced basal sphincter tone, account for a minority of reflux episodes [45–50]. Pensabene et al. reported that absent LES tone is the most common mechanism of reflux of gastric contents into the esophagus in a subgroup of NIC. Transient LES relaxation, the most common known event associated with acid reflux in healthy premature infants, as well as in older children and in adults, seems to be an uncommon mechanism in NIC with undetectable LES [51], but no data exist regarding the use of HRM in NIC.

Finally, HRM has facilitated in children the routine measurement and analysis of physiological parameters not normally appreciated during a conventional manometric evaluation. Although HRM study protocols and normative data are well established in adults [15, 38, 52], pediatric data are sparse. HRM is simple to use and easy to learn for those with a basic knowledge of conventional manometry. No sleeve sensor is required (an electronic "virtual-sleeve" provides an identical recording if required) and it has several advantages over conventional esophageal manometry [25]. HRM may prove to have clinical advantages in pediatric patients as it has in adults, but further proof of its usefulness in these subjects will be required. Current limitations of HRM in pediatrics relate largely to the pneumohydraulic perfusion of a catheter having multiple microlumina and the need for fastidious maintenance of this system to ensure accurate recordings. Recent development of a 36-sensor solid state catheter having circumferential pressure transducers embedded along its length has eliminated water perfusion, allows sampling of the entire esophagus without catheter repositioning, and has simplified HRM in adults [32].

References

1. Clark JH. Anatomy and physiology of the esophagus. In: Wyllie R, Hyams JS, editors. Pediatric gastrointestinal disease, pathophysiology, diagnosis and management. Philadelphia, PA: WB Saunders; 1993. p. 311–7.
2. Grand RJ, Watkins JB, Torti FM. Development of the human gastrointestinal tract, a review. Gastroenterology. 1976;70:790–810.
3. Grybowski JD. The swallowing mechanism of the neonate: I. Esophageal and gastric motility. Pediatrics. 1965;35:445–52.
4. Grybowski JD, Thayer WR, Spiro HM. Esophageal motility in infants and children. Pediatrics. 1963;31:382–95.
5. Cucchiara S, Borrelli O, Di Nardo G. Esophageal motility. In: Walker WA et al., editors. Walker's pediatric gastrointestinal disease, 5th ed. BC Decker Inc: Hamilton; 2008. p. 47–58.

6. Kahrilas PJ, Dodds WJ, Dent J, et al. Upper esophageal function during belching. Gastroenterology. 1986;91:133–40.
7. Moroz SP, Espinoza J, Cumming WA, Diamant NE. Lower esophageal sphincter function in children with and without gastresophageal reflux. Gastroenterology. 1976;71:236–41.
8. Kahrilas PJ, Clouse RE, Hogan WJ. An American Gastroenterological Association Medical Position statement on the clinical use of esophageal manometry. Gastroenterology. 1994;107:1865–84.
9. Newell SJ, Sarkar PK, Durbin GM, Booth IW, McNeish AS. Maturation of the lower esophageal sphincter in the preterm baby. Gut. 1988;29:167–72.
10. Savarino E, Tutuian R. Combined multichannel intraluminal impedance and manometry testing. Dig Liver Dis. 2008;40:167–73.
11. Gilger MA, Boyle JT, Sondheimer JM, Colletti RB. A Medical Position Statement of the North American Society for Pediatric Gastroenterology and Nutrition: indications for pediatric esophageal manometry. J Pediatr Gastroenterol Nutr. 1997;24:616–8.
12. Fung KP, Math MV, Ho CO, Yap KM. Midazolam as a sedative in esophageal manometry: a study of the effect on esophageal motility. J Pediatr Gastroenterol Nutr. 1992;15:85–8.
13. Vanderhoof JA, Rappaport PJ, Paxson CL. Manometric diagnosis of lower esophageal sphincter incompetence in infants: use of a small, single-lumen perfused catheter. Pediatrics. 1978;62:805–8.
14. Orenstein SR, Giarrusso VS, Proujansky R, Kocoshis SA. The Santmyer swallow: a new useful infant reflex. Lancet. 1988;1:345–6.
15. Fox MR, Bredenoord AJ. Esophageal high-resolution manometry: moving from research into clinical practice. Gut. 2008;57:405–23.
16. Spechler SJ, Castell DO. Classification of esophageal motility abnormalities. Gut. 2001;49:145–51.
17. Pandolfino JE, Kahrilas PJ. AGA technical review on the clinical use of esophageal manometry. Gastroenterology. 2005;128:209–24.
18. Nayar DS, Khandwala F, Achkar E, et al. Esophageal manometry: assessment of interpreter consistency. Clin Gastroenterol Hepatol. 2005;3:218–24.
19. Reidel WL, Clouse RE. Variations in clinical presentation of patients with esophageal contraction abnormalities. Dig Dis Sci. 1985;30:1065–71.
20. Achem SR, Crittenden J, Kolts B, et al. Long-term clinical and manometric follow-up of patients with nonspecific esophageal motor disorders. Am J Gastroenterol. 1992;87:825–30.
21. Swift GL, Alban-Davies H, McKirdy H, et al. A long-term clinical review of patients with esophageal pain. Q J Med. 1991;81:937–44.
22. Clouse RE, Staiano A, Alrakawi A. Development of a topographic analysis system for manometric studies in the gastrointestinal tract. Gastrointest Endosc. 1998;48:395–401.
23. Clouse RE, Prakash C. Topographic esophageal manometry: an emerging clinical and investigative approach. Dig Dis Sci. 2000;18:64–74.
24. Fox M. High resolution manometry—an introduction. Guy's and St Thomas' NHS Foundation Trust: London; 2006, p. 1–10.
25. Fox M, Hebbard G, Janiak P, Brasseur JG, Ghosh S, Thumshirn M, Fried M, Schwizer W. High-resolution manometry predicts the success of esophageal bolus transport and identifies clinically important abnormalities not detected by conventional manometry. Neurogastroenterol Motil. 2004;16:533–42.
26. Ghosh SK, Janiak P, Schwizer W, Hebbard GS, Brasseur JG. Physiology of the esophageal pressure transition zone: separate contraction waves above and below. Am J Physiol Gastrointest Liver Physiol. 2006;290:G568–76.
27. Tutuian R, Castell DO. Combined multichannel intraluminal impedance and manometry clarifies esophageal function abnormalities: study in 350 patients. Am J Gastroenterol. 2004;99:1011–9.
28. Ghosh SK, Pandolfino JE, Zhang Q, Jarosz A, Shah N, Kahrilas PJ. Quantifying Esophageal Peristalsis with High-Resolution Manometry: a study of 75 asymptomatic volunteers. Am J Physiol Gastrointest Liver Physiol. 2006;290:G988–97.
29. Staiano A, Clouse RE. Detection of incomplete lower esophageal sphincter relaxation with conventional point-pressure sensors. Am J Gastroenterol. 2001;96:3258–67.
30. Clouse RE, Staiano A, Alrakawi A, Haroian L. Application of topographical methods to clinical esophageal manometry. Am J Gastroenterol. 2000;95:2720–30.
31. Williams RB, Pal A, Brasseur JG, Cook IJ. Space-time pressure structure of pharyngo-esophageal segment during swallowing. Am J Physiol Gastrointest Liver Physiol. 2001;281:G1290–300.
32. Staiano A, Boccia G, Miele E, Clouse RE. Segmental characteristics of esophageal peristalsis in paediatric patients. Neurogastroenterol Motil. 2008;20:19–26.
33. Clouse RE, Staiano A. Topography of the esophageal peristaltic pressure wave. Am J Physiol. 1991;261:G677–84.
34. Clouse RE, Staiano A. Topography of esophageal motility in patients with normal and high-amplitude esophageal peristalsis. Am J Physiol. 1993;265:G1098–107.
35. Clouse RE, Alrakawi A, Staiano A. Intersubject and interswallow variability in the topography of esophageal motility. Dig Dis Sci. 1998;43:1978–85.
36. Staiano A, Boccia G, Salvia G, Zappulli D, Clouse RE. Development of esophageal peristalsis in preterm and term neonates. Gastroenterology. 2007;132:1718–25.
37. Fox M, Menne D, Stutz B, Fried M, Schwizer W. The effects of tegaserod on esophageal function and bolus transport in healthy volunteers: studies using concurrent high-resolution manometry and videofluoroscopy. Aliment Pharmacol Ther. 2006;24:1017–27.
38. Goldani HA, Staiano A, Borrelli O, Thapar N, Lindley KJ. Pediatric esophageal high-resolution manometry: utility of a standard protocol and size-adjusted pressure topography parameters. Am J Gastroenterol. 2010;105:460–7.

39. Breumelhof R, Timmer R, van Hees PA, Obertop H, Smout AJ. Low-amplitude distal esophageal spasm as a cause of severe dysphagia for solid food. Am J Gastroenterol. 1996;91:143–6.
40. Pouderoux P, Shi G, Tatum RP, Kahrilas PJ. Esophageal solid bolus transit: studies using concurrent videofluoroscopy and manometry. Am J Gastroenterol. 1999;94:1457–63.
41. Jolley SG, Johnson DG, Roberts CC, Herbst JJ, Matlak ME, McCombs A, Christian P. Patterns of gastresophageal reflux in children following repair of esophageal atresia and distal tracheo-esophageal fistula. J Pediatr Surg. 1980;15:857–62.
42. Cheng W, Poon KH, Lui VCH, Yong JL, Law S, So KT, et al. Esophageal atresia and achalasia-like esophageal dysmotility. J Pediatr Surg. 2004;39:1581–3.
43. Dutta HK, Grover VP, Dwivedi SN, Bhatnagar V. Manometric evaluation of postoperative patients of esophageal atresia and tracheo-esophageal fistula. Eur J Pediatr Surg. 2001;11:371–6.
44. Ceriati E, De Peppo F, Ciprandi G, Marchetti P, Silveri M, Rivosecchi M. Surgery in disabled children: general gastroenterological aspects. Acta Paediatr Suppl. 2006;95:34–7.
45. Dent J, Holloway RH, Toouli J, Dodds WJ. Mechanisms of lower esophageal sphincter incompetence in patients with symptomatic gastresophageal reflux. Gut. 1988;29:1020–8.
46. Dent J, Dodds WJ, Friedman RH, Sekiguchi T, Hogan WJ, Arndorfer RC, et al. Mechanism of gastresophageal reflux in recumbent asymptomatic human subjects. J Clin Invest. 1980;65:256–67.
47. Mittal RK, Holloway RH, Penagini R, Blackshaw LA, Dent J. Transient lower esophageal sphincter relaxation. Gastroenterology. 1995;109:601–10.
48. Werlin SL, Dodds WJ, Hogan WJ, Arndorfer RC. Mechanisms of gastresophageal reflux in children. J Pediatr. 1980;97:244–9.
49. Cucchiara S, Bortolotti M, Minella R, Auricchio S. Fasting and postprandial mechanisms of gastresophageal reflux in children with gastresophageal reflux disease. Dig Dis Sci. 1993;38:86–92.
50. Kawahara H, Dent J, Davidson G. Mechanisms responsible for gastresophageal reflux in children. Gastroenterology. 1997;113:399–408.
51. Pensabene L, Miele E, Del Giudice E, Strisciuglio C, Staiano A. Mechanisms of gastresophageal reflux in children with sequelae of birth asphyxia. Brain Dev. 2008;30:563–71.
52. Pandolfino JE, Ghosh SK, Rice J, Clarke JO, Kwiatek MA, Kahrilas PJ. Classifying esophageal motility by pressure topography characteristics: a study of 400 patients and 75 controls. Am J Gastroenterol. 2008;103:27–37.

Antroduodenal Manometry

9

Osvaldo Borrelli, Valentina Giorgio, and Nikhil Thapar

Introduction

Antroduodenal manometry (ADM) is a diagnostic tool that provides both qualitative and quantitative assessment of foregut motor function by recording intraluminal pressure changes within the gastric antrum and proximal small intestine. Specifically, such pressure readings provide a measure of coordination and contractile activity of the foregut. Since first manometric recordings, methodological improvements have steadily occurred, progressing ADM manometry from a purely research technique to an investigation commonly performed in adults and children for definitive clinical purposes. A substantial development has been the ability of the recording equipment to digitize on line manometric recordings so that the latter can be easily analyzed by computer programs. Although the test is still performed in highly specialized motility centers, ADM has provided an improved understanding of the pathophysiology of neuromuscular disorder of the stomach and small intestine.

Normal Motility

In healthy individuals the primary function of the small intestine is the absorption of nutrients, and the motor pattern is programmed to promote this function by assuring a timely propulsion of luminal contents and avoiding stasis or excessively rapid transit of luminal contents. Under physiologic conditions, the motor activity of the antrum and the small intestine is characterized by patterns of organized motor activity in the fasting and postprandial periods [1].

Fasting or interdigestive gastrointestinal motility comprises a sequence of three main components or phases with a combined total average duration of about 100 min (50–180 min), which together constitute the so-called migrating motor complex (MMC) (Fig. 9.1) [2, 3]. Phase III of the MMC, the most distinctive and well-studied pattern of gastrointestinal motor activity, is a

O. Borrelli, M.D., Ph.D. (✉)
Division of Neurogastroenterology & Motility, Department of Paediatric Gastroenterology, ICH University College of London, Great Ormond Street Hospital for Children, London, UK
e-mail: borreo@gosh.nhs.uk

V. Giorgio
Division of Neurogastroenterology & Motility, Department of Paediatric Gastroenterology, Great Ormond Street Hospital for Children, London, UK

N. Thapar, B.Sc.(hon), B.M.(hon), M.R.C.P., M.R.C.P.C.H., Ph.D.
Gastroenterology Unit, University College London, Institute of Child Health, Division of Neurogastroenterology and Motility, London, UK

Department of Paediatric Gastroenterology, Great Ormond Street Hospital for Children, London, UK

C. Faure et al. (eds.), *Pediatric Neurogastroenterology: Gastrointestinal Motility and Functional Disorders in Children*, Clinical Gastroenterology,
DOI 10.1007/978-1-60761-709-9_9,

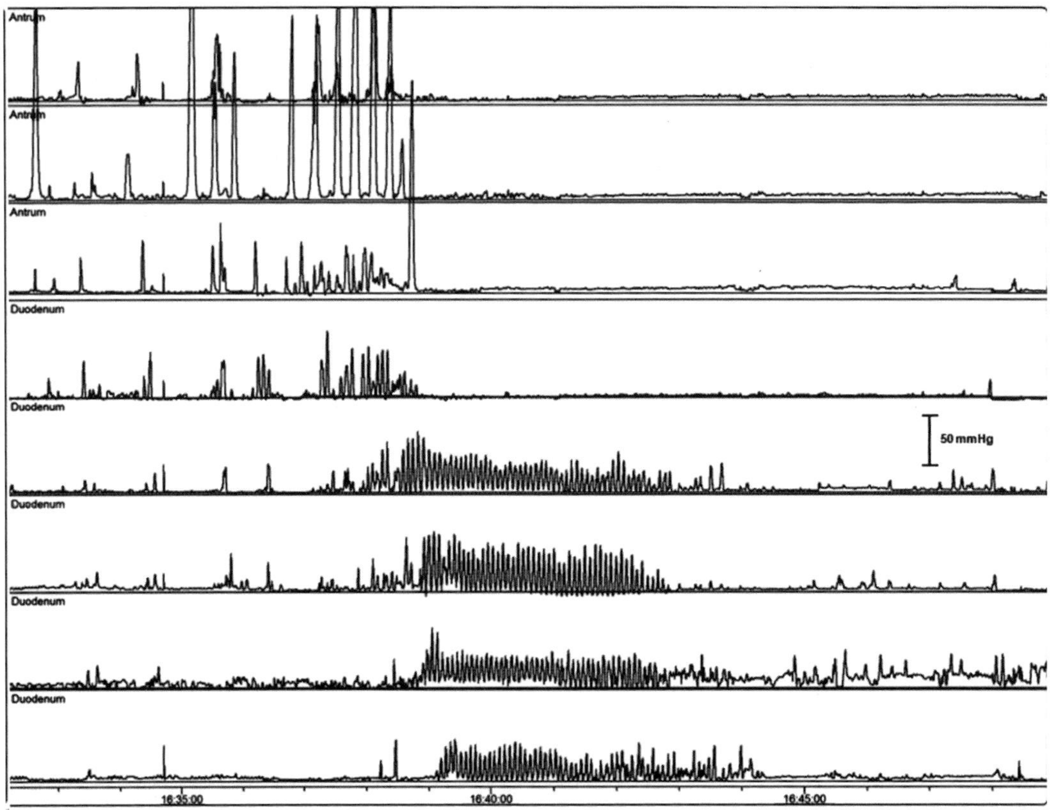

Fig. 9.1 Normal Migrating Motor Complex recorded in a child with recurrent vomiting. All three phases (Phase I, Phase II and Phase III) are well represented. The phase III is seen starting in the antrum and migrating aborally along the duodenum. A period of quiescence (phase I) follows phase III; the latter is preceded by intermittent phasic activity (phase II)

characteristic burst of high amplitude rhythmic contractions of at least 2 min duration occurring at the maximum frequency allowed by the underlying myoelectrical rhythm for a given segment of the gastrointestinal tract [4]. For instance in the antrum the contractions occur at a rate of 2–3 per minute, whereas in the proximal small bowel this increases to 10–14 per minute. In children, phase III, may begin anywhere from the stomach to the ileum, but in about 70% it starts in the gastric antrum, 18% in the proximal duodenum, 10% in the distal duodenum, and 1% in the proximal jejunum [2, 3]. Migration is a basic requisite of phase III activity, which usually propagates aborally over various lengths of the small intestine; however, only 50% of these propagate beyond the middle jejunum, and only 10% reach the distal ileum [5]. The duration of phase III progressively increases in the aboral direction ranging between 2 and 5 min in the duodenum and 10–20 min the distal ileum [2, 6–8]. Conversely, the propagation velocity of phase III decreases from 5 to 10 cm/min in the proximal small bowel to about 0.5–1 cm/min in the distal ileum [1, 2, 7]. The average amplitude of single contractions is at least 40 mmHg in the antrum and 20 mmHg in the small intestine. Finally, the mean interval between episodes of phase III varies with age. It ranges between 25 and 45 min in newborn, approximately 60 min in children less than 2 years, and 85–110 min in adolescent and adults [3, 8–12]. Significant variation occurs between subjects and within the same individuals [2, 13, 14]. Phase III activity is usually succeeded by quiescence or phase I, which is defined as less than three pressure waves every 10 min [15]. Phase I is followed by a period (Phase II) of irregular contractions (more than three pressure waves every 10 min), which represent in the small intestine about 70–80% of the whole cycle. Phases I and III of the MMC require an intact enteric nervous system (ENS) with modulation by the central nervous system and gastrointestinal regulatory peptides [5, 16, 17]. For instance, endogenous motilin blood concentration peaks during late phase II and phase III of the MMC cycle [18, 19]. However, motilin is not required for initiation or aboral migration of Phase III in the small bowel, but seems to be involved in the antral participation of phase III [20, 21]. Conversely, Phase II activity seems to rely more on extrinsic modulation of CNS, given it is suppressed during sleep and abolished after vagotomy [5, 16]. The importance of MMC is highlighted by the fact that its absence is associated with bacterial overgrowth [1]. Indeed, the pulsatile flow ahead of phase III is of clinical importance for clearing secretion, debris and microbes during the interdigestive period, and colonization of the foregut with gram-negative bacteria is observed when phase III is impaired or absent [22]. For this reason phase III has been termed the "gastrointestinal housekeeper." MMC cycles do not occur in the intestine of premature infants age less than 34 weeks, which instead show a pattern of clustered phasic contractions lasting between 1 and 20 min and occurring every 4–35 min. As post-conceptional age increases, this activity becomes longer and the frequency of occurrences decreases. By term, well-defined cyclical fasting motor activity is present with distinct phase I, II and III activity, with the latter showing less variability in term of length and intervals [11, 23].

Following the ingestion of food, the MMC cycle is interrupted and replaced by a pattern of regular antral contractions associated with apparently uncoordinated contractions of variable amplitude in the small intestine, termed "postprandial" or "fed" pattern (Fig. 9.2) [5, 16, 24]. These phasic contractions also show variable frequency and propagation. Typical postprandial contractions usually propagate over a shorter distance than those of phase III, and almost 80% of them propagate less than 2 cm [24]. These minute movement of postprandial contractions are devoted to mixing and grinding of the nutrient chyme, stirring, spreading, and exposing the intestinal contents to a larger surface, and thus promoting its optimal absorption. Moreover, minute aboral transport is also sufficient in preventing bacterial colonization. Thus, normal postprandial motor activity is a compromise between optimal absorption and adequate clearance. The postprandial period lasts from the time of the evident increase in frequency and/or amplitude of contractions occurring after the introduction of a meal to the onset of the following phase III, and is affected by the amount of calories as well as by the composition of the meal [25]. For instance, fats induce a more prolonged fed pattern than protein and carbohydrates. Extrinsic neural control is a prerequisite for a normal postprandial pattern, since persisting MMC activity after meal intake has been reported after vagal cooling [26, 27]. Neural reflexes, endocrine and paracrine mechanisms also play also a key role [17]. In small infants less 32 week's post-conceptional age, who usually receive only small volumes of enteral feeding, the fasting pattern is not disrupted by either the bolus or continuous feeding. Between 31 and 35 week's post-conceptional age, the larger volumes of enteral feeding induce a degree of postprandial activity, but it is only over 35 week's post-conceptional age that a disruption of cyclical activity can be seen with feeds [10].

The presence of other distinct motility patterns has been identified in both healthy individual and patients. *Discrete clustered contractions (DCCs)* or *cluster of contractions (CCs)* are defined as the presence of 3–10 pressure waves of slow frequency, each having a significantly higher amplitude and duration compared to isolated individual contractions [15, 28]. They propagate aborally for less than 30 cm at rate of 1–2 cm/s and usually show a rhythmic pattern with regular intervals of quiescence lasting at least 30 s (Fig. 9.3) [3]. DCC are usually recorded

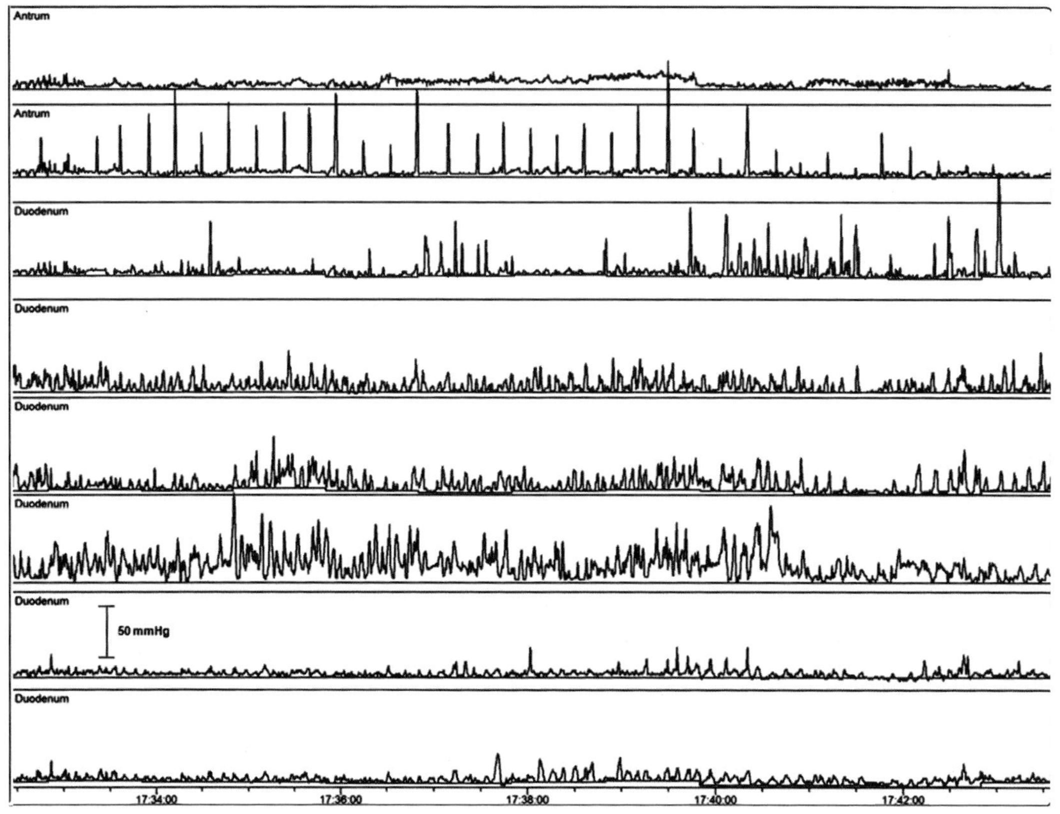

Fig. 9.2 Normal postprandial activity characterized by irregular but persistent phasic activity. Note the normal antral activity during the fed state

during phase II, although are occasionally also seen during the postprandial period (phase III-like activity) [3, 14, 28, 29]. Postprandially, clusters of contractions seem to occur in association with mechanical obstruction or intestinal pseudo-obstruction, and they are characteristically non-propagated [30]. *Bursts of contractions* are defined as sequences of intense irregular pressure waves, which do not correspond to the definition for phase III or for DCC (Fig. 9.4). They can be clearly distinguished from background pressure wave activity during both phase II and the postprandial period. Short bursts of propagating contractions have been described in healthy individuals, whereas sustained bursts of contractions confined to one limited segment (non-propagated) lasting for a period of >30 min and associated with tonic intermittent baseline pressure elevation are considered an abnormal neuropathic pattern [21, 31, 32]. *Giant migrating contractions* or *prolonged intestinal contractions* are pressure waves of prolonged duration (>20 s) and large amplitude more than 30 mmHg. In healthy individuals they occur primarily in the distal ileum and propagate uninterruptedly and rapidly with highly propulsive force over long distance in aboral direction in the small intestine and colon [33, 34]. "*r*" *waves* are simultaneous increases in pressure throughout all the recording sensors, usually associated with regurgitation or frank emesis, and represent the manometry correlate of the abdominal wall contraction in patients with rumination syndrome.

Technical Aspects

Manometry is by nature a highly technical evaluation. When knowledgeably used, manometric examination provides an accurate description of

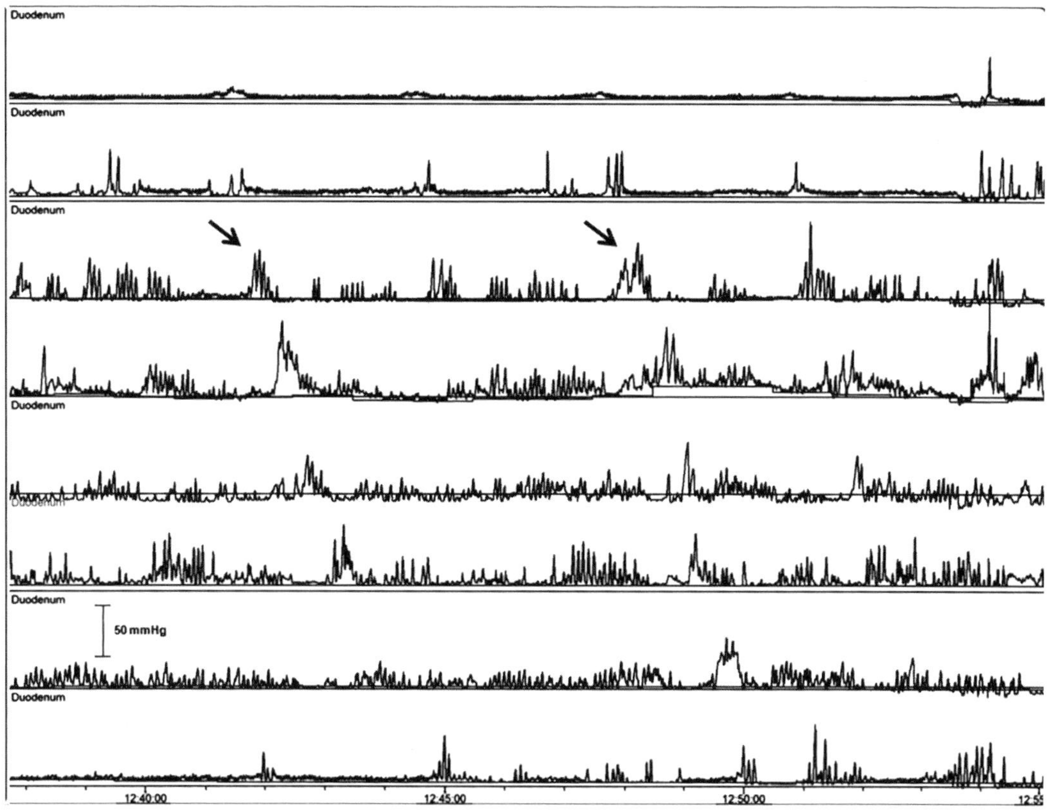

Fig. 9.3 Discrete cluster of contractions (DCCs) (*arrows*) recorded in the duodenum and jejunum during the postprandial period in a normal child. DCCs are defined as the presence of 3–10 pressure waves of slow frequency, which can propagate aborally for less than 30 cm

intestinal neuromuscular function but only if physical principles and equipment characteristics are respected. In general, manometric data are reliable only if the methodology used to acquire them is accurate.

A manometric apparatus set-up consists of a pressure sensor and transducer combination that detects the gastric and small intestine pressure complex and transduces it into an electrical signal, and a recording device to amplify, record and store that electrical signal. The pressure sensor/transducer components of a manometric assembly function as a matched pair and are available in two general designs: either water perfused catheters connected to a pneumohydraulic perfusion pump and to volume displacement transducers, or strain gauge transducers with solid state circuitry [35].

Low Compliance Perfused Manometric System

The water infusion system includes a catheter composed of small capillary tubes, a low compliance hydraulic capillary infusion pump and external transducers. In adults, the small capillary tubes usually have an internal diameter of approximately 0.4–0.8 mm and an opening or port at a known point along the length of the catheter. In adults, the most commonly used catheters have an overall diameter of 4.5 mm [35]. In children in order to reduce the diameter of the catheter smaller capillary tubes (with internal diameters of 0.35 mm) are utilized; moreover the study is performed at lower infusion rates [36]. The manometric probes are usually tailored to the child's size, and the distance between the recording ports should be decided

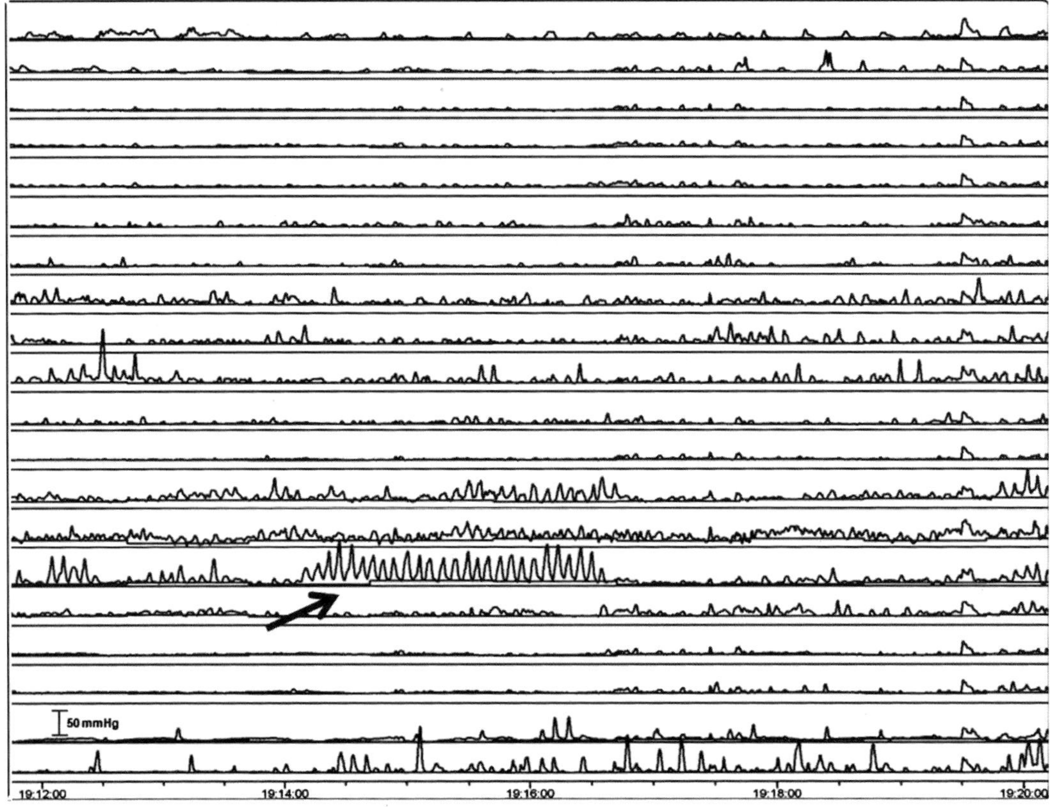

Fig. 9.4 Short burst of contractions (*arrow*) recorded in the proximal jejunum during phase II lasting more than 2 min. These can be clearly distinguished from background pressure wave activity during phase II. The recording was performed with a 20-channel manometric catheter (side holes 2.5 cm apart)

based on the purpose of the investigation [35]. Since one antral recording site is insufficient to provide an accurate recording of antral motor activity due to its continuous forward and backward movement, the manometric catheter should have at least five recording ports with the two most proximal side holes spaced 0.5–1.5 cm apart positioned 1 cm proximal to the pylorus to provide measurements of antral activity, while the remaining side holes positioned in the small intestine and spaced 2.5–5 cm apart in infants and toddlers and 5–10 cm apart in children and adolescents [35, 36]. Each capillary tube is connected to an external transducer. The infusion pump, a simple and essential device for stationary manometry, perfuses the capillary tubes providing a constant flow rate without increasing the compliance of the manometric system. When a catheter port is occluded (e.g., by a muscular contraction), there is a pressure rise in the water filled tubes that is transmitted to the external transducers. High-fidelity recordings of intraluminal pressure are achieved by infusion rates from 0.1 to 0.4 mL/min, even if they may provide an unacceptable amount of water to small babies or premature infants. In order to overcome this problem perfusion rates as low as 0.02 mL/min have been successfully used [37]. Furthermore, for prolonged studies the use of a balanced saline solution should be considered.

A device activating the pressure transducers, storing their signals, and displaying the latter in such a way to allow immediate interpretation and analysis is needed. The personal computer has become the heart of any manometry system. It interfaces with purposed-designed electronic modules that activate and receive signals from pressure transducers, whereas commercially available software programs are essential for acquiring, displaying and storing pressure recording data. Actually, the technical adequacy of different commercially available device recording systems is quite comparable. Probably the dominant consideration that should determine the choice of a system is the level of technical assistance and the training available locally to support the user.

The required characteristics of the manometric recording apparatus are defined by the magnitude of the pressure to be recorded and the frequency content and waveform of foregut contractile waves. It has been shown that the frequency response of manometric systems required to reproduce foregut pressure waves with 98% accuracy is of 0–4 Hz (maximal recordable d*P*/d*t*: 300 mmHg/s). Most of commercially available manometric systems can provide a pressure rise rate of 300–400 mmHg/s, which is adequate for faithful recordings in the gastric antrum and small intestine.

Solid-State Manometric System

The main alternative to the water-perfused manometric system is a manometric assembly incorporating strain gauge sensors and solid state electronic elements [38]. In this system, the manometric probe contains miniature strain gauge pressure transducers built into the catheter at a fixed location along its length, so that pressure changes directly influence the transducers to generate electrical output signals. The probe can be plugged into a small box containing the electronics, which is then connected to the recording device and to a personal computer. In the ambulatory system the recording devices are blind and need to be connected to a personal computer with the appropriate software to display and analyze the recording. The main advantage of using solid-state catheters is that the pressures are recorded directly from the area and are unrelated to the relative position of the subject; therefore manometric studies may also be performed with the subjects in the upright position. This, and the fact that it does not require water perfusion, makes solid-state catheters suitable for long-term ambulatory monitoring of the intraluminal pressure [39]. It has been calculated that for a given number of pressure recording points on a recording assembly, solid-state catheters are 20 times more expensive than a perfused manometric assembly. In the last years the improvement in miniaturizing transducers has allowed the production of solid-state catheter with up to 36 recording channels with an external diameter comparable to that of the water perfused manometric catheter used in small infants and children. However, there is still a very little experience in pediatric patients.

High Resolution Manometry

Manometric techniques have improved in a stepwise fashion from few pressure recording channels to the development of high-resolution manometry (HRM), which is a relatively recent technique that enables more detailed definition, both in term of space and time, of pressure profiles along segments of the gut [40]. This has been achieved by a combination of new manometric assemblies allowing intraluminal pressure to be recorded from up to 72 pressure sensors spaced less than 2 cm. At the same time, advances in computer processing allow pressure data to be presented in real time as a compact, visually intuitive "spatiotemporal plot" of gastric and small intestine pressure activity. HRM recordings may reveal the complex functional anatomy of the foregut, and recent studies suggest that spatiotemporal plots may provide objective measurements of the intraluminal pressure profile in the small intestine, and improve the sensitivity and specificity of manometric recording by removing much of the ambiguity usually encountered using line plot analysis [41]. However, further efforts to define the role of HRM in the diagnosis and management of neuromuscular disorders are needed.

Methodological Aspects

Preparation of the Patient

Before starting the ADM manometric recording it is important to assess patient information with regard to medical history, symptoms, medication, and allergies. Any drug with a known effect on gastrointestinal motility should be discontinued at least 72 h before the study.

It is important to emphasize that ADM manometry in children is performed in a different fashion to that in adults due to differences in size, cooperation, and neurological and developmental maturation. Performing manometric studies in children require great patience from the operator. The parents should be present during the testing in order to settle the child, and to provide the child with a model of cooperative behavior with the physician. The cooperation can also be improved by the use of age-appropriate relaxation techniques. For example, infants may relax with swaddling and the use of a pacifier. Having a favorite toy can comfort toddlers. School age and older children benefit when equipment is shown and explained prior to the procedure. ADM manometry is best performed without sedation [36]. However, in many children sedation is necessary, and midazolam has been shown to be effective with no or minimal influence on pressure measurement [42]. It is advisable to wait for complete child recovery from any drug effect before starting the motility tests. Finally, before starting the procedure it is important to obtain and verify signed informed consent and necessary to check that the fasting period has been of adequate duration. In healthy children an overnight fast is enough, whereas in infants at least 4 h are necessary to avoid nausea, vomiting and aspiration. In children on parenteral nutrition, the latter should be stopped 12 h before the studies, due to the effect of nutrients on hormones, which may affect the intestinal motility [17]. Similarly, blood glucose levels should be carefully assessed, since hyperglycemia inhibits gastric emptying and reduce the occurrence of phase III [43, 44].

Study Procedure

The manometric catheter can be placed either nasally or orally, but there is broad consensus that studies are better tolerated when the catheter is introduced through the nose. The catheter can also be placed through an existing gastrostomy, or jejunostomy. The manometric probe should be positioned deep enough in the small intestine in order to avoid its falling back into the stomach as a consequence of postprandial gastric distension or duodenal contraction. The tube placement can be performed either fluoroscopically or endoscopically [45]. Under fluoroscopy the probe placement usually requires high skill to pass the pyloric region, which may be easier with a firm probe rather than a soft, flexible one. The former, however, is more difficult to advance beyond the duodenal bulb due to its acute angle. Moreover, hard probe may cause great discomfort during the recording time especially for young children. The addition of a weighted probe tip may facilitate the placement as it utilizes gravity in addition. The probe can be also advanced through the pylorus using an endoscope and biopsy forceps, taking care to use as little air as possible to insufflate the bowel, given over-inflation may affect gastrointestinal motility and provoke a backward movement of the manometric probe. In some center the manometric recording is performed the day after the tube placement and following check radiology to ascertain catheter position with correction if necessary.

During the manometric recording using a water-perfused system, the patients usually maintain the same position (supine), whereas using portable solid state equipment the patients are encouraged to perform daily activities when possible [35]. Ambulatory manometry is usually performed for 24 h, whereas for stationary manometry, recording must be carried out until a phase III and/or clear-cut abnormalities are recorded. However, it is generally advisable to perform a fasting recording for at least 4–6 h (one or two MMCs), and postpradial recording for at least 90 min [36]. The type and the size of meal should be adjusted according to patient's age and preference. In older children the test meal should be at least 400 kcal, in order to ensure an adequate postprandial response in the small intestine lasting at least 90–120 min [25, 36]. In younger children the test meal should provide at least 10 kcal/kg. The meal should be balanced with at least 30% of calories as fat calories. However, in

Table 9.1 Manometric features associated with gastrointestinal motility disorders

Interdigestive or fasting period
• Absence of phase III
• Short intervals between phase III
• Abnormal phase III – Stationary – Retrograde
• Non migrating burst of contraction
• Sustained simultaneous cluster of contractions
• Low amplitude contraction
Postprandial or fed period
• Failure to switch to postprandial period
• Postprandial hypomotility – Low frequency of contraction – Low amplitude of contraction
• Non migrating cluster of contraction

some cases is impossible to give predetermined volume to a patient, e.g., one with severe gastrointestinal dysmotility and inability to tolerate oral or enteral feeding. Finally, if no phase III is recorded during fasting, a drug stimulation test should be performed using erythromycin (1 mg/kg over a period of 30 min), which is able to induce a gastric phase III and allows assessment of its migration in the small intestine [46, 47].

Analysis of Manometric Recording

Both qualitative and quantitative analysis of the ADM tracings should be performed. Qualitative analysis includes the recognition of specific motor patterns as well as the overall characteristics of the fasting period (typical cycling pattern of the MMC, characteristics of phase III activity including the numbers found, migration pattern, mean amplitude, mean peak velocity, and intervals) and fed period (presence of change in motility after test meal). Quantitative analysis includes the calculation of distal antral and duodenal motility indexes (MI), expressing the contractile activity as the natural logarithm of the area under the manometric pressure peaks above a threshold pressure. Computerized data evaluation, including wave identification algorithms, artifact removal and algorithms for detection of propagated activity offer an improved degree of objectivity in the analysis of pressure tracing and can facilitate the quantitative analysis of relevant parameters [48].

A normal motility pattern is defined as the presence of at least one MMC per 24 h of recording (it has been shown that almost 95% of normal children have phase III within 4 h fasting study), conversion to the fed pattern without return of MMC for at least 2 h after a 400-kcal meal, distal postprandial contractility (MI per 2 h >13.67), small intestinal contraction >20 mmHg, and absence of abnormal findings described in Table 9.1 [49]. Therefore, the presence and characteristics of the MMC and its response to nutrients is used as a marker of enteric neuromuscular function.

Based on the findings of abnormal manometric features different clinic-pathophysiological categories of abnormalities can be recognized [35, 49]. In patients with *enteric neuropathy* the motor activity is typically disorganized and/or uncoordinated. The most compelling finding is represented by the absence of a MMC during a sufficient recording time (ideally 24 h); however, this scenario is a rare event in patient with enteric neuropathy. More common findings include the presence of retrograde or uncoordinated phase III activity (Fig. 9.5), increased frequency of phase III (in adults and older children>1 MMC cycle per hour) (Fig. 9.6), presence of non-propagated bursts and sustained uncoordinated phasic activity, antral hypomotility, inability to establish a fed pattern after a test meal, and presence of phase III-like activity in the fed period. In patients with *enteric myopathy* the normal manometric patterns are usually preserved, but the amplitude of contractions in both preprandial and postprandial periods do not exceed 20 mmHg (Fig. 9.7); however, low amplitude contractions may also represent a consequence of gut dilatation proximal to an obstructive segment. For this reason, the absence of dilated loops is a prerequisite for a diagnosis of enteric myopathy. In patients with *mechanical obstruction* multiple simultaneous giant contractions as well as the presence of simultaneous DCCs in the postprandial period are frequently reported.

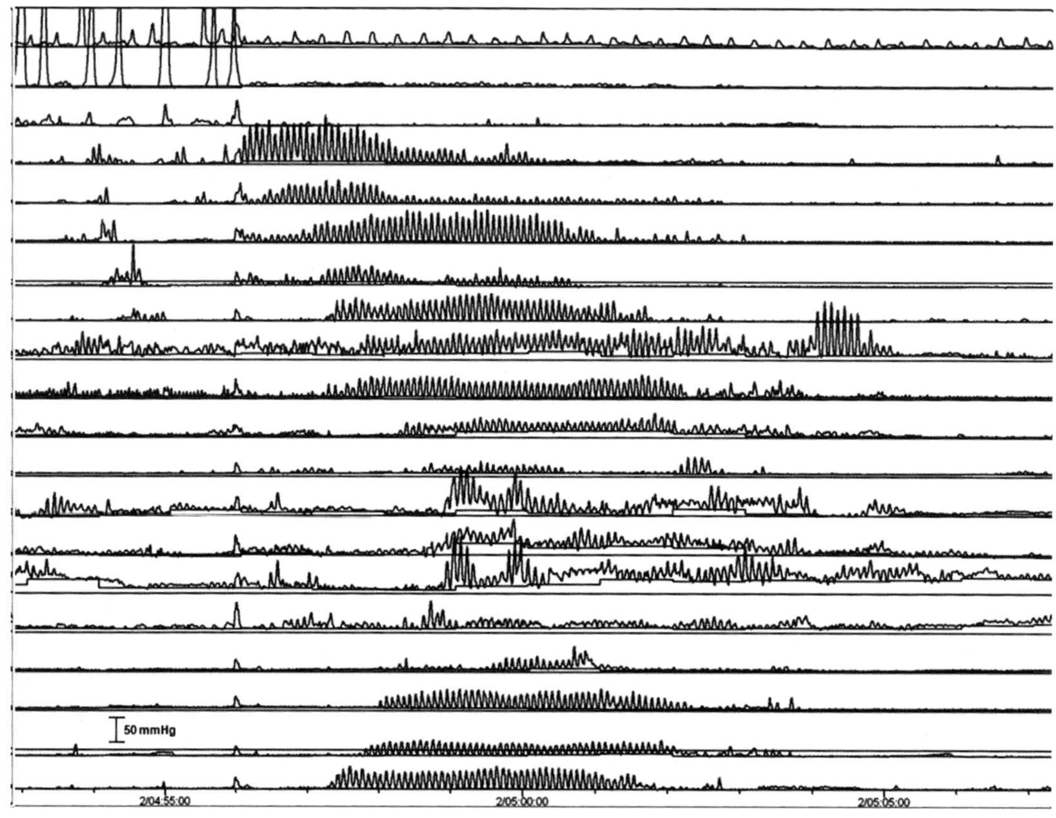

Fig. 9.5 Abnormal propagation of phase III in a child with chronic intestinal pseudo-obstruction. Note the presence of retrograde contractions in the proximal jejunum meeting, in the distal duodenum, the activity front migrating from the antrum (*arrow image*). The recording was performed with a 20-channel manometric catheter (side holes 2.5 cm apart). The first two channels are localized in the antrum

In neonates the presence of high amplitude retropropagated contractions should raise the suspicion of mechanical obstruction. In children with *CNS abnormalities* it has been show an abnormal frequency and propagation of phase III, increase proportion of non-propagated DCCs, antral hypomotility, abnormal proportion between periods of phase I and II activity, and altered postprandial pattern duration with the presence of phase III-like activity [50]. Finally, in adult patients with *postvagotomy syndrome* the most common manometric findings are an increased frequency of MMC, the absence of antral phase III and the presence of antral hypomotility after test meal, and an altered postprandial pattern duration with a rapid return of MMC activity.

Reference Values

Before interpreting the recorded data and deciding whether abnormalities of gastric and small intestine motor activity are present, it should be of pivotal importance to define the limits of normality. Unfortunately, the lack of normal controls is an important limiting factor for the establishment of normal motility patterns, making the interpretation of manometric recording data difficult and subjective and occasionally leading to over-interpretation. However, some control data have been published. Although, each center performing ADM manometry should have an own set of normal values, it is suggested that "normal" ranges proposed by one group could be used by another

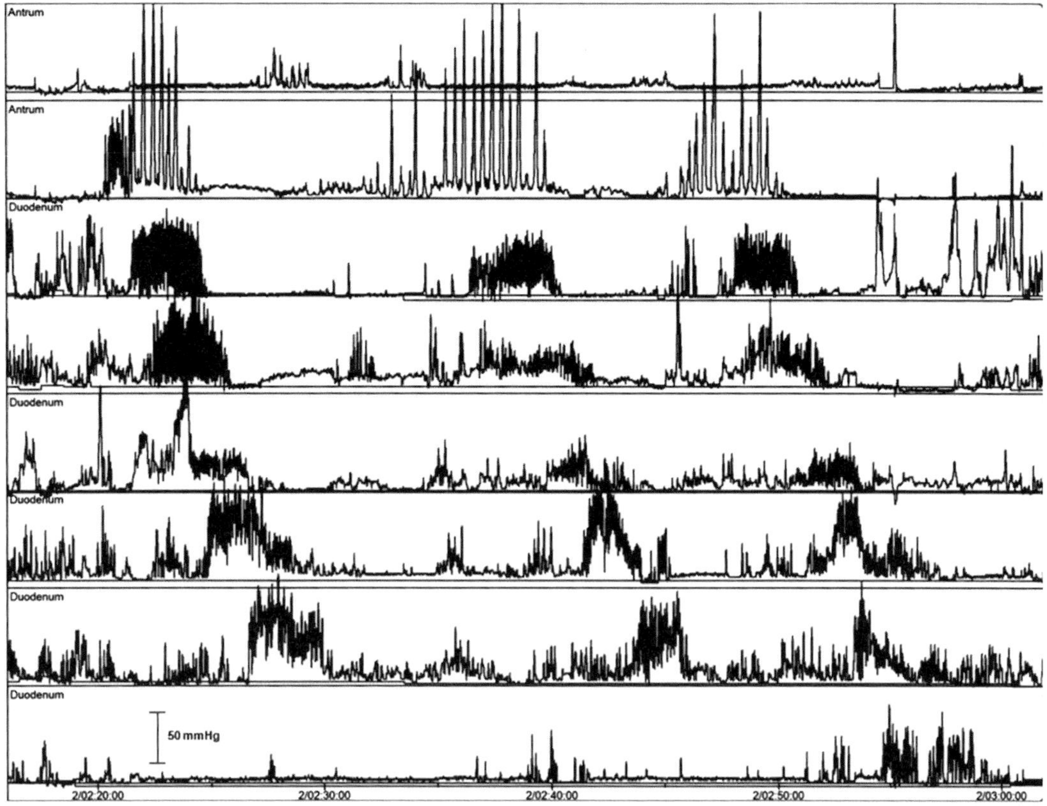

Fig. 9.6 Short intervals of phase III activity in a child with chronic intestinal pseudo-obstruction. The phase IIIs were separated by intervals of only 10–20 min. Note also the tonic component within phases III, which are defined as an elevation of the baseline more than 10 mmHg for longer than 1 min

if the investigation is performed and interpreted in the same way.

Indications

Although ADM manometry is well tolerated by patients with otherwise undiagnosed gut motility disorders unresponsive to conventional therapies and whose quality of life is substantially impaired (by symptom severity and the diagnostic uncertainty), it is a rather cumbersome procedure to perform, not always easy to interpret, and practically useful in the clinical management of only a minority of patients. For instance, it has been shown in children that there is an excellent interobserver agreement for the number of fasting phase III and their measurement, while the interobserver agreement for the detection of other motor abnormalities, such as sustained phasic contraction and postprandial simultaneous clusters, is significantly low [51]. Therefore, given small bowel manometry requires expertise and dedicated equipment and personnel, it should be restricted to a limited number of referral centers with a specific interest in the field.

ADM manometry serves to clarify a clinical diagnosis of abnormal motility or exclude a GI motility disorders. There are only few indications for the test (Table 9.2). Manometry is indicated in children with suspected chronic intestinal pseudo-obstruction in order to verify the diagnosis, clarify the pathogenesis and optimize clinical management [52]. For instance, the presence of a myopathic pattern is an indicator of a poor response to enteral feeding, whereas the presence of MMC predicts clinical response to prokinetics therapy and success of enteral feeding [53, 54].

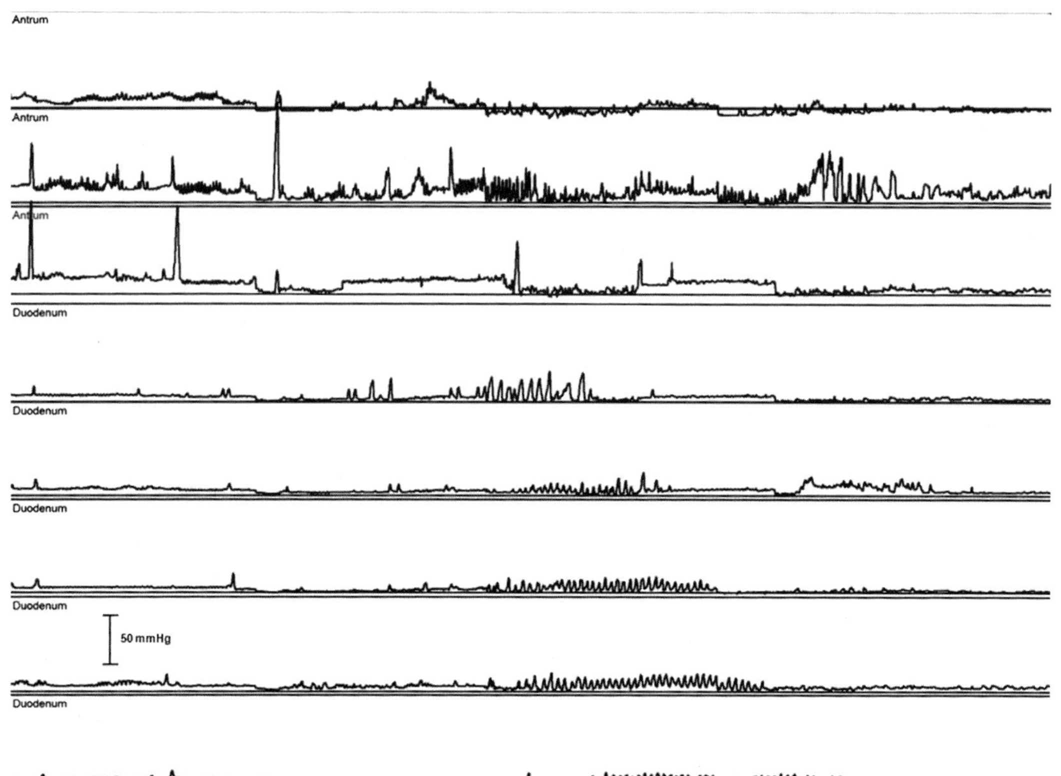

Fig. 9.7 Manometric tracing in a child with enteric myopathy. Note the low amplitude but normal propagation of the phase III and the paucity of other contractile activity in the small intestine

Table 9.2 Clinical indication for antroduodenal manometry

1. Clarify the diagnosis in patients with unexplained nausea, vomiting or symptoms suggestive of upper GI dysmotility
2. Differentiate between neuropathic vs. myopathic gastric or small bowel dysfunction in pts with chronic intestinal pseudo-obstruction.
3. Identify generalized dysmotility in patients with colonic dysmotility (e.g., chronic constipation), particularly prior to subtotal colectomy
4. Confirm diagnosis in suspected chronic intestinal pseudo-obstruction syndromes when the diagnosis is unclear on clinical or radiological grounds
5. Assess for possible mechanical obstruction when clinical features suggest, but radiological studies do not reveal, obstruction
6. Determine which organs need to be transplanted (isolated vs. multi-visceral transplantation) in patients with chronic intestinal pseudo-obstruction being considered for intestinal transplantation
7. Confirm a diagnosis of rumination syndrome

Manometric assessment may allow determination of the extent of disease (localized or diffuse) and the optimal route for nutritional support (gastric, enteric, or parenteral). ADM may be useful in determining the suitability of intestinal transplantation for children with chronic intestinal pseudo-obstruction [54]. Severe gastric or duodenal motor abnormalities seem to compromise the postoperative course of the intestinal graft recipient. In patients with intractable constipation, ADM manometry should be performed if surgery is being considered; given patients with small bowel dysmotility have generally a poor outcome after the surgery. ADM is also indicated in patients with recurrent subocclusive episodes, in order to differentiate a pseudo-obstructive syndrome from a mechanical obstruction, which is sometimes overlooked also by an experienced radiologist [55]. Manometry is indicated in the investigation of children with severe unexplained gastrointestinal symptoms, such as vomiting, nausea, abdominal distension and abdominal pain who fail to respond to any therapy, and in this context the test helps to differentiate between vomiting and rumination [56, 57]. This is covered elsewhere in the book. Finally, an entirely normal study in children suspected clinically of having a severe dysmotility syndrome may help to redirect the diagnostic effort, and may result in the consideration of other diagnoses such as fabricated induced illness (formerly Munchausen's by proxy syndrome) [58, 59].

Conclusion

ADM provides relevant physiological information on the neuromuscular activity of the foregut and is useful in diagnosing and guiding the management of enteric neuromuscular disorders. Because of the complexity in performing and analyzing ADM, it requires considerable experience and skills that may only be available in referral centers with a specific interest in the field of GI motility. The development of recording equipment and advanced computer analysis that are in progress appear to have the potential to substantially improve our understanding of normal and abnormal foregut neuromuscular function.

References

1. Vantrappen G, Janssens J, Hellemans J, Ghoos Y. The interdigestive motor complex of normal subjects and patients with bacterial overgrowth of the small intestine. J Clin Invest. 1977;59:1158–66.
2. Dooley CP, Di Lorenzo C, Valenzuela JE. Variability of migrating motor complex in humans. Dig Dis Sci. 1992;37:723–8.
3. Kellow JE, Borody TJ, Phillips SF, Tucker RL, Haddad AC. Human interdigestive motility: variations in patterns from esophagus to colon. Gastroenterology. 1986;91:386–95.
4. Kellow JE, Delvaux M, Azpiroz F, Camilleri M, Quigley EM, Thompson DG. Principles of applied neurogastroenterology: physiology/motility-sensation. Gut. 1999;45 Suppl 2:17–24.
5. Quigley EM. Gastric and small intestinal motility in health and disease. Gastroenterol Clin North Am. 1996;25:113–45.
6. Tomomasa T, Kuroume T, Arai H, Wakabayashi K, Itoh Z. Erythromycin induces migrating motor complex in human gastrointestinal tract. Dig Dis Sci. 1986;31:157–61.
7. Lindberg G, Iwarzon M, Stål P, Seensalu R. Digital ambulatory monitoring of small-bowel motility. Scand J Gastroenterol. 1990;25:216–24.
8. Cucchiara S, Bortolotti M, Colombo C, et al. Abnormalities of gastrointestinal motility in children with nonulcer dyspepsia and in children with gastroesophageal reflux disease. Dig Dis Sci. 1991;36:1066–73.
9. Tomomasa T, Itoh Z, Koizumi T, Kuroume T. Nonmigrating rhythmic activity in the stomach and duodenum of neonates. Biol Neonate. 1985;48:1–9.
10. Berseth CL, Ittmann PI. Antral and duodenal motor responses to duodenal feeding in preterm and term infants. J Pediatr Gastroenterol Nutr. 1992;14:182–6.
11. Ittmann PI, Amarnath R, Berseth CL. Maturation of antroduodenal motor activity in preterm and term infants. Dig Dis Sci. 1992;37:14–9.
12. Piñeiro-Carrero VM, Andres JM, Davis RH, Mathias JR. Abnormal gastroduodenal motility in children and adolescents with recurrent functional abdominal pain. J Pediatr. 1988;113:820–5.
13. Husebye E, Skar V, Aalen OO, Osnes M. Digital ambulatory manometry of the small intestine in healthy adults. Estimates of variation within and between individuals and statistical management of incomplete MMC periods. Dig Dis Sci. 1990;35:1057–65.
14. Husebye E, Engedal K. The patterns of motility are maintained in the human small intestine throughout the process of aging. Scand J Gastroenterol. 1992;27:397–404.
15. Husebye E. The patterns of small bowel motility: physiology and implications in organic disease and functional disorders. Neurogastroenterol Motil. 1999;11:141–61.
16. Sarna SK, Otterson MF. Small intestinal physiology and pathophysiology. Gastroenterol Clin North Am. 1989;18:375–404.
17. Fox-threlkeld FET. Motility and regulatory peptides. In: Kumar D, Windgate D, editors. An illustrated guide to gastrointestinal motility. 2nd ed. Edinburgh: Churchill Livingstone; 1993. p. 78–94.
18. Vantrappen G, Janssens J, Peeters TL, Bloom SR, Christofides ND, Hellemans J. Motilin and the interdigestive migrating motor complex in man. Dig Dis Sci. 1979;24:497–500.
19. Chung SA, Rotstein O, Greenberg GR, Diamant NE. Mechanisms coordinating gastric and small intestinal MMC: role of extrinsic innervation rather than motilin. Am J Physiol. 1994;267:G800–9.

20. Janssens J, Vantrappen G, Peeters TL. The activity front of the migrating motor complex of the human stomach but not of the small intestine is motilin-dependent. Regul Pept. 1983;6:363–9.
21. Luiking YC, Akkermans LM, van der Reijden AC, Peeters TL, van Berge-Henegouwen GP. Differential effects of motilin on interdigestive motility of the human gastric antrum, pylorus, small intestine and gallbladder. Neurogastroenterol Motil. 2003;15:103–11.
22. Husebye E, Skar V, Høverstad T, Iversen T, Melby K. Abnormal intestinal motor patterns explain enteric colonization with gram-negative bacilli in late radiation enteropathy. Gastroenterology. 1995;109:1078–89.
23. Bisset WM, Watt JB, Rivers RP, Milla PJ. Ontogeny of fasting small intestinal motor activity in the human infant. Gut. 1988;29:483–8.
24. Sarna SK, Soergel KH, Harig JM, et al. Spatial and temporal patterns of human jejunal contractions. Am J Physiol. 1989;257:G423–32.
25. Soffer EE, Adrian TE. Effect of meal composition and sham feeding on duodenojejunal motility in humans. Dig Dis Sci. 1992;37:1009–14.
26. Hall KE, el-Sharkawy TY, Diamant NE. Vagal control of canine postprandial upper gastrointestinal motility. Am J Physiol. 1986;250:G501–10.
27. Thompson DG, Ritchie HD, Wingate DL. Patterns of small intestinal motility in duodenal ulcer patients before and after vagotomy. Gut. 1982;23:517–23.
28. Summers RW, Anuras S, Green J. Jejunal manometry patterns in health, partial intestinal obstruction, and pseudoobstruction. Gastroenterology. 1983;85:1290–300.
29. Ouyang A, Sunshine AG, Reynolds JC. Caloric content of a meal affects duration but not contractile pattern of duodenal motility in man. Dig Dis Sci. 1989;34:528–36.
30. Camilleri M. Jejunal manometry in distal subacute mechanical obstruction: significance of prolonged simultaneous contractions. Gut. 1989;30:468–75.
31. Stanghellini V, Camilleri M, Malagelada JR. Chronic idiopathic intestinal pseudo-obstruction: clinical and intestinal manometric findings. Gut. 1987;28:5–12.
32. McRae S, Younger K, Thompson DG, Wingate DL. Sustained mental stress alters human jejunal motor activity. Gut. 1982;23:404–9.
33. Sarna SK. Giant migrating contractions and their myoelectric correlates in the small intestine. Am J Physiol. 1987;253:G697–705.
34. Sood MR, Cocjin J, Di Lorenzo C, Narasimha Reddy S, Flores AF, Hyman PE. Ileal manometry in children following ileostomies and pull-through operations. Neurogastroenterol Motil. 2002;14:643–6.
35. Camilleri M, Hasler WL, Parkman HP, Quigley EM, Soffer E. Measurement of gastrointestinal motility in the GI laboratory. Gastroenterology. 1998;115:747–62.
36. Di Lorenzo C, Hillemeier C, Hyman P, et al. Manometry studies in children: minimum standards for procedures. Neurogastroenterol Motil. 2002;14:411–20.
37. Omari T, Bakewell M, Fraser R, Malbert C, Davidson G, Dent J. Intraluminal micromanometry: an evaluation of the dynamic performance of micro-extrusions and sleeve sensors. Neurogastroenterol Motil. 1996;8:241–5.
38. Wilson P, Perdikis G, Hinder RA, Redmond EJ, Anselmino M, Quigley EM. Prolonged ambulatory antroduodenal manometry in humans. Am J Gastroenterol. 1994;89:1489–95.
39. Bortolotti M, Annese V, Coccia G. Twenty-four hour ambulatory antroduodenal manometry in normal subjects. Neurogastroenterol Motil. 2000;12:231–8.
40. Dinning PG, Arkwright JW, Gregersen H, O'Grady G, Scott SM. Technical advances in monitoring human motility patterns. Neurogastroenterol Motil. 2010;22:366–80.
41. Desipio J, Friedenberg FK, Korimilli A, Richter JE, Parkman HP, Fisher RS. High-resolution solid-state manometry of the antropyloroduodenal region. Neurogastroenterol Motil. 2007;19:188–95.
42. Castedal M, Björnsson E, Abrahamsson H. Effects of midazolam on small bowel motility in humans. Aliment Pharmacol Ther. 2000;14:571–7.
43. Rayner CK, Samsom M, Jones KL, Horowitz M. Relationships of upper gastrointestinal motor and sensory function with glycemic control. Diabetes Care. 2001;24:371–81.
44. Kuo P, Wishart JM, Bellon M, Smout AJ, Holloway RH, Fraser RJ, et al. Effects of physiological hyperglycemia on duodenal motility and flow events, glucose absorption, and incretin secretion in healthy humans. J Clin Endocrinol Metab. 2010;95:3893–900.
45. Camilleri M. Perfused tube manometry. In: Kumar D, Windgate D, editors. An illustrated guide to gastrointestinal motility. 2nd ed. Edinburgh: Churchill Livingstone; 1993. p. 183–99.
46. Di Lorenzo C, Flores AF, Tomomasa T, Hyman PE. Effect of erythromycin on antroduodenal motility in children with chronic functional gastrointestinal symptoms. Dig Dis Sci. 1994;39:1399–404.
47. Faure C, Wolff VP, Navarro J. Effect of meal and intravenous erythromycin on manometric and electrogastrographic measurements of gastric motor and electrical activity. Dig Dis Sci. 2000;45:525–8.
48. Andrioli A, Wilmer A, Coremans G, Vandewalle J, Janssens J. Computer-supported analysis of continuous ambulatory manometric recordings in the human small bowel. Med Biol Eng Comput. 1996;34:336–43.
49. Camilleri M, Bharucha AE, Di Lorenzo C, Hasler WL, Prather CM, Rao SS, et al. American Neurogastroenterology and Motility Society consensus statement on intraluminal measurement of gastrointestinal and colonic motility in clinical practice. Neurogastroenterol Motil. 2008;20:1269–82.
50. Werlin SL. Antroduodenal motility in neurologically handicapped children with feeding intolerance. BMC Gastroenterol. 2004;4:19.
51. Connor FL, Hyman PE, Faure C, Tomomasa T, Pehlivanov N, Janosky J, et al. Interobserver variability in antroduodenal manometry. Neurogastroenterol Motil. 2009;21:500–7.
52. Hyman PE, Di Lorenzo C, McAdams L, Flores AF, Tomomasa T, Garvey 3rd TQ. Predicting the clinical

response to cisapride in children with chronic intestinal pseudo-obstruction. Am J Gastroenterol. 1993 Jun;88(6):832–6.
53. Di Lorenzo C, Flores AF, Buie T, Hyman PE. Intestinal motility and jejuna feeding in children with chronic intestinal pseudo-obstruction. Gastroenterology. 1995;108:1379–85.
54. Soffer EE. Small bowel motility: ready for prime time? Curr Gastroenterol Rep. 2000;2:364–9.
55. Frank JW, Sarr MG, Camilleri M. Use of gastroduodenal manometry to differentiate mechanical and functional intestinal obstruction: an analysis of clinical outcome. Am J Gastroenterol. 1994;89:339–44.
56. Khan S, Hyman PE, Cocjin J, Di Lorenzo C. Rumination syndrome in adolescents. J Pediatr. 2000;136:528–31.
57. Tack J, Blondeau K, Boecxstaens V, Rommel N. Review article: the pathophysiology, differential diagnosis and management of rumination syndrome. Aliment Pharmacol Ther. 2011;33:782–8.
58. Cucchiara S, Borrelli O, Salvia G, Iula VD, Fecarotta S, Gaudiello G, et al. A normal gastrointestinal motility excludes chronic intestinal pseudoobstruction in children. Dig Dis Sci. 1999;44:2008–13.
59. Hyman PE, Bursch B, Beck D, DiLorenzo C, Zeltzer LK. Discriminating pediatric condition falsification from chronic intestinal pseudo-obstruction in toddlers. Child Maltreat. 2002;7:132–7.

Colonic Manometry

10

Brian P. Regan, Alejandro Flores, and Carlo Di Lorenzo

Introduction

The main functions of the colon are absorption of water and electrolytes, mixing of contents of the colon with distal propulsion, and storage of fecal waste until a socially appropriate time for defecation. These functions are achieved through slow net distal propulsion, continuous mixing, and exposure to mucosal surfaces. The process by which this happens is an organized pattern with specific actions at different regions of the colon. Much is known about in vitro activity on a cellular level of this process; however, there are still unanswered questions regarding in vivo activity, in part due to the lack of a suitable animal model. For many years studies in human subjects were also limited due to the difficulty to place manometry catheters into the proximal colon. Colonic manometry is the most direct means of assessing colonic motility, and the current state of knowledge of this diagnostic technique is shared in this chapter.

B.P. Regan, D.O. (✉) • A. Flores, M.D.
Pediatric Gastroenterology, Tufts Medical Center, 800 Washington Street, Boston 02111, USA
e-mail: bregan@tuftsmedicalcenter.org

C. Di Lorenzo, M.D.
Division of Pediatric Gastroenterology, Nationwide Children's Hospital, The Ohio State University, Columbus, OH, USA

Normal Physiology of Colonic Motility

It has been hypothesized that defecation has two phases, the first being an involuntary phase during which fecal content is transported to the rectum, followed by a second voluntary phase. During the voluntary phase, intra-abdominal pressure increases, with descent of the pelvic floor and straightening of the anorectal angle. Rectal pressure then increases, resulting in internal anal sphincter relaxation, followed by expulsion of stool when the external anal sphincter relaxes [1]. Normal colorectal motility involves the coordinated activity of the muscular structures, the enteric nervous system, the interstitial cells of Cajal (ICC) and the autonomic nervous system made up of the sympathetic and parasympathetic nervous systems.

The neural input controlling the function of the colon and rectum includes the enteric nervous system, the autonomic, composed of sympathetic and parasympathetic nervous system, and the extrinsic spinal sensory nerves. The enteric nervous system affects the majority of the gut neural function. The autonomic nervous system impacts the gut function primarily through mediation of the enteric nervous system. The myenteric plexus controls the motor function with innervation to the circular muscle layers and the taeniated longitudinal muscle layers of the colon. Sensory input affecting motility is accomplished via intrinsic sensory neurons which are activated by stretch

C. Faure et al. (eds.), *Pediatric Neurogastroenterology: Gastrointestinal Motility and Functional Disorders in Children*, Clinical Gastroenterology,
DOI 10.1007/978-1-60761-709-9_10, © Springer Science+Business Media New York 2013

and by muscle tension and via input from chemical and mechanical receptors within the mucosal epithelium, reacting to intraluminal chemical stimuli [2, 3]. The autonomic nervous system, via the sympathetic nervous systems, directly innervates smooth muscle but large amount of its influence is indirectly mediated by influences on enteric neuronal circuits. Norepinephrine acts via alpha-2 receptors causing presynaptic inhibition of enteric motor reflexes [4]. The parasympathetic nervous system is influenced primary by vagal efferents to the upper colon. There is little or no vagal effect beyond in the distal colon where sacral parasympathetic influences come into play. The sacral parasympathetic pathways are identified as being responsible for the distal colonic activity in defecation [5].

How to Perform the Study

Colonic contractile function in children traditionally has been measured using catheters located within the colonic lumen, with pressure sensitive ports placed along the catheter length. Most pediatric studies have been done using water perfused catheters; however, solid state probes are available as well. The spacing between recording sites on the catheter is variable but usually ranges 5–15 cm, based upon the age of the child and the length of the colon to be studied. Each port is connected via a separate lumen (channel) to individual strain gauge pressure transducers allowing multichannel studies. Perfusion is at a constant flow rate and is achieved by use of distilled water at constant pressure [6]. Contraction of the colonic wall occludes the manometric ports and impedes the flow of water. Resistance to flow at each port is measured as pressure changes. The advantages of this system include its simplicity and the relatively inexpensive components. The catheters are fully autoclavable, allowing easy sterilization. The major disadvantage of this system is the need to be linked to an infusion pump and recording equipment which precludes ambulatory studies. The amount of water infused during prolonged studies needs to be monitored carefully especially in small infants in order to reduce the risk for water intoxication.

Solid state catheters include multiple microtransducers linked to a flexible, pressure sensitive diaphragm. They have been shown to give higher readings in the presence of amplitudes <100 mmHg and lower reading with amplitudes >100 mmHg. An opposite trend was found for the duration of contractions when compared with the more traditional water perfused assembly [7]. Using solid state catheters, the transmitted signals can be recorded by a portable digital recorder allowing ambulatory studies to capture more representative time periods for analysis. Disadvantages include the higher cost and the relative fragility of the transducers.

Catheter Placement

Placement of colonic catheters constitutes one of the most challenging portions of the testing in children. In pediatrics, the placement is always done transanally, in a retrograde fashion, except in the presence of ostomies which may allow placement of the catheter from the ostomy in an antegrade fashion into the more distal colon. Colonoscopic placement requires bowel preparation which some studies have suggested may affect basal motor activity [8, 9]. Different endoscopic techniques can be used for the placement. A biopsy forceps can be passed through the biopsy channel grasping the manometry catheter via a suture loop placed at the catheter tip. The catheter is advanced along with the colonoscope to the desired location, the forceps is opened, and the scope is then slowly retracted suctioning as much air as possible. Recently, it has been suggested that the catheter is clipped to the colonic mucosa, making it less likely to be dislodged during the manometry testing (Figs. 10.1 and 10.2) [10]. This can be easily accomplished grabbing the suture loop with a hemostasis clipping device that is then deployed when the catheter is released. Once the test is complete, a gentle pull allows the easy removal of the catheter. An alternate trans-rectal placement technique uses a guidewire passed though the biopsy channel, and left in place with removal of the colonoscope.

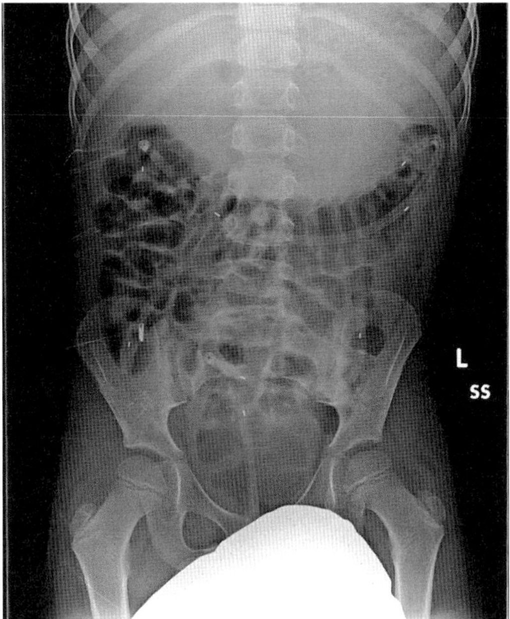

Fig. 10.1 Abdominal radiograph showing a colonic motility catheter placed with its tip in the ascending colon. The *arrow* shows an endoscopic clip holding the catheter in place

The manometry catheter is then advanced over this guidewire with fluoroscopic assistance. It should be emphasized that in children the endoscopic placement is always done under sedation or general anesthesia and the endoscopies are often very challenging due to the presence of very dilated colons, at times poorly cleansed, especially when performed in children with years of severe constipation. Fluoroscopic placement of the catheter in the proximal colon may also be achieved by skilled interventional radiologists, obviating the need for general anesthesia but exposing the patient to more radiation [11].

Study Protocol

There is variability in study protocols with no prospective data indicating superiority of any specific one. Studies of relatively short duration, approximately 4–8 h, are usually adequate to evaluate response to stimuli; however, more physiologic studies lasting 24 h in ambulating subjects provide more physiologic data. Most of the pediatric literature has been generated using the shorter duration studies with water perfused catheters. Short duration tests, also known as provocation studies, are used to assess response to stimuli such as food, sleep, and medications. Response to food is the most powerful physiologic stimulus. After eating, there is an increase in phasic and tonic motor activity, known as the gastro-colonic response. The early response is most intense in the distal colon. A second peak in motility is seen after 50–110 min lasting up to 3 h. Increased motor activity following a meal may be regarded as an indication of the integrity of the neurohumoral control of colonic motility. Intraluminal bisacodyl instillation is typically done after the postprandial portion of the testing and it induces high amplitude propagated contractions (HAPC) in normal individuals [12, 13]. Absent response has been associated with colonic inertia and myenteric plexus damage in adults and children [14, 15]. Stimulation with other drugs, such as neostigmine, is not routinely done in children.

Pediatric studies are initiated after the effect of the sedation or the anesthesia used to the place the catheter has resolved. Typical protocols in pediatrics start with fasting unstimulated motility testing for 1 h. The child is then offered a large, age-appropriate meal, and postprandial motility is measured for at least one more hour. Changes with sleep and wake and symptoms experienced by the child are noted if occurring during the study. Pharmacologic provocation is then performed with 0.2 mg/kg of bisacodyl (max 10 mg), infused through the motility catheter into the most proximal portion of the colon. It is particularly informative to observe the child's reaction to the onset of the urge to defecate associated with the administration of bisacodyl. At times, the child's attempts to withhold are finally recognized as such by the parents once the experienced medical providers observing the study point out that behavior to the parents. Thus, it is imperative that a nurse or a physician is in the room with the child undergoing the test at all times.

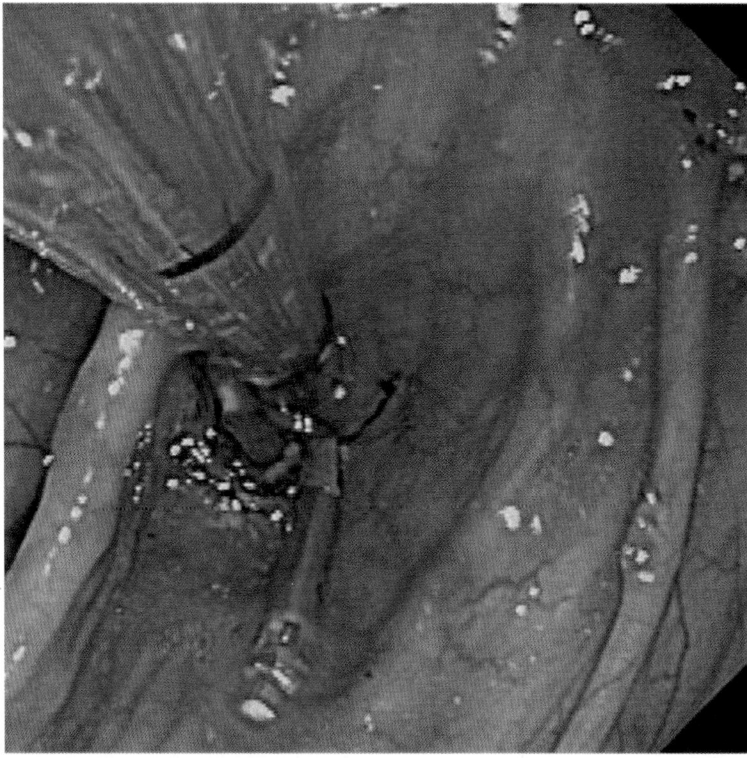

Fig. 10.2 Endoscopic image of a colonic motility catheter clipped to a fold in the cecum. The suture material tied to the tip of the catheter is shown attached to an endoscopic clip

Identifiable Motility Patterns

High amplitude propagating contraction (Fig. 10.3) constitute a motor pattern found in patients with normal colonic motility and are defined as contractions with an amplitude greater than 80 mmHg, have a duration greater than 10 s, and propagate over at least 30 cm, stopping at the junction between sigmoid colon and rectum. They typically occur following meals, upon awakening, and can be induced by bisacodyl, glycerin and other colonic irritants. They are more common in younger children [16] and in patients who have had a distal colonic resection, such as in patients after surgery for Hirschsprung's disease [17]. Recent studies have also shown that propagated contractions of varied amplitude can also be induced by saline infusion and distention of the right colon [18, 19].

Low amplitude propagating contractions (LAPC), in contrast to HAPC, are defined as having an amplitude of less than 50 mmHg. They occur 45–120 times per 24 h and are typically 5–40 mmHg in amplitude. They occur significantly more during the day than at night, and much like HAPC, increase following meals and after waking [20, 21]. The function of LAPC is poorly understood. They are likely to be associated with lesser propulsive movement of intraluminal contents, and have been reported to be involved with the transport of less viscous colonic contents, such as fluid or gas [22].

An increase in colonic motility, often measured as the "motility index" (a parameter which takes in account both frequency and amplitude of contractions), is expected after ingestion of a meal. Such contractions are both tonic and phasic in nature and may be difficult to quantify especially when the postprandial period is associated with motion artifacts. Evaluation of postprandial changes in colonic tone using the electronic barostat, a frequent feature of colonic manometries performed in adults, is not

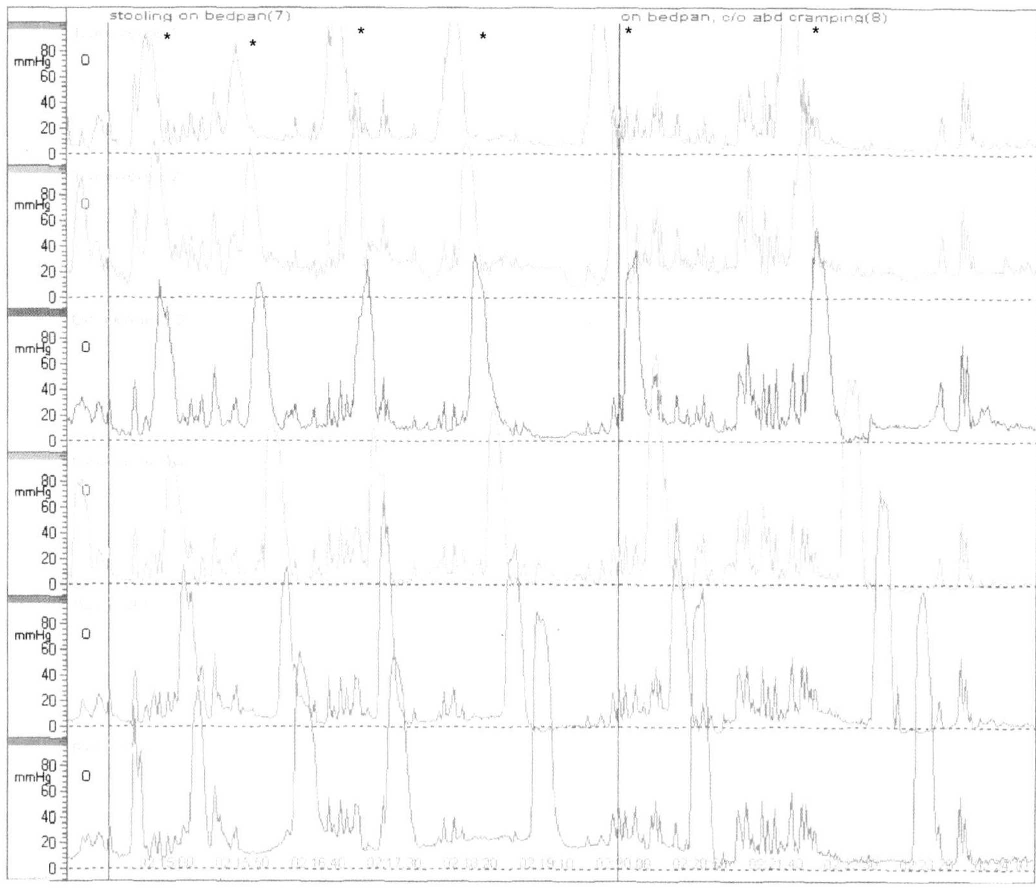

Fig. 10.3 Example of a cluster of six high amplitude propagating contractions (HAPC), indicated with *asterisks*, associated with the urge to defecate

commonly done in the pediatric patient [23]. Visual interpretation of the gastrocolonic response produces the maximum variability in interindividual interpretation of the test. On the other hand, there seems to be great concordance among different investigators in the recognition of the HAPC pattern. The median agreement regarding the overall interpretation of the colonic manometry in children being either normal or abnormal is 87% [24].

Indications the Study [23]

1. Intractable constipation
   (a) Assessment of patients with severe constipation, unresponsive to medical therapy, with no evidence of an evacuation disorder.
   (b) Guide surgical interventions including placement of diverting stoma, resection of a portion of the colon, or formation of a conduit for administration of antegrade enemas.
   (c) Evaluate the function of the disconnected colon before possible closure of a diverting ostomy.
2. Chronic intestinal pseudo-obstruction
   (a) Evaluation if the colon is involved in the disease.
   (b) Help plan which organs to transplant before a small bowel transplant.
3. Hirschsprung's disease and repaired imperforate anus
   (a) Clarify the pathophysiology of persistent symptoms after removal of the aganglionic segment and repair of anorectal malformations.

Intractable Constipation

Most children with constipation suffer from functional constipation, a condition related to a maladaptive response to a painful or frightening defecation. A small proportion of children with constipation have symptoms which are severe and unresponsive to aggressive medical and behavioral therapy. The lack of response can lead to frustration, distrust with the medical team and loss of self-esteem for the child. Colonic manometry is indicated for the evaluation of such children in order to discriminate normal colonic motility from abnormal colonic motor function [25, 26] which may be associated with colonic neuromuscular disease. This information can then be used to guide management [27]. Resection of colonic segments found to have abnormal motor function leads to improvement in symptoms [28, 29]. Interestingly, there seems to be little or no correlation between manometric findings and histopathologic abnormalities, suggesting that our current ability to study the morphology and function of the enteric neuromusculature is limited [30].

A study by Villareal et al. used HAPC as a marker for intact neuromuscular colonic function [31]. The colonic manometry pattern, namely the failure to demonstrate colonic HAPC, directed the providers to the formation of a defunctioning ostomy (ileostomy or colostomy). In patients who had evidence of a dilated colon with abnormal motility patterns, repeat manometry testing after a period of decompression (5–30 months) led to an improved motor function. Aspirot et al. evaluated the effect of chronic use of antegrade enemas on colonic motility in children and adolescents with severe constipation [32]. Although only few patients were included in the study, all those with abnormal manometry prior to cecostomy placement showed improvement in colonic motility after using antegrade enema for at least 1 year. The patients evaluated were selected due to consideration of removal of their cecostomy tubes, in view of their clinical improvement. Colonic manometry may be also used to predict positive response to antegrade enema. Retrospective studies have indicated that patients with HAPC and an intact gastrocolonic response are more likely to do well when receiving antegrade enemas [33, 34]. The propagated contractions seem to be essential to propel colonic contents during antegrade irrigation. However, the motor response is still not a guarantee for success, as even some patients with HAPC have had a poor outcome, indicating that motility pattern is important, but there are additional factors, such as compliance with the infusion schedule and anorectal and pelvic floor function, possibly playing a role.

Chronic Intestinal Pseudo-Obstruction

Chronic intestinal pseudo-obstruction (CIPO) is a heterogeneous group of disorders what vary in cause, severity, course, and response to treatment. Di Lorenzo et al. studied patients with CIPO, and found a subgroup of patients with chronic constipation as part of their CIPO symptomatology had abnormal HAPC, absent gastrocolonic response or total lack of identifiable colonic motor activity [35]. A thorough manometry evaluation including colonic manometry needs to be performed during the evaluation for possible isolated small bowel or multivisceral transplantation in children with CIPO, in order to assess which organs need to be transplanted and if a permanent diverting ileostomy needs to be planned [36].

Hirschsprung's Disease and Anorectal Malformations

After resection of the abnormally innervated bowel in Hirschsprung's disease, a large percentage of patients continue to struggle with abnormal defecation patterns [37]. Colonic manometry testing allows classification of symptomatic patients post-Hirschsprung's surgery into four groups, each with different

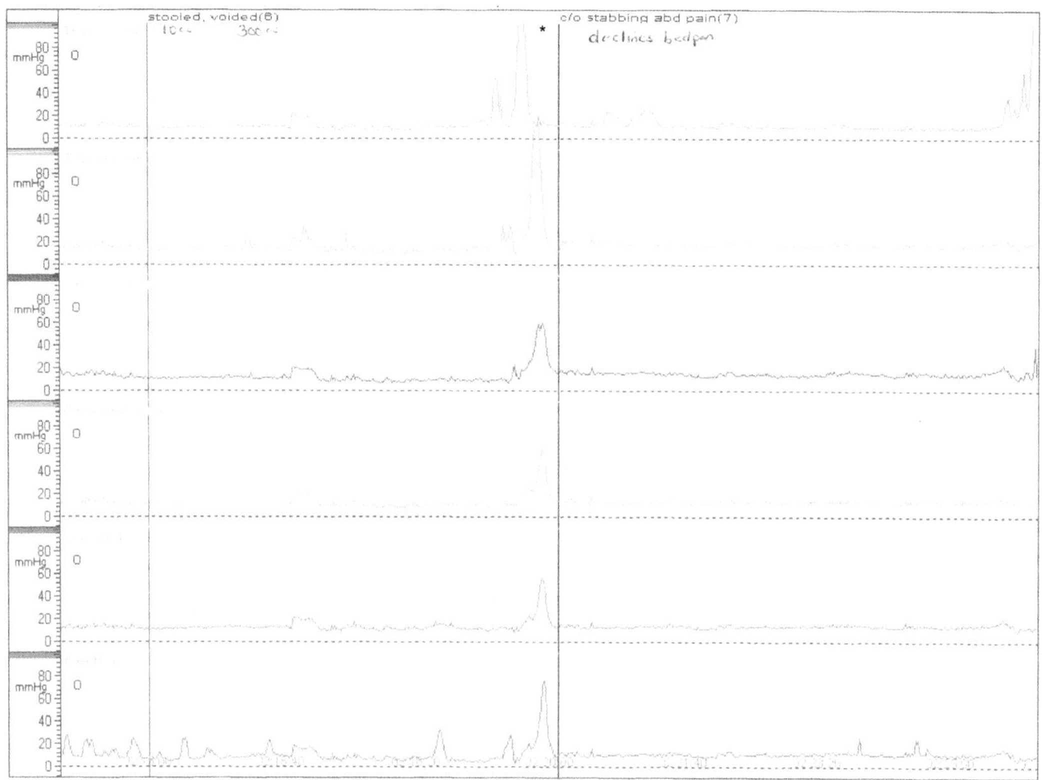

Fig. 10.4 Example of non-propagating HAPC, indicated by *asterisks*. The contractions appear to be propagating only in the proximal colon (*top two* recording channels)

physiology [38]. Each category and physiologic process directs different therapy: (1) The first group of patients has HAPC which progress through the neorectum all the way to the anal verge. The amplitude of the HAPC exceeds that of the voluntary contraction of the external anal sphincter. The result is incontinence or rectal pain as the patient attempts to retain the stool. (2) The second group has normal colonic motility with fear of defecation and stool withholding. The negative experience related to attempting defecation before surgical removal of the aganglionic segment may result in fecal retention after surgery. Identification of normal colonic manometry pattern in these children provides reassurance in the diagnosis and more confidence in the behavioral and medical treatment plan. (3) Abnormal colonic manometry with lack of HAPC, poorly propagating HAPCs (Fig. 10.4) or simultaneous increases in pressure in the distal colon (Fig. 10.5) may be due to a neuropathic motility disorders proximal to the aganglionic segment, possibly associated with intestinal neuronal dysplasia [39], or to a common cavity phenomenon. (4) Finally, a small number of patients with defecation disorders post-surgery for Hirschsprung's disease have normal colonic motility and a hypertensive anal sphincter. Successful treatment options for this subset of patients have included myectomy, which leads to irreversible destruction of the internal anal sphincter, and botulinum toxin injection to the hypertensive anal sphincter [40–42].

Similar findings have been reported in children with continence disorders after anorectal malformations repair. Heikenen et al. have reported that propagation of excessive numbers of HAPCs into the neorectum as well as internal anal sphincter dysfunction can contribute to fecal incontinence in these children [43].

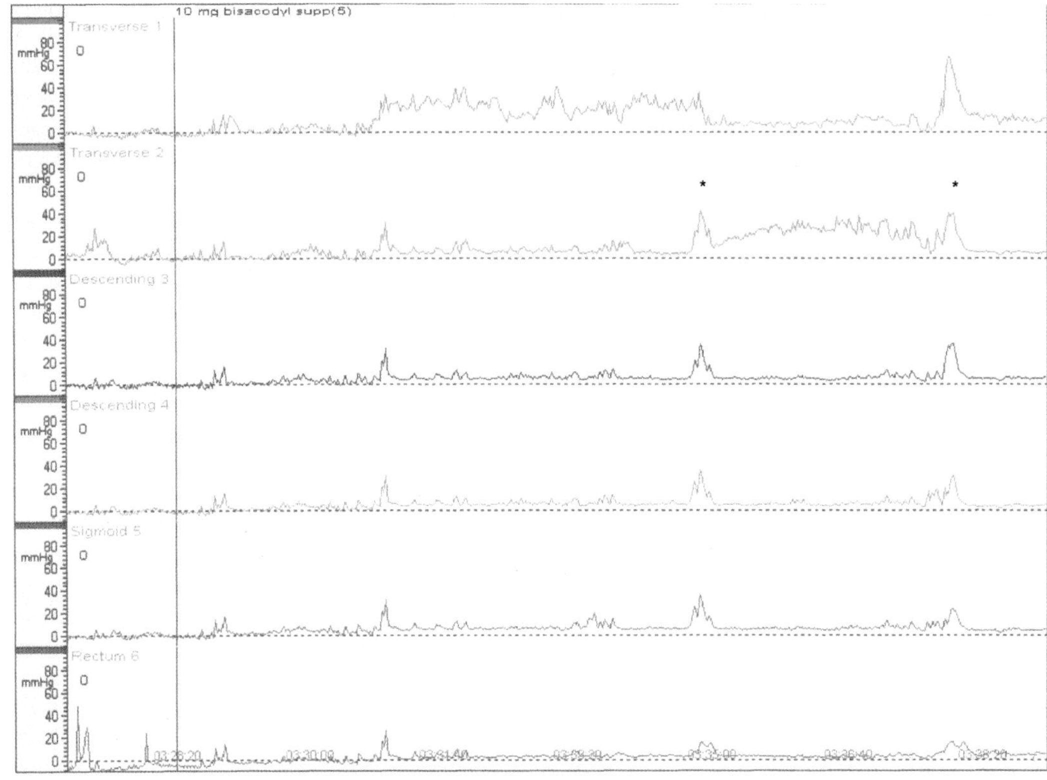

Fig. 10.5 Example of simultaneous increases in pressure in the distal colon, indicated by *asterisks*

Variations on Colonic Manometry Testing

Ambulatory 24 h Colonic Manometry

A limitation of traditional colonic manometry studies is the duration of the study. There is a well-established circadian variation in colonic manometry which is missed during short studies [21, 44–46]. Twenty-four hour colonic manometry has been proposed as a better test which evaluates a time period felt to be more representative of the patient's environment, eating and sleeping patterns. It has been performed in children using water perfused probes [47] but it is best done using solid state probes which do not confine the patient to a restricted environment. Solid state probes have been placed via colonoscopy with clips adhering to multiple sites of colonic wall. The probe is then taped to the gluteal region and connected to a portable recorder. The patient is allowed to ambulate, eat and defecate in a hospital setting for 24-h with continuous manometric measurement. It is unclear how much the additional information collected during a 24-h study changes clinical management compared to a shorter study with meal ingestion and pharmacological stimulation.

Wireless Motility Capsule

This tool has been approved by the US Food and Drug Administration (FDA) for measurement of gastric emptying and whole gut transit time. Once swallowed, this fairly sizable capsule is capable of measuring intraluminal pH, pressure and temperature throughout the entire gastrointestinal tract. Data is transmitted to a data receiver and downloads to a computer for analysis. Gastric emptying is measured by timing the point from ingestion to the point where the pH rises above pH 6, indicating the capsule has left the acid environment of the stomach and has entered the more neutral pH of the duodenum [48]. Because it has a single pressure measurement, propagation of motor activity cannot be defined. In addition, the gastric emptying time for the capsule most probably reflects the gastric emptying of a large non-digestible solid, which is different from the emptying of a digestible solid [49]. Wireless pH motility capsule has been found to be useful in evaluating colonic transit, and has been validated in adults as an alternative to radiopaque markers as a tool to assess colonic transit [50]. The exact role of the wireless pressure capsule in the evaluation of children with possible colonic dysmotility is still under investigation.

High Resolution Colonic Manometry

High resolution manometry is well established in esophageal and anorectal evaluation. Similar technology is being developed for colonic assessment and has been tested primarily in adults [51–53]. The spacing of the sensors is 1 cm interval as opposed to the greater than 5 cm in traditional catheters. The recorded data is transmitted to advanced computer hardware and software used in recording and analyzing the data. rospective studies are needed to provide standards for the application of this technology, and determine its utility in clinical practice. Although the authors are aware of preliminary studies on the use of colonic HRM in children, at the current time there is limited published data in this age group. It is likely that this will evolve in the near future

Conclusion

Much information has been garnered in the field of colonic motility in the past decade and pediatric studies have been at the forefront of clinical investigations. Colonic manometry has asserted itself as a standard diagnostic test in pediatrics and represents one of the rare instances of a manometric technique more commonly used in children than in adults. There are now clearly defined indications for its use and meaningful clinical decisions that are determined by its results. Colonic manometry is best performed in specialized centers by investigators with a special expertise in motility and who are comfortable in evaluating children with complex biopsychosocial disturbances. Better understanding on how to perform and interpret the test continues to occur and new techniques, such as high resolution fiber optic manometry and wireless motility capsule [54], are emerging which will hopefully continue to increase knowledge in the field of colonic motility disorders.

References

1. Sarna SK. Physiology and pathophysiology of colonic motor activity (1). Dig Dis Sci. 1991;36:827–62.
2. Kunze WA, Furness JB. The enteric nervous system and regulation of intestinal motility. Annu Rev Physiol. 1999;61:117–42.
3. Costa M, Brookes SJ, Steele PA, Gibbins I, Burcher E, Kandiah CJ. Neurochemical classification of myenteric neurons in the guinea-pig small intestine. Neuroscience. 1996;75:949–67.
4. Wilson AJ, Llewellyn-Smith IJ, Furness JB, Costa M. The source of the nerve fibres forming the deep muscular and circular muscle plexuses in the small intestine of the guinea-pig. Cell Tissue Res. 1987;247:497–504.
5. De Groat WC, Krier J. The sacral parasympathetic reflex pathway regulating colonic motility and defaecation in the cat. J Physiol. 1978;276:481–500.
6. Arndorfer RC, Stef JJ, Dodds W, Lineham JH, Hogan WJ. Improved infusion system for intraluminal esophageal manometry. Gastroenterology. 1977;73:23–7.
7. Liem O, Burgers RE, Connor FL, Benninga MA, Reddy SN, Mousa HM, Di Lorenzo C. Solid-state vs water-perfused catheters to measure colonic high-amplitude propagating contractions. Neurogastroenterol Motil. 2012;24:345–e167.
8. Dinoso VP, Murthy SNS, Goldstein J, Rosner B. Basal motor activity of the distal colon: a reappraisal. Gastroenterology. 1983;85:637–42.
9. Lemann M, Fluorie B, Picon L, Coffin B, Jian R, Rambaud JC. Motor activity recorded in the unprepared colon of healthy humans. Gut. 1995;37:649–53.
10. Rao SS, Singh S, Sadeghi P. Is endoscopic mucosal clipping useful for preventing colonic manometry probe displacement? J Clin Gastroenterol. 2010;44:620–4.
11. van den Berg MM, Hogan M, Mousa HM, Di Lorenzo C. Colonic manometry catheter placement with primary fluoroscopic guidance. Dig Dis Sci. 2007;52:2282–6.
12. Bassotti G, Crowell MC, Whitehead WE. Contractile activity of the human colon: lessons from 24 hours study. Gut. 1993;34:129–33.

13. Preston DM, Lennard-Jones JE. Pelvic motility and reponse to intraluminal bisacoldyl in slow transit constipation. Dig Dis Sci. 1985;30:289–94.
14. Kamm MA, Van Der Sijp JR, Lennard-Jones JE. Observations on the characteristics of stimulated defaecation in severe idiopathic constipation. Int J Colorectal Dis. 1992;7:197–201.
15. Stanton MP, Hutson JM, Simpson D, Oliver MR, Southwell BR, Dinning P, Cook I, Catto-Smith AG. Colonic manometry via appendicostomy shows reduced frequency, amplitude, and length of propagating sequences in children with slow-transit constipation. J Pediatr Surg. 2005;40:1138–45.
16. Di Lorenzo C, Flores AF, Hyman PE. Age-related changes in colon motility. J Pediatr. 1995;127:593–6.
17. Kaul A, Garza JM, Connor FL, Cocjin JT, Flores AF, Hyman PE, Di Lorenzo C. Colonic hyperactivity results in frequent fecal soiling in a subset of children after surgery for Hirschsprung disease. J Pediatr Gastroenterol Nutr. 2011;52:433–6.
18. Liem O, van den Berg MM, Mousa HM, Youssef NN, Langseder AL, Benninga MA, Di Lorenzo C. Distention of the colon is associated with initiation of propagatedcontractionsinchildren.Neurogastroenterol Motil. 2010;22:19–23.
19. Gomez R, Mousa H, Liem O, Hayes J, Di Lorenzo C. How do antegrade enemas work? Colonic motility in response to administration of normal saline solution into the proximal colon. J Pediatr Gastroenterol Nutr. 2010;51:741–6.
20. Bassotti G, Clementi M, Antonelli E, Pelli MA, Tonini M. Low amplitude propagated contractile waves: a relevant propulsive mechanism of human colon. Dig Liver Dis. 2001;33:36–40.
21. Rao SSC, Sadeghi P, Beaty J, Kavlock R, Ackerson K. Ambualtory 24 h colonic manometry in healthy humans. Am J Physiol Gastrointest Liver Physiol. 2001;280:G629–39.
22. Scott SM. Manometric techniques for the evaluation of colonic motor activity: current status. Neurogastroenterol Motil. 2003;15:483–509.
23. Camilleri M, Bharucha AE, Di Lorenzo C, Hasler WL, Prather CM, Rao SS, Wald A. American neurogastroenterology and motility society consensus statement of intraluminal measurement of gastrointestinal and colonic motility in clinical practice. Neurogastroenterol Motil. 2008;20:1269–82.
24. Sood MR, Mousa H, Tipnis N, Di Lorenzo C, Werlin S, Fernandez S, Liem O, Simpson P, Rudolph C. Interobserver variability in the interpretation of colon manometry studies in children. J Pediatr Gastroenterol Nutr. 2012; In press.
25. Di Lorenzo C, Flores A, Reddy N, Hyman P. Use of colonic manometry to differentiate causes of intractable constipation in children. J Pediatr. 1992;5:690–5.
26. Baker SS, Liptak GS, Colletti RB, Croffie JM, Di Lorenzo C, Ector W, Nurko S. Constipation in infants and children:evaluation and treatment. A medical position statement of the North American Society for Pediatric Gastroenterology and Nutrition. J Pediatr Gastroenterol Nutr. 1999;29:612–26.
27. Pensabene L, Youssef NN, Griffiths JM, Di Lorenzo C. Colonic manometry in children with defecatory disorders. Rose in diagnosis and management. Am J Gastroenterol. 2003;98:1052–7.
28. Youssef NN, Pensabene L, Barksdale Jr E, Di Lorenzo C. Is there a role for surgery beyond colonic aganglionosis and anorectal malformations in children with intractable constipation? J Pediatr Surg. 2004;39:73–7.
29. Christison-Lagay ER, Rodriguez L, Kurtz M, St Pierre K, Doody DP, Goldstein AM. Antegrade colonic enemas and intestinal diversion are highly effective in the management of children with intractable constipation. J Pediatr Surg. 2010;45:213–9.
30. van den Berg MM, Di Lorenzo C, Mousa HM, Benninga MA, Boeckxstaens GE, Luquette M. Morphological changes of the enteric nervous system, interstitial cells of cajal, and smooth muscle in children with colonic motility disorders. J Pediatr Gastroenterol Nutr. 2009;48:22–9.
31. Villareal J, Sood M, Zangen T, Flores A, Michel R, Reddy N, Di Lorenzo C, Hyman P. Colonic diversion for intractable constipation in children: colonic manometry helps guide clinical decisions. J Pediatr Gastroenterol Nutr. 2001;33:588–91.
32. Aspirot A, Fernandez S, Di Lorenzo S, Skaggs B, Mousa H. Antegrade enemas for defecation disorders: do they improve the colonic motility? J Pediatr Surg. 2009;44:1575–80.
33. van den Berg MM, Hogan M, Di Caniano DA, Lorenzo C, Benninga MA, Mousa HM. Colonic manometry as predictor of cecostomy success in children with defecation disorders. J Pediatr Surg. 2006;41:730–6.
34. Youssef NN, Barksdale Jr E, Griffiths JM, Flores AF, Di Lorenzo C. Management of intractable constipation with antegrade enemas in neurologically intact children. J Pediatr Gastroenterol Nutr. 2002;34:402–5.
35. Di Lorenzo C, Flores AF, Reddy SN, Snape Jr WJ, Bazzocchi G, Hyman PE. Colonic manometry in children with chronic intestinal pseudo-obstruction. Gut. 1993;34:803–7.
36. Sigurdsson L, Reyes J, Kocoshis SA, Mazariegos G, Abu-Elmagd KM, Bueno J, Di Lorenzo C. Intestinal transplantation in children with chronic intestinal pseudo-obstruction. Gut. 1999;45:570–4.
37. Catto-Smith AG, Trajanovska M, Taylor RG. Long-term continence after surgery for Hirschsprung's disease. J Gastroenterol Hepatol. 2007;22:2273–82.
38. Lorenzo D, Solzi GF, Flores A, Schwankovsky L, Hyman P. Colonic motility after surgery for Hirschsprung's disease. Am J Gastroenterol. 2000;95:1759–64.
39. Schmittenbecher PP, Sacher P, Cholewa D, Haberlik A, Menardi G, Moczulski J, Rumlova E, Schuppert

W, Ure B. Hirschsprung's disease and intestinal neuronal dysplasia—a frequent association with implications for the postoperative course. Pediatr Surg Int. 1999;15:553–8.
40. Blair GK, Murphy JJ, Fraser GC. Interal sphincterotomy in post pull through Hirschsprung's disease. J Pediatr Surg. 1996;31:843–5.
41. Patrus B, Nasr A, Langer JC, Gerstle JT. Intrasphincteric botulinum toxin decreases the rate of hospitalization for postoperative obstructive symptoms in children with Hirschsprung disease. J Pediatr Surg. 2011;46:184–7.
42. Foroutan HR, Hosseini SM, Banani SA, Bahador A, Sabet B, Zeraatian S, Banani SJ. Comparison of botulinium toxin injection and posterior anorectal myectomy in treatment of internal anal sphincter achalasia. Indian J Gastroenterol. 2008;27:62–5.
43. Heikenen JB, Werlin SL, Di Lorenzo C, Hyman PE, Cocjin J, Flores AF, Reddy SN. Colonic motility in children with repaired imperforate anus. Dig Dis Sci. 1999;44:1288–92.
44. Narducci F, Bassotti G, Gaburri M, Morelli A. Twenty-four hour manometric recordings of colonic motor activity in healthy man. Gut. 1987;28:17–25.
45. Hagger R, Kumar D, Benson M. Periodic colonic motor activity identified by 24-h pancolonic ambulatory manometry in humans. Neurogastroenterol Motil. 2002;14:271–8.
46. Frexinos J, Bueno L, Fioramonti J. Diurnal changes in myoelectric spiking activity of the human colon. Gastroenterology. 1985;88:1104–10.
47. King SK, Catto-Smith AG, Stanton MP, Sutcliffe JR, Simpson D, Cook I, Dinning P, Hutson JM, Southwell BR. 24-Hour colonic manometry in pediatric slow transit constipation shows significant reductions in antegrade propagation. Am J Gastroenterol. 2008;103:2083–91.
48. Rao SS, Kuo B, McCallum RW, Chey WD, DiBaise JK, Hasler WL, Koch KL, Lackner JM, Miller C, Saad R, Semler JR, Sitrin MD, Wilding GE, Parkman HP. Investigation of colonic and whole-gut transit with wireless motility capsule and radiopaque markers in constipation. Clin Gastroenterol Hepatol. 2009;7:537–44.
49. Kuo B, McCallum RW, Koch KL, Sitrin MD, Wo JM, Chey WD, Hasler WL, Lackner JM, Katz LA, Semler JR, Wilding GE, Parkman HP. Comparison of gastric emptying of a nondigestible capsule to a radio-labelled meal in healthy and gastroparetic subjects. Aliment Pharmacol Ther. 2008;27:186–96.
50. Camilleri M, Thorne NK, Ringel Y, Hasler WL, Kuo B, Esfandyari T, Gupta A, Scott SM, McCallum RW, Parkman HP, Soffer E, Wilding GE, Semler JR, Rao SS. Wireless pH-motility capsule for colonic transit: prospective comparison with radiopaque markers in chronic constipation. Neurogastroenterol Motil. 2010;22:874–82.
51. Arkwright JW, Blenman NG, Underhill ID, Maunder SA, Szczesniak MM, Dinning PG, Cook IJ. In-vivo demonstration of a high resolution optical fiber manometry catheter for diagnosis of gastrointestinal motility disorders. Opt Express. 2009;17:4500–8.
52. Arkwright JW, Underhill ID, Maunder SA, Blenman N, Szczesniak MM, Wiklendt L, Cook IJ, Lubowski DZ, Dinning PG. Design of a high-sensor count fibre optic manometry catheter for in-vivo colonic diagnostics. Opt Express. 2009;17:22423–31.
53. Dinning PG, Arkwright JW, Gregersen H, o'grady G, Scott M. Technical advances in monitoring human motility patterns. Neurogastroenterol Motil. 2010;22:366–80.
54. Dinning PG, Scott SM. Novel diagnostics and therapy of colonic motor disorders. Curr Opin Pharmacol. 2011;11:624–9.

Anorectal Manometry

11

Minou Le-Carlson and William Berquist

Introduction

Fecal continence and defecation are achieved through a coordinated sequence of events involving the relaxation and contraction of abdominal musculature, as well those muscles that form and surround the anorectal canal. Anorectal manometry (ARM) is an objective way to assess the function of such muscles, thereby allowing the diagnosis of abnormalities and the subsequent application of appropriately tailored treatments. Pediatric patients typically referred for ARM testing include those with severe constipation refractory to medical management, anorectal pain especially with defecation and/or fecal incontinence. Constipation in children is generally characterized by less than 3 bowel movements weekly, as well as hard, often painful stools that are difficult to pass [1, 2]. Fecal incontinence is the inappropriate leakage of stool which is often secondary to stool withholding, although can be non-retentive in nature. Constipation and incontinence can be highly distressing conditions for patients and their families constituting approximately 3% of all pediatric outpatient visits [3]. However, given the significant overlap of symptomatology among the different functional and non-functional causes of anorectal dysfunction, diagnosis is often not possible based on history and exam alone. Indeed, anal achalasia, Hirschsprung's disease (HD), and pelvic floor dyssynergia can all present similarly with constipation but can require highly varied forms of therapy—botulinum toxin injection, surgery, and biofeedback, respectively. By characterizing the underlying pathology of similarly presenting symptoms through ARM, appropriate forms of management can be applied to help patients gain normal or near normal stool function. Equally as important, ARM also offers providers an objective way to educate patients and families regarding the underlying pathophysiology of these often chronic and consuming conditions.

M. Le-Carlson, M.D. (✉)
Pediatric Gastroenterology, Hepatology and Nutrition, Pediatrics Department, Stanford University Medical Center, Lucile Packard Children's Hospital, 750 Welch Road, Suite 116, Palo Alto, CA 94304, USA
e-mail: minoule@stanford.edu

W. Berquist, M.D.
Gastroenterology Division, Pediatrics Department, Stanford University, Lucile Packard Children's Hospital, Stanford, CA, USA

Anatomy/Physiology

The major structures of the anorectal canal include the internal anal sphincter (IAS), external anal sphincter (EAS) and the levator ani complex including the puborectalis sling (Fig. 11.1a). The IAS, located proximally and most medial to the central lumen, envelopes the canal and is involved in involuntary or reflexive muscular contraction. Distal and lateral to the IAS, the skeletal muscles of the EAS form an additional layer of circumferential musculature that is under voluntary control

C. Faure et al. (eds.), *Pediatric Neurogastroenterology: Gastrointestinal Motility and Functional Disorders in Children*, Clinical Gastroenterology,
DOI 10.1007/978-1-60761-709-9_11,

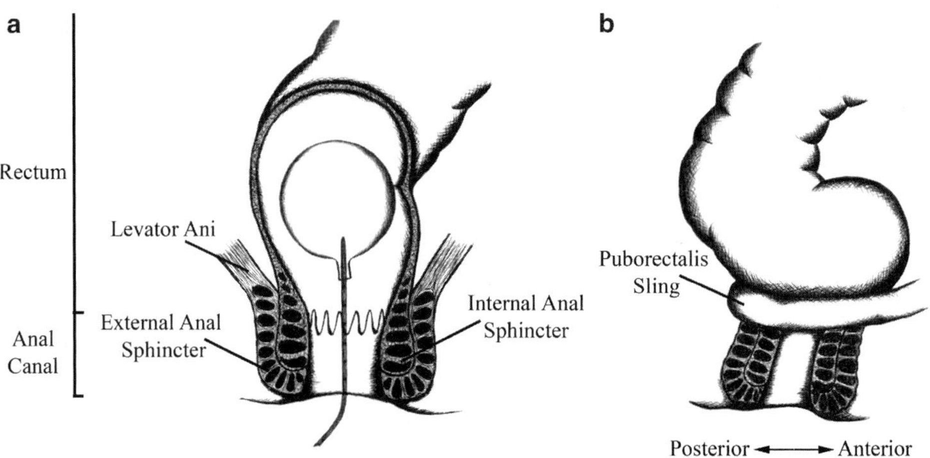

Fig. 11.1 (**a**) Anterior–posterior view of the anorectal canal with ARM catheter and inflated balloon in place. (**b**) Lateral view with puborectalis sling angulating anorectal canal. Figures drawn by Minou Le-Carlson

[4–6]. There is considerable overlap of the two anal sphincters such that differentiation on ARM often is not possible, particularly in younger children as the anorectal canal does not extend beyond a few centimeters in length [7]. The levator ani complex is composed of a group of muscles that acts to support and lift the pelvic floor. Part of this complex, the puborectalis, loops posteriorly around the rectum forming a sling that angulates the anorectal canal. The degree of this angle, typically 85–105° at rest, plays an important role in controlling anorectal function by narrowing to support continence and widening to permit the passage of stool (Fig. 11.1b) [4].

During normal function, the passage of stool into the rectum leads to the involuntary relaxation of the IAS to accommodate the stool burden, referred to as the rectoanal inhibitory reflex (RAIR), as well as to the urge to defecate. Simultaneous contraction of the EAS and puborectalis muscles counters this action to increase distal anorectal pressures, decrease the anorectal angle and ultimately, prevent forward propulsion of stool and dissipate the urge to defecate. When defecation is permissible in both a practical and appropriate social context, an increase in intra-abdominal pressure coupled with the relaxation of the EAS and puborectalis muscle allows forward propagation and evacuation of stool and ultimately, the urge to defecate is relieved [4–6].

Methods/Technique

There are several forms of ARM available including conventional water perfusion, sleeve catheter, water and air filled balloon catheter, as well as high-resolution or solid-state manometry. The more widely used water-perfusion manometry (WPM) and high-resolution manometry (HRM) will be reviewed here. WPM involves a flexible catheter with multiple side-holes either circumferentially or spirally arranged along the length in a staggered configuration to permit continuous perfusion of water typically at rates of 0.1–0.5 mL/min (Fig. 11.2a) [5]. HRM involves a catheter with channels positioned several millimeters apart, each composed of multiple sensing points arranged in a circumferential pattern which accumulatively allow retrieval of more than a hundred of data points (Fig. 11.2b, see also Fig. 11.4a). Newly emerged is the high resolution, three-dimensional ARM which configures a multidimensional view of the anorectal canal (Fig. 11.2c) [8]. The utility and practical advantages of this method over other forms of ARM, however, have yet to be well established clinically. All methods include an inflatable balloon positioned at the tip for measurement of rectal distention and balloon expulsion. The comparable advantages and disadvantages of each system are debatable. Generally, the simplicity and cost

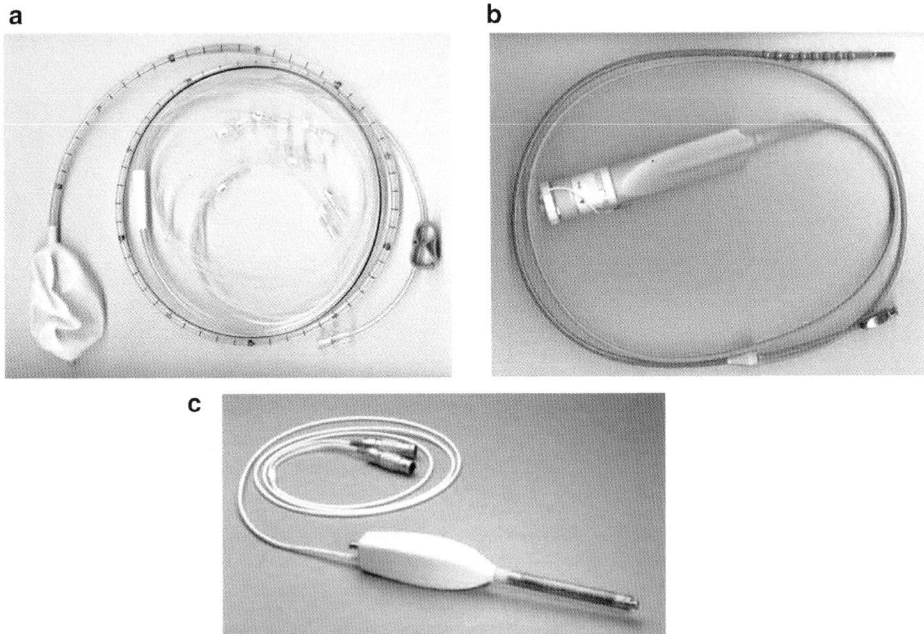

Fig. 11.2 (**a**) Water-perfusion catheter (Medical Measurement Systems). (**b**) High-resolution catheter (Medical Measurement Systems). (**c**) Three-dimensional high-resolution catheter (Sierra Scientific Instruments). Printed with permission from Medical Measurement Systems

are major advantages of WPM, while maintenance of the narrow fluid channels—susceptible to leakage and occlusion—can be a drawback. Meanwhile, HRM offers substantially higher anatomic detail of the anorectal canal allowing some differentiation between internal and external rectal sphincters and increased appreciation of asymmetric anatomy—potential advantages when surgical intervention is being considered. Additionally, given its circumferentially located sensors, HRM requires less catheter manipulation after placement in the canal, thereby minimizing sensor migration. The major downsides to HRM are most notably the cost and cleaning, as well as temperature sensitivity and potentially longer downtime when repairs are needed.

Prior to the procedure, children should attempt to defecate or if concerns for large rectal burden, an enema or suppository should be administered several hours prior to the study. For younger babies, no bowel preparation is required [9, 10]. A digital rectal exam should precede the ARM study to assess stool content, as well as overall anatomy and patient's ability to follow commands. If possible, any home medications with the potential to modify muscle activity should be held including opioids and anticholinergics. Ideally, patients should be in the lateral position with knees flexed slightly towards the chest, awake and actively participating in the study particularly to evaluate rectal sensitivity and defecatory dynamics. While most ARM procedures are done without anesthetics, when they cannot be avoided the provider must always factor the potential impact of such drugs towards the interpretation of study outcomes. Limited studies have demonstrated that ketamine and midazalom do not significantly impact resting anal pressure or RAIR [11, 12]. Propofol has also been shown to have no effect on RAIR, but there is evidence to suggest an alteration of resting pressures in an adult study [13]. As with all studies of motility, the impact of anesthesia on ARM is not fully characterized. Additionally, some providers concurrently perform ARM and electromyography (EMG) for an enhanced investigation of pelvic floor activity. During EMG, external surface electrodes are placed near the anus to capture the

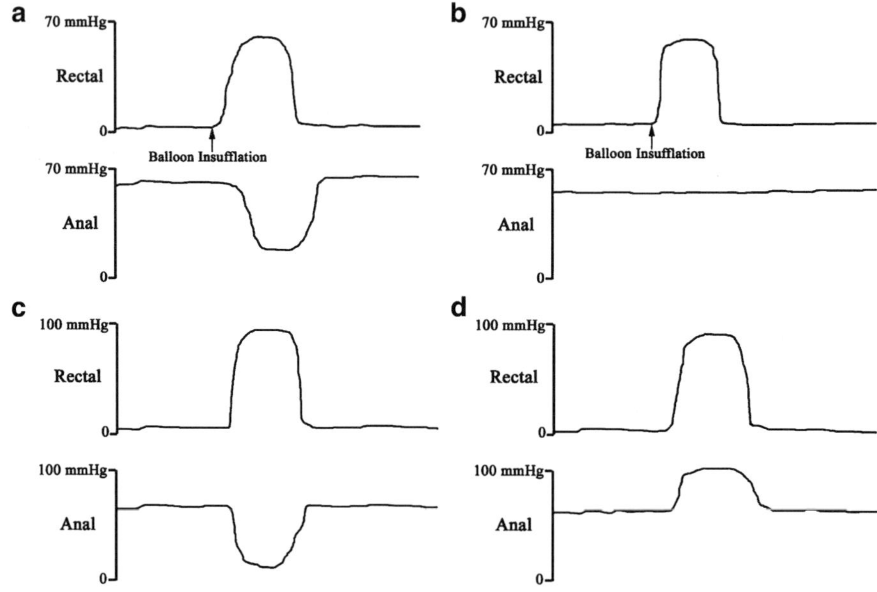

Fig. 11.3 (**a**) Normal RAIR. (**b**) Absent RAIR in an HD patient. (**c**) Normal balloon expulsion with normal EAS relaxation. (**d**) Dyssynergia with abnormal EAS contraction

electrical activity of the striated muscles of the region (EAS and levator ani) and to highlight the ability of such muscles to relax and contract appropriately [14].

Some of the key measurable values of routine ARM in pediatrics include the following: basal or resting anal pressure, maximal squeeze pressure, anal canal length, RAIR, conscious rectal sensation, initial urge to defecate, and defecatory dynamics:

1. Basal or resting anal sphincter pressure—A measure of the canal at rest which is reflective of overall muscle tone from both the EAS and IAS, with a >75% contribution from the latter [15]. There are several techniques for obtaining the anal resting pressure in WPM, including the station pull-through for circumferentially arranged and continuous withdrawal for spirally arranged catheters [5, 15].
2. Maximal squeeze pressure—By maximally squeezing or tightening the anal sphincter when directed, the patient produces a force on the catheter called the maximal squeeze pressure. Specifically, it is defined as the highest pressure increase over the average resting pressure (or the average of at least three of the highest pressures).
3. Anal canal length—The length of the anal canal is determined by the distance between the anal verge and the location of ≥5 mmHg pressure increase above rectal pressure.
4. RAIR—It is the reflexive relaxation of the IAS with stimulation with either stool accommodation or balloon inflation. To obtain the RAIR, the balloon is rapidly inflated and either rapidly deflated or left distended for a short period (10–20 s). No clear standard has been accepted as the criteria qualifying an intact reflex, although both a drop of ≥5 mmHg or ≥15% from resting pressure have been proposed (Fig. 11.3a, also see Fig. 11.4b) [5]. A dose response should be observed with both the overall degree and duration of such reflex increasing with increasing volumes of balloon inflation. Patients should be instructed not to provide voluntary squeeze during balloon inflation, as it may artificially affect the degree of the RAIR. Careful consideration must be made to ensure stable position of the catheter during this particular test, as movement within

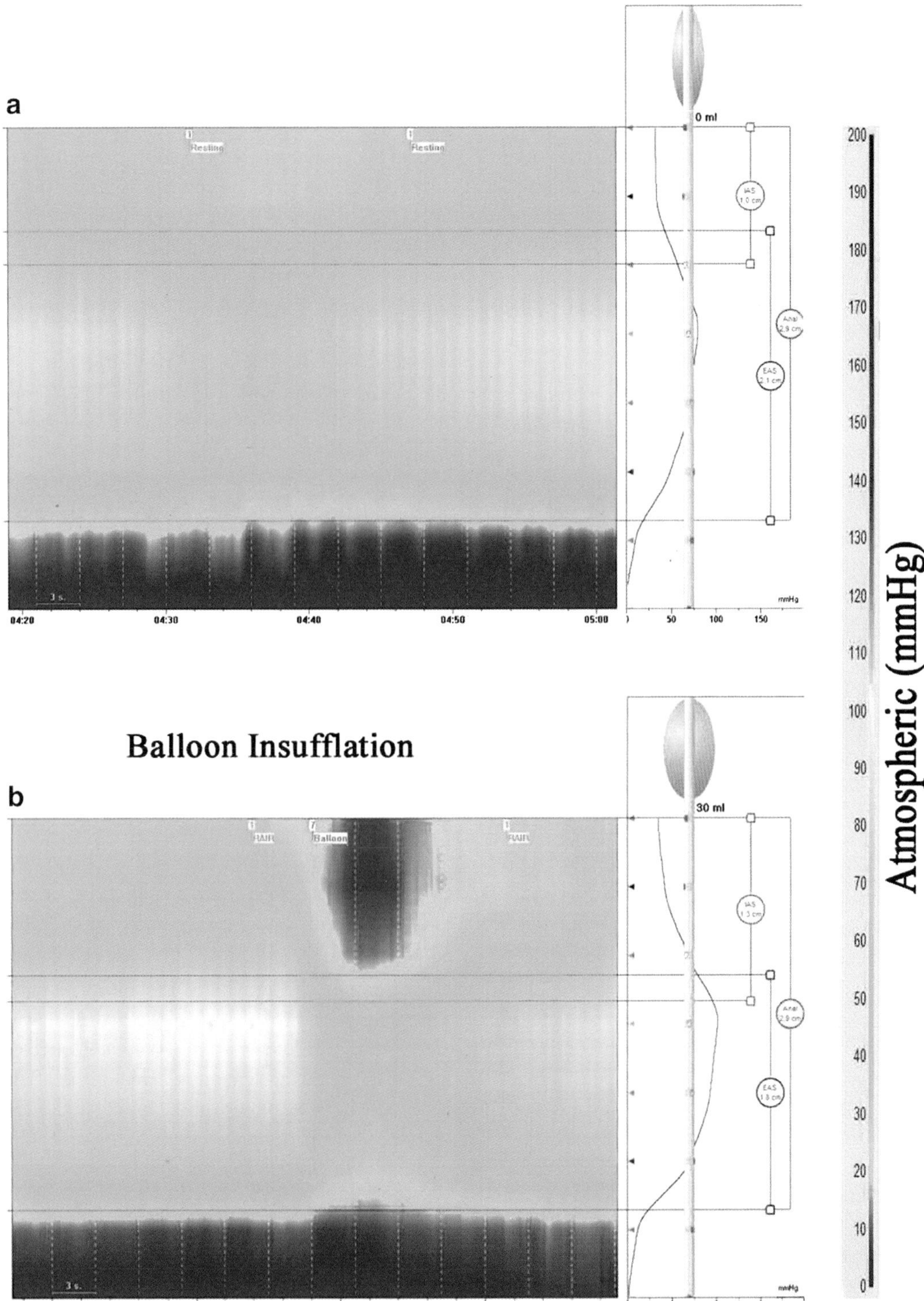

Fig. 11.4 High resolution ARM. (**a**) Normal at rest. (**b**) Normal RAIR. Printed with permission from Medical Measurement Systems

the canal can lead to a drop in pressure and subsequently, an inaccurate interpretation of an intact reflex. Of note, such catheter movement can be detected in HRM but may be missed with WPM.

5. Conscious rectal sensation and initial urge to defecate—Conscious rectal sensation has many variations in the literature including transient rectal sensation or conscious sensitivity threshold. Essentially, it is the smallest balloon volume that elicits a sensory response by the patient. In relation, the initial urge to defecate is the minimal balloon volume that the patient perceives as a need to defecate.
6. Balloon expulsion or defecatory dynamics—As the patient attempts to expel the balloon, often at varying volumes, the dynamic coordination of muscle contraction and relaxation can be assessed for evidence of dyssynergia by the balloon expulsion test [9, 10, 15].

Noticeably lacking are age-specific, normative ranges for the above measurements in the pediatric population. Table 11.1 lists several references for key measurements for various age groups using WPM, although differences in methodology and equipment certainly need to be acknowledged. HRM data in healthy pediatric subjects has not been published. Although there appears to be good correlation between methods, the absolute values obtained in HRM have been suggested to be relatively higher than those of WPM [16, 17]. Ultimately, given the lack of sufficient pediatric control data or standards, as well as the wide range of techniques and equipment, it is essential to always correlate data obtained by ARM with patient symptoms.

Diseases of the Anorectal Canal

Hirschsprung's Disease

Any patient with severe constipation presenting in infancy, constipation refractory to standard medical interventions, and of course, intestinal obstruction should be considered for HD. In HD, neural crest cell migration abnormally arrests leading to aganglionosis of the distal enteric plexuses, which in ARM is manifested by an absent RAIR (Fig. 11.3b) [18]. The absence of RAIR is suggestive but not diagnostic of HD. Such patients should then undergo a full-thickness rectal biopsy to detect the absence of ganglion cells, the universally accepted standard to confirm the diagnosis of HD. A systematic review by Lorijn et al. analyzed 22 studies of the three commonly used diagnostic studies to workup HD including rectal suction biopsy, ARM, and contrast enema, and found the sensitivity and specificity of the former to be 93% and 98%, respectively. In this study, ARM reached diagnostic accuracy similar to rectal suction biopsy with a sensitivity of 91% and specificity of 94% with both being far superior to contrast enema with a sensitivity of 70% and specificity of 83% [19]. There exists data that suggests detecting HD through ARM in younger children is inconsistent and unreliable with a 26% error rate in neonates in one study [20]. Such findings may reflect the technical challenges of choosing an appropriate catheter in terms of size and type, and of correct positioning of such a probe within the short, developing anorectal canal of neonates. Studies have suggested that the sleeve catheters, and air rather than balloon insufflation, yield the most reliable results in this younger age group [21, 22]. Based on the above information, ARM is considered an accurate, noninvasive screening test for HD particularly in children >1 year [23]. Beyond playing a role in just the initial diagnosis, ARM can be useful in patients with HD who have undergone surgery by characterizing the activity of the anorectal canal following pull-through surgery, which can vary among the different surgical techniques depending on the residual aganglionic rectum and IAS [24]. ARM can also help guide various treatment options such as sphincter myectomy or botulinum toxin injection [25, 26].

Anal Achalasia

ARM can also help in the diagnosis of anal achalasia. Patients with anal achalasia can present similarly to HD both clinically with intractable constipation and incontinence, and in ARM test-

Table 11.1 References for normal manometric measurements

	Technique	Healthy controls, *N*=	Ages	Anal resting tone (mmHg)	Rectal pressure (mmHg)	Anal canal length (cm)	Threshold of RAIR (mL)	Sensation threshold (mL)	Critical volume (mL)	Maximal squeeze pressure (mmHg)
Benninga [40]	WPM	13	8–16 years	55 ± 16			18 ± 10	19 ± 12	131 ± 31	182 ± 61
Hyman [5]	Not specified	20	5–16 years	67 ± 12		3.3 ± 0.8				140 ± 52
		16	>5 years				11 ± 5	14 ± 7	101 ± 39	
Kumar [7]	WPM	30	<1 month (GA 34–39 weeks)	31 ± 11		1.7 ± 0.3	10 ± 4			
		30	1–16 months	42 ± 9		1.9 ± 0.6	14 ± 10			
		30	18 month to 12 years	43 ± 9		3.0 ± 0.5	25 ± 12			
Li [41]	Not Specified	10	5–15 years					28 ± 11	117 ± 46	
Sutphen [42]	WPM	27	~7–12 years					30 ± 12	96 ± 38	142 ± 47
Benninga [21]	Sleeve, WPM	22	Neonates (PMA 30–33 weeks)	32 ± 4[a]	9 ± 2		1.6 ± 0.3[b]			
De Lorijn [22]	Sleeve, WPM	16	Neonates (PMA 27–30 weeks)	25 ± 11[a]	7 ± 5		3.4 ± 1.6[b]			

GA gestational age, PMA postmenstrual age
[a]Anal sphincter pressure
[b]Air insufflation

ing with the absence of an intact RAIR. Anal achalasia is differentiated from HD, however, by the presence of ganglion cells on rectal biopsy. In patients with anal achalasia, also referred to as ultrashort HD, the IAS fails to properly relax for reasons that are not well characterized [27]. Similar to postsurgical HD patients above, treatment approaches are geared towards inducing IAS relaxation either through the injection of botulinum toxin or internal sphincter myectomy. Both approaches have demonstrated good outcomes in pediatric studies [25, 28]. An interesting subset of anorectal motility dysfunction is found in patients with food-allergy related constipation. Studies have shown hypertensive resting anal pressures and partial relaxation on rectal distention, somewhat similar to anal achalasia, which improves with allergen food elimination [29].

Neuromuscular Disease

Neuromuscular disease can also be associated with anorectal dysfunction. Patients with conditions such as myotonic dystrophy, Duchenne muscular dystrophy and congenital myopathy commonly present with constipation, fecal incontinence and fecal impaction which can even progress to megacolon and/or chronic intestinal obstruction. While there are no specific findings on ARM that can diagnosis neuromuscular disease, there are several patterns that can be supportive of such a diagnosis. Consistent with the overall presentation of weakness, patients with neuromuscular disease often demonstrate low anal resting and squeeze pressures [5]. Additionally, patients with neuromyopathy often have an intact RAIR but will often lack a normal dose response, as the degree and duration of the relaxation will fail to increase with increasing balloon volumes [30]. Also notable in this subset of patients is an exaggerated rebound contraction following the RAIR [31]. Patients with spinal cord lesions such as tethered cord have notable variations in ARM such as anal spasms with balloon dilatation and a left-shifted RAIR dose–response curve. Thus, ARM may be helpful to identify which patients with intractable constipation may be at increased risk of spinal cord lesions requiring further investigation with MRI [32]. Lastly, ARM can be helpful in the management of patients with imperforate anus by assessing postsurgical sensory and functional capabilities. Successful management can be challenging for patients with neuromyopathic disease. Stool softeners, though helpful in improving constipation, have the tendency to worsen incontinence. However, establishing a scheduled toileting regimen in conjunction with intermittent stimulants or enemas to empty bowel contents can be an effective approach for patients with neuromuscular disease [5].

Dyssynergic Defecation

Chronic functional constipation is a common problem in the pediatric population and is believed to represent up to 95% of all cases of constipation in children [3]. Dyssynergia, perhaps the most prevalent form of pediatric functional constipation, occurs when the abdominal, anorectal and pelvic floor muscles are not properly coordinated during attempted defecation. Again, in order for effective stooling to occur, a rise in the propulsive forces of the rectum must be countered by the relaxation of the EAS and subsequent drop in anal pressures to permit forward passage of stool (Fig. 11.3c). Typically, dyssynergia is a learned behavior resulting from withholding tendencies of constipated children with a history of painful, dry bowel movements—in children most commonly characterized by a paradoxical tightening of the EAS with defecation (Fig. 11.3d) [33]. Dyssynergia describes the pathophysiologic correlate of functional retentive constipation where such withholding behavior initiates a vicious cycle of firm stool accumulation, impaction, over flow incontinence and ultimately, worsening intractable constipation. Pediatric dyssynergic defecation is identifiable by ARM through the balloon expulsion test, which evaluates the dynamic defecatory process. Four distinct patterns of dyssynergia have been identified, each defined by two parameters: rectal pressures (appropriate versus insufficient increase) and anal sphincter pressures (anal contraction versus incomplete relaxation). Additional ARM findings often associated with dyssynergia include evidence of sensory dysfunction with elevated minimal sensory and urge to defecate thresholds [34]. If dyssynergia is diagnosed through ARM, patients and families can be offered reassurance that symptoms are of a functional and treatable cause with therapy directed towards stool softening and biofeedback therapy. Biofeedback involves the use of auditory or visual sensory displays, often provided by EMG, which represent anorectal activity allowing patients to see and react to their anorectal and abdominal muscle actions. Biofeedback has shown to be highly effective in improving bowel function in several adult randomized-controlled trials [35–38]. Studies in children have not shown the same level of efficacy with biofeedback but pediatric studies are limited [33, 39] (Fig. 11.4).

Conclusion

ARM is a safe, well-tolerated procedure that is highly useful in the investigation of anorectal canal abnormalities. Patients who typically benefit from ARM include those with severe constipation, fecal incontinence and anorectal pain—symptoms which are often chronic and quite distressing for patients and their families. There is a wide range of techniques and specific tests that can be performed during ARM such that each individual study needs to be tailored to the patient based on their age, capacity for participation, symptoms and information that is desired to be obtained. Data ascertainable by ARM includes resting, active, reflexive, and sensory threshold pressures of the anorectal canal, as well as overall dynamic function and anal canal length. Such data can help rule out both HD and anal achalasia, and support the diagnosis of anorectal canal neuromyopathy and pediatric dyssynergia. Fundamental, however, is correlating ARM finding with the patient's symptomatology. When appropriately applied, ARM creates a highly informative, descriptive picture of anorectal function that elucidates underlying pathophysiology and offers customized treatment interventions to help patients gain normalized stool function.

References

1. Hyman PE, Milla PJ, Benninga MA, et al. Childhood functional gastrointestinal disorders: neonate/toddler. Gastroenterology. 2006;130(5):1519–26.
2. Rasquin A, Di Lorenzo C, Forbes D, et al. Childhood functional gastrointestinal disorders: child/adolescent. Gastroenterology. 2006;130(5):1527–37.
3. Loening-Baucke V. Constipation in children. Curr Opin Pediatr. 1994;6(5):556–61.
4. Schuster atlas of gastrointestinal motility in health and disease. 2nd ed. Hamilton, ON: B.C. Decker; 2002.
5. Pediatric gastrointestinal motility disorders. 1st ed. New York: Academy Professional Information Services, Inc; 1994.
6. Practical guide to anorectal testing. 1st ed. New York: Igaku-Shoin Medical Publishers, Inc; 1990.
7. Kumar S, Ramadan S, Gupta V, et al. Manometric tests of anorectal function in 90 healthy children: a clinical study from Kuwait. J Pediatr Surg. 2009;44(9):1786–90.
8. Rao SSC. Advances in diagnostic assessment of fecal incontinence and dyssynergic defecation. Clin Gastroenterol Hepatol. 2010;8(11):910–9.
9. Rao SSC, Azpiroz F, Diamant N, et al. Minimum standards of anorectal manometry. Neurogastroenterol Motil. 2002;14(5):553–9.
10. Di Lorenzo C, Hillemeier C, Hyman P, et al. Manometry studies in children: minimum standards for procedures. Neurogastroenterol Motil. 2002;14(4):411–20.
11. Paskins JR, Lawson JO, Clayden GS. The effect of ketamine anesthesia on anorectal manometry. J Pediatr Surg. 1984;19(3):289–91.
12. Pfefferkorn MD, Croffie JM, Corkins MR, Gupta SK, Fitzgerald JF. Impact of sedation and anesthesia on the rectoanal inhibitory reflex in children. J Pediatr Gastroenterol Nutr. 2004;38(3):324–7.
13. Liu T, Yi C, Chen C, Liu H, Chen T. Influence of intravenous propofol sedation on anorectal manometry in healthy adults. Am J Med Sci. 2009;337(6):429–31.
14. Scott SM, Gladman MA. Manometric, sensorimotor, and neurophysiologic evaluation of anorectal function. Gastroenterol Clin North Am. 2008;37(3):511–38. vii.
15. Diamant NE, Kamm MA, Wald A, Whitehead WE. AGA technical review on anorectal testing techniques. Gastroenterology. 1999;116(3):735–60.
16. Puglia M, Fachnie E, Bercik P. A Comparison of high resolution and water-perfused manometry for anorectal disorders. Canadian Digestive Disease Week Abstract; 2009.
17. Jones MP, Post J, Crowell MD. High-resolution manometry in the evaluation of anorectal disorders: a simultaneous comparison with water-perfused manometry. Am J Gastroenterol. 2007;102(4):850–5.

18. Heanue TA, Pachnis V. Enteric nervous system development and Hirschsprung's disease: advances in genetic and stem cell studies. Nat Rev Neurosci. 2007;8(6):466–79.
19. de Lorijn F, Kremer LCM, Reitsma JB, Benninga MA. Diagnostic tests in Hirschsprung disease: a systematic review. J Pediatr Gastroenterol Nutr. 2006;42(5):496–505.
20. Meunier P, Marechal JM, Mollard P. Accuracy of the manometric diagnosis of Hirschsprung's disease. J Pediatr Surg. 1978;13(4):411–5.
21. Benninga MA, Omari TI, Haslam RR, et al. Characterization of anorectal pressure and the anorectal inhibitory reflex in healthy preterm and term infants. J Pediatr. 2001;139(2):233–7.
22. de Lorijn F, Omari TI, Kok JH, Taminiau JAJM, Benninga MA. Maturation of the rectoanal inhibitory reflex in very premature infants. J Pediatr. 2003;143(5):630–3.
23. de Lorijn F, Reitsma JB, Voskuijl WP, et al. Diagnosis of Hirschsprung's disease: a prospective, comparative accuracy study of common tests. J Pediatr. 2005;146(6):787–92.
24. Mishalany HG, Woolley MM. Postoperative functional and manometric evaluation of patients with Hirschsprung's disease. J Pediatr Surg. 1987;22(5):443–6.
25. Chumpitazi BP, Fishman SJ, Nurko S. Long-term clinical outcome after botulinum toxin injection in children with nonrelaxing internal anal sphincter. Am J Gastroenterol. 2009;104(4):976–83.
26. Blair GK, Murphy JJ, Fraser GC. Internal sphincterotomy in post-pull-through Hirschsprung's disease. J Pediatr Surg. 1996;31(6):843–5.
27. Doodnath R, Puri P. Internal anal sphincter achalasia. Semin Pediatr Surg. 2009;18(4):246–8.
28. De Caluwé D, Yoneda A, Akl U, Puri P. Internal anal sphincter achalasia: outcome after internal sphincter myectomy. J Pediatr Surg. 2001;36(5):736–8.
29. Borrelli O, Barbara G, Di Nardo G, et al. Neuroimmune interaction and anorectal motility in children with food allergy-related chronic constipation. Am J Gastroenterol. 2009;104(2):454–63.
30. Lecointe-Besancon I, Leroy F, Devroede G, et al. A comparative study of esophageal and anorectal motility in myotonic dystrophy. Dig Dis Sci. 1999;44(6):1090–9.
31. Eckardt VF, Nix W. The anal sphincter in patients with myotonic muscular dystrophy. Gastroenterology. 1991;100(2):424–30.
32. Siddiqui A, Rosen R, Nurko S. Anorectal manometry may identify children with spinal cord lesions. J Pediatr Gastroenterol Nutr. 2011;53(5):507–11.
33. Loening-Baucke V. Biofeedback treatment for chronic constipation and encopresis in childhood: long-term outcome. Pediatrics. 1995;96(1 Pt 1):105–10.
34. Rao SSC. Dyssynergic defecation and biofeedback therapy. Gastroenterol Clin North Am. 2008;37(3):569–86. viii.
35. Rao SSC, Seaton K, Miller M, et al. Randomized controlled trial of biofeedback, sham feedback, and standard therapy for dyssynergic defecation. Clin Gastroenterol Hepatol. 2007;5(3):331–8.
36. Chiarioni G, Whitehead WE, Pezza V, Morelli A, Bassotti G. Biofeedback is superior to laxatives for normal transit constipation due to pelvic floor dyssynergia. Gastroenterology. 2006;130(3):657–64.
37. Chiarioni G, Salandini L, Whitehead WE. Biofeedback benefits only patients with outlet dysfunction, not patients with isolated slow transit constipation. Gastroenterology. 2005;129(1):86–97.
38. Heymen S, Scarlett Y, Jones K, et al. Randomized, controlled trial shows biofeedback to be superior to alternative treatments for patients with pelvic floor dyssynergia-type constipation. Dis Colon Rectum. 2007;50(4):428–41.
39. van der Plas RN, Benninga MA, Büller HA, et al. Biofeedback training in treatment of childhood constipation: a randomised controlled study. Lancet. 1996;348(9030):776–80.
40. Benninga MA, Wijers OB, van der Hoeven CW, et al. Manometry, profilometry, and endosonography: normal physiology and anatomy of the anal canal in healthy children. J Pediatr Gastroenterol Nutr. 1994;18(1):68–77.
41. Li Z, Dong M, Wang Z. Functional constipation in children: investigation and management of anorectal motility. World J Pediatr. 2008;4(1):45–8.
42. Sutphen J, Borowitz S, Ling W, Cox DJ, Kovatchev B. Anorectal manometric examination in encopretic-constipated children. Dis Colon Rectum. 1997;40(9):1051–5.

Esophageal pH and Impedance Monitoring

12

Rachel Rosen and Eric Chiou

Introduction

Gastroesophageal reflux disease (GERD) is defined by the reflux of gastric contents into the esophagus resulting in well-defined symptoms and complications [1, 2]. In many cases, GERD can be diagnosed based on history alone; however, when patients present with atypical complaints or do not respond to medical therapy, objective testing may be necessary to assess the frequency and duration of acid reflux, or to document the association between gastroesophageal reflux (GER) and specific symptoms. Diagnostic techniques designed to discriminate between physiologic and pathologic reflux have been developed.

Esophageal pH monitoring, which employs a pH electrode to detect acid reflux in the distal esophagus, was first introduced in 1969 [3]. Over the years the advantages and limitations of traditional, catheter-based esophageal pH monitoring have become better understood, with a subsequent evolution to newer diagnostic techniques. Wireless methods to detect acidic contents in the esophagus have now become available (Bravo pH capsule) and pharyngeal probes have recently been introduced (Restech). Additionally, multichannel intraluminal impedance with pH (MII-pH) has been introduced as a novel method to measure acid and non-acid reflux. In the present chapter, we will discuss the technical details, clinical indications and applications of these diagnostic techniques for the dynamic detection of reflux episodes.

R. Rosen, M.D., M.P.H. (✉)
Harvard Medical School, Center for Motility and Functional Gastrointestinal Disorders Children's Hospital Boston, 300 Longwood Avenue, Boston, MA 02115, USA
e-mail: rachel.rosen@childrens.harvard.edu

E. Chiou, M.D.
Center for Motility and Functional Gastrointestinal Disorders Children's Hospital Boston, 300 Longwood Avenue, Boston, MA 02115, USA

Catheter-Based Esophageal pH-Monitoring

Catheter-based esophageal pH monitoring is the most widely available and commonly used method to document abnormal acid exposure and correlate symptoms with acid reflux episodes. Testing quantifies the frequency and duration of acid reflux episodes, usually over an 18–24 h period. Most ambulatory catheter-based pH probes contain a small antimony electrode connected to a portable data logger that records intraesophageal pH, as well as events during the study, such as symptoms, meals, position changes, and activity. The methodology of esophageal pH monitoring has become relatively standardized with specific guidelines for use in children [4, 5].

C. Faure et al. (eds.), *Pediatric Neurogastroenterology: Gastrointestinal Motility and Functional Disorders in Children*, Clinical Gastroenterology,
DOI 10.1007/978-1-60761-709-9_12,

Electrode Placement

Appropriate placement of the pH electrode relative to the lower esophageal sphincter (LES) is very important in order to gather accurate data. At higher distances above the LES, there is a linear decrease in acid exposure time, which decreases the sensitivity of the test. Adult protocols typically recommend that the pH electrode be positioned 5 cm above the superior margin of the LES in order to decrease the risk of slipping into the stomach during swallow-induced shortening of the esophagus [6]. Stationary esophageal manometry, usually performed as a separate procedure, is optimal for determination of LES location. In children however, this additional invasive procedure is not routinely performed. Strobel's formula may be used to approximate the esophageal length for initial placement of the pH electrode above the LES [length from nares to LES (cm) = 5 + 0.252(height)] [7]. In the absence of manometry however, fluoroscopy should be used to confirm placement of the sensor at the level of the third vertebral body above the diaphragm, according to recommendations from the Working Group of the European Society of Pediatric Gastroenterology and Nutrition [5].

Recording Conditions

The optimal duration of monitoring should be at least 18 h, including a day and a night period [5]. Shorter studies have been proposed (30 min, 2 h, 8 h, and 12 h studies) but no study period has been found to be sufficiently sensitive or reproducible to replace the 24 h studies [8, 9]. Instructions for feeding and activity during the study should represent a balance between maintaining a degree of standardization and recreating a normal lifestyle with minimal restrictions. Although a strict standardized diet is generally not necessary, a minimum of three meals should be included. Meal periods are routinely excluded from the analysis because the pH probe cannot differentiate swallowed acidic contents from refluxate [10, 11]. Documentation of patient position and activity during the study should also be recorded since the effect of body position on different patterns of GER has been well reported; acid reflux is more common in the supine and right lateral positions than the prone or left lateral positions [4, 12]. Depending on the aim of the study, H_2-blockers and proton-pump inhibitors should be stopped at least 3 or 7 days prior to the study, respectively. Adult data in healthy volunteers suggests that intragastric pH returns to baseline within 2–4 days after stopping acid suppression [13].

Definitions and Criteria

After the study is completed, data is downloaded from the data logger and analyzed with computer software. A reflux episode is usually defined as a drop in pH below 4 that lasts for more than 5 s [14]. The reflux index, which is the percentage of time of the entire duration of the investigation with pH <4 is generally considered the single most important variable in clinical practice for both adults and children [4, 6]. A pH of 4 is generally accepted as the optimum cutoff in both children and adults, based on early studies of correlating acid exposure with heartburn [15–17]. The threshold of pH < 4 also provides the best discrimination between subjects with proven reflux disease (the presence of esophagitis) and asymptomatic controls [6, 18, 19]. However, there is significant overlap between the reflux profiles of patients with and without symptoms and in patients with and without esophagitis because there are many possible criteria that define pathologic reflux, including the number of episodes greater than 5 min, the longest reflux episode, the percentage of time pH < 4, and the total number of reflux events. Several scores have been proposed, including the DeMeester score and the Boix-Ochoa score, but the current gold standard for reporting pH monitoring results is the reflux index, which is the percentage of time of the entire duration of the investigation with pH < 4 [4, 6].

Normal Ranges

Normative data are essential to guide interpretation of pH monitoring results and distinguish between physiologic versus pathologic reflux. Published pediatric data is rather limited, however, due to the difficulty in obtaining data from truly healthy and asymptomatic volunteers. In some studies, "normals" were obtained from children hospitalized for GER evaluations who turned out to be asymptomatic during the time of pH monitoring [20] or were found to have other causes for their gastrointestinal symptoms [21]. Overall, studies suggest that physiologic acid reflux is a common occurrence in infants during the first year of life, with decreased acid exposure found in older children and adults [20–24]. Based on the available data, the North American Society for Pediatric Gastroenterology, Hepatology, and Nutrition (NASPGHAN) has established guidelines that define the upper limit of normal of the reflux index up to 12% in the first year of life and up to 6% thereafter [4].

Diagnostic Accuracy and Reproducibility

The estimated sensitivity of pH monitoring for predicting esophagitis in children is good, ranging from 83 to 100%, but the severity of reflux as measured by pH monitoring has not been found to necessarily correlate with the severity of symptoms [15, 25]. For children with non-erosive reflux disease (NERD), the clinical utility of pH monitoring has not been well studied. In adults, there is significant overlap between patients with NERD and normal patients; approximately 40% of adults with NERD had pathologic reflux but 60% did not, making the differentiation of normal patients from NERD patients difficult based on reflux burden alone [26, 27].

Reports on intrasubject reproducibility of esophageal pH results in children have had varied results. Vandenplas et al. studied infants and children over two consecutive 24-h periods; the correlation coefficients for the reflux index and number of reflux episodes between day 1 and day 2 were 0.95 and 0.98, respectively [28]. In contrast, the correlation coefficient for the reflux index reported by Mahajan and colleagues was only 0.62 between day 1 and day 2 [29]. In another study, 9 out of 30 children had discordant (normal versus abnormal) results between the two recording days, yielding an overall reproducibility of 70% [30]. Hampton et al found that there was discordance between day 1 and day 2 studies in 62% of infants. An additional study was done in the pediatric population comparing the amount of reflux in children who has pH monitoring with and without anesthesia; Hampton et al found that there was discordance between day 1 and day 2 studies in 62% of infants. An additional study was done in the pediatric population comparing the amount of reflux in children who has pH monitoring with and without anesthesia; McCallion et al found that the reproducibility of the percent time pH<4 was 85%. [31, 32]. Overall, there appears to be some degree of day-to-day variability among patients; whether these differences are clinically significant is debatable. When the clinical picture is unclear, consideration should be given for repeat testing.

The next question to ask is whether obtaining pH probe results translate into improvement in clinical outcome. Malfroot et al. found that 75% of patients with abnormal pH monitoring experienced symptomatic improvement in their pulmonary symptoms suggesting that it accurately measures pathologic reflux [33]. A randomized control trial of acid suppression in children with pathologic reflux by pH monitoring showed that between 69 and 74% of patients with pathologic reflux experience symptomatic improvement with acid suppression, suggesting that pH probe accurately predicts clinical response [34]. There is very limited data on the impact of this test on clinical outcome; the majority of data is on the correlation of esophagitis with clinical outcome and since there is a correlation between esophagitis and pH abnormalities, it may be reasonable to assume that there is a correlation between reflux burden and symptom improvement but there are few studies to support this directly.

Symptom Correlation

In addition to the quantification of reflux, 24-h esophageal pH monitoring also provides the opportunity to assess the temporal relationship between episodes of reflux and onset of symptoms. This may be especially helpful for patients with nonspecific or extraesophageal symptoms. Lam et al. found that using a two minute time window was best for correlation of chest pain with reflux, although the optimal time window for symptom–reflux association may vary depending on the particular symptom of interest [35].

Several statistical methods have been developed to better quantify the association of symptoms and reflux episodes but there is no conclusive data proving one index to be superior to the others. The symptom index (SI) is defined as the percentage of symptom episodes that are related to reflux, with a score of ≥50% suggesting a positive relationship between symptom and reflux [36, 37]. A second approach is the symptom sensitivity index (SSI), which divides the number of reflux episodes associated with symptoms by the total number of reflux episodes [38]. An arbitrary cutoff of 10% or higher is commonly used to indicate a significant association between symptoms and reflux episodes. The SI may overestimate the relationship between reflux and symptoms when there are a high number of reflux episodes, and the SSI is more likely to be positive when the number of symptom episodes is high. More recently, the symptom association probability (SAP) has been introduced. Using Fisher's exact test, this method expresses the statistical likelihood that the patient's symptoms are related to reflux [39]. By statistical convention, SAP ≥95% indicates that the probability that the observed association between reflux and the symptom occurred by chance is <5%.

While these indices are helpful for research, it is essential to determine if these indices predict symptom response to acid suppression. Taghavi et al. found that the SSI and the SAP predicted a response to acid suppression but this was an imperfect relationship. Although patients with a positive relationship between symptoms and reflux have been shown to more likely to respond to medical and surgical therapy, further prospective validation studies are needed [40, 41]. Unfortunately, all of these indices rely on the patient to accurately record symptoms immediately as they occur. Additionally, while these may suggest a temporal association, they do not always prove causality.

Pharyngeal pH Monitoring

Proving causality is even more difficult in the patient with extraesophageal manifestations of reflux (hoarseness, recurrent pneumonia, otitis media, and sinusitis) as there is an often unsatisfactory correlation between esophageal reflux and extraesophageal symptoms. As a result, the measurement of oropharyngeal acidification has been proposed as a more accurate indicator of proximal reflux than dual channel pH probes. The Restech Dx-pH probe (Respiratory Technology Corp., San Diego, CA) is a recently introduced, transnasal, oropharyngeal pH sensor. Besides being less invasive than traditional catheters, the antimony-based sensor is also designed to measure the pH of both liquid and aerosolized droplets in the posterior oropharynx. Investigators have recently proposed the use of less acidic pH thresholds or relative drops in pH to identify episodes of reflux in the posterior oropharynx, based on the hypothesis that the threshold of pH <4 may be too stringent and insensitive and that pH changes above 4 may be damaging to laryngeal tissue [42, 43].

The clinical validity of these alternative criteria, however, is not yet established. A previous study which employed pharyngeal pH monitoring found that 92% of pharyngeal pH decreases of 1–2 pH units and 66% of pH <4 events were artifactual or independent of esophageal acidification [44]. Moreover, recent studies which combined the Restech oropharyngeal pH probe with concurrent esophageal pH monitoring in adults have also found inconsistencies between oropharyngeal and distal esophageal pH data, with higher numbers of non-correlating oropharyngeal pH events during sleep and supine periods [45, 46].

Chiou et al., who used the Restech probe in children, found that a high proportion of oropharyngeal pH events did not correlate with distal reflux by pH-MII, especially with the use of alternative pH criteria and during supine periods [47]. One reason for this finding may be that decreased salivary flow during sleep leads to drying of the oropharyngeal pH electrode and subsequently false readings. This phenomenon was initially described by Wiener et al. as "pharyngeal pseudo-reflux" in reference to artifacts with a gradual descent to pH <4 without a corresponding fall in esophageal pH [48]. The utility of pharyngeal monitoring is still questionable and additional studies are underway to validate its use.

Wireless pH Monitoring

One of the main limitations to all of the catheter-based tests is that patient discomfort can be significant, such that their typical eating and activity patterns are altered to the point that the study may not be representative of a "typical" day for the patient. To overcome this limitation, a wireless method has recently been devised. The Bravo pH system (Medtronic, Shoreview, MN) consists of an antimony electrode contained within a small capsule which is pinned to the mucosal wall of the distal esophagus during an upper GI endoscopy and transmits pH data wirelessly to a portable receiver using radiotelemetry. The capsule can remain in place for up to 4 or more days but typically is in place for at least 2 days allowing for extended recording. In adults, the capsule is placed 6 cm above the squamocolumnar junction, with placement confirmation by endoscopy [49]. There are currently no specific guidelines for placement in children. Adult series have reported significant chest discomfort, early detachment of the capsule, perforation, and the need for endoscopic removal of the capsule but because of the small case series in pediatrics, the extent of Bravo complications in children is still largely unknown [49–51].

In published studies of children older than 4 years old, pH monitoring with the Bravo capsule was better tolerated than the transnasal catheter in terms of appetite, activity, and satisfaction, with no significant complications other than mild chest discomfort [52–54]. Because of the prolonged recording, using this technique there is additional opportunity for the correlation of symptoms with reflux, particularly symptoms that do not typically occur on a daily basis.

Only one study to date has compared the Bravo capsule side-by-side with a simultaneous transnasal pH catheter in children. Croffie and colleagues found no significant difference in the reflux index obtained by the two devices on day 1; on day 2, however, the median reflux index recorded by the Bravo capsule was significantly higher compared to day 1 of both the capsule and catheter [54]. The clinical significance of this is unclear, with only one patient having discordant (abnormal versus normal) results between the 2 days of recording.

Several pediatric studies have compared the pH results between day 1 and day 2 of the Bravo studies. In a study of Bravo in 23 children, Gunnarsdottir et al. found no statistically significant differences in the reflux profiles between the first 24 h and the entire 48-h recording but 7 children received a different classification (normal versus abnormal) between day 1 and 2 [55]. In a series of 145 Bravo studies in children, there were significantly more long duration events and a higher percentage of time that the pH was less than 4 in the upright position on day 1 compared to day 2 [52]. Currently, there is no consensus on whether the interpretation of the results should rely on the first or the second day or average of the days; outcome studies are needed to make this determination.

Currently, Bravo is a reasonable alternative for patients that cannot tolerate a catheter-based system, but the need for anesthesia for placement (and the resultant associated costs) combined with the need to stop acid suppression therapy may limit its utility in becoming the gold standard reflux tool [51, 56].

Proximal Esophageal pH Monitoring

Proximal esophageal pH monitoring is designed to assess the proximal extent of acid reflux and its relationship with oropharyngeal and respiratory symptoms. Studies employing dual-probe pH monitoring of both the distal and proximal esophagus have provided mixed results in terms of sensitivity and specificity for extra-esophageal manifestations of reflux, intra-subject reproducibility and prediction of response to therapy [57, 58]. Additionally, there is poor correlation between the acidification in the proximal sensor with the acidification in the distal esophagus raising the question of whether the proximal acidification has any significance in the absence of distal acidification. In pediatrics, because there are a limited number of catheter sizes and a wide range of esophageal lengths, it is difficult to ensure that the proximal sensor is uniformly in the same location without compromising distal sensor location. Furthermore, it is unclear which pH level produces damage to bronchial, laryngeal and pharyngeal tissue and while the literature is based on a pH cutoff of 4, non-acid reflux with pH 4–7 may also play a clinically significant role in aerodigestive diseases [59, 60]. At the current time however, the clinical advantage of proximal esophageal pH monitoring in children is not yet clearly proven and more studies are needed to validate their use.

Multichannel Intraluminal Impedance (pH-MII)

MII-pH uses sensors distributed throughout the esophagus to measure resistance to flow rather than pH changes alone. The advantages of pH-MII are the following: (1) the sensors are able to determine the directionality of flow so that reflux events can be distinguished from swallows; (2) multiple sensors throughout the esophagus allows for accurate determination of refluxate height; (3) the sensors, which do not rely on pH, are able to detect non-acid reflux which is common in the pediatric population, in the acid suppressed patient and in the postprandial period [61–63]; and (4) because liquid and gas have different impedances, the sensors can differentiate the composition of the refluxed material.

Traditionally, there are seven impedance sensors placed in series which generate six impedance waves, one for each pair of adjacent sensors (Fig. 12.1). Sensors are distributed throughout the esophagus at different spacing depending on the size of the catheter that is used (infant for ages 0–2, pediatric for ages 2–10 and adult for children older than 10). Since the impedance sensors cannot differentiate between acid versus non-acid material, a distal pH sensor has been added to the catheter allowing the clinician to determine whether the flow across the catheter is acidic, weakly acidic, or non-acidic, depending on the pH value.

The pH-MII catheter is inserted through the nose and the catheter is positioned so the distal pH sensor is at the third vertebral body above the diaphragmatic angle (Fig. 12.2) [5]. Studies are performed for 24 h and, as with pH studies, meals are conventionally excluded from analyses. Typically, when performing pH studies, acid suppression medications are stopped a minimum of 48 h prior to testing because the pH probe cannot detect non-acid reflux, which is prevalent in the acid suppressed patient [64]. Since the pH-MII catheter can detect acid and non-acid reflux, the studies can be performed off or on acid suppression therapy, although adult studies suggest that symptom correlation may be improved if medications are stopped prior to pH-MII testing [65].

Definitions

A liquid episode is defined as a drop in impedance to 50% of the baseline value or below, with a subsequent recovery back to 50% of the baseline value. This drop in impedance needs to be visualized in at least the distal two channels to be considered "reflux." Gas reflux is defined as simultaneous increases in impedance to greater than 8,000 Ω in two or more channels. Mixed reflux has components of both liquid and gas. There are three types of reflux episodes that can be detected: (1) acid reflux events detected by both the impedance and the pH-sensor, (2) non-acid reflux events, which are detected only by the impedance sensors, and (3) pH-only events, which are detected only by the pH sensor, without any impedance changes. In some studies, non-acid reflux is further subdivided into weakly acidic reflux (pH 4–7) and alkaline reflux (pH>7). The importance of pH-only events is still questionable

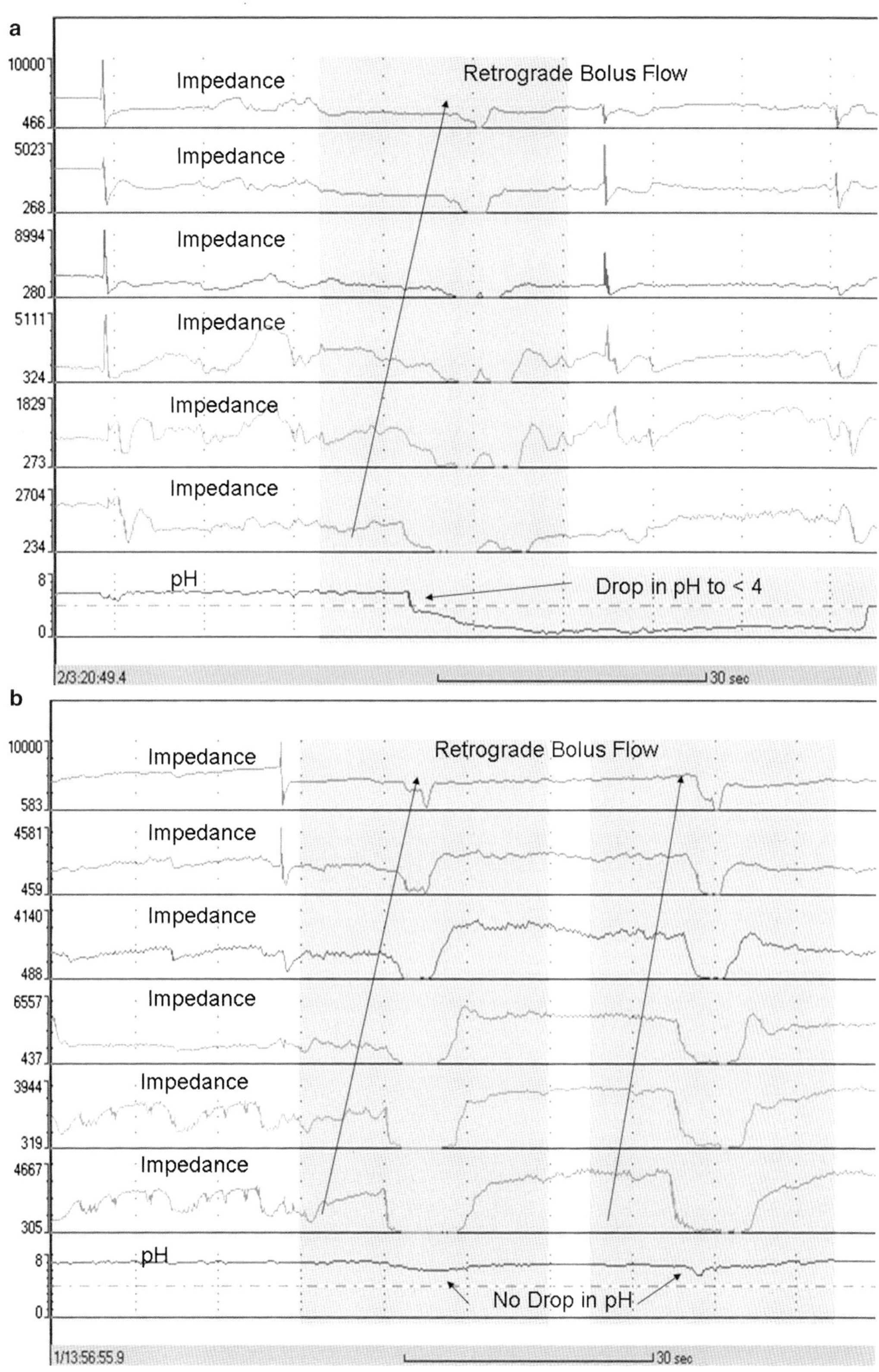

Fig. 12.1 Examples of retrograde bolus movement up the esophagus across six areas of the esophagus indicating an acid (**a**) and non-acid (**b**) reflux episode. The episodes are categorized as acid or non-acid depending on if there is a pH drop to less than 4 during the impedance-detected episode

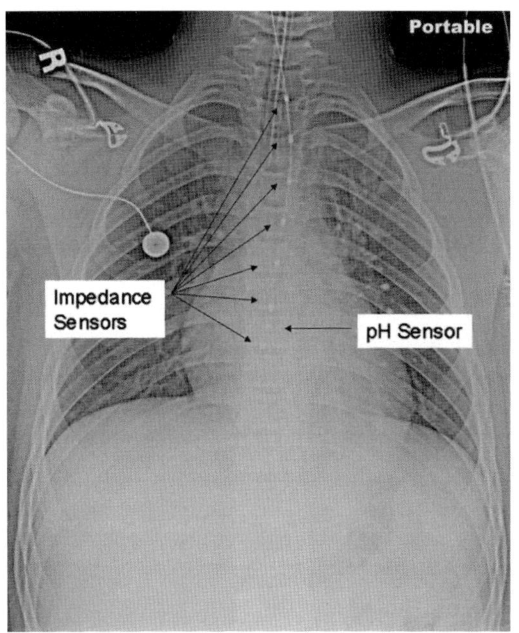

Fig. 12.2 Chest X-ray showing placement of an impedance catheter. The catheter is positioned such that pH electrode is at the third vertebral body above the diaphragmatic angle

and the current theory is that pH only episodes represent very distal reflux that does not meet criteria for an impedance detected event (i.e., the reflux does not reach the required three impedance sensors).

Interpretation

The interpretation of impedance tracings is time-consuming and in most research laboratories is still done by hand even though there is commercially available analysis software. Roman et al. studied the concordance of the automated software (Sandhill Scientific) to detect reflux events compared to a manual scoring of the events. Agreement between visual and automated analysis was good (Kendall's coefficient $W>0.750$, $P<0.01$) for all parameters. They also analyzed symptom detection, and concluded that despite good agreement with manual analysis, automatic analysis overestimated the number of non-acid reflux events [66]. Manual analysis remains the gold standard to detect an association between symptoms and non-acid reflux events [66]. Hemmink et al. determined the sensitivity of the automated software (Medical Measurement Systems) and found that sensitivity of the software was 73±4%. Additionally, the automated software incorrectly determined a symptom association 16–20% of the time, depending on the symptom index used [67]. There are selected populations where the impedance software is particularly inaccurate; manual interpretation is critical in the presence of esophagitis or if there is a motility disorder, such as achalasia or esophageal atresia, all of which lower impedance baselines. The low impedance baseline results in significant underestimations of the amount of reflux present.

Sensitivity

Impedance sensors have been shown to accurately detect boluses in the esophagus down to 0.1 ml using fluoroscopy [68, 69]. The difficulty in determining the sensitivity of pH-MII is which gold standard technique should be used as the basis for comparison; the pediatric studies have used reflux detected by any device (pH-MII and pH probe) as the gold standard. Rosen et al. found that the sensitivity of pH-MII was 76±13% compared to the pH probe whose sensitivity was 80±18%. When patients taking acid suppression were studied, the sensitivity of the pH probe dropped to 47±36% whereas the sensitivity of pH-MII in medicated patients was 80±21% [70]. Francavilla et al. found that the sensitivity of pH-MII was 86±12%, that this sensitivity was higher in infants compared to children as infants have more non-acid reflux events, and that impedance resulted in a higher symptom index, symptom sensitivity index, and symptom association probability than the pH probe [71]. Wenzl et al. found that in untreated infants, the sensitivity of pH-MII to detect acid reflux events was 54% compared to the pH probe [72]. Failure of pH-MII to report reflux events detected by pH probe primarily occurs when (1) there is a persistent drop in pH less than 4 even after the bolus had been cleared by impedance, (2) the pH hovers around

4 with multiple drops to less than 4, or (3) pH drops are associated with swallows.

Reproducibility

Dalby et al. performed 48 h impedance studies in 30 children to determine the degree of variability between the first and second day of recording [73]. The authors found that the reproducibility for the total number of reflux events in each patient between different days was better than the reproducibility for the number of acid or non-acid events individually. On a population basis, there was no significant difference between the median total number, acid or non-acid events between day 1 and day 2 [73]. Results from adult studies support this pediatric study. Aanen et al., in a study of 21 adults, found that the number of acid, weakly acidic, and total events was similar between the 2 days with a Kendall's *W* value ranging from 0.9 to 0.92, where a value of 1 indicates perfect concordance. Additionally, the reproducibility of symptom indices using the SAP, SI and SSI was 0.9, 0.73, and 0.86 respectively [74]. Similarly Zerbib et al. found, in 27 adults, that there was good reproducibility for the number, acidity and composition of reflux events (Kendall's *W*-values=0.72–0.85) [75].

Normal Values

One of the current limitations to pH-MII monitoring is the lack of normal pediatric values to differentiate physiologic from pathologic reflux. Adult normal values have been published. Shay et al. conducted a multicenter study of 60 healthy volunteers and found that the upper limit of normal for total, acid, weakly acid, and non-acid reflux were 73, 55, 26, and 1, respectively [76]. Zerbib et al. found similar numbers in normal adults with the upper limit of normal for healthy adults for total, acid, weakly acid, and non-acid reflux were 75, 50, 33, and 15, respectively [75].

Normal preterm infant values differ significantly from adults; the upper limit for total number of reflux events was 100 of which up to 52% can be acid and up to 98% can be non-acid [61]; the study, however, was performed with nasogastric tubes in place which can stent open the Lower Esophageal Sphincter and increase the number of reflux events by more than 50%, suggesting that these values may be artificially high [77]. In contrast, in a small study of older children ($n=10$, patients with normal pH recording and normal esophageal biopsies and no gastrointestinal symptoms), the 95th percentile for total events was 69, a value very similar to adult data [78]. Obviously, larger studies are needed to confirm the range of normal values in children. Because normal cut-off values are not available in pediatrics, the main role of impedance is to correlate symptoms with reflux events.

Symptom Association

Given the lack of normative data to determine normal pH-MII in children, the most important use of the technique has been to study the temporal association between symptoms and reflux. There is significant debate in the adult literature about the optimal way to correlate reflux with symptoms but the literature is clear that pH-MII is superior to pH monitoring alone when evaluating symptom correlation [59, 65, 79, 80]. The rates of symptom index (SI), symptom sensitivity index (SSI), and the symptom association probability (SAP) positivity have been studied using MII-pH. In adults, Aanen et al. found that the SAP and the SSI were the most reproducible indices in patients who had two impedance studies separated by a minimum of 1 week [74]. Similarly, Brendenoord et al. found that the SAP was the most frequently positive index followed by the SI and then the SSI. They also found that the addition of pH-MII over a standard pH probe increased the number of patients with a positive SI and SAP but did not increase the number of patients with a positive SSI [79].

In pediatrics, Rosen et al. studied 28 children taking acid suppression therapy for intractable respiratory symptoms; in these patients, more patients had a positive SI for respiratory symptoms using MII-pH than pH probe alone but there was no difference in the number of patients with a positive SSI when MII-pH was used compared to a standard pH probe [59]. In contrast, Thilmany et al. found that the rate of positivity for the SI was higher for acid reflux episodes whereas the rate of positivity of SSI was higher for non-acid reflux episodes suggesting that the value of pH-MII may differ depending on what symptom index is used [81]. Loots et al. studied 50 children undergoing pH-MII testing and found that uniformly pH-MII resulted in a higher symptom association, regardless of the index used, compared to pH probe and that the SAP was the most frequently positive symptom index [82].

One of the limitations of symptom indices is that they only represent a significant temporal relationship rather than a true cause and effect relationship. The normal cut off values, therefore, represent statistical definitions and are not linked to clinical outcomes; the normal values of 50% for the SI, 10% for the SSI and 95% for the SAP were not generated by investigating clinical outcomes. Rosen et al. looked at the value of the SI and the SSI in predicting fundoplication outcome. They found that neither a positive SI nor an SSI predicted fundoplication results and, using ROC curves, there was no clear cut off value for either index predicting outcome [83]. These data suggest that a temporal association alone does not prove causality which is the key limitation to all of the symptom indices. A second limitation of the symptom indices is the time lag between when a symptom occurs and when the patient actually records the symptom. In a study by Sifrim et al., there was an average delay of 28 s between the time when a patient coughed and when they actually recorded a cough on the symptom log [84]. Furthermore, patients only recorded, on average, 38% of coughs on the log [84]. To address this limitation, impedance sensors can be paired with pressure sensors which measures esophageal pressure spikes occurring when a patient coughs. Coughs appear as simultaneous high pressure spikes in the esophagus and this allows for precise correlation between reflux and cough without the possibility for recording error. Because the placement of two catheters can be uncomfortable, new technologies are on the horizon to measure cough-reflux associations less invasively.

Proximal Reflux

One of the advantages of MII-pH is that the multiple sensors can detect full column reflux which is extremely important when determining the impact of reflux on the airways. Rosen et al. found that, in children with severe respiratory symptoms, full column reflux is more highly associated with respiratory symptoms than distal reflux [59]. The importance of full column reflux in the generation of symptoms is further supported by Jadcherla et al. who found that acid reflux events reaching the proximal esophagus were four times more likely to be associated with symptoms that distal events [85]. The next step is to determine whether full column reflux predicts clinical outcome. Rosen et al. found that full column reflux events, rather than total reflux burden, predicted a positive surgical outcome after fundoplication [86]. In other studies, the relationship between full column reflux and symptoms is less clear. Condino et al. found that, in asthmatic children, proximal reflux was not a predictor of symptom generation [80]. Because extraesophageal symptoms represent the consequences of a heterogeneous grouping of diseases, it is often difficult to determine a definitive relationship between full column events and symptoms, but it is becoming increasingly clear that full column reflux may be an important component of a pH-MII report.

Impedance and Clinical Outcome

The role of impedance in improving clinical outcomes is uncertain at this time. Several adult studies have shown that pH-MII may predict a clinical response to therapy [87, 88]. There is only a single pediatric study which investigated the role of how pH-MII testing changed clinical outcome. For each pH-MII done for clinical reasons, Rosen et al. gave the results of the pH portion of the test and asked the referring gastroenterologist how the pH results changed management. The MII portion of the test was then given to the ordering clinician who was again asked how this result changed clinical management. Out of 50 impedances ordered by 23 attendings, the MII portion of the test changed the clinical management of the patient 22% of the time. Whether this change in management results in patient improvement is unknown.

The Future for MII

Currently, evidence indicates that pH-MII has replaced the gold standard pH-only monitoring for the evaluation of reflux in a research setting. It also seems to be the new gold standard for the evaluation of patients with persistent symptoms in the postprandial period and for patients with persistent symptoms despite acid suppression therapy. The utility of the technology is limited by the time-consuming nature of the study interpretation and a paucity of evidence to prove that it improves clinical outcomes over a standard pH monitoring.

Acknowledgment This work was supported in part by NIH NIDDK073713 (R.R.).

References

1. Vakil N, van Zanten SV, Kahrilas P, Dent J, Jones R. The Montreal definition and classification of gastroesophageal reflux disease: a global evidence-based consensus. Am J Gastroenterol. 2006;101:1900–20.
2. Sherman PM, Hassall E, Fagundes-Neto U, et al. A global, evidence-based consensus on the definition of gastroesophageal reflux disease in the pediatric population. Am J Gastroenterol. 2009;104:1278–95.
3. Spencer J. Prolonged pH recording in the study of gastro-oesophageal reflux. Br J Surg. 1969;56:912–4.
4. Rudolph C, Mazur L, Liptak G, et al. Guidlines for evaluation and treatment of gastroesophageal reflux in infants and children: recommendations of the North American Society for Pediatric Gastroenterology and Nutrition. J Pediatr Gastroenterol Nutr. 2001;32:S1–31.
5. Vandenplas Y, Belli D, Boige N. A standardized protocol for the methodology of esophageal pH monitoring and interpretation of the data for the diagnosis of gastro-esophageal reflux. J Pediatr Gastroenterol Nutr. 1992;14:467–71.
6. Hirano I, Richter J. ACG practice guidelines: esophageal reflux testing. Am J Gastroenterol. 2007;102:668–85.
7. Strobel C, Byrne W, Ament M, Euler A. Correlation of esophageal lengths in children with height: application to the Tuttle test without prior esophageal manometry. J Pediatr. 1979;94:81–4.
8. Jolley SG, Tunell WP, Carson JA, Smith EI, Grunow J. The accuracy of abbreviated esophageal pH monitoring in children. J Pediatr Surg. 1984;19:848–54.
9. Tolia V, Kauffman RE. Comparison of evaluation of gastroesophageal reflux in infants using different feedings during intraesophageal pH monitoring. J Pediatr Gastroenterol Nutr. 1990;10:426–9.
10. Wo JM, Castell DO. Exclusion of meal periods from ambulatory 24-hour pH monitoring may improve diagnosis of esophageal acid reflux. Dig Dis Sci. 1994;39:1601–7.
11. Ter RB, Johnston BT, Castell DO. Exclusion of the meal period improves the clinical reliability of esophageal pH monitoring. J Clin Gastroenterol. 1997;25:314–6.
12. Tobin JM, McCloud P, Cameron DJ. Posture and gastro-oesophageal reflux: a case for left lateral positioning. Arch Dis Child. 1997;76:254–8.
13. Bell N, Karol MD, Sachs G, Greski-Rose P, Jennings DE, Hunt RH. Duration of effect of lansoprazole on gastric pH and acid secretion in normal male volunteers. Aliment Pharmacol Ther. 2001;15:105–13.
14. van Wijk MP, Benninga MA, Omari TI. Role of the multichannel intraluminal impedance technique in infants and children. J Pediatr Gastroenterol Nutr. 2009;48:2–12.
15. Cucchiara S, Staiano A, Gobio Casali L, Boccieri A, Paone F. Value of the 24 hour intraoesophageal pH monitoring in children. Gut. 1990;31:129–33.
16. Vandenplas Y, Franckx-Goossens A, Pipeleers-Marichal M, Derde M, Sacre-Smits L. Area under pH 4: advantages of a new parameter in the interpretation of esophageal pH monitoring data in infants. J Pediatr Gastroenterol Nutr. 1989;9:34–9.
17. Wenner J, Johansson J, Johnsson F, Oberg S. Optimal thresholds and discriminatory power of 48-h wireless esophageal pH monitoring in the diagnosisof GERD. Am J Gastroenterol. 2007;102:1862–9.
18. Steiner SJ, Gupta SK, Croffie JM, Fitzgerald JF. Correlation between number of eosinophils and reflux index on same day esophageal biopsy and 24 hour esophageal pH monitoring. Am J Gastroenterol. 2004;99:801–5.
19. Black D, Haggitt R, Orenstein S, Whitington P. Esophagitis in infants. Morphologic histological diagnosis and correlation with measures of gastroesophageal reflux. Gastroenterology. 1990;98:1408–14.
20. Boix-Ochoa J, Lafuenta J, Gil-Vernet J. Twenty-four hour esophageal pH monitoring in gastroesophageal reflux. J Pediatr Surg. 1980;15:74–8.
21. Cucchiara S, Santamaria F, Minella R, et al. Simultaneous prolonged recordings of proximal and distal intraesophageal pH in children with gastroesophageal reflux disease and respiratory symptoms. Am J Gastroenterol. 1995;90:1791–6.
22. Euler A, Byrne W. Twenty-four-hour esophageal intraluminal pH probe testing: a comparative analysis. Gastroenterology. 1981;80:957–61.

23. Sondheimer J. Continuous monitoring of distal esophageal pH: a diagnostic test for gastroesophageal reflux in infants. J Pediatr. 1980;96:804–7.
24. Vandenplas Y, Goyvaerts H, Helven R, et al. Gastroesophageal reflux, as assessed by 24-hour pH monitoring, in 509 healthy infants screened for SIDS-risk. Pediatrics. 1991;88:834–40.
25. Salvatore S, Hauser B, Vandemaele K, Novario R, Vandenplas Y. Gastroesophageal reflux disease in infants: how much is predictable with questionnaires, pH-metry, endoscopy and histology? J Pediatr Gastroenterol Nutr. 2005;40:210–5.
26. Savarino E, Zentilin P, Tutuian R, et al. The role of nonacid reflux in NERD: lessons learned from impedance-pH monitoring in 150 patients off therapy. Am J Gastroenterol. 2008;103:2685–93.
27. Bredenoord AJ, Hemmink GJ, Smout AJ. Relationship between gastro-oesophageal reflux pattern and severity of mucosal damage. Neurogastroenterol Motil. 2009;21:807–12.
28. Vandenplas Y, Helven R, Goyvaerts H, et al. Reproducibility of continuous 24 hour oesophageal pH monitoring in infants and children. Gut. 1990;31:374–7.
29. Mahajan L, Wyllie RLO, et al. Reproducibility of 24-hour intraesophageal pH monitoring in pediatric patients. Pediatrics. 1998;101:260–3.
30. Nielsen R, Kruse-Andersen S, Husby S. Low reproducibility of 2 × 24-hour continuous esophageal pH monitoring in infants and children: a limiting factor for interventional studies. Dig Dis Sci. 2003;48:1495–502.
31. Hampton F, MacFadyen U, Simpson H. Reproducibility of 24 hour oeosophageal pH studies in infants. Arch Dis Child. 1990;65:1249–54.
32. McCallion WA, Gallagher TM, Boston VE, Potts SR. Effect of general anaesthesia on prolonged intraoesophageal pH monitoring. Arch Dis Child. 1995;73:235–8.
33. Malfroot A, Vandenplas Y, Verlinden M, Piepsz A, Dab I. Gastroesophageal reflux and unexplained chronic respiratory disease in infants and children. Pediatr Pulmonol. 1987;3:208–13.
34. Gunasekaran T, Gupta S, Gremse D, et al. Lansoprazole in adolescents with gastroesophageal reflux disease: pharmacokinetics, pharmacodynamics, symptom relief efficacy, and tolerability. J Pediatr Gastroenterol Nutr. 2002;35 Suppl 4:S327–35.
35. Lam H, Breumelhof R, Roelofs J, Van Berge Henegouwen G, Smout A. What is the optimal time window in a symptom analysis of 24-hour esophageal pressure and pH data? Dig Dis Sci. 1994;39:402–9.
36. Ward B, Wu W, Richter J, et al. Ambulatory 24-hour esophageal pH monitoring. Technology searching for a clinical application. J Clin Gastroenterol. 1986;8:59–67.
37. Singh S, Richter JE, Bradley LA, Haile JM. The symptom index. Differential usefulness in suspected acid-related complaints of heartburn and chest pain. Dig Dis Sci. 1993;38:1402–8.
38. Breumelhof R, Smout A. The symptom sensitivity index: a valuable additional parameter in 24-hour esophageal pH monitoring. Am J Gastroenterol. 1991;86:160–4.
39. Weusten B, Roelofs J, Akkermans L, Van Berge Henegouwen G, Smout A. symptom-association probability: an improved method for symptom analysis of 24-hour esophageal pH data. Gastroenterology. 1994;107:1741–5.
40. Taghavi S, Ghasedi M, Saberi-Firoozi M, et al. Symptom association probability and symptom sensitivity index: preferable but still suboptimal predictors of response to high dose omeprazole. Gut. 2005;54:1067–71.
41. Diaz S, Aymerich R, Clouse RE. The symptom association probability (SAP) is superior to the symptom index (SI) for attributing symptoms to gastroesophageal reflux: validation using outcome from laparoscopic antireflux surgery (LARS). Gastroenterology. 2002;122:A75.
42. Wiener GJ, Tsukashima R, Kelly C, et al. Oropharyngeal pH monitoring for the detection of liquid and aerosolized supraesophageal gastric reflux. J Voice. 2009;23:498–504.
43. Ayazi S, Lipham JC, Hagen JA, et al. A new technique for measurement of pharyngeal pH: normal values and discriminating pH threshold. J Gastrointest Surg. 2009;13:1422–9.
44. Williams R, Ali G, Wallace K. Esophagopharyngeal acid regurgitation: dual pH monitoring criteria for its detection and insights into mechanisms. Gastroenterology. 1999;117:1051–61.
45. Golub JS, Johns III MM, Lim JH, DelGaudio JM, Klein AM. Comparison of an oropharyngeal pH probe and a standard dual pH probe for diagnosis of laryngopharyngeal reflux. Ann Otol Rhinol Laryngol. 2009;118:1–5.
46. Chheda NN, Seybt MW, Schade RR, Postma GN. Normal values for pharyngeal pH monitoring. Ann Otol Rhinol Laryngol. 2009;118:166–71.
47. Chiou E, Rosen R, Nurko S. Correlation of changes in oropharyngeal pH with gastroesophageal reflux events in children. J Pediatr Gastroenterol Nutr. 2009;49:E36.
48. Wiener G, Koufman J, Wu W, et al. Chronic hoarseness secondary to gastroesophageal reflux disease: documentation with 24-h ambulatory pH monitoring. Am J Gastroenterol. 1989;84:1503–8.
49. Pandolfino JE, Richter JE, Ours T, Guardino JM, Chapman J, Kahrilas PJ. Ambulatory esophageal pH monitoring using a wireless system. Am J Gastroenterol. 2003;98:740–9.
50. Lacy B, Edwards S, Paquette L, Weiss J, Kelley M, Ornvold K. Tolerability and clinical utility of the Bravo pH capsule in children. J Clin Gastroenterol. 2009;43(6):514–9.
51. Fajardo NR, Wise JL, Locke GR, Murray JA, Talley NJ. Esophageal perforation after placement of wireless Bravo pH probe. Gastrointest Endosc. 2006;63:184–5.

52. Souza AL, Morley-Fletcher A, Nurko S, Rodriguez L. BRAVO wireless pH in children: is there an effect of anesthesia? Gastroenterology. 2009;136:A-510.
53. Gunnarsdottir A, Stenstrom P, Arnbjornsson E. Wireless esophageal pH monitoring in children. J Laparoendosc Adv Surg Tech. 2008;18:443–7.
54. Croffie J, Fitzgerald J, Molleson J, et al. Accuracy and tolerability of the Braco catheter-free pH capsule in patients between the ages of 4 and 18 years. J Pediatr Gastroenterol Nutr. 2007;45:559–63.
55. Gunnarsdottir A, Stenstrom P, Arnbjornsson E. 48-hour wireless oesophageal pH-monitoring in children: are two days better than one? Eur J Pediatr Surg. 2007;17:378–81.
56. Pandolfino J, Kahrilas P. Prolonged pH monitoring: Bravo capsule. Gastrointest Endosc Clin North Am. 2005;15:307–18.
57. Toila V, Vandenplas Y. Systematic review: the extra-oesophageal symptoms of gastro-oesophageal reflux disease in children. Aliment Phamacol Ther. 2009;29:258–72.
58. Vaezi MF, Richter JE, Stasney CR, et al. Treatment of chronic posterior laryngitis with esomeprazole. Laryngoscope. 2006;116:254–60.
59. Rosen R, Nurko S. The importance of multichannel intraluminal impedance in the evaluation of children with persistent respiratory symptoms. Am J Gastroenterol. 2004;99:2452–8.
60. Patterson N, Mainie I, Rafferty G, et al. Nonacid reflux episodes reaching the pharynx are important factors associated with cough. J Clin Gastroenterol. 2009;43:414–9.
61. Lopez-Alonso M, Moya MJ, Cabo JA, et al. Twenty-four-hour esophageal impedance-pH monitoring in healthy preterm neonates: rate and characteristics of acid, weakly acidic, and weakly alkaline gastroesophageal reflux. Pediatrics. 2006;118:e299–308.
62. Mitchell DJ, McClure BG, Tubman TR. Simultaneous monitoring of gastric and oesophageal pH reveals limitations of conventional oesophageal pH monitoring in milk fed infants. Arch Dis Child. 2001;84:273–6.
63. Sifrim D, Holloway R, Silny J, Tack J, Lerut A, Janssens J. Composition of the postprandial refluxate in patients with gastroesophageal reflux disease. Am J Gastroenterol. 2001;96:647–55.
64. Vela MF, Camacho-Lobato L, Srinivasan R, Tutuian R, Katz PO, Castell DO. Simultaneous intraesophageal impedance and pH measurement of acid and nonacid gastroesophageal reflux: effect of omeprazole. Gastroenterology. 2001;120:1599–606.
65. Hemmink GJ, Bredenoord AJ, Weusten BL, Monkelbaan JF, Timmer R, Smout AJ. Esophageal pH-impedance monitoring in patients with therapy-resistant reflux symptoms: 'on' or 'off' proton pump inhibitor? Am J Gastroenterol. 2008;103:2446–53.
66. Roman S, des Bruley Varannes S, Pouderoux P, et al. Ambulatory 24-h oesophageal impedance-pH recordings: reliability of automatic analysis for gastro-oesophageal reflux assessment. Neurogastroenterol Motil. 2006;18:978–86.
67. Hemmink GJ, Bredenoord AJ, Aanen MC, Weusten BL, Timmer R, Smout AJ. Computer analysis of 24-h esophageal impedance signals. Scand J Gastroenterol. 2011;46(3):271–6.
68. Imam H, Shay S, Ali A, Baker M. Bolus transit patterns in healthy subjects: a study using simultaneous impedance monitoring, videoesophagram, and esophageal manometry. Am J Physiol Gastrointest Liver Physiol. 2005;288:G1000–6.
69. Peter CS, Wiechers C, Bohnhorst B, Silny J, Poets CF. Detection of small bolus volumes using multiple intraluminal impedance in preterm infants. J Pediatr Gastroenterol Nutr. 2003;36:381–4.
70. Rosen R, Lord C, Nurko S. The sensitivity of multichannel intraluminal impedance (MII) compared to pH probe in the detection of gastroesophgeal reflux in children. Clin Gastroenterol Hepatol. 2006;4:167–72.
71. Francavilla R, Magista AM, Bucci N, et al. Comparison of esophageal pH and multichannel intraluminal impedance testing in pediatric patients with suspected gastroesophageal reflux. J Pediatr Gastroenterol Nutr. 2010;50:154–60.
72. Wenzl TG, Moroder C, Trachterna M, et al. Esophageal pH monitoring and impedance measurement: a comparison of two diagnostic tests for gastroesophageal reflux. J Pediatr Gastroenterol Nutr. 2002;34:519–23.
73. Dalby K, Nielsen RG, Markoew S, Kruse-Andersen S, Husby S. Reproducibility of 24-hour combined multiple intraluminal impedance (MII) and pH measurements in infants and children. Evaluation of a diagnostic procedure for gastroesophageal reflux disease. Dig Dis Sci. 2007;52:2159–65.
74. Aanen MC, Bredenoord AJ, Numans ME, Samson M, Smout AJ. Reproducibility of symptom association analysis in ambulatory reflux monitoring. Am J Gastroenterol. 2008;103:2200–8.
75. Zerbib F, des Varannes SB, et al. Normal values and day-to-day variability of 24-h ambulatory oesophageal impedance-pH monitoring in a Belgian-French cohort of healthy subjects. Aliment Pharmacol Ther. 2005;22:1011–21.
76. Shay S, Tutuian R, Sifrim D, et al. Twenty-four hour ambulatory simultaneous impedance and pH monitoring: a multicenter report of normal values from 60 healthy volunteers. Am J Gastroenterol. 2004;99:1037–43.
77. Peter CS, Wiechers C, Bohnhorst B, Silny J, Poets CF. Influence of nasogastric tubes on gastroesophageal reflux in preterm infants: a multiple intraluminal impedance study. J Pediatr. 2002;141:277–9.
78. Rosen R, Furuta G, Fritz J, Donovan K, Nurko S. Role of acid and nonacid reflux in children with eosinophilic esophagitis compared with patients with gastroesophageal reflux and control patients. J Pediatr Gastroenterol Nutr. 2008;46:520–3.
79. Bredenoord AJ, Weusten BL, Timmer R, Conchillo JM, Smout AJ. Addition of esophageal impedance monitoring to pH monitoring increases the yield of

symptom association analysis in patients off PPI therapy. Am J Gastroenterol. 2006;101:453–9.
80. Condino AA, Sondheimer J, Pan Z, Gralla J, Perry D, O'Connor JA. Evaluation of gastroesophageal reflux in pediatric patients with asthma using impedance-pH monitoring. J Pediatr. 2006;149:216–9.
81. Thilmany C, Beck-Ripp J, Griese M. Acid and non-acid gastro-esophageal refluxes in children with chronic pulmonary diseases. Respir Med. 2007;101: 969–76.
82. Loots CM, Benninga MA, Davidson GP, Omari TI. Addition of pH-impedance monitoring to standard pH monitoring increases the yield of symptom association analysis in infants and children with gastroesophageal reflux. J Pediatr. 2009;154:248–52.
83. Rosen R, Levine P, Lewis J, Mitchell P, Nurko S. Reflux events detected by pH-MII do not determine fundoplication outcome. J Ped Gastroenterol Nutrit 2010 Mar;50(3):251–5.
84. Sifrim D, Dupont L, Blondeau K, Zhang X, Tack J, Janssens J. Weakly acidic reflux in patients with chronic unexplained cough during 24 hour pressure, pH, and impedance monitoring. Gut. 2005;54:449–54.
85. Jadcherla SR, Gupta A, Fernandez S, et al. Spatiotemporal characteristics of acid refluxate and relationship to symptoms in premature and term infants with chronic lung disease. Am J Gastroenterol. 2008;103:720–8.
86. Rosen R, Levine P, Lewis J, Mitchell P, Nurko S. Reflux events detected by pH-MII do not determine fundoplication outcome. J Pediatr Gastroenterol Nutr. 2010;50:251–5.
87. Mainie I, Tutuian R, Agrawal A, Adams D, Castell DO. Combined multichannel intraluminal impedance-pH monitoring to select patients with persistent gastro-oesophageal reflux for laparoscopic Nissen fundoplication. Br J Surg. 2006;93:1483–7.
88. Becker V, Bajbouj M, Waller K, Schmid RM, Meining A. Clinical trial: persistent gastro-oesophageal reflux symptoms despite standard therapy with proton pump inhibitors—a follow-up study of intraluminal-impedance guided therapy. Aliment Pharmacol Ther. 2007;26:1355–60.

Barostat and Other Sensitivity Tests 13

Christophe Faure

Introduction

Visceral sensitivity is a complex phenomenon that is regarded as a key pathophysiological factor in children with functional gastrointestinal disorders. In recent years, novel techniques have been developed in adults and adapted to children allowing the measurement of visceral sensory thresholds of stomach and colon. This chapter reviews the barostat technique and the satiety drinking tests. Functional cerebral imaging and other chemical stimulations that have not been yet used in pediatric subjects are not discussed.

Barostat

Principles

The barostat is a computer-driven air pump connected to a double-lumen catheter on which a highly compliant balloon or bag is securely fixed. The balloon is introduced in a hollow organ (in children rectum or stomach) and is used to measure tone, compliance and sensory threshold (Fig. 13.1). The principle of the barostat is to maintain a constant pressure within the air-filled bag inserted in the organ: when the organ relaxes, the air-pump inflates the balloon to compensate for the decrease in pressure; when the organ contracts, the system withdraws air and deflates the balloon so that the intraballoon pressure does not change. Because in barostat studies the function of the bag is to isolate a segment of the digestive tract without interfering with its function and its motility, the compliance of the balloon or bag should be "infinite" and its volume must be greater than the range of volumes used during the study (rectal bags: length 11 cm, maximal capacity: 600 mL, gastric bags: maximal diameter 17 cm, maximal capacity: 1,200 mL). Polyethylene bags rather than latex balloons are recommended.

Because visceral sensitivity relies on wall pressure and not on volume of the organ [1, 2], sensory thresholds should be expressed as pressure. Moreover, reproducibility of pressures measurements between laboratories and between subjects is higher than volumes because the pressure scale compensates for differences in bag shape, smooth muscle compliance, and contractile activity of the organs [3].

Procedure

Technical recommendations for measurements of sensory threshold and compliance have been published in adults and the general principles also

C. Faure, M.D. (✉)
Division of Pediatric Gastroenterology, Department of Pediatrics, Sainte-Justine University Health Center, Université de Montréal, 3175 Côte Sainte-Catherine, Montréal, H3T1C5, QC, Canada
e-mail: christophe.faure@umontreal.ca

C. Faure et al. (eds.), *Pediatric Neurogastroenterology: Gastrointestinal Motility and Functional Disorders in Children*, Clinical Gastroenterology,
DOI 10.1007/978-1-60761-709-9_13, © Springer Science+Business Media New York 2013

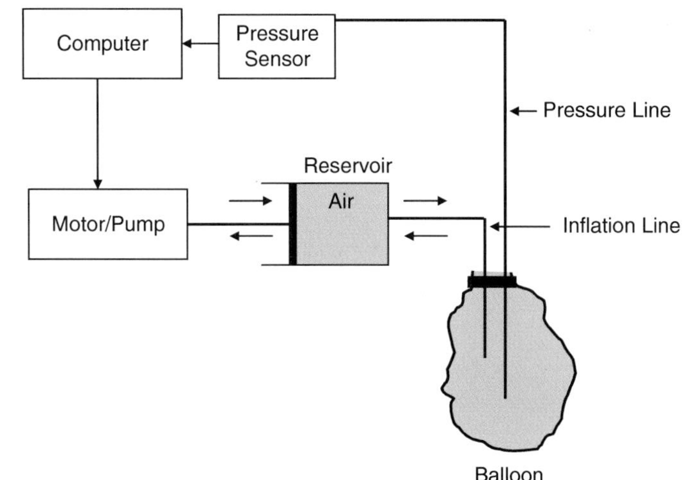

Fig. 13.1 Schematic diagram of a barostat and catheter

apply to practice in children [3]. However, sensory threshold assessment requires an adequate cooperation for the report of sensations and feelings by the subject. Children younger than 7–8 years may not be able to relate adequately their sensations during the test. Age appropriate explanation about the equipment and sequence of the procedure must be offered to the child. Because psychological state modulation results in changed sensation at a given stimulus in healthy adult subjects [4], environment during the barostat study should be as quiet as possible in order to minimize the external influences and standardize the procedure.

For rectal sensitivity studies in children, most authors do not clean extensively the colon but rather suggest to the child to go to the bathroom before the study. When studying rectal compliance in children with constipation, cleansing of the rectum with an enema should be done on the day before the barostat study. Because meals may interfere with colonic and gastric tone, a 4–6-h fasting period prior to the study is recommended. All medications affecting pain or gastrointestinal motility should be discontinued at least 48 h prior to the test.

For rectal studies, the patient lies in the left lateral position and the catheter is gently inserted into the rectum. For gastric studies, the device is inserted orally. The catheter is then secured with tape and 5–10 min is allowed for adaptation before beginning the procedure. The barostat bag is slowly inflated with 30 mL of air and the pressure is allowed to equilibrate for 3 min. The average bag pressure during the last 15 s defines the individual operating pressure (IOP) also called the minimal distending pressure (MDP) which is the minimum pressure required to overcome surrounding mechanical forces and inflate the bag with 30 mL of air.

Various distension protocols have been described [3]. In children the ascending method of limits (AML) without [5–7] or with [8–13] tracking has been the most applied. In the AML the barostat is programmed to deliver phasic intermittent stimuli starting at the IOP progressively increased in 2–4 mmHg steps lasting 60 s followed by 60 s deflation. When the first sensation of pain is reported, the study can be stopped (the sensory threshold is determined) or can be prolonged (tracking) by subsequent distensions randomly adjusted up or down depending on the response to the previous distension (if the subject reports pain, the next distension will be decreased or kept the same; if the subject reports no pain, the next distension will be increased or kept the same). The threshold is determined by averaging the pressures at which pain had been indicated after a series of measures (usually 3) (Fig. 13.2). A 4–5-point scale [6, 10] is used as a verbal descriptor for sensations felt during the barostat procedure. The AML is vulnerable to psychological biases (fear of pain) because the stimuli are predictable to the subject. The tracking technique is believed to be more reliable because it is less vulnerable to psychological bias (the stimuli is unpredictable) and because there are multiple determinations of the threshold. On the other

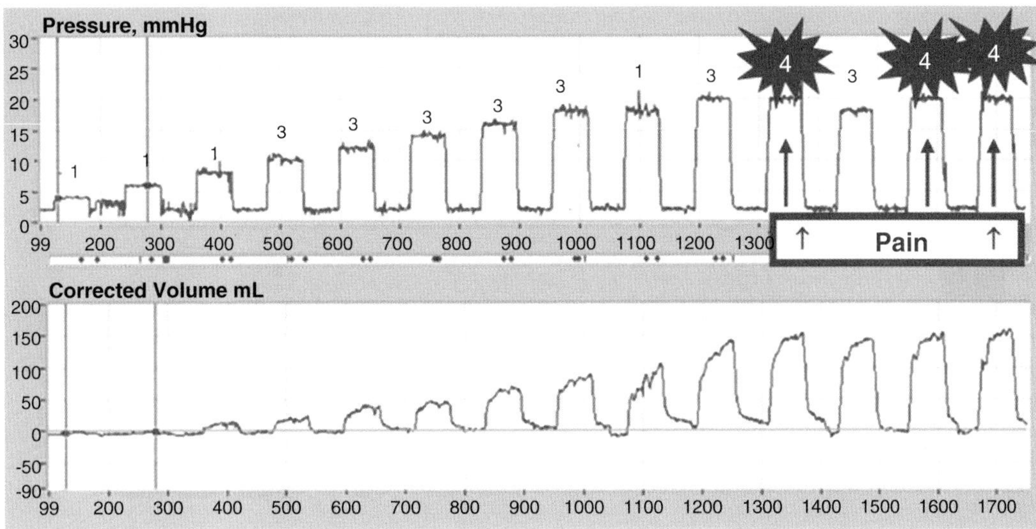

Fig. 13.2 Ascending method of limits with tracking. Rectal barostat tracing in an 11-year old girl with IBS. Verbal scale: 1—*gas or first sensation*, 2—*need to go to the bathroom*, 3—*urge to go to the bathroom*, 4—*pain*

hand, the tracking technique necessitates delivering multiple painful stimuli, making it less suitable for use in children. Nevertheless, the tracking method has been used successfully without any adverse event by several pediatric groups [8–13]. Of note the majority of children tested report that the pain sensation felt during the barostat is notably lower than the pain felt in the *real life*.

Measurements

Sensory Thresholds

The visceral sensory threshold can be separated into two components: the *perceptual sensitivity* (the ability to detect intraluminal distension) and the *response bias* (how the sensation is reported). The perceptual sensitivity allows discrimination between two distensions and reflects the ability of the organ to detect and transduce the stimulus to the central nervous system. The response bias (or perceptual response) is the reporting behavior (intensity, painfulness), a cognitive process influenced by past experience and psychological state. The tools currently used (distending protocols, methods for reporting subjects' response) are not able to accurately measure separately the two components. Adult studies have shown that the threshold measurement is responsive to changing environments or perturbations and psychological modulation resulting in changed sensation at a given stimulus in healthy subjects [4]. In children, there are few data regarding the influence of psychological state or trait on sensory threshold assessment. One pediatric study found that rectal sensory threshold did not correlate with the *state* of anxiety, suggesting that the anxiety generated by the procedure itself is not sufficient to bias the child's response to distension [10]. Results can be expressed as sensory thresholds, i.e., the first pressure that triggers a given sensation (urge to defecate, pain), or in intensity of sensation triggered by stimuli at fixed pressure.

Compliance

The compliance reflects the ability of a hollow organ to adapt to an imposed distension. It is expressed in mL/mmHg. It is defined as the pressure–volume relationship, represented by a sigmoid shape, composed of an initial reflex relaxation followed by a linear section and a final plateau phase. Compliance is calculated according to a nonlinear model fitting the pressure–volume curves. Pressure–volume curves are constructed with average computed volumes during each consecutive pressure step (when equilibration of the volume is reached, typically after 30–45 s).

Compliance is calculated as the maximum slope of the pressure–volume curves [3, 9, 12, 14–18]. Normal pediatric values have been published for rectal compliance by two different groups (16 mL/mmHg, range 12–20 mL/mmHg in 22 healthy volunteers aged 12±2.6 years [16]; 8.7 mL/mmHg, range 6.0–14 mL/mmHg in ten control children aged 13.7 years [12]). Alteration of gastric compliance has been reported in eight children after Nissen fundoplication [17].

Tone and Accommodation

The volume of air entering or withdrawn from the balloon is an indirect measurement of tone of the organ. Changes in volume in response to a meal (accommodation) can thus be easily measured by subtracting preprandial from postprandial balloon volumes. Rectal volume response to feeding (decrease of 25±3% from 88±8 mL before the meal to 66±7 mL after the meal) has been reported in healthy children [6]. In the stomach, no data have been reported in children but they been described in young adults [18].

Qualitative and Quantitative Assessment of the Sensations

Sensations elicited during the barostat test, painful or not, must be rated (intensity) and qualitatively reported. Visual analog scales can be used by children aged 6–7 years or older to rate sensations such as urgency or pain [9, 11, 12] and are easier to use than verbal descriptors in this population. Rating separately pain from unpleasantness is difficult in children. Qualitative evaluation of the pain has been conducted by using validated human body diagrams [10, 19] and questionnaires inquiring about the similarity of the induced pain and the typical pain felt in the real life [9, 13].

Clinical Relevance of Barostat Measurements

Functional Gastrointestinal Disorders

Rectal Sensitivity Measurement

Using the rectal barostat, several independent groups have reported that 75–100% of children with irritable bowel syndrome (IBS) have rectal hypersensitivity when compared to control children [6, 8–10, 13]. In adults affected by IBS, the prevalence of visceral hypersensitivity varies from 20% [20] to 94% [21] across studies suggesting that rectal hypersensitivity is a more reliable diagnostic marker of IBS in children than in adults. This has been confirmed in a prospective study that included children with abdominal pain for whom rectal sensory threshold was measured prior to any other diagnostic procedures [9]. In the 51 children included, rectal sensory threshold was lower in the functional gastrointestinal disorders (FGID) group than in the organic disease group (25.4 mmHg vs. 37.1 mmHg; $P=0.0002$) and 77% of the children with FGID displayed rectal hypersensitivity. At the cutoff of 30 mmHg, the rectal sensory threshold of pain measurement for the diagnosis of FGID had a sensitivity of 94% and a specificity of 77%. Rectal compliance has not been found different between IBS and control subjects [6, 8, 9, 11, 13]. Children with functional dyspepsia (FD) have normal rectal sensitivity suggesting that visceral hypersensitivity is organ specific [10].

Data regarding visceral sensitivity in children with functional abdominal pain (FAP) according to Rome criteria are less clear with discrepancies (sensory threshold similar to controls [6] or similar to IBS [10]) among authors.

Gastric Sensitivity Measurement

Because of the invasiveness of gastric barostat, the pathophysiology of functional dyspepsia has been studied scarcely in children. A subset of children with recurrent abdominal pain studied by gastric barostat using a latex balloon was reported to have hypersensitivity at the gastric level [13]. More recently, 16 dyspeptic children were extensively studied using gastric barostat [18]. Compliance was similar between patients and controls (69.5±8.9 mL/mmHg). Pressures at the discomfort threshold were significantly lower in dyspeptic children compared with young healthy controls. Accommodation to a meal was also significantly lower in dyspeptic children. Hypersensitivity to gastric distension was present in 56% (9/16) of patients and impaired accommodation in 11 (69%). When studied by gastric barostat, children with IBS seem to have normal gastric sensitivity [13].

Somatic Projections and Reproducibility of the Visceral Pain

Somatic referral induced by rectal distension differs in IBS, FAP and FD children.

In normal children without any gastrointestinal complaints and in dyspeptic patients rectal distension-induced sensations refer to the S3 dermatome (perineal area). In IBS and FAP, children refer their sensation to aberrant sites compared to the controls, i.e., with abdominal projections to dermatomes T8 to L1 [10]. However, similar results have been obtained in barostat study of children with organic diseases suggesting that subjects with protracted complaints of abdominal pain not related to FGID may have in contrast to "true" controls an abnormal perceptual response to distension (i.e., abnormal interpretation and sensation in response to rectal distension) [9]. The reproduction of pain during rectal distension is frequent in IBS and FAP children but is not predictive of a diagnosis of FGID as compared to organic diseases [9].

Constipation

In constipated children a high rectal compliance (>20 mL/mmHg) is present in a majority (58%) of patients suggesting that in order to reach the intrarectal pressure threshold that triggers the sensation of the need to defecate, a larger stool volume is required. In contrast to previous studies which had used different methodologies, it has now been reported that only 10% of the patients have a true rectal hyposensitivity [15, 16]. Whether the abnormal rectal compliance is primitive or secondary to fecal impaction is uncertain although there is no difference in compliance between groups with and without impaction [16]. Moreover, rectal emptying by regularly using enemas does not normalize compliance [15].

Satiety Drinking Tests

Because gastric barostat studies are more invasive than rectal barostat tests, less invasive methods of measuring gastric sensitivity have been developed. A satiety drinking test using a liquid meal has been validated in adults and has been correlated to gastric barostat measurements [22]. Subjects are studied after an overnight fast. A peristaltic pump fills one of two beakers at a rate of 15 mL/min with a liquid meal (Nutridrink [23], Ensure [24]). The children are instructed to drink the meal at the filling rate, thereby alternating the beakers by filling and emptying. Every 5 min, they score their satiety using a graphic rating scale, graded 0–5 (1 = no sensation, 5 = maximum sensation). Satiety is defined and explained to the children as the opposite of desire to eat. Children are asked to cease the meal intake when a score of 5 is reached. The maximal tolerated volume has been thought to reflect gastric accommodation. This method has been used in a large group of 59 children aged 5–15 years for which normal values have been published [23]. Adolescents with FD have been shown to develop increased symptoms 30 min after reaching maximum satiation [24].

Role of Visceral Sensitivity Measurement in Clinical Practice

By providing an objective criterion in addition to the clinical symptoms of FGID, the determination of a low sensory threshold may give a pathophysiological explanation to pediatric patients and their parents, making it possible for them to understand the nature and mechanisms underlying the symptoms and providing effective reassurance. Children with IBS or FAP symptoms with a normal rectal sensory threshold of pain should be carefully reexamined to exclude other diagnoses. Rectal hypersensitivity has been reported in children with inactive Crohn's disease suffering from protracted abdominal pain, suggesting that rectal barostat may be useful to recognize FGID in such patients [12]. Whether measurement of visceral sensitivity impacts the outcome of patients with FGID (number of procedures ordered by the physician, long-term prognosis, and response to drugs) is unknown.

References

1. Camilleri M. Testing the sensitivity hypothesis in practice: tools and methods, assumptions and pitfalls. Gut. 2002;51:34i–40. 10.1136/gut.51.suppl_1.i34.
2. Distrutti E, Azpiroz F, Soldevilla A, Malagelada JR. Gastric wall tension determines perception of gastric distention. Gastroenterology. 1999;116:1035–42.
3. Whitehead WE, Delvaux M. Standardization of barostat procedures for testing smooth muscle tone and sensory thresholds in the gastrointestinal tract. The Working Team of Glaxo-Wellcome Research, UK. Dig Dis Sci. 1997;42:223–41.
4. Ford MJ, Camilleri M, Zinsmeister AR, Hanson RB. Psychosensory modulation of colonic sensation in the human transverse and sigmoid colon. Gastroenterology. 1995;109:1772–80.
5. Vlieger AM, van den Berg MM, Menko-Frankenhuis C, Bongers ME, Tromp E, Benninga MA. No change in rectal sensitivity after gut-directed hypnotherapy in children with functional abdominal pain or irritable bowel syndrome. Am J Gastroenterol. 2010;105:213–8.
6. Van Ginkel R, Voskuijl WP, Benninga MA, Taminiau JA, Boeckxstaens GE. Alterations in rectal sensitivity and motility in childhood irritable bowel syndrome. Gastroenterology. 2001;120:31–8.
7. van den Berg MM, Voskuijl WP, Boeckxstaens GE, Benninga MA. Rectal compliance and rectal sensation in constipated adolescents, recovered adolescents and healthy volunteers. Gut. 2008;57:599–603.
8. Iovino P, Tremolaterra F, Boccia G, Miele E, Ruju FM, Staiano A. Irritable bowel syndrome in childhood: visceral hypersensitivity and psychosocial aspects. Neurogastroenterol Motil. 2009;21:940–e74.
9. Halac U, Noble A, Faure C. Rectal sensory threshold for pain is a diagnostic marker of irritable bowel syndrome and functional abdominal pain in children. J Pediatr. 2010;156:60–5.e1.
10. Faure C, Wieckowska A. Somatic referral of visceral sensations and rectal sensory threshold for pain in children with functional gastrointestinal disorders. J Pediatr. 2007;150:66–71.
11. Castilloux J, Noble A, Faure C. Is visceral hypersensitivity correlated with symptom severity in children with functional gastrointestinal disorders? J Pediatr Gastroenterol Nutr. 2008;46:272–8.
12. Faure C, Giguere L. Functional gastrointestinal disorders and visceral hypersensitivity in children and adolescents suffering from Crohn's disease. Inflamm Bowel Dis. 2008;14:1569–74.
13. Di Lorenzo C, Youssef NN, Sigurdsson L, Scharff L, Griffiths J, Wald A. Visceral hyperalgesia in children with functional abdominal pain. J Pediatr. 2001;139:838–43.
14. Fox M, Thumshirn M, Fried M, Schwizer W. Barostat measurement of rectal compliance and capacity. Dis Colon Rectum. 2006;49:360–70.
15. van den Berg, Bongers MEJ, Voskuijl WP, Benninga MA. No role for increased rectal compliance in pediatric functional constipation. Gastroenterology. 2009; 137:1963–69.
16. Voskuijl WP, van Ginkel R, Benninga MA, Hart GA, Taminiau JA, Boeckxstaens GE. New insight into rectal function in pediatric defecation disorders: disturbed rectal compliance is an essential mechanism in pediatric constipation. J Pediatr. 2006;148:62–7.
17. Mousa H, Caniano DA, Alhajj M, Gibson L, Di Lorenzo C, Binkowitz L. Effect of Nissen fundoplication on gastric motor and sensory functions. J Pediatr Gastroenterol Nutr. 2006;43:185–9.
18. Hoffman I, Vos R, Tack J. Assessment of gastric sensorimotor function in paediatric patients with unexplained dyspeptic symptoms and poor weight gain. Neurogastroenterol Motil. 2007;19:173–9.
19. Savedra MC, Tesler MD, Holzemer WL, Wilkie DJ, Ward JA. Pain location: validity and reliability of body outline markings by hospitalized children and adolescents. Res Nurs Health. 1989;12:307–14.
20. Camilleri M, McKinzie S, Busciglio I, Low PA, Sweetser S, Burton D, Baxter K, Ryks M, Zinsmeister AR. Prospective study of motor, sensory, psychologic, and autonomic functions in patients with irritable bowel syndrome. Clin Gastroenterol Hepatol. 2008;6:772–81.
21. Mertz H, Naliboff B, Munakata J, Niazi N, Mayer E. Altered rectal perception is a biological marker of patients with irritable bowel syndrome. Gastroenterology. 1995;109:40–52.
22. Tack J, Caenepeel P, Piessevaux H, Cuomo R, Janssens J. Assessment of meal induced gastric accommodation by a satiety drinking test in health and in severe functional dyspepsia. Gut. 2003;52:1271–7.
23. Hoffman I, Vos R, Tack J. Normal values for the satiety drinking test in healthy children between 5 and 15 years. Neurogastroenterol Motil. 2009;21:517–20.e6.
24. Chitkara DK, Camilleri M, Zinsmeister AR, Burton D, El-Youssef M, Freese D, Walker L, Stephens D. Gastric sensory and motor dysfunction in adolescents with functional dyspepsia. J Pediatr. 2005;146:500–5.

14 Radionuclide Transit Tests

Lorenzo Biassoni, Keith J. Lindley,
and Osvaldo Borrelli

Scintigraphic techniques are well established methods in the assessment of motility throughout the gastrointestinal tract [1, 2]. However, although research has expanded our understanding of the gastrointestinal physiology and our available clinical tools, in the last decade the routine clinical application of scintigraphy for assessing gastrointestinal motility has been relative static as the technical advantages achieved have not gained widespread clinical acceptance. For instance, scintigraphy is the gold standard for measuring gastric motility, but its application is usually limited to measuring total gastric emptying time although several data support the clinical value of evaluating both antral and fundal motor function in patients with dyspeptic symptoms. Moreover, small bowel and colonic transit scintigraphic studies are still performed only in selected specialized centers.

Scintigraphic tests are attractive as a means of providing exquisite gastrointestinal function under physiological conditions with a set of low-cost procedures that are easy to perform, well tolerated and not operator-dependent [3]. The radiation burden is smaller than conventional radiology, and, as γ-cameras are linked to digital computers, quantification is relatively easy. However, the main pitfalls of most scintigraphic tests are still the lack of standardization of the technique and the poor image processing.

As in adults, scintigraphic tests in infants and children usually require a modest amount of cooperation; however, some aspects of pediatric nuclear medicine are unique due to differences in organ size, cooperation and neurological and developmental maturation. Performing scintigraphy in children require great patience and skills from the radiographers who interact with the child and family at the time of the examination [4]. A fully explanation of the procedure to both child and parents is mandatory, including the length of time they will need to be in the hospital. The parents should be present during the test in order to support the child during the examination. The cooperation of the child can also be improved by the use of age-appropriate relaxation and distraction techniques. For example, infants relax with swaddling and use of a pacifier. Having a favorite toy can comfort toddlers. School age and older children may find it helpful to listen to a full explanation of the function of the different pieces of equipment before starting the procedure. Furthermore, immobilization of the child during the test is an essential part to obtain high-quality images; this is often challenging, and in some instances sedation may have to be considered.

L. Biassoni, M.Sc., F.R.C.P.
Nuclear Medicine, Department of Radiology, Great Ormond Street Hospital for Children,
London, UK

K.J. Lindley, M.D., Ph.D. • O. Borrelli, M.D., Ph.D. (✉)
Division of Neurogastroenterology & Motility,
Department of Paediatric Gastroenterology,
ICH University College of London, Great Ormond Street Hospital for Children, London, UK
e-mail: borreo@gosh.nhs.uk

C. Faure et al. (eds.), *Pediatric Neurogastroenterology: Gastrointestinal Motility and Functional Disorders in Children*, Clinical Gastroenterology,
DOI 10.1007/978-1-60761-709-9_14, © Springer Science+Business Media New York 2013

Finally, the administered activity of the radiopharmaceutical depends on the child's body weight or body surface.

Radiopharmaceuticals

Tracers used in gastrointestinal motility studies have to be nonabsorbable and stable in the gastric acidity. For esophageal transit, gastroesophageal reflux (GER) and gastric emptying studies the main tracers utilized are ^{99m}Tc sulfur colloid or ^{99m}Tc nanocolloid. For instance, for a gastric emptying study these tracers are used for both the liquid phase, as they bind well to milk, and for the solid phase, as they have a good affinity for the protein matrix of the egg white. The maximal limit of the activity that can be administered varies according to the different countries, ranging between 18 and 74 MBq [5, 6]. In the UK, the maximal limit is 40 MBq for studies evaluating oesophageal motility and GER: this activity gives a maximal radiation burden of 0.9 mSv. For gastric emptying studies the maximal activity is 12 MBq, which gives a radiation burden of approximately 0.3 mSv.

^{99m}Tc diethyl-triamine-pentacetic acid (DTPA) is used as a tracer for the liquid phase of the gastric emptying, for small bowel transit and colonic studies. The maximal administered activity varies between 18 and 37 MBq. ^{99m}Tc macroaggregates of albumin (MAA) can be used in the liquid phase of the gastric emptying study.

With regard to the small bowel and colon transit studies, ^{111}In-DTPA is frequently used as a tracer for the liquid phase. The administered activity varies between 5.55 and 18.5 MBq. The maximal administered activity in the UK is 10 MBq, which gives a radiation burden of approximately 3 mSv.

Esophageal Transit

Esophageal transit scintigraphy is a non invasive method to qualitatively and quantitatively assess esophageal motility. It is fast, easy to perform with minimal radiation exposure. However, since its introduction by Kazam several protocols have been used without standardization, thus limiting its widespread use [7]. Some protocols used in adults are applicable to older children able to of swallow a bolus on command. Some variations have been introduced for assessing esophageal motility in young children and infants [8, 9]. This test provides imaging and quantitative data on the transit of a radiolabeled bolus through the esophagus. It can be used for the diagnosis of organic and functional esophageal disorders and is especially valuable when performed serially to evaluate the effect of medical or surgical treatments [10].

The procedure is performed after a fast of at least 3 h in infants and 6 h in children. Any medication with a known effect on esophageal motility should be discontinued at least 72 h before the testing. ^{99m}Tc sulfur colloid is routinely used for esophageal transit scintigraphy. In adults, the majority of the studies have been performed using a liquid bolus, whereas only few studies have used a semisolid bolus [11, 12]. A semisolid bolus requires more intense peristalsis to complete the transport over the distal half of the esophagus and this can increase the sensitivity of the test [13]. Because of the difficulty in reaching a consensus on the viscosity and the type of the semisolid bolus, as well as the difficulty of keeping the bolus viscosity constant to avoid its fragmentation, the liquid bolus is still routinely used for assessing esophageal motility abnormalities. In infants and children a dose of at least 150 μ(mu)Ci (5.55 MBq) is added to 10 mL bolus of milk or water. In the case of milk allergy a substitute may be used.

Infants can lie on a slightly inclined collimator. Older children can sit up with their back to the collimator. It is essential to turn the head of the bottle fed infants to the side, to avoid superimposition of the radioactivity in the bottle over the upper esophagus. Older children can be fed with a cup or with a straw. Before the administration of the radiolabeled bolus an external small radioactive marker is placed over the cricoid cartilage as anatomical landmark. After a practice swallow with unlabeled liquid, the radioactive bolus is placed in the mouth and swallowed on command followed by a dry bolus at least 30 s later. Since some swallows are not completely propagated even in healthy subjects, 4–6 swallows should be obtained. The patient's position during the study can affect the results due to the effect of gravity. Performing the study with the patient in an upright position may be more physiologic. Eliminating the force of gravity by performing the study with the patient in the supine position is more practical in infants and young children and more efficient in exposing motility disorders.

A large-field-of-view γ(gamma)-camera fitted with a low-energy high-sensitivity collimator is usually used due to high temporal resolution required for quantitative studies. Dynamic images in 128 × 128 matrix must be acquired in a rapid sequence. Because many of the events occur in a short time, images should be acquired at 4–10 frames per second for 60 s. The field of view of the γ(gamma)-camera must include the entire esophageal tract including the mouth and the gastric fundus. An additional 10 min static acquisition is obtained when the patient is asked to dry swallow, in order to measure the clearance from the esophagus. If a large residual remains in the esophagus delayed static images are obtained at 30 and 60 min. A Co-57 transmission image may be taken immediately or at 10 min following completion of the dynamic acquisition when the anatomical location of the tracer is uncertain (gastric fundus versus esophagus).

Once the study has been completed, the images are reviewed in a one-to-one single-frame analysis and then played back in a cine display mode. This procedure depicts the dynamics of the swallowing and swallowing-related esophageal motor pattern, and helps to identify aberrant patterns. For instance the adynamic pattern is characterized by slow progression or even stopping of the bolus along the esophagus, such as in achalasia and scleroderma, whereas the uncoordinated pattern is characterized by random disorganized retrograde/antegrade contractions throughout the esophagus as occur in patients with diffuse esophageal spasm [14–16]. This visual pattern corresponds to multiple peaks of the time–activity curves as determined by the quantitative assessment of the esophageal transit. Esophageal transit can be measured quantitatively with time and retention parameters. The esophagus is divided into upper, middle and lower zones. Equal regions of interest (ROI) are placed on each zone and a fourth ROI is placed over the stomach. Time–activity curves for the proximal, mid and distal parts of the esophagus are generated. The curves allow quantitative and qualitative assessment of the bolus transit. Condensed dynamic images that summarize the whole deglutition event into one single image may also be used. A condensed dynamic image displays the profile of the swallowing event side by side on the *y*-axis, along with the time on the *x*-axis. The total transit time is usually calculated as the period between the first appearance of the marker in the proximal esophagus and the time needed to obtain 90% radioactivity clearance from the distal esophagus. The residual 10% of the marker is ignored in order to avoid any potential overlap with the marker contained in the fundus. Besides total and segmental transit times, a clearance rate at time t is usually obtained with the following formula: $C = (E_{max} - E_t)/E_{max} \times 100\%$, where E_{max} is the maximal esophageal radioactivity and E_t is the radioactivity at time 0 [9, 11, 12]. In healthy adults and in children, the pharyngeal transit is quite rapid requiring less than 1 s. The normal transit time through the esophagus is typically less than 10 s, ranging from 3.4 ± 1 s for infants, 4.6 ± 1.9 for children aged 8–16 years, 5.5 ± 1.1 for adults [17].

The sensitivity and specificity of the esophageal scintigraphy to detect esophageal disorders vary widely depending on the technique used and the esophageal disorder investigated. No diagnostic benefit of esophageal scintigraphy has been shown in patients with normal peristalsis even in the presence of severe motor abnormalities as nutcracker esophagus or isolated hypertensive lower esophageal sphincter (LES) [18–20]. On the other hand, several studies have shown its ability in detecting abnormalities of esophageal peristalsis, such as achalasia, scleroderma, esophageal atresia, and diffuse esophageal spasm [14, 21–23]. However, it still represents an ancillary test when compared to esophageal manometry.

The main indications for esophageal transit scintigraphy are the evaluation of esophageal motility in patients who cannot tolerate manometry, the lack of availability of esophageal manometry, equivocal manometric results, and follow-up of patients with esophageal motor disorders such as achalasia and scleroderma (for instance, to assess the efficacy of surgical or medical therapy).

Gastroesophageal Reflux and Aspiration

GER scintigraphy has been widely used for the evaluation of GER in children [8, 24–28]. It is easy to perform, is well tolerated and requires minimum patient's cooperation. It also entails a low radiation burden. Advantages of GER scintigraphy include the ability to detect pulmonary aspiration and to evaluate gastric emptying in the same study [29, 30].

In young infants the radioactive milk or formula should replace the normally scheduled feeding, while older children should fast at least 4 h prior to the test. The tracer used is ^{99m}Tc sulfur colloid or nanocolloid (or ^{99m}Tc DTPA) mixed with an appropriate volume (between 30 and 240 ml) of milk, or milk formula. The amount of activity administered is 0.55 MBq/kg, with a minimum activity of 7.4 MBq and a maximum of 40 MBq. The tracer is added to a portion of the patient's feeding (one third to one half of the normal milk or formula feeding volume). This volume is introduced into the stomach by oral feeding or alternatively by nasogastric tube (which should be removed after feeding) or by gastrostomy tube when used for routine feedings. A second tracer free volume is then given to complete the meal. The tracer free volume has an important role of clearing residual tracer from the oropharynx and esophagus prior to imaging. The volume of the feeding varies according to the patient's age and weight. In most cases the desired volume is similar to the volume the patient is given for regular meals. The times of beginning and completing feeding should be recorded.

There is no single universally accepted protocol for this study. Most protocols however share the same basic principles. After feeding, the child is positioned supine on the γ(gamma)-camera couch. Young infants should be burped when possible prior to imaging. Restraints (sand bags and Velcro straps) may be used to secure young children to the imaging bed and prevent motion. Dynamic images are acquired from the posterior view with the stomach and chest in the field of view at a frame rate variable between 10 and 30 s/frame for 60 min [31]. Any event during the acquisition (motion, coughing, vomiting, reflux), is recorded, with the time when it happens. The dynamic images are followed by anterior and posterior static views of the chest with the stomach out of the field of view. These images are recorded on a 256×256 matrix over 3–5 min. It is important to perform the dynamic study over 60–120 min because a significant number of GER episodes can be missed by limiting the study to 60 min. The supine position is more sensitive than the prone position to detect GER [32].

New appearance of tracer in the esophagus indicates a reflux episode. Placing markers over the shoulders, suprasternal notch, and xiphoid is helpful in determining the level of reflux in the esophagus or oropharynx and in localizing possible activity within the lungs. The interpretation can be enhanced by generating time–activity curves from ROIs placed over the esophagus. GER episodes are seen as sharp spikes in the curves. Patient motion during the study can introduce significant artifacts in the curves. Images should always be inspected for motion prior to interpretation and motion correction should be applied when necessary. Visual inspection of the images in conjunction with curve interpretation and viewing of the study in cine mode is the most accurate way to read the study.

The presence of GER can be quantified using the formula: $R = E(t) - E(b) \times 100/\mathrm{Go}$, where R is the percentage of reflux material into the esophagus, $E(t)$ the esophageal count at time t, $E(b)$ the para-esophageal background counts, Go the gastric counts at the beginning of the study. R and $E(t)$ may refer to the entire organ and the individual regions [33]. According to this formula, the presence of a reflux >5% is considered abnormal [27].

Sensitivity and specificity of a 1-h scintigraphy for the diagnosis of GERD are 15–59% and 83–100%, respectively, when compared with 24-h esophageal pH monitoring [26, 28, 34, 35]. Interestingly, scintigraphy has been shown to be more sensitive in the detection of reflux beyond the first postprandial hour as compared to pH monitoring, which usually fails to detect some types of reflux, especially when little or no acid is present in the refluxate [28]. Evidence of pulmonary aspiration is usually assessed through images obtained up to 24 h after administration of the radionuclide [29, 30]. However, a negative test does not exclude the possibility of infrequently occurring aspiration. Following the introduction of multichannel intraluminal impedance and pH (MII-pH) monitoring that can characterize the reflux episodes as acid or non-acid, as well as the level reached by the refluxate, nuclear scintigraphy is not recommended in the routine diagnosis and management of GER disease (GERD) in infants and children [36].

Gastric Emptying Study

Children with gastric motor disorders may present with a wide array of foregut symptoms from nausea and vomiting to early satiety and abdominal distension of varying severity. Although there is a poor correlation between severity of symptoms and the degree of gastric emptying, assessment of gastric emptying in some circumstances helps to guide treatment decisions [37]. Measurement of gastric emptying is generally indicated when morphologic investigations fail to reveal the cause of dyspeptic symptoms, in diabetics with poor control of the disease and in severe GERD unresponsive to medical treatment [38–41]. Meaningful quantification of gastric emptying requires standardization of study techniques and standardization of the test meal. Standardization is essential for inter- and intra-subject comparisons. Gastric emptying scintigraphy is the most widely accepted technique in clinical practice and is regarded as the gold standard [42]. It is a physiologic, noninvasive, low cost technique to evaluate gastric emptying based on imaging and quantification of a radiolabeled test meal.

Several protocols for gastric emptying are used in clinical practice. These vary in the meal content, volume, and imaging technique. A solid test meal is considered more reliable than a liquid meal for measuring gastric emptying. Solid meals are used in older children and adolescents. In infants milk or milk formula is the natural and only practical choice for a test meal. Medications that affect gastric motility should be discontinued for an appropriate period prior to the test depending on the pharmacokinetics of the drugs, unless the purpose of the study is to evaluate the effect of specific drugs on gastric motility. Furthermore, fasting blood glucose should be within normal range, due to the well-known effect of hyperglycemia on the gastric motor activity [43].

The child has to be kept nil by mouth for approximately 4 h. Young infants should miss a normal feeding just prior to the test. The meal (either liquid or solid or both) has to be introduced within 10–15 min. The tracer of choice is either ^{99m}Tc nanocolloid or sulfur colloid or ^{99m}Tc-DTPA, mixed with an appropriate volume of liquid (between 30 and 240 ml, according to age) [24]. The liquid used can be milk or formula, orange or apple juice. The radioisotope is added to the meal and a second tracer-free volume is added to complete the desired feeding volume. Oral feeding is preferred but feeding through a nasogastric tube or gastrostomy tube is occasionally required. The gastric emptying study with a liquid feed is performed preferentially in children up to 2 years of age. In older children the liquid phase is used in addition to the solid phase.

After completion of the feeding, the patient is placed in the supine position and continuous dynamic images of the stomach and chest are recorded on a 128×128 matrix, 30 s/frame, for 60–120 min. Images are obtained in the anterior and posterior projections using a dual head camera. Static images of the chest and abdomen using a 256×256 matrix at 60 min are acquired. If gastric emptying is delayed, additional images should be obtained at hourly intervals up to 4 h [44, 45]. A ROI is placed around the stomach, as seen in the immediate post-feeding image. A time–activity curve, corrected for decay, is generated from the stomach ROI. Motion correction should be applied when required. Care should be taken not to include bowel activity in the gastric ROI. Gastric emptying can be expressed as a percentage of the initial activity remaining at a specific time point (residual) or as the activity emptied by the stomach at these times. It can also be expressed as the half-emptying time ($t½$). The pattern of the emptying curve is important, including the presence and the duration of the lag phase (seen in solid gastric emptying), which can provide evidence on abnormalities in gastric motility. Milk usually empties in an exponential or bi-exponential manner [24].

Some features of the protocol are subject to variability and warrant further discussion. The duration of the study is not well standardized, although several studies in adults support the superiority of a longer, 4 h study rather than 2-h study [44, 45]. Geometrical mean of the anterior and posterior counts, acquired simultaneously with a dual detector camera, is recommended to correct for the artifacts produced by the non-uniform attenuation of the radiotracer within the stomach, with the fundus situated more posteriorly and the antrum more anteriorly. Continuous data recording is preferable over recording data only at discrete time intervals, as it gives information on the lag phase and may be helpful in identifying patterns of rapid gastric emptying.

A major problem with gastric emptying scintigraphy in children is the lack of age related normal values derived from large groups of normal controls. Normal children cannot be studied as control subjects due to ethical considerations. Pooling data from different institutions to establish a normal range is problematic due to lack of standardization of the study technique and the test meal. Given these limitations, it is best for individual laboratories to establish their own normal range. For milk, a residual of 36–68% at 1 h was reported in infants, and 42–56% in a small number of older children [46]. The normal range for liquid gastric emptying residuals with ^{99m}Tc sulfur colloid labeled dextrose at 1 h in children less than 2 years of age can range between 27 and 81%, and in children 2 years of age or over 11–47% [47]. The range of normal values for solid gastric emptying in children has not been established. In a small series of 11 normal control children, 5–11 years old, solid gastric emptying values corresponded well to those described in adults [48]. Using the anterior imaging projection, normal control values can be used as a guide. These values expressed as a percentage of gastric residuals are 60–82% at 1 h and 25–55% at 2 h. An example of delayed gastric emptying with GOR is shown in Fig. 14.1.

At the end of the dynamic acquisition further imaging is performed at 2 h to assess for further gastric emptying. It is expected that no significant activity persist in the stomach by 2 h with a liquid feed. This delayed imaging acquisition is performed in the same way as the remainder of the study, to allow comparison with the previous imaging and extrapolation of the time activity curve to the delayed images.

Gastric emptying with a solid test meal is the preferred method to assess gastric emptying in older children and adolescents. It is important that the radioactive label remains firmly attached to the solid phase. A stable label can be achieved by mixing and cooking ^{99m}Tc sulfur colloid with a whole egg (82% bound at 3 h) or with the egg white (95% bound at 3 h). A stable label can also be obtained with fat free egg substitutes. The consensus guidelines for the gastric emptying study using a solid meal recommend a meal based on egg whites, two slices of toasted white bread, jam or jelly and water. The guidelines specify the details of how to cook the meal, with the amount of the different ingredients. The tracer of choice is ^{99m}Tc sulfur or nanocolloid, as it sticks well to the egg white. If the child is intolerant to eggs, a different meal should be used. It is important that every effort is made to follow the standardized meal as this allows comparison with an established normal range and between results from different centers. A detailed record of the time it takes to ingest the meal (or if any portion of it has not be eaten) should be kept.

At the time of reporting, it is very important to have a detailed clinical history including possible previous surgical procedures, current medications, and current symptoms. The clinical question that motivates the examination should be clear. Symptoms occurring during the examination (cough, vomit) should be documented, with the time when they occurred. The type of meal given, the amount, the imaging protocol, the technique of acquisition, should be described in

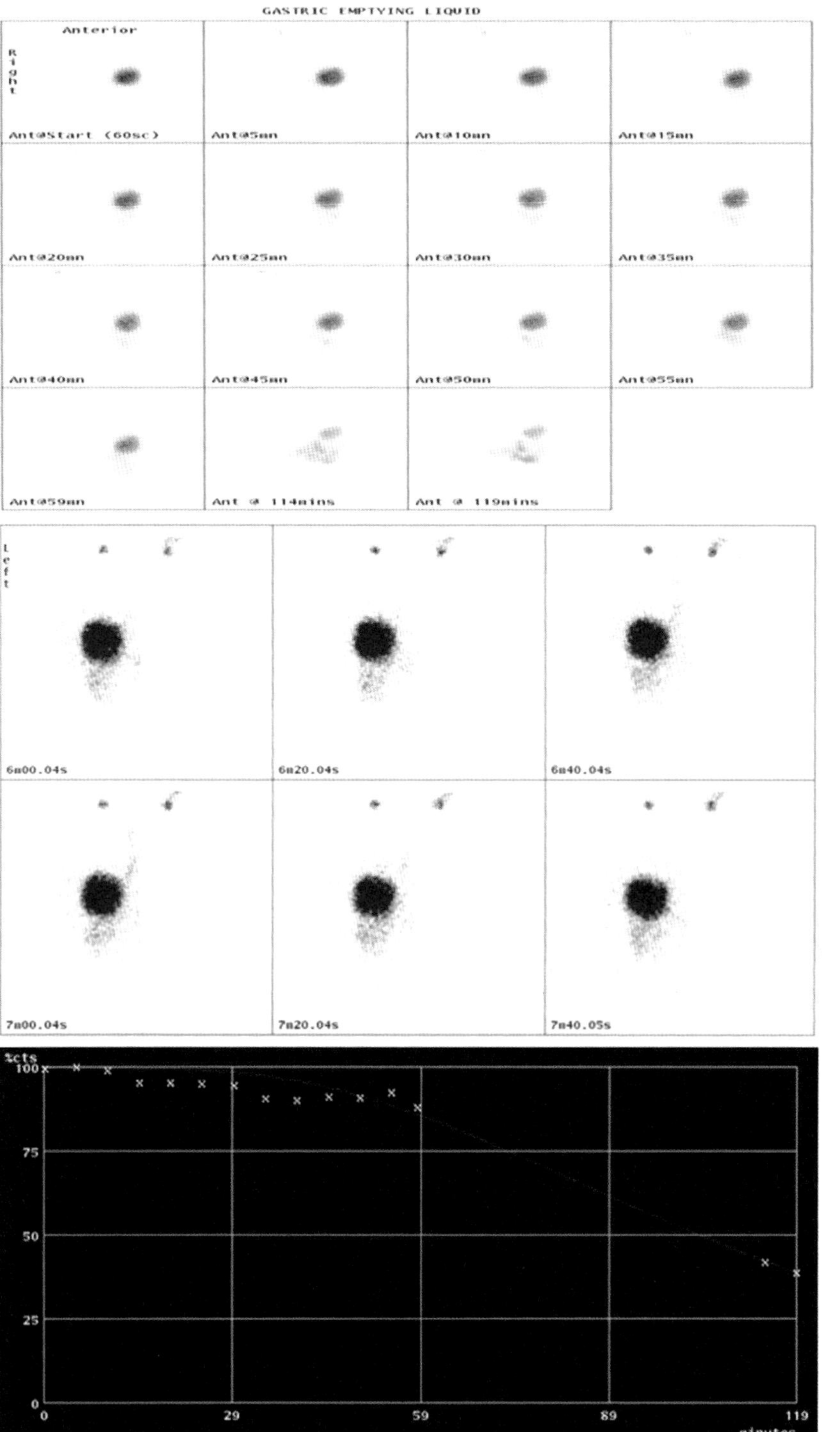

Fig. 14.1 Twenty-two-months-old girl complaining of difficulties in feeding. A gastric emptying study with liquid feed was performed. Images were acquired at a frame rate of 20 s/frame over 60 min. A delayed acquisition for 1 min at the same rate was performed. 15 MBq Tc-99m-nanocolloid mixed with 150 ml of milk was given through the gastrostomy tube. There are multiple episodes of gastroesophageal reflux (GER) reaching the upper third of the oesopagus during the first 40 min of the dynamic study. At the end of the 60 min acquisition only 10% of the administered tracer leaves the stomach. By 2 h, approximately 60% of tracer has left the stomach, with 40% of the initial gastric content still seen. The appearances are compatible with a severely delayed gastric emptying for liquids and several episodes of GER

the report. The percentage of tracer retained in the stomach at specific times in comparison to the normal reference values should be mentioned. A description of the different patterns of gastric emptying (i.e., tracer remaining within the antrum or fundus, possible dysmotility) may be helpful.

Possible sources of error include a nonstandard meal, poor labeling of the meal, nausea caused by the meal, vomit after the ingestion of the meal, ingestion of food just before the study, overlap of small bowel activity over the stomach, prolonged time to ingest the meal, and GER. Furthermore, although a delayed gastric emptying can be found in up to 70% of patients with functional dyspepsia, it does not prove that symptoms are due to gastroparesis, as well as both rapid and delayed gastric emptying cause similar symptoms [49].

Small Intestine Transit Scintigraphy

Assessment of small bowel transit time is largely dependent on gastric emptying time and complex movements of the chyme into the small intestine [50]. In adults, small bowel scintigraphy is not commonly used outside research settings, and it is usually performed as part of whole gut transit study. To our knowledge in children there are only few published data regarding this issue. The study involves the ingestion of either a solid (meals or capsule) or liquid (water) materials labeled with ^{99m}Tc or ^{111}In (see colonic transit study) [51–53]. The commonest scintigraphic method for assessing small bowel transit is to measure orocecal transit time, defined as the time taken for 10% of small bowel radioactivity to accumulate into the cecum [54–56]. Thus, it is a very laborious method since it requires multiple image taken every 10 min until 10% of the activity reaches the colon. A valid surrogate for the 10% activity is the percentage of the administered activity in the terminal ileum at 6 h after meal ingestion. Normative data in adults are limited, thus the test seems to be diagnostic only if extreme value are present. Identification of abnormal small bowel transit through scintigraphy has been shown to modify both initial diagnosis and clinical management, although its analysis needs to be interpreted with caution, keeping in mind that both delayed colonic transit and gastric emptying can affect small bowel transit. No data are available in children.

Colonic Transit Scintigraphy

Two techniques are used to evaluate motility through the GI tract, both of which involve irradiation of the subjects: transit of radiopaque (plastic) markers viewed by x-ray and transit of radioisotope viewed by γ(gamma)-camera (scintigraphy). Together, with the assessment of rectal evacuation dynamics and rectal sensation, the radioisotope studies of colonic transit represent the cornerstone investigations in patients with chronic constipation. These investigations have led to constipation being conceptualized in three broad and overlapping categories: normal transit constipation, slow transit constipation, and evacuation disorders. Transit studies per se address the question of whether the patient has a normal or delayed colonic transit.

Colonic transit scintigraphy is a safe and noninvasive method for the quantitative evaluation of overall and regional colonic transit [57]. It has been shown to correlate with radiopaque markers [58–62]. The radioisotope can be given orally either in a nonabsorbable form together with a test meal (radiolabeled mixed meal), or in a nondigestible capsules. As the images are captured on a γ-camera there is no increase of radiation exposure with multiple scans, as the radiation burden is the same irrespective of the number of times the patient is imaged. It has been shown that the total amount of radiation exposure is similar to two abdominal x-rays [63]. This test offers reproducible and accurate performance across a spectrum of disorders, linking colonic transit measurement to symptoms and disease processes, and demonstrating response to treatment [57].

The patient should use their usual method of bowel emptying 2 days before the study and should not use any further stool softeners, laxative, enemas, and suppositories until the end of the study. The procedure is performed after a fast of at least 6 h in children. The isotope (^{99m}Tc or ^{111}In) can be given orally in a nonabsorbable form with a test meal, or in a capsule coated with pH sensitive material that dissolves in the colon or terminal ileum [64, 65]. ^{111}In labeled tracers are the most widely used in this clinical setting. Because the test is relatively new in clinical practice, there are many different protocols. A standardized protocol of acquisition has not been agreed yet. In the single-isotope test meal, ^{99m}Tc phytate colloid is suspended in 20 ml of milk. The dose is determined according to body's weight based on an adult dose of 250 MBq. The dual isotope test meal consists of a sandwich of two ^{99m}Tc sulfur colloid labeled scrambled eggs and 300 ml of water labeled with ^{111}In-DTPA. The meal is consumed by the patient at the start of the study. The rationale for utilizing radiolabeled liquids for the small intestine and colonic transit studies is the reduction of variability in small intestine and colonic transit that might be caused by delayed gastric emptying for solids. In general, the liquid component of a test meal leaves the stomach much more rapidly than the solid component. In a different single and dual method ^{111}In-Cl$_3$ (0.1 mCi) mixed with a slurry of 5 mg of activated charcoal is delivered within a coated capsule. The slurry is evaporated to dryness on a hotplate at 90 °C, and the dried charcoal is placed into a size 1 gelatine capsule and coated with pH-sensitive methacrylate. Luminal pH increases in the distal ileum and the capsule opens to release its contents into the cecum. Markers placed on the patient's anterior superior iliac spine facilitated identification of the small bowel, in order to ascertain that the capsule had emptied from the stomach before feeding the ^{99m}Tc sulfur colloid-labeled test meal.

Imaging is performed with the patient in upright position using a large γ-camera equipped with a medium energy collimator. During dual isotope test images are acquired immediately after ingestion of the meal every 30 min for 2 h to measure gastric emptying of solid and liquids. Afterwards, the images are usually taken at 4, 6, 24, and 48 h. There is a consensus that images at 24 and 48 h give a good summary of colonic transit with acceptable specificity and high sensitivity for detecting motility disorders, although in selected circumstances images can be taken at 72 h and possibly up to 96 h [66]. Anterior and posterior images are obtained for an acquisition time up to 400 s on a 256×256 matrix. The pulse height analyzer of the γ(gamma)-camera is centered on 140 keV with a window of ±20% to detect counts from Tc-99 m and on two peaks (173 and 247 keV) ±20% to detect counts from In-111. An example of colonic scintigraphy in a patient with slow transit constipation is shown in Fig. 14.2.

The analysis of colonic transit is performed drawing different colonic ROIs on both the anterior and the posterior images in order to quantify the geometric center (GC) which represents the weighted average of radioactivity over specific regions of the bowel and determines the median point of radioactivity for each time point. The number of ROIs varies from 5 to 7, including the segment referring to the expelled stools (Fig. 14.3). For instance, Southwell and coworkers defined six colonic ROIs each with a numerical values: (1) Small Intestine, (2) Cecum-Ascending Colon, (3) Transverse Colon, (4) Descending Colon, (5) Rectosigmoid Colon, and (6) Excreted Stools [66]. The geometric center is calculated as the sum of the products of the proportion of ^{111}In counts in each region and its weighting factor from the following equation: GC: Σ(Sigma)^n fraction of activity in ROI^n×n, where n is the number of each region (1–5, 1–7, or 1–8, based on the method applied). A low GC indicates that the center of the activity is in the proximal colon, and a higher GC indicates that it has progresses on the left side of the colon has been eliminated in the stool. In adults, based on the method, the normal mean (±1 SD) GC values range between 2.67±1.09 to 4.6±1.5 at 24 h, 3.89±0.15 to 6.1±1.0 at 48 h, and 6.6±0.19 at 72 h [59, 67]. In children, the normal mean±SD GC values are 3.9±1.1 at 24 h, and 5.2±0.9 at 48 h [68]. Of note, as a summary of the colonic transit some researchers also utilize the emptying of ascending colon expressed as *t*½ (time for 50% emptying), which is significantly correlated with stools consistency.

Three categories of colonic transit could be readily distinguished also by visual assessment of

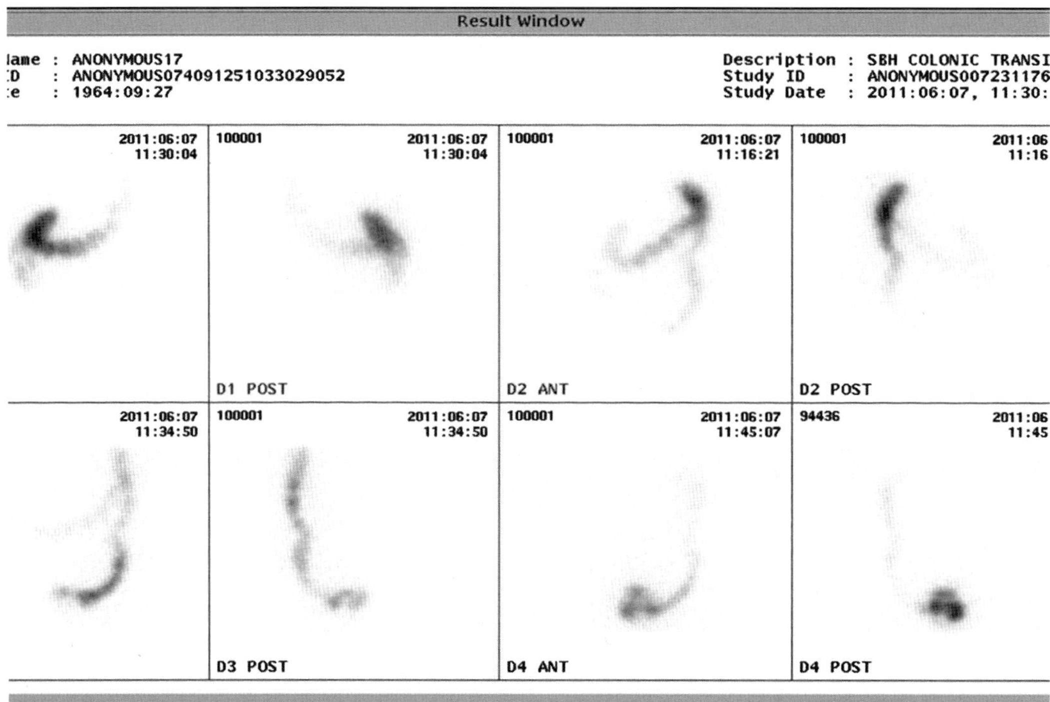

Fig. 14.2 Colonic transit study of a patient with severe slow transit chronic constipation. The study was performed following the administration of 3 MBq In-111 chloride as a liquid. Imaging was obtained on day 1 6 h after tracer ingestions and subsequently on days 2, 3, and 4. The images show slow progression of the tracer throughout the whole of the colon, not just in a specific portion of it

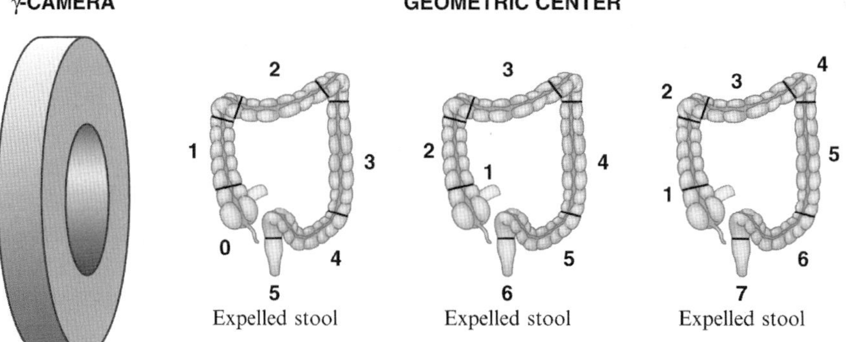

Fig. 14.3 To quantitate colon transit, the geometric center (GC) has been defined to measure the progression of colonic activity. To calculate the GC, the colon is divided into anatomic regions each with a numerical value. The number of Regions of Interest (ROIs) used in different studies varies from 5 to 7, including the segment referring to the expelled stools

the acquired images. In normal studies, the tracer reaches the cecum in 6 h, and is largely excreted by 48 h. Slow colonic transit is identified when the tracer reaches the cecum at 6 h, but most radioactivity is retained in the proximal colon and transverse colon at 24, 36 and 48 h. In children with outlet obstruction or functional fecal retention, the tracer reaches the rectosigmoid by 24 to 36 h but is not passed at 48 h. In children and adolescent with refractory functional constipation, slow transit in the proximal colon occurs in 20–50% and outlet obstruction in 22–55% with some children presenting both [69].

In quantifying colonic transit, the colonic transit scintigraphy can influence management of patients with refractory constipation who might benefit from different treatment strategies. For instance, by using colonic scintigraphy the degree of efficacy of several prokinetics drugs can be evaluated. Also, the type of surgery or stoma positioning may be determined by identifying the site of delay [57]. Unfortunately, although colonic transit scintigraphy should be recommended in all patients with refractory abnormal bowel habit, its availability is limited to a selected number of centers.

Acknowledgments We thank Dr. Alex Green for his help and expertise in providing high quality illustrations.

References

1. Camilleri M, Hasler WL, Parkman HP, Quigley MM, Soffer E. Measurement of gastrointestinal motility in the GI laboratory. Gastroenterology. 1998;115:747–62.
2. Rao SSC, Camilleri M, Hasler WL, et al. Evaluation of gastrointestinal transit in clinical practice: position paper of the American and European Neurogastroenterology and Motility Societies. Neurogastroenterol Motil. 2011;23:8–23.
3. Odunsi ST, Camilleri M. Selected interventions in nuclear medicine: gastrointestinal motor functions. Semin Nucl Med. 2009;39:186–94.
4. Ljung B. The child in diagnostic nuclear medicine. Eur J Nucl Med. 1997;24:683–90.
5. Lassmann M, Biassoni L, Monsieurs M, et al. The new EANM paediatric dosage card. Eur J Nucl Med Mol Imaging. 2007;34:796–8.
6. Gelfand MJ, Parisi MT, Treves ST. Pediatric Nuclear Medicine Dose Reduction Workgroup. Pediatric radiopharmaceutical administered doses: 2010 North American consensus guidelines. J Nucl Med. 2011;52:318–22.
7. Kazem I. A new scintigraphic technique for the study of the esophagus. AJR. 1972;115:681–8.
8. Rudd TG, Christie DL. Demonstration of gastroesophageal reflux in children by radionuclide gastroesophagography. Radiology. 1979;131:483–6.
9. Mariani G, Boni G, Barreca M, et al. Radionuclide gastroesophageal motor studies. J Nucl Med. 2004;45:1004–28.
10. Kochan P, Maurer A, Parkman H, et al. Clinical role of esophageal and gastroesophageal reflux scintigraphy. J Nucl Med. 2002;43:162P.
11. Tatsch K, Voderholzer WA, Weiss MJ, Schrottle W, Hahn K. Re-appraisal of quantitative esophageal scintigraphy by optimizing results with ROC analyses. J Nucl Med. 1996;37:1799–805.
12. Tatsch K. Multiple swallow test for quantitative and qualitative evaluation of esophageal motility disorders. J Nucl Med. 1991;32:1365–70.
13. Mughal MM, Marples M, Bancewicz J. Scintigraphic assessment of esophageal motility: what does it show and how reliable is it? Gut. 1986;27:946–53.
14. Holloway RH, Lange RC, Plankey MW, McCallum RW. Detection of esophageal motor disorders by radionuclide transit studies: a reappraisal. Dig Dis Sci. 1989;34:905–12.
15. Edenbrandt L, Theander E, Hogstrom M, et al. Esophageal scintigraphy in normal subjects and patients with systemic sclerosis. J Nucl Med. 1995; 36:1533–37.
16. Stacey B, Patel P. Oesophageal scintigraphy for the investigation of dysphagia: in and out of favour—underused when available. Eur J Nucl Med Mol Imaging. 2002;29:1216–20.
17. Warrington C, Charron M. Pediatric gastrointestinal nuclear medicine. Semin Nucl Med. 2007;37: 269–85.
18. de Caestecker JS, Blackwell JN, Adam RD, Hannan WJ, Brown J, Heading RC. Clinical value of radionuclide esophageal transit measurement. Gut. 1986;27:659–66.
19. Stier AW. Image processing in esophageal scintigraphy: topography of transit times. Dis Esophagus. 2000;13:152–60.
20. Howarth D, Oldfield G, Booker J, Tan P. Esophageal dysfunction in patients with atypical chest pain investigated with esophageal scintigraphy and myocardial perfusion imaging: an outcome study. J Nucl Cardiol. 2003;10:490–7.
21. Taillefer R, Jadliwalla M, Pellerin E, et al. Radionuclide esophageal transit study in the detection of esophageal motor dysfunction: comparison with motility studies (manometry). J Nucl Med. 1990;31:1921–6.
22. Geatti O, Shapiro B, Fig LM, et al. Radiolabelled semisolid test meal clearance of esophageal involvement in scleroderma and Sjo¨gren syndrome. Am J Physiol Imaging. 1991;6:65–73.
23. Cozzi F, Zucchetta P, Durigon N, et al. Esophageal dysmotility in scleroderma patients with different forms of disease and ANA patterns: a scintigraphic study in 100 cases. Reumatismo. 2003;55:86–92.
24. Heyman S. Gastric Emptying in children. J Nucl Med. 1998;39:865–9.
25. Heyman S, Kirkpatrick JA, Winter HS, Treves S. An improved radionuclide method for the diagnosis of gastroesophageal reflux and aspiration in children (milk scan). Radiology. 1979;131:479–82.
26. Blumhagen JD, Rudd TG, Christie DL. Gastroesophageal reflux in children: radionuclide gastroesophagography. AJR Am J Roentgenol. 1980; 135:1001–4.
27. Heyman S. Gastroesophageal reflux, esophageal transit, gastric emptying, and pulmonary aspiration. In:

Treves ST, editor. Pediatric nuclear medicine. New York: Springer-Verlag; 1994. p. 430–52.
28. Vandenplas Y, Derde MP, Piepsz A. Evaluation of reflux episodes during simultaneous esophageal pH monitoring and gastroesophageal reflux scintigraphy in children. J Pediatr Gastroenterol Nutr. 1992;14:256–60.
29. Thomas EJ, Kumar R, Dasan JB, et al. Gastroesophageal reflux in asthmatic children not responding to asthma medication: a scintigraphic study in 126 patients with correlation between scintigraphic and clinical findings of reflux. Clin Imaging. 2003;27:333–6.
30. Ravelli AM, Panarotto MB, Verdoni L, Consolati V, Bolognini S. Pulmonary aspiration shown by scintigraphy in gastroesophageal reflux-related respiratory disease. Chest. 2006;130:1520–6.
31. Reyhan M, Yapar AF, Aydin M, et al. Gastroesophageal scintigraphy in children: a comparison of posterior and anterior imaging. Ann Nucl Med. 2005;19:17–21.
32. Blumenthal I, Lealman GT. Effect of posture on gastro-oesophageal reflux in the newborn. Arch Dis Child. 1982;57:555–6.
33. Maurer AH, Parkman HP. Update on gastrointestinal scintigraphy. Semin Nucl Med. 2006;36:110–8.
34. Seibert JJ, Byrne WJ, Euler AR, Latture T, Leach M, Campbell M. Gastroesophageal reflux–the acid test: scintigraphy or the pH probe? AJR Am J Roentgenol. 1983;140:1087–90.
35. Arasu TS, Wyllie R, Fitzgerald JF, et al. Gastroesophageal reflux in infants and children—comparative accuracy of diagnostic methods. J Pediatr. 1980;96:798–803.
36. Vandenplas Y, Rudolph CD, Di Lorenzo C, et al. North American Society for Pediatric Gastroenterology Hepatology and Nutrition, European Society for Pediatric Gastroenterology Hepatology and Nutrition. Pediatric gastroesophageal reflux clinical practice guidelines: joint recommendations of the North American Society for Pediatric Gastroenterology, Hepatology, and Nutrition (NASPGHAN) and the European Society for Pediatric Gastroenterology, Hepatology, and Nutrition (ESPGHAN). J Pediatr Gastroenterol Nutr. 2009;49:498–547.
37. Tack J, Bisschops R, Sarnelli G. Pathophysiology and treatment of functional dyspepsia. Gastroenterology. 2004;127:1239–55.
38. Sýkora J, Malán A, Záhlava J, et al. Gastric emptying of solids in children with H. pylori-positive and H. pylori-negative non-ulcer dyspepsia. J Pediatr Gastroenterol Nutr. 2004;39:246–52.
39. Spiroglou K, Xinias I, Karatzas N, et al. Gastric emptying in children with cerebral palsy and gastroesophageal reflux. Pediatr Neurol. 2004;31:177–82.
40. Argon M, Duygun U, Daglioz G, et al. Relationship between gastric emptying and gastroesophageal reflux in infants and children. Clin Nucl Med. 2006;31:262–5.
41. Caldaro T, Garganese MC, Torroni F, et al. Delayed gastric emptying and typical scintigraphic gastric curves in children with gastroesophageal reflux disease: could pyloromyotomy improve this condition? J Pediatr Surg. 2011;46:863–9.
42. Abell TL, Camilleri M, Donohoe K, et al. American Neurogastroenterology and Motility Society and the Society of Nuclear Medicine. Consensus recommendations for gastric emptying scintigraphy: a joint report of the American Neurogastroenterology and Motility Society and the Society of Nuclear Medicine. Am J Gastroenterol. 2008;103:753–63.
43. Camilleri M, Bharucha AE, Farrugia G. Epidemiology, mechanisms, and management of diabetic gastroparesis. Clin Gastroenterol Hepatol. 2011;9:5–12.
44. Guo JP, Maurer AH, Urbain JL, et al. Extending gastric emptying scintigraphy from two to four hours detects more patients with gastroparesis. Dig Dis Sci. 2001;46:24–9.
45. Ziessman HA, Bonta DV, Goetze S, et al. Experience with a new simplified and standardized four-hour gastric emptying protocol. J Nucl Med. 2007;48:568–72.
46. Seibert JJ, Byrne WJ, Euler AR. Gastric emptying in children: unusual patterns detected by scintigraphy. AJR. 1983;141:49–51.
47. Rosen PR, Treves S. The relationship of gastroesophageal reflux and gastric emptying in infants and children: concise communication. J Nucl Med. 1984;25:571–4.
48. Montgomery M, Escobar-Billing R, Hellstrom PM, et al. Impaired gastric emptying in children with repaired esophageal atresia: a controlled study. J Pediatr Surg. 1998;33:476–80.
49. Sarnelli G, Caenepeel P, Geypens B, Janssens J, Tack J. Symptoms associated with impaired gastric emptying of solids and liquids in functional dyspepsia. Am J Gastroenterol. 2003;98:783–8.
50. Tack J, Janssen P. Gastroduodenal motility. Curr Opin Gastroenterol. 2010;26:647–55.
51. Read NW, Al-Janabi MN, Holgate AM, et al. Simultaneous measurement of gastric emptying, small bowel residence and colonic filling of a solid meal by the use of the gamma camera. Gut. 1986;27:300–8.
52. Malagelada J, Robertson JS, Brown ML, et al. Intestinal transit of solid and liquid components of a meal in health. Gastroenterology. 1984;7:1255–63.
53. Maurer AH, Krevsky B. Whole-gut transit scintigraphy in the evaluation of small-bowel and colon transit disorders. Semin Nucl Med. 1995;25:326–38.
54. Argenyi EE, Soffer EE, Madsen MT, et al. Scintigraphic evaluation of small bowel transit in healthy subjects: inter- and intrasubject variability. Am J Gastroenterol. 1995;90:938–42.
55. Miller MA, Parkman HP, Urbain JL, et al. Comparison of scintigraphy and lactulose breath hydrogen test for assessment of orocecal transit: lactulose accelerates small bowel transit. Dig Dis Sci. 1997;42:10–8.
56. Charles F, Camilleri M, Phillips SF, et al. Scintigraphy of the whole gut: clinical evaluation of transit disorders. Mayo Clin Proc. 1995;70:113–8.

57. Camilleri M. Scintigraphic biomarkers for colonic dysmotility. Clin Parmacol Ther. 2010;87:748–53.
58. van der Sijp JR, Kamm MA, Nightingale JM, et al. Radioisotope determination of regional colonic transit in severe constipation: comparison with radio opaque markers. Gut. 1993;34:402–8.
59. Cremonini F, Mullan BP, Camilleri M, Burton DD, Rank MR. Performance characteristics of scintigraphic transit measurements for studies of experimental therapies. Aliment Pharmacol Ther. 2002;16:1781–90.
60. Lundin E, Graf W, Garske U, et al. Segmental colonic transit studies: comparison of a radiological and a scintigraphic method. Colorectal Dis. 2007;9:344–51.
61. Stivland T, Camilleri M, Vassallo M, et al. Scintigraphic measurement of regional gut transit in idiopathic constipation. Gastroenterology. 1991;101:107–15.
62. Degen LP, Phillips SF. Variability of gastrointestinal transit in healthy women and men. Gut. 1996;39:299–305.
63. Sutcliffe JR, King S, Hutson JM, Southwell B. What is new in radiology and pathology of motility disorders in children? Semin Pediatr Surg. 2010;19:81–5.
64. Bonapace ES, Maurer AH, Davidoff S, Krevsky B, Fisher RS, Parkman HP. Whole gut transit scintigraphy in the clinical evaluation of patients with upper and lower gastrointestinal symptoms. Am J Gastroenterol. 2000;95:2838–47.
65. Burton DD, Camilleri M, Mullan BP, Forstrom LA, Hung JC. Colonic transit scintigraphy labeled activated charcoal compared with ion exchange pellets. J Nucl Med. 1997;38:1807–10.
66. Southwell BR, Clarke MC, Sutcliffe J, Hutson JM. Colonic transit studies: normal values for adults and children with comparison of radiological and scintigraphic methods. Pediatr Surg Int. 2009;25:559–72.
67. Krevsky B, Maurer AH, Niewiarowski T, Cohen S. Effect of verapamil on human intestinal transit. Dig Dis Sci. 1992;37:919–24.
68. Cook BJ, Lim E, Cook D, et al. Radionuclear transit to assess sites of delay in large bowel transit in children with chronic idiopathic constipation. J Pediatr Surg. 2005;40:478–83.
69. Chitkara DK, Bredenoord AJ, Cremonini F, et al. The role of pelvic floor dysfunction and slow colonic transit in adolescents with refractory constipation. Am J Gastroenterol. 2004;99:1579–84.

Electrogastrography, Breath Tests, Ultrasonography, Transit Tests, and SmartPill

15

Leonel Rodriguez

Electrogastrography

Electrogastrography (EGG) is a noninvasive test that records the gastric myoelectrical activity through cutaneous leads. The basis of the test is to identify the normal rhythmicity of the stomach of 3 cycles per minute (range 2–4) which reliably corresponds to the slow wave generated by the gastric pacemaker, confirmed by simultaneous electrode recordings from gastric mucosa and serosa and skin in animals and humans [1–3]. Values above and below this range are called tachygastria and bradygastria, respectively (Fig. 15.1). The variables evaluated include the dominant frequency, the dominant power (amplitude in decibels), the percentage of normal frequency and the percentage of coupling. The rhythmicity from other organs (like heartbeat and respiration) is filtered out during the recording and motion artifact can be either analyzed visually or via a motion sensor and then manually excluded. The signal from all recordings is then selected and then the EGG parameters are computed based on spectral analysis. This allows an objective interpretation of the results. Since the first recording of an electrogastrogram in 1921 by Alvarez [4] multiple improvements to the technique have been applied with the advances of technology. In the early stages, most of the investigations on EGG were focused on its role on diagnosing peptic ulcer disease and gastric cancer and the physiological changes caused by gastric surgery. Over the last two decades the focus has expanded to evaluate symptoms more than conditions. The first report of the use of EGG in children occurred in 1976, when Disembaeva et al. reported the normal patterns of EGG in healthy children [5], followed by a report from Mirutko et al. describing its potential applicability on the evaluation and management of peptic ulcer disease [6]. The field of pediatric EGG exploded in the 1990s, when the technique was evaluated in multiple disorders and symptoms.

Developmental Aspects

The gastric rhythm of three contractions per minute seems to be irregular or absent at birth and matures over time [7, 8]. Although some have reported no difference between term and preterm infants [9], there seems to be agreement that the rhythmicity reaches adult characteristics in late childhood [7, 10].

L. Rodriguez, M.D., M.S. (✉)
Gastroenterology Division, Department of Medicine, Harvard Medical School, Children's Hospital, 300 Longowood Avenue, Boston, MA 02493, USA
e-mail: leonel.rodriguez@childrens.harvard.edu

C. Faure et al. (eds.), *Pediatric Neurogastroenterology: Gastrointestinal Motility and Functional Disorders in Children*, Clinical Gastroenterology,
DOI 10.1007/978-1-60761-709-9_15,

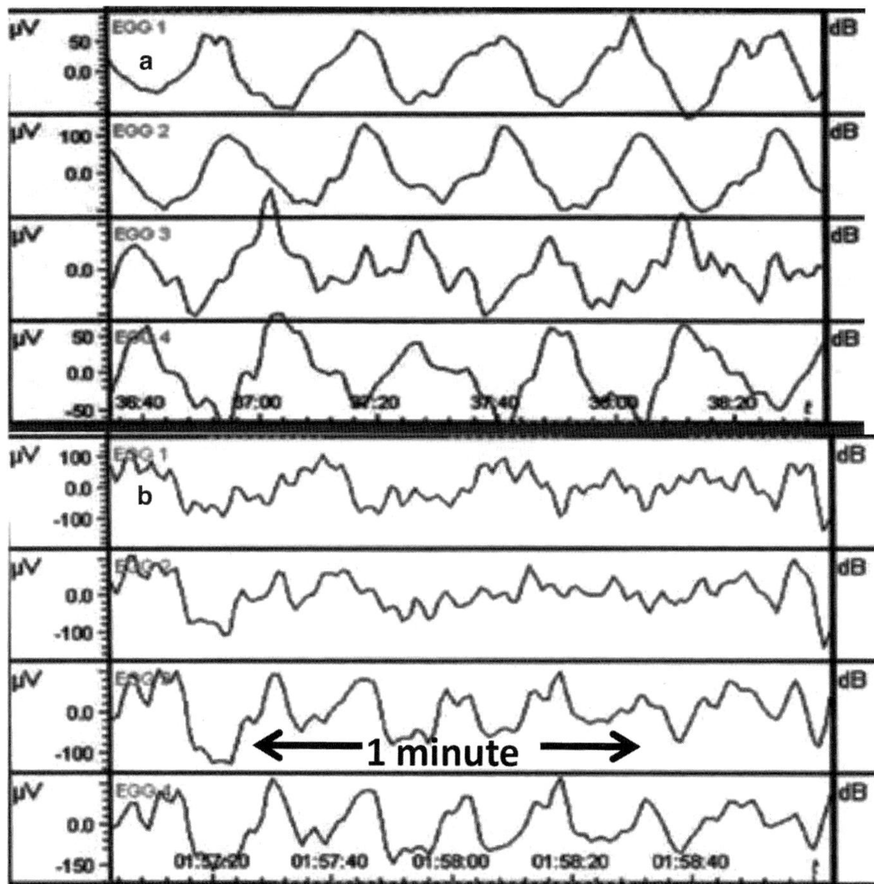

Fig. 15.1 Electrogastrogram parts of two electrogastrogram studies. (**a**) Shows normogastria or normal gastric rhythm of 3 cpm and (**b**) shows tachygastria with a rhythm of 5 cpm

Normal Values

Multiple studies have attempted to develop norms for children, unfortunately with different methodologies. The largest study evaluating normal values was done by Riezzo et al. in 114 healthy children aged 6–12 years, reporting a gastric rhythm in the 2.0–4.0 cpm range with a significant increase in postprandial dominant frequency and power [11]. Another study with 55 healthy volunteers age 6–18 years showed a mean dominant frequency 2.9±0.40 cycles per minute preprandially and 3.1±0.35 postprandially, 80%±13% preprandial normogastria and 85%±11% postprandial normogastria [12]. These normative values were independent from age, gender, BMI [11, 12], and position [13]. A recent study demonstrated that the adult norms reported by the American Neurogastroenterology and Motility Society can be used in children and adolescents when same methodology is applied [14]. Among the factors that may affect the values of the test are the meal content and position. For infants, breast feeding compared to formula feeding [15] and for adults solid meals compared to liquid meals [16] are associated with higher dominant frequency and power.

Clinical Applications

EGG has been regarded as substitute to other more invasive tests, like the gastric emptying by scintigraphy and the antroduodenal manometry, and also for others noninvasive but associated to operator dependent concerns, like ultrasonography. However, most studies have not used the same methodology in terms of number and position of electrodes, recording time, test meals and analytical software, limiting the validity of the test. Multiple studies in healthy adults as well as adults with specific disorders have shown no significant correlation between the findings on the EGG and the gastric emptying by scintigraphy, and small series in children have replicated those findings [17]. EGG is not useful to discriminate between the three phases of the myoelectric migrating complex in adults [18] but is helpful differentiating children with normal or abnormal antroduodenal manometry although there is significant overlap in EGG results with significant artifact from movement leading to inability to interpret data in up to 12% of patients [19]. Also, EGG findings do not correlate with ultrasonographic findings of gastric emptying and motility [20]. Rather than a substitute for these studies, EGG should be seen more as an adjunct in the evaluation of patients with functional and motility gastrointestinal disorders.

Functional Gastrointestinal Disorders

Although some have reported that EGG may not be helpful to differentiate functional abdominal pain from gastritis [21], others have reported significant EGG abnormalities in children with functional dyspepsia and functional abdominal pain [22–24] particularly in children with more severe pain [22]. Also, EGG does not seem to be a helpful tool to differentiate functional abdominal pain from peptic disease since chronic gastritis does not seem to be associated with gastric dysrhythmias [21, 25].

Gastroesophageal Reflux

EGG has been extensively used to assess the potential role of gastric myoelectrical abnormalities in GER. In children, myoelectrical abnormalities associated with delayed gastric emptying seem to be associated with severe GER [26].

Chronic Intestinal Pseudo-Obstruction

In children EGG has been reported to be abnormal [27] showing significant difference in the values of either preprandial dominant frequency with tachygastria or the postprandial value of 3 cpm compared to normal subjects [28].

Eating Disorders

Gastric myoelectrical abnormalities seem more common in bulimia than anorexia nervosa [29] and EGG is normal in the early stages of anorexia nervosa [30].

Effect of Medications on Gastric Myoelectrical Activity

Prokinetic agents domperidone [31] and cisapride [32] unlike erythromycin [33] were effective in normalizing gastric myoelectrical activity in children. General anesthesia has been associated with significant gastric dysrhythmias that return to baseline about an hour after anesthesia is stopped [34]. EGG has been helpful to elucidate the potential mechanism of chemotherapy induced emesis. EGG overall findings do not differ before and after chemotherapy, but tachygastria was noticed only during emesis episodes preceded by normal myoelectrical activity [35].

Surgery

Nissen fundoplication may increase gastric myoelectrical abnormalities in neurologically impaired children; this could explain in part the postoperative retching in some [36].

Strengths: Noninvasive, easy to perform, can be performed at bedside, no radiation required, not operator dependent.
Limitations: Methodology nonstandardized, motion artifact significant limitation.

Breath Tests

The most common indications for breath testing (BT) include assessment for lactose intolerance and evaluation of small bowel bacterial overgrowth. The first is assessed by the elevated levels of expired hydrogen in response to lactose ingestion and the second by the early rise of expired hydrogen after an oral challenge with glucose or lactulose.

Recently, BT has been used as a noninvasive and nonradioactive alternative to the gold standard test for gastric emptying with scintigraphy and also to assess whole gut transit (WGT). For this purpose, 13C is used to label the substrate used for the oral challenge. The test is based on measuring the ratios of Carbon 12 (12C) and Carbon 13 (13C). Both isotopes naturally exist in normal breath, 99% as 12C and about 1% as 13C. This ratio is changed by the test meal enriched with 13C resulting in enriched expired $13CO_2$. The exhalation of $13CO_2$ in patients' breath over time reflects the emptying of the substrate from the stomach. The substrates used for the evaluation of gastric emptying are 13C-octanoic acid for solids and 13C-sodium acetate for liquids. Recently the 13C-Spirulina platensis breath test has been validated compared to scintigraphy for gastric emptying in healthy volunteers [37–39]. Lactulose has been classically used in the evaluation of WGT, but due to concerns of inherent acceleration of WGT by increasing the osmolality of the gut contents, other substrates have been used, including lactose 13C-ureide breath test and more recently inulin that has been found to be the most reliable substrate since does not seem to affect gastric emptying [40, 41]. The 13C is typically measured in breath by continuous flow isotope ratio mass spectrometry, although some have also suggested the non-dispersive infrared spectrometry (IRMS) as a feasible method [42, 43]. The test relies on normal small intestine absorption, liver metabolism and pulmonary excretion to validate the results. An important concern is the reported high inter [44] and intrasubject [44, 45] variability and significant variability associated with the meal caloric content [46] in adult healthy volunteers, although some have reported very little intrasubject variability in critically ill subjects [47], making the test particularly attractive for that population. 13C-Octanoic acid has been reported as feasible [48], reliable and reproducible in preterm [49, 50] and term infants [51] and relatively independent from milk amount in preterm newborns in the first hours of life [50]. In children, BT was poorly reproducible in healthy children for gastric emptying of both liquids [52] and solids [53] and a high day-to-day variability has been reported in the evaluation of WGT [54]. The 13C-octanoic acid BT in children does not seem to be affected by osmolality, volume or density but reducing osmolality and increasing volume increases gastric emptying in preterm infants [55]. It is important to take into account the meal utilized for the study in children, as human milk [51] and hydrolyzed formulas [56] empty faster than partially and non-hydrolyzed formula. Another significant concern is the potential overestimation of the GE by the 13C-octanoic BT due to gastric processing of the substrate. A correction factor of approximately 60 min has been classically added and validated in infants [57] while others have suggested the use of the Wagner-Nelson method [58]. BT with 13C-sodium acetate for liquids and semisolids [59] and 13C-octanoic acid for solid meals [60] have been validated for gastric emptying compared to scintigraphy. In adults, both the 13C-sodium acetate [61] and 13C-octanoic acid [62] do not seem to be affected by age, gender or BMI.

Clinical Applications

Gastric Emptying

Functional Gastrointestinal Disorders

BT does not correlate with scintigraphy in functional dyspepsia [63] and could not discriminate between healthy volunteers and subjects with dyspeptic symptoms [64].

Gastroparesis

In children, the ½ emptying of 13C-sodium acetate correlates with the time to empty half of radioisotope in children with gastroparesis symptoms [65, 66] and also discriminates between healthy volunteers and children with gastroparesis symptoms [65]. BT has also been reported also as feasible in neurologically impaired children with GER [67]. BT can be done at the bedside, which makes it useful for special situations like in mechanically ventilated patients in the intensive care unit [68]. In the evaluation of diabetic gastroparesis in adults, 13C-octanoic acid BT was useful to discriminate between subjects with normal or delayed gastric emptying using scintigraphy as the gold standard [69].

Whole Gastrointestinal Transit

BT has demonstrated a constant WGT after the first month of age when a weight adapted dose of lactulose is given [70]. The lactose-[13C] ureide breath test has been reported useful to evaluate WGT in children older than 8 months [71]. Lactulose BT has been reported reproducible in healthy volunteers [72] and useful in the evaluation of small bowel transit in patients with anorexia nervosa [73].

Strengths: Noninvasive, low cost, safe, office based, not operator dependent, no radiation required, useful in particular situations (pregnancy, intensive care setting and infants).
Limitations: Requires normal intestinal, liver and pulmonary functions, poorly reproducible in children and adults, certain equipment may be expensive (IRMS).

Ultrasonography

Ultrasonography (US) is a noninvasive technique that can be used to evaluate gastric emptying and receptive accommodation, antral contractility, transpyloric flow, and gastric anatomical changes (volume and wall width) during meal and therapy challenges. US has been useful to demonstrate trituration of solids to small size particles and retention of larger particles with linear emptying of liquids [74] and antral motility coordination with pylorus flow [75] during normal conditions. Antral waves noticed in US correlate with peristaltic waves seen in antroduodenal manometry, with 99% propagating aborally and 68% becoming lumen occlusive at the site of the ultrasound marker [76]. It has been also useful to evaluate duodenogastric reflux in healthy volunteers [77] as well as in subjects with gastric ulcers [78]. The reproducibility in the assessment of gastric emptying is controversial with some reporting significant intra and interobserver variability [79, 80] while others report differing findings [81, 82], but there is a common agreement on the significant day-to-day variability [81]. More recently, 3D US has been used to assess gastric emptying with good correlation with scintigraphy in healthy subjects [83], but more studies are needed to validate the test.

Developmental Aspects

US is invaluable for the evaluation of fetal gastrointestinal physiology demonstrating evidence of gastric emptying by 12–13 weeks [84] with gastric filling and emptying by 20 weeks with an important change in gastric volume by 25 weeks [85]. The frequency of these emptying cycles reaches up to a periodicity of 35–55 min by about 35 weeks [86] and demonstrates a clear normalization along pregnancy with cycles of longer duration and stronger power along the third trimester [87]. Gastric accommodation also seems to develop over time with preterm infants showing delayed gastric distention with feeds at 26 weeks, followed by a subsequent improvement by the time full feeds are tolerated and almost immediate gastric distention with feeds by 32 weeks [88].

Clinical Applications

Gastric Emptying

Most common technique requires measurements by the same observer after fasting and at regular 30-min intervals postprandially. The emptying time is the time at which the antral area or volume returns to a basal value [89], although others have also reported the half emptying time. US has shown a strong correlation with scintigraphy in assessing gastric emptying of liquids in healthy adult volunteers at rest [90, 91] and after exercise [92] as well as in subjects with diabetic gastroparesis [93]. In children, US has shown good correlation with scintigraphy with discordances associated to overlapping of duodenum and stomach during scintigraphy and shadowing of the gastric antrum by air [94]. Establishing a safe preoperative fasting time has been another use of US in children after ingesting liquids [95] and in adults before undergoing anesthesia [96] and endoscopy [97]. US is reliable in assessing gastric emptying in preterm infants with a good correlation with intragastric volume [98] and particularly in very low birth weight infants with nasal continuous positive airway pressure [99]. US is also useful during pregnancy when radiation should be avoided. Another advantage is that allows for simultaneous assessment of gallbladder emptying [100]. US reliably assess changes in gastric emptying in response to use of prokinetic agents like domperidone [101–103], metoclopramide [104], cisapride [105], mosapride [106], and erythromycin [107].

Gastric Receptive Accommodation

US has emerged as an attractive alternative to the more invasive barostat to assess gastric accommodation. The test demonstrates no significant intra and interobserver variability but moderate day-to-day variability in healthy adult volunteers [108]. It has been reported as a reliable tool to assess gastric accommodation in subjects with functional dyspepsia [109], children with recurrent abdominal pain [110] and after therapy with prokinetic agents like mosapride [111].

Antral Motility

A novel use of the US is to characterize the antroduodenal motility associated with transpyloric fluid movement in healthy volunteers [112] and in subjects with GER symptoms [113]. Some have suggested an advantage of US by allowing a simultaneous observation of antral contractions and gastric emptying, and have reported a good correlation between antral hypomotility and delayed gastric emptying in patients with dyspepsia [114].

Strengths: Noninvasive, no radiation required, readily available, non-expensive.
Limitations: Reliable for assessment of liquids only, different and nonstandardized methodologies, requires certain expertise, operator dependent, obesity and presence of air impair study (gaseous distention is common in gastrointestinal motility disorders).

Transit Studies

Several tests have been developed to assess gastrointestinal transit as an alternative to other more invasive and expensive tests associated with radiation, like scintigraphy transit studies. Here we describe tests to assess transit in different segments of the gastrointestinal tract.

Gastric Emptying

Paracetamol Absorption Test

The rate of paracetamol absorption measured by serial serum levels after oral ingestion has been used in multiple research studies as an indirect and noninvasive test to assess gastric emptying of liquids. The test has low interindividual variability [115] with good correlation with scintigraphy [116, 117] although recent studies have questioned this correlation [118]. It is not widely used in clinical practice due to the technical requirements of frequent blood draws, the cost of the assays as well as lack of sensitivity to assess gastric emptying in clinical situations [119, 120]. Its use has been relegated mostly to pharmacokinetic studies [121] and in special situations where radiation, mobilization, or meal intake is a limitation, like patients in the intensive care units [120] and during pregnancy [122].

Epigastric Impedance

It is a noninvasive method for the assessment of gastric emptying/transit by measuring electrical impedance through skin electrodes. It is comparable to scintigraphy [123]. The method has been revised and improved by adding applied potential tomography to generate images of the electrical impedance of tissues and estimate gastric emptying and/or transit [124, 125]. Despite being an attractive noninvasive alternative its use has not spread and recommended due to low reproducibility from significant motion artifact [126, 127] and inconsistency of the impedance changes compared to phasic contractions obtained from applied potential tomography [128].

Radiopaque Markers

Extensively used in the evaluation of transit in the gastrointestinal tract due to their low cost, minimal radiation exposure and uncomplicated performance and interpretation. Despite the good agreement between gastric transit of radiopaque markers (ROM) to emptying measured by US [129] the test is not widely used due to the lack of standard methodologies and availability of other more reliable tests.

Intestinal Transit

Carmine dye, pellets and radiopaque markers have been used in the evaluation of intestinal

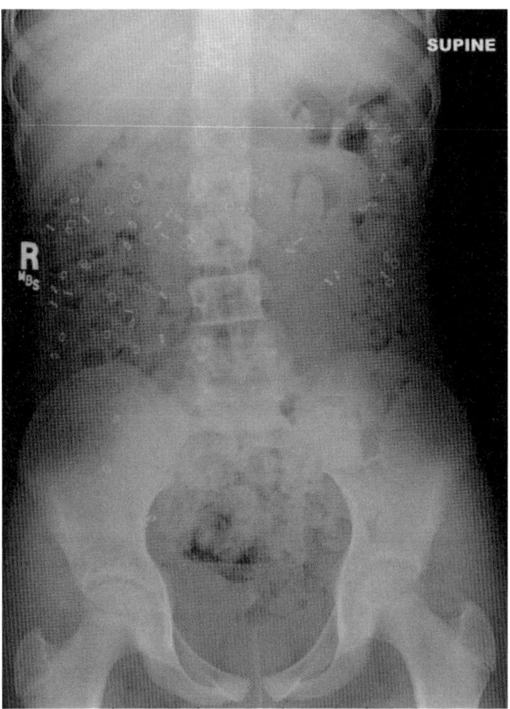

Fig. 15.2 Radiopaque marker study. This abdominal film was obtained on day 4 after ingesting three daily capsules with 24 markers each. Note the retention of all markers

transit with poor correlation with the gold standard scintigraphy. Small intestine transit is best assessed by scintigraphy and wireless motility capsule or breath testing when the former are not available.

Colon Transit

Multiple protocols have been developed using ROM to evaluate colonic transit, ranging from laborious protocols with multiple abdominal films to a simplified protocol with a single capsule and single abdominal film and the segmental transit Metcalf protocol (Fig. 15.2). The main drawback for the ROM studies is the lack of standardization between the multiple methods and the centers performing the studies. The simplified protocol requires a single capsule with ROM ingested on the first day followed by an abdominal film on the fifth day. Retention of >5 rings is considered abnormal, and this protocol is used mostly to simply assess for normal vs. abnormal colonic transit. The Metcalf protocol is used for the same purpose with the added information on segmental transit, providing a broader extent of information. In this method, three sets of distinctive ROM are ingested on 3 consecutive days followed by an abdominal film on the fourth day. This method has shown good correlation with the transit values obtained with other methods with multiple films. The normal values for the test are: total colonic transit 35.0±2.1 h, right colon 11.3±1.1 h, left colon 11.4±1.4 h and rectosigmoid colon 12.4±1.1 h with overall shorter transit in men and no effect by age [130]. Norms by the Metcalf protocol in children have been established: total colonic transit time 37.8±6.2 h, 10.8±3.5 h for the right colon, 12.2±2.7 h for the left and 14.7±2.1 h for the rectosigmoid [131]. The Metcalf protocol has been used to discriminate between constipated and non-constipated adolescents showing a statistically significant difference for the total colonic transit time and in both the right and left colon transit times [132]. Transit measured by ROM seems to be faster than colonic transit measured by scintigraphy [133]. ROM transit studies show similar transit times in young adults and children [133] but segmental transit seems to be different, with faster transit time in the right and left colon and most of the transit in the colon spent in the rectosigmoid in children compared to adults [134]. In regard to clinical applications in children, ROM transit studies have been helpful to define pediatric slow transit constipation [135] and to demonstrate correlation between colonic transit and severity of symptoms [136], slower colonic transit in constipated children without soiling compared to those with soiling [137], rectosigmoid transit delay in low variety and global delay in high variety anorectal malformations [138], constipation in neurologically impaired children associated with slow colonic transit rather than fecal retention [139] and response to therapy for constipation [140].

Strengths: Readily available, minimal radiation, noninvasive, easy to interpret, inexpensive.
Limitations: Multiple methodologies not standardized

SmartPill

This novel device offers the ability to simultaneously measure contractility and transit. The SmartPill or wireless motility capsule (WMC) measures 26.8×11.7 mm and has three sensors: pressure (to measure contractility), pH (to measure transit from stomach to small bowel and from small bowel to colon) [141] and temperature (to assess exit from the body). After ingesting the capsule orally with a standard meal, the patient is discharged and wears the recording device for 3–5 days. The most important uses of this device are to record pressures and measure transit simultaneously in different segments of the gastrointestinal tract. In this regard, it has been used to evaluate gastric residence time (GRT), small bowel transit (SBT), and colonic transit (CT) as well as whole gut transit (WGT) (Fig. 15.3). Perhaps the most significant contributions of the WMC in gastrointestinal physiology are the reaffirmation of the concept that non-digestible solids empty from the stomach primarily with the return of the phase III of the migrating motor complex (MMC) when the fed state is over and the pylorus is completely open. No less important is the novel finding of the emptying of non-digestible solids in some subjects associated with high amplitude antral contractions and not associated with the phase III of the MMC [142]. Since the WMC is an equivalent to a non-digestible solid, in healthy volunteers the gastric residence time correlates moderately with the gastric emptying of digestible solids by scintigraphy and it is not surprising that there is a stronger correlation with emptying at 4 h than at 2 h [142, 143]. The WMC has been also useful to demonstrate the lack of effect of proton pump inhibitors on antral and small bowel motility and transit [144]. A great concern with transit studies with scintigraphy is the significant daily variability, which also potentially applies to the WMC. This has not been addressed in humans, but animal studies have shown a significant variability of GRT by WMC and gastric emptying by scintigraphy with important intraindividual variability [145] and an inverse relationship between GRT and body weight [146]. At present, there are no reports yet of the utility of the WMC in children.

Clinical Applications

Gastric Emptying

Gastric residence time of the WMC correlates with the gastric emptying by scintigraphy with higher sensitivity at 4 h than at 2 h [143]. The WMC also has been useful to discriminate between healthy subjects and patients with diabetic gastroparesis by the GRT [143] and to measure contractility assessed by number of contractions and motility index in antrum and small bowel [147]. WMC has proven to be important in classifying motility disorders by region and diagnosing generalized motility disorders with good agreement with conventional motility studies [148].

Constipation

WMC is useful to measure contractility pressures in different segments of the gastrointestinal tract, including colon. Colonic contractility is poorly characterized in adult patients with constipation and constipation-IBS. WMC has been instrumental in the evaluation of colonic contractility and transit simultaneously in adults, demonstrating greater pressures in distal compared to proximal colon in healthy individuals and increased motor activity in constipated patients with normal or moderately delayed transit, emphasizing the importance of segmental evaluations of the colon [149]. In regard to CTT, the WMC has been validated for CTT and WGT by the simplified as well as by the Metcalf protocol. For the Metcalf protocol, a recent large multicenter study evidenced that although the transit was significantly different by WMC and ROM the agreement for delayed transit was 80% and for normal transit was 91% with an overall device agreement of 87% [150]. The WMC with the simplified method showed slower GRT, SBT, CT and WGT in subjects with constipation compared to controls. Interestingly CTT was slower in women than men and, more importantly, showed upper gastrointestinal transit delay in subjects with constipation [151]. Also WMC demonstrated that stool form predicts delayed vs. normal transit in adults in contrast to stool frequency [152] and reiterated the concept of a more generalized gastrointestinal dysmotility in patients with gastroparesis by evidencing also delayed CTT [153]. WMC has been also validated with scintigraphy

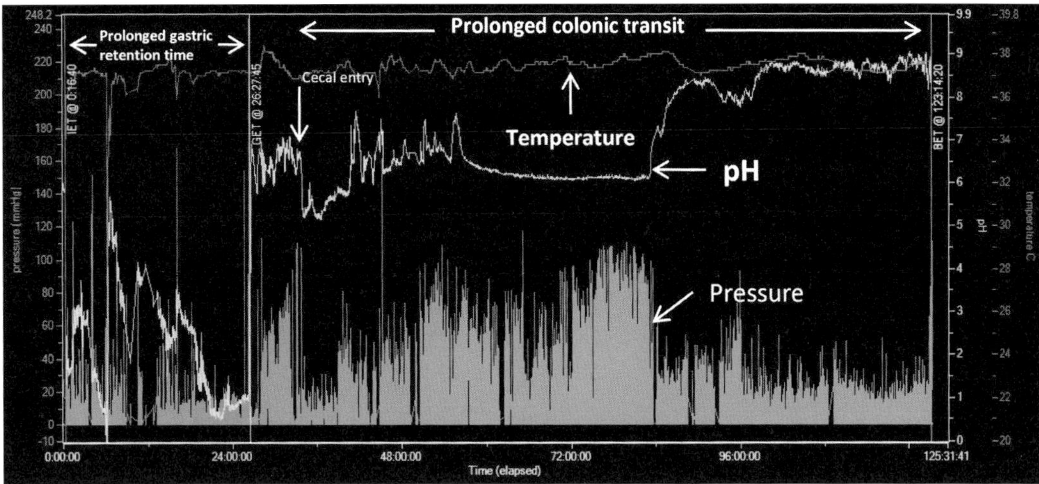

Fig. 15.3 SmartPill tracing Notice the prolonged gastric residency time as well as significantly prolonged colonic transit. Courtesy of Dr. Braden Kuo and Dr. Margarita Brun

for the evaluation of gastric emptying, colonic and whole gut transit (WGT) in healthy subjects as well as patients with constipation [154]. In regard to therapy outcome studies, the only study available so far has demonstrated a possible positive effect of increasing dietary fiber on CTT and WGT [155].

Strengths: Allows evaluation of transit of whole GI tract and pressure measurements simultaneously, not operator dependent, ambulatory.

Limitations: Cost, availability, requires expertise in interpretation, risk of capsule retention causing obstruction, capsule size limits use in children, no studies have been done in children.

References

1. Hamilton JW, et al. Human electrogastrograms. Comparison of surface and mucosal recordings. Dig Dis Sci. 1986;31(1):33–9.
2. Mintchev MP, Kingma YJ, Bowes KL. Accuracy of cutaneous recordings of gastric electrical activity. Gastroenterology. 1993;104(5):1273–80.
3. Chen JD, Schirmer BD, McCallum RW. Serosal and cutaneous recordings of gastric myoelectrical activity in patients with gastroparesis. Am J Physiol. 1994;266(1 Pt 1):G90–8.
4. Alvarez WC. The electrogastrogram and what it shows. JAMA. 1922;78:1116–9.
5. Disenbaeva LG, Khorunzhii GB. Motor function of the stomach in healthy children, 3–15 years of age, according to electrogastrography. Pediatriia. 1976;3:21–4.
6. Mirutko DD. Electrogastrography in chronic gastroduodenitis in children. Pediatriia. 1989;7:110.
7. Chen JD, et al. Patterns of gastric myoelectrical activity in human subjects of different ages. Am J Physiol. 1997;272(5 Pt 1):G1022–7.
8. Patterson M, Rintala R, Lloyd DA. A longitudinal study of electrogastrography in normal neonates. J Pediatr Surg. 2000;35(1):59–61.
9. Precioso AR, Pereira GR, Vaz FA. Gastric myoelectrical activity in neonates of different gestational ages by means of electrogastrography. Rev Hosp Clin Fac Med Sao Paulo. 2003;58(2):81–90.
10. Cheng W, Tam PK. Gastric electrical activity normalises in the first decade of life. Eur J Pediatr Surg. 2000;10(5):295–9.
11. Riezzo G, Chiloiro M, Guerra V. Electrogastrography in healthy children: evaluation of normal values, influence of age, gender, and obesity. Dig Dis Sci. 1998;43(8):1646–51.
12. Levy J, et al. Electrogastrographic norms in children: toward the development of standard methods, reproducible results, and reliable normative data. J Pediatr Gastroenterol Nutr. 2001;33(4):455–61.
13. Safder S, et al. Gastric electrical activity becomes abnormal in the upright position in patients with postural tachycardia syndrome. J Pediatr Gastroenterol Nutr. 2010;51(3):314–8.
14. Friesen CA, et al. An evaluation of adult electrogastrography criteria in healthy children. Dig Dis Sci. 2006;51(10):1824–8.
15. Riezzo G, et al. Gastric electrical activity in normal neonates during the first year of life: effect of feeding with breast milk and formula. J Gastroenterol. 2003;38(9):836–43.

16. Friesen CA, et al. Autonomic nervous system response to a solid meal and water loading in healthy children: its relation to gastric myoelectrical activity. Neurogastroenterol Motil. 2007;19(5):376–82.
17. Barbar M, et al. Electrogastrography versus gastric emptying scintigraphy in children with symptoms suggestive of gastric motility disorders. J Pediatr Gastroenterol Nutr. 2000;30(2):193–7.
18. Geldof H, van der Schee EJ, Grashuis JL. Electrogastrographic characteristics of interdigestive migrating complex in humans. Am J Physiol. 1986;250(2 Pt 1):G165–71.
19. Di Lorenzo C, et al. Is electrogastrography a substitute for manometric studies in children with functional gastrointestinal disorders? Dig Dis Sci. 1997;42(11):2310–6.
20. Pfaffenbach B, et al. The significance of electrogastrographically determined amplitudes—is there a correlation to sonographically measured antral mechanical contractions? Z Gastroenterol. 1995;33(2):103–7.
21. Uscinowicz M, Jarocka-Cyrta E, Kaczmarski M. Electrogastrography in children with functional abdominal pain and gastritis. Pol Merkur Lekarski. 2005;18(103):54–7.
22. Friesen CA, et al. Electrogastrography in pediatric functional dyspepsia: relationship to gastric emptying and symptom severity. J Pediatr Gastroenterol Nutr. 2006;42(3):265–9.
23. Devanarayana NM, de Silva DG, de Silva HJ. Gastric myoelectrical and motor abnormalities in children and adolescents with functional recurrent abdominal pain. J Gastroenterol Hepatol. 2008;23(11):1672–7.
24. Cucchiara S, et al. Electrogastrography in non-ulcer dyspepsia. Arch Dis Child. 1992;67(5):613–7.
25. Friesen CA, et al. Chronic gastritis is not associated with gastric dysrhythmia or delayed solid emptying in children with dyspepsia. Dig Dis Sci. 2005;50(6):1012–8.
26. Cucchiara S, et al. Gastric electrical dysrhythmias and delayed gastric emptying in gastroesophageal reflux disease. Am J Gastroenterol. 1997;92(7):1103–8.
27. Devane SP, et al. Gastric antral dysrhythmias in children with chronic idiopathic intestinal pseudoobstruction. Gut. 1992;33(11):1477–81.
28. Bracci F, et al. Role of electrogastrography in detecting motility disorders in children affected by chronic intestinal pseudo-obstruction and Crohn's disease. Eur J Pediatr Surg. 2003;13(1):31–4.
29. Diamanti A, et al. Gastric electric activity assessed by electrogastrography and gastric emptying scintigraphy in adolescents with eating disorders. J Pediatr Gastroenterol Nutr. 2003;37(1):35–41.
30. Ravelli AM, et al. Normal gastric antral myoelectrical activity in early onset anorexia nervosa. Arch Dis Child. 1993;69(3):342–6.
31. Franzese A, et al. Domperidone is more effective than cisapride in children with diabetic gastroparesis. Aliment Pharmacol Ther. 2002;16(5):951–7.
32. Riezzo G, et al. Gastric emptying and myoelectrical activity in children with nonulcer dyspepsia. Effect of cisapride. Dig Dis Sci. 1995;40(7):1428–34.
33. Faure C, Wolff VP, Navarro J. Effect of meal and intravenous erythromycin on manometric and electrogastrographic measurements of gastric motor and electrical activity. Dig Dis Sci. 2000;45(3):525–8.
34. Cheng W, Chow B, Tam PK. Electrogastrographic changes in children who undergo day-surgery anesthesia. J Pediatr Surg. 1999;34(9):1336–8.
35. Cheng W, Chan GC, Tam PK. Cytotoxic chemotherapy has minimal direct effect on gastric myoelectric activity in children with 5HT(3) antagonist prophylaxis. Med Pediatr Oncol. 2000;34(6):421–3.
36. Richards CA, et al. Nissen fundoplication may induce gastric myoelectrical disturbance in children. J Pediatr Surg. 1998;33(12):1801–5.
37. Lee JS, et al. A valid, accurate, office based non-radioactive test for gastric emptying of solids. Gut. 2000;46(6):768–73.
38. Viramontes BE, et al. Validation of a stable isotope gastric emptying test for normal, accelerated or delayed gastric emptying. Neurogastroenterol Motil. 2001;13(6):567–74.
39. Szarka LA, et al. A stable isotope breath test with a standard meal for abnormal gastric emptying of solids in the clinic and in research. Clin Gastroenterol Hepatol. 2008;6(6):635–43. e1.
40. Clegg M, Shafat A. Gastric emptying and orocaecal transit time of meals containing lactulose or inulin in men. Br J Nutr. 2010;104(4):554–9.
41. Geboes KP, et al. Inulin is an ideal substrate for a hydrogen breath test to measure the orocaecal transit time. Aliment Pharmacol Ther. 2003;18(7):721–9.
42. Schadewaldt P, et al. Application of isotope-selective nondispersive infrared spectrometry (IRIS) for evaluation of [13C]octanoic acid gastric-emptying breath tests: comparison with isotope ratio-mass spectrometry (IRMS). Clin Chem. 1997;43(3):518–22.
43. Braden B, Caspary WF, Lembcke B. Nondispersive infrared spectrometry for 13CO2/12CO2-measurements: a clinically feasible analyzer for stable isotope breath tests in gastroenterology. Z Gastroenterol. 1999;37(6):477–81.
44. Korth H, et al. Breath hydrogen as a test for gastrointestinal transit. Hepatogastroenterology. 1984;31(6):282–4.
45. Choi MG, et al. [13C]octanoic acid breath test for gastric emptying of solids: accuracy, reproducibility, and comparison with scintigraphy. Gastroenterology. 1997;112(4):1155–62.
46. Peracchi M, et al. Influence of caloric intake on gastric emptying of solids assessed by 13C-octanoic acid breath test. Scand J Gastroenterol. 2000;35(8):814–8.
47. Deane AM, et al. Intrasubject variability of gastric emptying in the critically ill using a stable isotope breath test. Clin Nutr. 2010;29(5):682–6.

48. Veereman-Wauters G, et al. The 13C-octanoic acid breath test: a noninvasive technique to assess gastric emptying in preterm infants. J Pediatr Gastroenterol Nutr. 1996;23(2):111–7.
49. Barnett C, et al. Reproducibility of the 13C-octanoic acid breath test for assessment of gastric emptying in healthy preterm infants. J Pediatr Gastroenterol Nutr. 1999;29(1):26–30.
50. Pozler O, et al. Development of gastric emptying in premature infants. Use of the (13)C-octanoic acid breath test. Nutrition. 2003;19(7–8):593–6.
51. Van Den Driessche M, et al. Gastric emptying in formula-fed and breast-fed infants measured with the 13C-octanoic acid breath test. J Pediatr Gastroenterol Nutr. 1999;29(1):46–51.
52. Hauser B, et al. Variability of the 13C-acetate breath test for gastric emptying of liquids in healthy children. J Pediatr Gastroenterol Nutr. 2006;42(4):392–7.
53. Hauser B, et al. Variability of the 13C-octanoic acid breath test for gastric emptying of solids in healthy children. Aliment Pharmacol Ther. 2006;23(9):1315–9.
54. Murphy MS, Nelson R, Eastham EJ. Measurement of small intestinal transit time in children. Acta Paediatr Scand. 1988;77(6):802–6.
55. Ramirez A, Wong WW, Shulman RJ. Factors regulating gastric emptying in preterm infants. J Pediatr. 2006;149(4):475–9.
56. Staelens S, et al. Gastric emptying in healthy newborns fed an intact protein formula, a partially and an extensively hydrolysed formula. Clin Nutr. 2008;27(2):264–8.
57. Omari TI, et al. Is the correction factor used in the breath test assessment of gastric emptying appropriate for use in infants? J Pediatr Gastroenterol Nutr. 2005;41(3):332–4.
58. Sanaka M, et al. The Wagner-Nelson method makes the [13C]-breath test comparable to radioscintigraphy in measuring gastric emptying of a solid/liquid mixed meal in humans. Clin Exp Pharmacol Physiol. 2007;34(7):641–4.
59. Braden B, et al. The [13C]acetate breath test accurately reflects gastric emptying of liquids in both liquid and semisolid test meals. Gastroenterology. 1995;108(4):1048–55.
60. Choi MG, et al. Reproducibility and simplification of 13C-octanoic acid breath test for gastric emptying of solids. Am J Gastroenterol. 1998;93(1):92–8.
61. Hellmig S, et al. Gastric emptying time of fluids and solids in healthy subjects determined by 13C breath tests: influence of age, sex and body mass index. J Gastroenterol Hepatol. 2006;21(12):1832–8.
62. Keller J, et al. Influence of clinical parameters on the results of 13C-octanoic acid breath tests: examination of different mathematical models in a large patient cohort. Neurogastroenterol Motil. 2009;21(10):1039–e83.
63. Punkkinen J, et al. Measuring gastric emptying: comparison of 13C-octanoic acid breath test and scintigraphy. Dig Dis Sci. 2006;51(2):262–7.
64. Delbende B, et al. 13C-octanoic acid breath test for gastric emptying measurement. Eur J Gastroenterol Hepatol. 2000;12(1):85–91.
65. Gatti C, et al. Is the 13C-acetate breath test a valid procedure to analyse gastric emptying in children? J Pediatr Surg. 2000;35(1):62–5.
66. Braden B, et al. Measuring gastric emptying of semisolids in children using the 13C-acetate breath test: a validation study. Dig Liver Dis. 2004;36(4):260–4.
67. Okada T, et al. Delay of gastric emptying measured by 13C-acetate breath test in neurologically impaired children with gastroesophageal reflux. Eur J Pediatr Surg. 2005;15(2):77–81.
68. Ritz MA, et al. Delayed gastric emptying in ventilated critically ill patients: measurement by 13 C-octanoic acid breath test. Crit Care Med. 2001;29(9):1744–9.
69. Lee JS, et al. Toward office-based measurement of gastric emptying in symptomatic diabetics using [13C]octanoic acid breath test. Am J Gastroenterol. 2000;95(10):2751–61.
70. Vreugdenhil G, Sinaasappel M, Bouquet J. A comparative study of the mouth to caecum transit time in children and adults using a weight adapted lactulose dose. Acta Paediatr Scand. 1986;75(3):483–8.
71. Van Den Driessche M, et al. Lactose-[13C]ureide breath test: a new, noninvasive technique to determine orocecal transit time in children. J Pediatr Gastroenterol Nutr. 2000;31(4):433–8.
72. La Brooy SJ, et al. Assessment of the reproducibility of the lactulose H2 breath test as a measure of mouth to caecum transit time. Gut. 1983;24(10):893–6.
73. Hirakawa M, et al. Small bowel transit time measured by hydrogen breath test in patients with anorexia nervosa. Dig Dis Sci. 1990;35(6):733–6.
74. Brown BP, et al. The configuration of the human gastroduodenal junction in the separate emptying of liquids and solids. Gastroenterology. 1993;105(2):433–40.
75. Berstad A, et al. Volume measurements of gastric antrum by 3-D ultrasonography and flow measurements through the pylorus by duplex technique. Dig Dis Sci. 1994;39(12 Suppl):97S–100.
76. Hveem K, et al. Relationship between ultrasonically detected phasic antral contractions and antral pressure. Am J Physiol Gastrointest Liver Physiol. 2001;281(1):G95–101.
77. Hausken T, et al. Quantification of gastric emptying and duodenogastric reflux stroke volumes using three-dimensional guided digital color Doppler imaging. Eur J Ultrasound. 2001;13(3):205–13.
78. Fujimura J, et al. Quantitation of duodenogastric reflux and antral motility by color Doppler ultrasonography. Study in healthy volunteers and patients with gastric ulcer. Scand J Gastroenterol. 1994;29(10):897–902.

79. Gerards C, Tromm A, May B. Optimizing antrum planimetry for ultrasound determination of gastric emptying using emptying function reference lines. Ultraschall Med. 1998;19(2):83–6.
80. Ahluwalia NK, et al. Evaluation of human postprandial antral motor function using ultrasound. Am J Physiol. 1994;266(3 Pt 1):G517–22.
81. Irvine EJ, et al. Reliability and interobserver variability of ultrasonographic measurement of gastric emptying rate. Dig Dis Sci. 1993;38(5):803–10.
82. Ricci R, et al. Real time ultrasonography of the gastric antrum. Gut. 1993;34(2):173–6.
83. Gentilcore D, et al. Measurements of gastric emptying of low- and high-nutrient liquids using 3D ultrasonography and scintigraphy in healthy subjects. Neurogastroenterol Motil. 2006;18(12):1062–8.
84. Sase M, et al. Ontogeny of gastric emptying patterns in the human fetus. J Matern Fetal Neonatal Med. 2005;17(3):213–7.
85. Sase M, et al. Development of gastric emptying in the human fetus. Ultrasound Obstet Gynecol. 2000;16(1):56–9.
86. Devane SP, Soothill PW, Candy DC. Temporal changes in gastric volume in the human fetus in late pregnancy. Early Hum Dev. 1993;33(2):109–16.
87. Sase M, et al. Gastric emptying cycles in the human fetus. Am J Obstet Gynecol. 2005;193(3 Pt 2):1000–4.
88. Carlos MA, et al. Changes in gastric emptying in early postnatal life. J Pediatr. 1997;130(6):931–7.
89. Bolondi L, et al. Measurement of gastric emptying time by real-time ultrasonography. Gastroenterology. 1985;89(4):752–9.
90. Holt S, et al. Measurement of gastric emptying rate in humans by real-time ultrasound. Gastroenterology. 1986;90(4):918–23.
91. Marzio L, et al. Evaluation of the use of ultrasonography in the study of liquid gastric emptying. Am J Gastroenterol. 1989;84(5):496–500.
92. Marzio L, et al. Influence of physical activity on gastric emptying of liquids in normal human subjects. Am J Gastroenterol. 1991;86(10):1433–6.
93. Tympner F, Feldmeier J, Rosch W. Study of the correlation of sonographic and scintigraphic results in measuring stomach emptying. Ultraschall Med. 1986;7(6):264–7.
94. Gomes H, Hornoy P, Liehn JC. Ultrasonography and gastric emptying in children: validation of a sonographic method and determination of physiological and pathological patterns. Pediatr Radiol. 2003;33(8):522–9.
95. Sethi AK, et al. Safe pre-operative fasting times after milk or clear fluid in children. A preliminary study using real-time ultrasound. Anaesthesia. 1999;54(1):51–9.
96. Perlas A, et al. Ultrasound assessment of gastric content and volume. Anesthesiology. 2009;111(1):82–9.
97. Spahn TW, et al. Assessment of pre-gastroscopy fasting period using ultrasonography. Dig Dis Sci. 2009;54(3):621–6.
98. Newell SJ, Chapman S, Booth IW. Ultrasonic assessment of gastric emptying in the preterm infant. Arch Dis Child. 1993;69(1 Spec No):32–6.
99. Gounaris A, et al. Gastric emptying in very-low-birth-weight infants treated with nasal continuous positive airway pressure. J Pediatr. 2004;145(4):508–10.
100. Glasbrenner B, et al. Simultaneous sonographic study of postprandial gastric emptying and gallbladder contraction. Bildgebung. 1992;59(2):88–93.
101. Bateman DN, Gooptu D, Whittingham TA. The effects of domperidone on gastric emptying of liquid in man. Br J Clin Pharmacol. 1982;13(5):675–8.
102. Duan LP, Zheng ZT, Li YN. A study of gastric emptying in non-ulcer dyspepsia using a new ultrasonographic method. Scand J Gastroenterol. 1993;28(4):355–60.
103. Gounaris A, et al. Gastric emptying of preterm neonates receiving domperidone. Neonatology. 2010;97(1):56–60.
104. Tympner F, Rosch W. Ultrasound measurement of gastric emptying time values. Ultraschall Med. 1982;3(1):15–7.
105. Carroccio A, et al. Gastric emptying in infants with gastroesophageal reflux. Ultrasound evaluation before and after cisapride administration. Scand J Gastroenterol. 1992;27(9):799–804.
106. Kusunoki H, et al. Efficacy of mosapride citrate in proximal gastric accommodation and gastrointestinal motility in healthy volunteers: a double-blind placebo-controlled ultrasonographic study. J Gastroenterol. 2010;45(12):1228–34.
107. Costalos C, et al. Erythromycin as a prokinetic agent in preterm infants. J Pediatr Gastroenterol Nutr. 2002;34(1):23–5.
108. Gilja OH, et al. Monitoring postprandial size of the proximal stomach by ultrasonography. J Ultrasound Med. 1995;14(2):81–9.
109. Gilja OH, et al. Impaired accommodation of proximal stomach to a meal in functional dyspepsia. Dig Dis Sci. 1996;41(4):689–96.
110. Olafsdottir E, et al. Impaired accommodation of the proximal stomach in children with recurrent abdominal pain. J Pediatr Gastroenterol Nutr. 2000;30(2):157–63.
111. Kusunoki H, et al. Efficacy of mosapride citrate in proximal gastric accommodation and gastrointestinal motility in healthy volunteers: a double-blind placebo-controlled ultrasonographic study. J Gastroenterol. 2010;45(12):1228–34.
112. King PM, et al. Relationships of human antroduodenal motility and transpyloric fluid movement: non-invasive observations with real-time ultrasound. Gut. 1984;25(12):1384–91.
113. King PM, Pryde A, Heading RC. Transpyloric fluid movement and antroduodenal motility in patients with gastro-oesophageal reflux. Gut. 1987;28(5):545–8.
114. Kusunoki H, et al. Real-time ultrasonographic assessment of antroduodenal motility after ingestion of solid and liquid meals by patients with functional dyspepsia. J Gastroenterol Hepatol. 2000;15(9):1022–7.

115. Paintaud G, et al. Intraindividual variability of paracetamol absorption kinetics after a semi-solid meal in healthy volunteers. Eur J Clin Pharmacol. 1998;53(5):355–9.
116. Koizumi F, et al. Plasma paracetamol concentrations measured by fluorescence polarization immunoassay and gastric emptying time. Tohoku J Exp Med. 1988;155(2):159–64.
117. Maddern G, et al. Liquid gastric emptying assessed by direct and indirect techniques: radionuclide labelled liquid emptying compared with a simple paracetamol marker method. Aust N Z J Surg. 1985;55(2):203–6.
118. Naslund E, et al. Gastric emptying: comparison of scintigraphic, polyethylene glycol dilution, and paracetamol tracer assessment techniques. Scand J Gastroenterol. 2000;35(4):375–9.
119. Willems M, Quartero AO, Numans ME. How useful is paracetamol absorption as a marker of gastric emptying? A systematic literature study. Dig Dis Sci. 2001;46(10):2256–62.
120. Cohen J, Aharon A, Singer P. The paracetamol absorption test: a useful addition to the enteral nutrition algorithm? Clin Nutr. 2000;19(4):233–6.
121. Medhus AW, et al. Gastric emptying: the validity of the paracetamol absorption test adjusted for individual pharmacokinetics. Neurogastroenterol Motil. 2001;13(3):179–85.
122. Wong CA, et al. Gastric emptying of water in term pregnancy. Anesthesiology. 2002;96(6):1395–400.
123. Sutton JA, Thompson S, Sobnack R. Measurement of gastric emptying rates by radioactive isotope scanning and epigastric impedance. Lancet. 1985;1(8434):898–900.
124. Brown BH, Barber DC, Seagar AD. Applied potential tomography: possible clinical applications. Clin Phys Physiol Meas. 1985;6(2):109–21.
125. Nour S, et al. Measurement of gastric emptying in infants with pyloric stenosis using applied potential tomography. Arch Dis Child. 1993;68(4):484–6.
126. Smith HL, Hollins GW, Booth IW. Epigastric impedance recording for measuring gastric emptying in children: how useful is it? J Pediatr Gastroenterol Nutr. 1993;17(2):201–6.
127. Lange A, et al. Gastric emptying patterns of a liquid meal in newborn infants measured by epigastric impedance. Neurogastroenterol Motil. 1997;9(2):55–62.
128. Smout AJ, et al. Role of electrogastrography and gastric impedance measurements in evaluation of gastric emptying and motility. Dig Dis Sci. 1994;39(12 Suppl):110S–3.
129. Loreno M, et al. Gastric clearance of radiopaque markers in the evaluation of gastric emptying rate. Scand J Gastroenterol. 2004;39(12):1215–8.
130. Metcalf AM, et al. Simplified assessment of segmental colonic transit. Gastroenterology. 1987;92(1):40–7.
131. Bautista Casasnovas A, et al. Measurement of colonic transit time in children. J Pediatr Gastroenterol Nutr. 1991;13(1):42–5.
132. Zaslavsky C, da Silveira TR, Maguilnik I. Total and segmental colonic transit time with radio-opaque markers in adolescents with functional constipation. J Pediatr Gastroenterol Nutr. 1998;27(2):138–42.
133. Southwell BR, et al. Colonic transit studies: normal values for adults and children with comparison of radiological and scintigraphic methods. Pediatr Surg Int. 2009;25(7):559–72.
134. Arhan P, et al. Segmental colonic transit time. Dis Colon Rectum. 1981;24(8):625–9.
135. Benninga MA, et al. Colonic transit time in constipated children: does pediatric slow-transit constipation exist? J Pediatr Gastroenterol Nutr. 1996;23(3):241–51.
136. Papadopoulou A, Clayden GS, Booth IW. The clinical value of solid marker transit studies in childhood constipation and soiling. Eur J Pediatr. 1994;153(8):560–4.
137. Benninga MA, et al. Defaecation disorders in children, colonic transit time versus the Barr-score. Eur J Pediatr. 1995;154(4):277–84.
138. Rintala RJ, et al. Segmental colonic motility in patients with anorectal malformations. J Pediatr Surg. 1997;32(3):453–6.
139. Staiano A, Del Giudice E. Colonic transit and anorectal manometry in children with severe brain damage. Pediatrics. 1994;94(2 Pt 1):169–73.
140. Soares AC, Tahan S, Morais MB. Effects of conventional treatment of chronic functional constipation on total and segmental colonic and orocecal transit times. J Pediatr (Rio J). 2009;85(4):322–8.
141. Zarate N, et al. Accurate localization of a fall in pH within the ileocecal region: validation using a dual-scintigraphic technique. Am J Physiol Gastrointest Liver Physiol. 2010;299(6):G1276–86.
142. Cassilly D, et al. Gastric emptying of a non-digestible solid: assessment with simultaneous SmartPill pH and pressure capsule, antroduodenal manometry, gastric emptying scintigraphy. Neurogastroenterol Motil. 2008;20(4):311–9.
143. Kuo B, et al. Comparison of gastric emptying of a nondigestible capsule to a radio-labelled meal in healthy and gastroparetic subjects. Aliment Pharmacol Ther. 2008;27(2):186–96.
144. Michalek W, Semler JR, Kuo B. Impact of acid suppression on upper gastrointestinal pH and motility. Dig Dis Sci. 2011;56(6):1735–42.
145. Boillat CS, et al. Variability associated with repeated measurements of gastrointestinal tract motility in dogs obtained by use of a wireless motility capsule system and scintigraphy. Am J Vet Res. 2010;71(8):903–8.
146. Boillat CS, Gaschen FP, Hosgood GL. Assessment of the relationship between body weight and gastrointestinal transit times measured by use of a wireless motility capsule system in dogs. Am J Vet Res. 2010;71(8):898–902.
147. Kloetzer L, et al. Motility of the antroduodenum in healthy and gastroparetics characterized by wireless motility capsule. Neurogastroenterol Motil. 2010;22(5):527–33. e117.

148. Rao SS, et al. Diagnostic utility of wireless motility capsule in gastrointestinal dysmotility. J Clin Gastroenterol. 2011;45(8):684–90.
149. Hasler WL, et al. Heightened colon motor activity measured by a wireless capsule in patients with constipation: relation to colon transit and IBS. Am J Physiol Gastrointest Liver Physiol. 2009;297(6):G1107–14.
150. Camilleri M, et al. Wireless pH-motility capsule for colonic transit: prospective comparison with radiopaque markers in chronic constipation. Neurogastroenterol Motil. 2010;22(8):874–82. e233.
151. Rao SS, et al. Investigation of colonic and whole-gut transit with wireless motility capsule and radiopaque markers in constipation. Clin Gastroenterol Hepatol. 2009;7(5):537–44.
152. Saad RJ, et al. Do stool form and frequency correlate with whole-gut and colonic transit? Results from a multicenter study in constipated individuals and healthy controls. Am J Gastroenterol. 2010;105(2):403–11.
153. Sarosiek I, et al. The assessment of regional gut transit times in healthy controls and patients with gastroparesis using wireless motility technology. Aliment Pharmacol Ther. 2010;31(2):313–22.
154. Maqbool S, Parkman HP, Friedenberg FK. Wireless capsule motility: comparison of the SmartPill GI monitoring system with scintigraphy for measuring whole gut transit. Dig Dis Sci. 2009;54(10):2167–74.
155. Timm D, et al. The use of a wireless motility device (SmartPill(R)) for the measurement of gastrointestinal transit time after a dietary fibre intervention. Br J Nutr. 2010;105(9):1337–42.

Autonomic Nervous System Testing 16

Gisela Chelimsky and Thomas C. Chelimsky

Autonomic Nervous System Testing

The role of autonomic testing in pediatric functional gastrointestinal disorders is slowly taking shape. At the simplest level, the autonomic nervous system constitutes the link between the central control of gastrointestinal function and the enteric nervous system. So far, no clinical tests directly assess the portion of the autonomic nervous system that innervates the gastrointestinal tract. Current routine clinical testing is limited to examination of cardiac, vasomotor and sudomotor function, and based on the results of these tests in the appropriate clinical setting, the gastroenterologists or autonomic specialists must infer the potential role of the autonomic nervous system in the pathogenesis of gastrointestinal symptoms. The goal of this chapter is as follows:

1. To describe the current available autonomic testing and discuss the portion of the autonomic nervous system assessed by each test
2. Discuss the utility of these tests in clinical practice

Autonomic testing in children is becoming increasingly available, though at this time still only a few centers perform more than just a tilt table test. Although cardiologists may perform tilt table tests, this is seldom performed in patients with primarily gastrointestinal complaints. This chapter describes the tests done most commonly in autonomic function referral centers (summarized in Table 16.1 below).

Tests Currently Available

The most common tests can be divided in two categories:

1. Tests of cardiovascular autonomic function:
   (a) Deep breathing
   (b) Valsalva maneuver
   (c) Head up tilt table test
   (d) Handgrip
   (e) Cold pressor test
2. Tests of sudomotor autonomic function (sweating)
   (a) Quantitative sudomotor reflex test (QSART)
   (b) Thermoregulatory sweat test (TST)

The tests of cardiovascular autonomic function are particularly helpful in evaluating the branch of the autonomic nervous system involved (afferent baroreflex, or efferent sympathetic vs. parasympathetic), whereas the sweat tests provide information on lesion localization (central vs.

G. Chelimsky, M.D. (✉)
Division of Pediatric Gastroenterology, Medical College of Wisconsin, 8701 Watertown Plank Rd, Milwaukee, WI 53226, USA
e-mail: gchelimsky@mcw.edu

T.C. Chelimsky, M.D.
Neurology Department, Medical College of Wisconsin, Milwaukee, WI, USA

C. Faure et al. (eds.), *Pediatric Neurogastroenterology: Gastrointestinal Motility and Functional Disorders in Children*, Clinical Gastroenterology,
DOI 10.1007/978-1-60761-709-9_16, © Springer Science+Business Media New York 2013

Table 16.1 Tests of autonomic function

Autonomic test	Receptor	Afferent	Integrating center	Efferent signal
Deep breathing	Pulmonary stretch J-receptors	Vagus nerve	Nucleus tractus solitarius	Dorsal motor nucleus of the vagus (DMNX) to vagus nerve
Valsalva maneuver	Low-pressure atrial baroreceptors	Vagus nerve	Nucleus tractus solitarius	*Phase II:* 1. Inhibition of DMNX HR 2. Excitation VLM to descending sympathetics exiting at T1 vasoconstriction *Phase IV:* Reverse of 1 and 2
Tilt-table test	Low-pressure atrial baroreceptors	Vagus nerve	Nucleus tractus solitarius	1. Inhibition of DMNX to HR 2. Excitation of VML to descending sympathetics exiting at T1 vasoconstriction
Sudomotor axon reflex test	Nicotinic cholinergic	Sudomotor nerve	None	Sudomotor nerve (axon reflex)
Thermoregulatory Sweat test	Temperature sensors in the anterior hypothalamus and peripheral veins	Temperature C-fibers	Anterior hypothalamus	Descending projections from anterior and lateral hypothalamus to intermedio-lateral cell horn preganglionic spinal neurons postganglionic sudomotor axons

DMNX dorsal motor nucleus of the vagus, *VLM* ventrolateral medulla peripheral nervous system). At this time, the pediatric norms are not well defined [1], and therefore, norms are inferred from adult values. Other tests of autonomic function such as pupillometry and pharmacologic evaluation of the baroreflex also exist; these are even less commonly utilized, have even less clearly defined norms, and therefore are not described in this chapter.

Deep Breathing

This test assesses heart rate variability, a parasympathetic nervous system function. The test is performed by instructing the patient to breathe deeply and regularly at a rate of 6 breaths per minute for 1 min. This is repeated after a minute of rest. Values for this parameter are age-dependent and a reduction in heart rate variability is considered abnormal. The authors utilize the data published by Ingall et al. [1] as age-based norms in their laboratory. The presumed purpose of the reflex is to provide adequate blood volume to absorb incoming oxygen during deep inspiration. When an individual inhales deeply, both air and vascular spaces expand and requiring increased lung blood volume. This need is met through an increase in heart rate during inspiration, triggered by vagal parasympathetic inhibition. When the individual exhales, the heart rate decreases, due to parasympathetic excitation [2]. In teenage years, this heart variability may become very large, probably due to high vagal tone. The Nucleus Tractus Solitarius orchestrates this response to pulmonary stretch receptor afferents (J-receptors) [3] also accounting for baroreflex responses to blood pressure changes, and intrinsic central respiratory rhythms.

Valsalva Maneuver

The Valsalva maneuver (VM) (Fig. 16.1) evaluates cardiac parasympathetic, cardiac sympathetic, and vasomotor sympathetic functions in response to low pressure baroreceptor afferents from the right atrium and the great veins. The patient generates a continuous expiratory pressure of 40 mmHg for 15 s by blowing against a fixed resistance and then suddenly releases the pressure. This sudden high pressure in the chest cavity impedes venous return to the heart, and reduces ventricular filling and stroke volume. Phase I and III are mechanical phases unrelated to autonomic physiology. During Phase I, blood pressure rises for a few seconds as the held pressure is transmitted directly as a pressure wave through the vascular system. Phase II is mediated a sympathetic nervous system response to the decline in cardiac output, resulting in vasoconstriction and tachycardia to restore blood pressure. The lost cardiac output is reflected in a drop in systolic pressure, while vasoconstriction causes a rise in diastolic pressure, resulting in a marked reduction in pulse pressure. When the subject releases pressure, blood pressure drops transiently during the mechanical phase III. The dominant effect occurs when blood fills the heart again, reaching higher levels than baseline, due to thoracic pressure normalization in the face of continued vasoconstriction. The baroreflex triggers a relative bradycardia through sympathetic withdrawal and parasympathetic excitation. Since vasodilation is slow, the blood pressure overshoots temporarily before returning to baseline. The result is usually read as a ratio of the fastest heart rate during phase II and the slowest heart rate during phase IV. If the ratio is below the age-based normal value, one must determine if this is due to an inadequate bradycardia during phase IV or inadequate tachycardia during phase II. In most centers, results of this study are repeated three times, with the two largest responses included in the dataset [2]. The values vary with age and we currently utilize the pediatric values published by Ingall et al. [1].

Head Up Tilt

This test evaluates sympathetic vasomotor responses. The patient must remain supine for a minimum of 10 min to obtain reliable baseline values, and then passively tilted to 70°. The length of time of the tilt is varies greatly across centers, being 10 min in many neurologic autonomic centers, and up to 45 min when performed by cardiologists. No data are available to guide tilt duration in children. Currently, in our institution, we tilt children without history of syncope for 30 min and if there is a

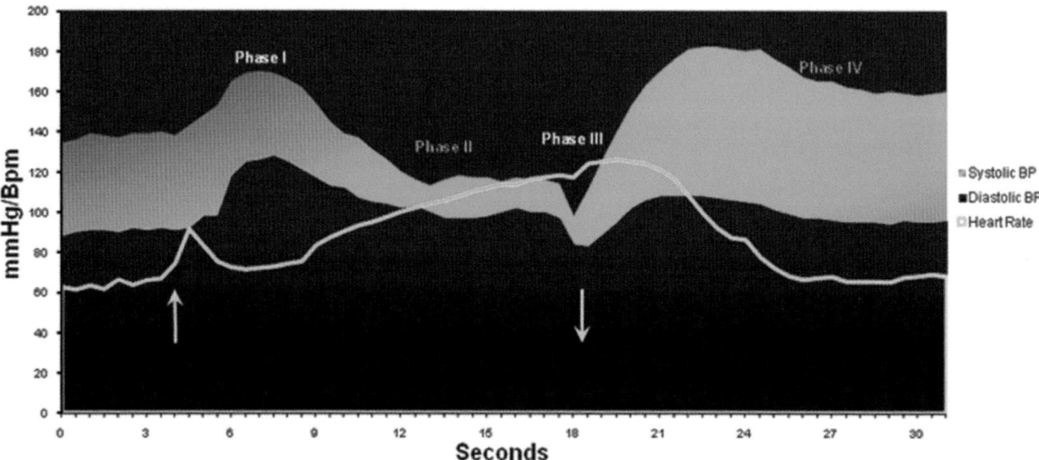

Fig. 16.1 Valsalva maneuver, showing the four phases and the blood pressure and heart rate changes of each phase

history of recurrent fainting the tilt is extended to 40 min. In our clinical experience, many subjects would be diagnosed as normal had the tilt table test been stopped at 10 min. The clinical significance is still unknown. A study performed by Carew et al. [4] in adolescents to adult age group (14–60 years) showed that 75% of the subjects develop a sustained increase in heart rate to fulfill the heart rate criteria for postural tachycardia syndrome (POTS) within the first 3 min of head-up tilt and by 7 min had developed the diagnostic criteria for POTS. None of the subjects in the control group had sustained tachycardia. Thirty six percent of the subjects with POTS developed reflex syncope between 7.4 and 32 min into the head-up tilt [4]. This frequency of syncope in POTS is remarkably similar to that found by Ojha et al. of 38% [5]. Based on these various data sources, children should be tilted for a minimum of 30 minutes, *or less if* they experience a presyncopal or syncopal event. During the test, all symptoms should be documented (and rated on a numeric rating scale) so they can later be correlated with vital sign changes. It is of particular importance if children replicate their gastrointestinal complaints during the upright portion of the tilt test, as they will often benefit from treatment aimed at orthostatic intolerance [6].

The tilt table test may demonstrate four patterns (Fig. 16.2): (a) normal response, (b) postural tachycardia syndrome (POTS), (c) orthostatic hypotension (OH), and (d) reflex syncope. In our clinical experience, children seldom demonstrate true orthostatic hypotension, *while* POTS and POTS associated with reflex syncope is the more common finding.

The Normal Response to a Tilt Table Test

A normal tilt response includes a mild increase in diastolic pressure by 5–10 mmHg, a mild decrease in systolic blood pressure of 5–10 mmHg and an increase in heart rate of about 10–20 bpm. A transient drop in blood pressure with reflex tachycardia within the first few minutes of tilt is common in healthy adolescents during tilt test [7].

Postural Tachycardia Syndrome

POTS is defined in adults as an increase in heart rate greater than 30 bpm within 10 min of becoming upright or to greater than 120 bpm, without a gradual drop in BP, and associated with orthostatic symptoms [8]. There are no pediatric norms. The mechanism involved in the pathogenesis of POTS symptoms is still unknown. However, the common final pathway is probably an excessive cardiovascular sympathetic activation perhaps secondary to abnormal blood volume distribution with venous pooling resulting in central hypovolemia and inadequate cardiac return [9].

Reflex Syncope

Other terms for this include neurally mediated syncope, vasovagal syncope, cardiogenic syncope,

Tilt Table Testing

	Orthostatic Hypotension	Postural Tachycardia	Reflex Syncope
Definition	Gradual sustained ↓ sBP>20 dBP>10 ≤3′	↑HR>30 in 10′ no ↓ BP	Sudden ↓ BP ± HR
BP / HR Pattern	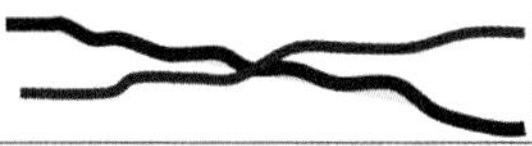	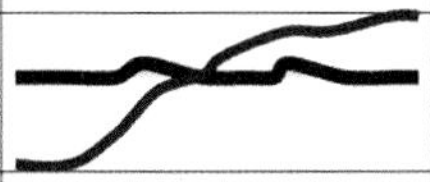	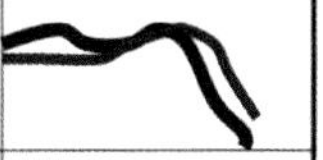
Physiology	Arterial denervation impacts ***diastole***	Venous return impacts ***systole***	Brainstem ***threshold***
CV reflexes	Usually abnormal	Usually normal	Usually nl
Associated Dysauton.	Structural Poor prognosis	Functional Good Prognosis	Functional

Fig. 16.2 This figure summarizes the different blood pressure (*black line*) and heart rate (*red line*) changes in the three orthostatic syndromes as well as the physiologic mechanism and a graphic description of the vital signs. (*nl* normal)

and vasodepressor syncope. It is defined as a temporary loss of consciousness caused by inadequate brain perfusion. It is produced by a sudden discharge from the medullary vasomotor center decreasing sympathetic tone and increasing vagal tone and leading to peripheral vasodilation, hypotension, and bradycardia. Subjects usually experience a brief episode of loss of consciousness followed by a relatively clear sensorium. It is important to note that syncope is a normal reflex that may occur in all subjects if enough strain is placed on orthostatic pressure maintenance (for example through the application of lower body negative pressure). Its probable function is the continued perfusion of the brain through gravitational mechanisms when the individual experiences severe loss of blood volume. Thus, the occurrence of syncope per se is not abnormal, but its occurrence at an inappropriate time is. POTS and syncope can coexist, being present in 30% of the children evaluated in our center.

Orthostatic Hypotension

Orthostatic hypotension is defined as sustained drop in blood pressure of greater than 20 mmHg systolic or 10 mmHg diastolic within 3 min of being upright, associated with symptoms. The underlying pathophysiology is an impaired efferent sympathetic signal to the arterioles with consequent vasoconstrictive insufficiency [10]. Figure 16.2 graphically summarizes the three orthostatic syndromes and their etiopathology.

Sustained (Static) Handgrip

This test evaluates sympathetic vasomotor function, sympathetic cardiac and parasympathetic function. After baseline recording, the patient is instructed to sustain a grip at 30% of their maximal grip strength for 3 min by squeezing a hand dynamometer. Heart rate and blood pressure are monitored continuously from the contralateral upper extremity. The maneuver results in both cardio-acceleration and an increase in blood pressure. In contrast to the tilt table test and the Valsalva maneuver, the afferent signal here originates from muscle and is related to lactate accumulation, in contrast to the former two tests where the initial afferent signal originates from the low-pressure baroreceptor in the right atrium. An early heart rate increase is due to vagal withdrawal and a later heart rate response is due to sympathetic activation. The blood pressure increase is due to both increased cardiac output and to sympathetically mediated arterial vasoconstriction [11].

Quantitative Sudomotor Reflex Test

This study evaluates for an autonomic neuropathy through the presence and function of postganglionic sudomotor axons. Though innervated by the sympathetic nervous system, acetylcholine is the post-gangliononic neurotransmitter to the sweat gland. The test is performed by applying a capsule with dual concentric chambers to the patient's skin. Acetylcholine from the outer chamber is iontophoresed into the skin, and via an axon reflex stimulates axons that innervate the local sweat glands. The axon reflex stimulates more distant sweat glands whose output is then measured in the area of the central chamber of the capsule. The capsules are usually placed from distal to proximal on two sites on the upper and lower extremities respectively, though other groups use three capsules in the lower extremity and one in the upper [11]. A reduced response indicates postganglionic sympathetic sudomotor impairment. The sudomotor reflex is preserved in central nervous system processes.

Thermoregulatory Sweat Test

This study helps differentiate a central disorder from a neuropathy or radiculopathy. It evaluates both preganglionic and postganglionic pathways. The patient dressed in a disposable swim-suit like garment is covered with a powder that changes color on contact with moisture. The subject is placed supine in a sauna-like enclosure, kept at an air temperature of 50 °C, with a relative humidity of 50%. The skin temperature is maintained between 38.5 and 39.5 °C. The skin may also be heated with infrared heaters. The test is interpreted based on the detection of areas of lack of sweat (anhidrosis) [12]. Usually a subject with central disorder will have lack of sweating all over the body, although sweating on hands and feet may be preserved. Reduced sweating in the toes, fingers with a distal to proximal gradient is suggestive of a peripheral process. If there is lack of sweating following a nerve root pattern, the study may suggest a radiculopathy.

Critical Steps in Preparation for All Autonomic Function Testing

Prior to testing, the patients should be asked to have a normal meal at the usual mealtime with plenty of fluid. They must also taper or stop all medications and dietary or nutritional supplements that may influence test results. This includes caffeine and passive or active exposure to nicotine. When the patient is unable to hold medications results need to be interpreted accordingly. Each center has protocols for when and which medications should be stopped. As a general guideline, α(alpha)- and β(beta)-receptor agonists and antagonists, pro- and anticholinergics (particularly phenothiazines and tricyclic agents) and mineralocorticoids (including fludrocortisone) must be discontinued at least 5 half lives prior to testing. Selective serotonin reuptake inhibitors (SSRI) and serotonin nonselective reuptake inhibitors (SNRI) agents should be discontinued 5–7 days prior to the testing.

Utility of Autonomic Testing in the Evaluation of Children with Functional Gastrointestinal Disorders and Motility Disorders

To date, autonomic testing in children has been deployed in limited ways, being primarily utilized in the evaluation of rare disorders such as Familial Dysautonomia. The utility of autonomic testing in functional gastrointestinal disorders (FGID) is just emerging. About 10 years ago the first case series was reported of children with FGID demonstrating a postural tachycardia in most subjects, and an autonomic neuropathy in many. The cardiac parasympathetic function was preserved in all the subjects [13]. A few case reports further supported this association and reported improvement of the gastrointestinal symptoms when treatment was aimed at the orthostatic intolerance [14, 15]. A few years later, Sullivan and collaborators reported tilt table results in 24 children with FGID [16]. These children had symptoms of abdominal pain (71%), nausea (56%) and vomiting (50%). The tilt table showed POTS in 4, POTS and neurally mediated hypotension (termed reflex syncope in this chapter) in 8 and neurally mediated hypotension alone in 12. In about half of the cases, the tilt table test reproduced the gastrointestinal complaints. Follow-up was available in 18/24. Twelve children were treated with fludrocortisone (4 had also sertraline) with either improvement or resolution of symptoms [16]. A retrospective study supported the concept that children that replicate the gastrointestinal symptoms during the tilt table test usually had POTS and often show improvement of gastrointestinal symptoms when treated with fludrocortisone [6].

This association was further explored by performing electrogastrography in subjects with and without POTS in the supine position and during the upright portion of the tilt test. The study found that in the upright position, children with POTS developed more gastric electrical abnormalities in the locations corresponding to the fundus and the antrum, while the opposite happened in the non-POTS group [17]. These findings suggested a possible mechanism for the association between orthostatic intolerance and the gastrointestinal symptoms. Further prospective, blinded studies will determine if treatment aimed at the orthostatic intolerance is superior to "conventional" treatment of FGID or to placebo. Against the concept of placebo response, most children have failed all "conventional" gastrointestinal treatments prior to referral to our center. Sullivan and collaborators reported that tilt table was performed after having symptoms for more than a year, sometime even 3 years (48%) and had failed gastric acid secretory blockers, antispasmodics, and prokinetics. Many of them (50%) had been referred to a psychiatrist or psychologist for their symptoms, having then resolution with fludrocortisone or sertraline [16]. One would not expect a placebo effect to be restricted to orthostatic agents.

Practitioners often wonder if anxiety may be the primary cause of the increase in heart rate during tilt table test. Masuki et al. attempted to answer that question by performing graded venous pooling with lower body negative pressure by wearing antishock trousers to −40 mmHg and sham venous pooling by inflating the trousers to −5 mmHg and vacuum pump activation without lower body negative pressure in subjects with POTS and in controls [18]. They also performed mental stress to determine if there were differences in the heart rate increase in the two groups. They demonstrated that only significant venous pooling caused a rise in heart rate in the POTS group, whereas the heart rate increase in response to "sham" venous pooling and mental stress was not significantly different between the two groups. These results suggest that the heart rate increase in patients with POTS is not related to anxiety, but rather to reduced venous return to the heart [18].

Although many of these studies are either retrospective or small series, evidence is slowly mounting for the role of autonomic dysfunction in children with FGID and hence a benefit of autonomic testing in the evaluation of children with FGID. Prospective studies are needed comparing different treatment modalities and determining if fludrocortisone, salt supplementation, beta blockers may be beneficial in these children.

References

1. Ingall TJ, McLeod JG, O'Brien PC. The effects of ageing on the autonomic nervous system function. Aust N Z J Med. 1990;20:570–7.
2. Freeman R. Noninvasive evaluation of heart rate: time and frequency domains. In: Low PA, Benarroch EE, editors. Clinical autonomic disorders. 3rd ed. Philadelphia: Lipincott Williams &Wilkins; 2008. p. 185–97.
3. Bonham AC, Coles SK, McCrimmon DR. Pulmonary stretch receptor afferents activate excitatory amino acid receptors in the nucleus tractus solitarii in rats. J Physiol. 1993;464:725–45.
4. Carew S, Cooke J, O'Connor M, et al. What is the optimal duration of tilt testing for the assessment of patients with suspected postural tachycardia syndrome? Europace. 2009;11:635–7.
5. Ojha A, McNeeley K, Heller E, Alshekhlee A, Chelimsky G, Chelimsky TC. Orthostatic syndromes differ in syncope frequency. Am J Med. 2010;123:245–9.
6. Safder S, Chelimsky TC, O'Riordan MA, Chelimsky G. Autonomic testing in functional gastrointestinal disorders: implications of reproducible gastrointestinal

complaints during tilt table testing. Gastroenterol Res Pract. 2009;2009:868496.
7. Stewart JM. Transient orthostatic hypotension is common in adolescents. J Pediatr. 2002;140:418–24.
8. Low PA, Sandroni P, Joyner MJ, Shen W. Postural tachycardia syndrome. In: Low PA, Benarroch EE, editors. Clinical autonomic disorders. 3rd ed. Philadelphia: Lippincott Williams &Walkins; 2008. p. 515–33.
9. Medow MS, Stewart JM. The postural tachycardia syndrome. Cardiol Rev. 2007;15:67–75.
10. Low PA, Fealey RD. Management of neurogenic orthostatic hypotension. In: Low PA, Benarroch EE, editors. Clinical autonomic disorders. 3rd ed. Philadelphia: Lippicott Williams & Walkins; 2008. p. 547–59.
11. Low PA, Sletten DM. Laboratory evaluation of autonomic failure. In: Low PA, Benarroch EE, editors. Clinical autonomic disorders. 3rd ed. Philadelphia: Lippicott Williams & Wilkins; 2008. p. 130–63.
12. Fealey RD. Thermoregulatory sweat test. In: Low PA, Benarroch EE, editors. Clinical autonomic disorders. 3rd ed. Philadelphia: Lippincott Williams & Wilkins; 2008. p. 244–63.
13. Chelimsky G, Boyle JT, Tusing L, Chelimsky TC. Autonomic abnormalities in children with functional abdominal pain: coincidence or etiology? J Pediatr Gastroenterol Nutr. 2001;33:47–53.
14. Chelimsky G, Chelimsky T. Treatment of autonomic dysfunction resolving gastrointestinal symptoms in a parent and child. J Auton Nerv Syst. 1999;9:238.
15. Chelimsky G, Chelimsky T. Familial association of autonomic and gastrointestinal symptoms. Clin Auton Res. 2001;11:383–6.
16. Sullivan S, Hanauer J, Rowe P, Barron D, Darbari A, Oliva-Hemker M. Gastrointestinal symptoms associated with orthostatic intolerance. J Pediatr Gastroenterol Nutr. 2005;40:425–8.
17. Safder S, Chelimsky TC, O'Riordan MA, Chelimsky G. Gastric electrical activity becomes abnormal in the upright position in patients with postural tachycardia syndrome. J Pediatr Gastroenterol Nutr. 2010;51(3):314–8.
18. Masuki S, Eisenach JII, Johnson CP, et al. Excessive heart rate response to orthostatic stress in postural tachycardia syndrome is not caused by anxiety. J Appl Physiol. 2007;102:896–903.

Part III

Disorders of Digestive Motility: Developmental and Acquired Anomalies of the Enteric Neuromuscular System

Pathology of Enteric Neuromusculature

17

Virpi Vanamo Smith

Introduction

Over many decades, pathology of enteric neuromuscular diseases has been elusive and continues to be a challenge to the histopathologist. Although the causes of intestinal pseudo-obstruction such as "an insufficient degree of intestinal muscular power and action as a physical cause for costiveness" were already recognised by Jacobi in 1869 [1], the pathology was not understood. Even after Harald Hirschsprung in 1886 first presented his detailed necropsy findings on two infants (aged 11 and 8 months) for the Gesellschaft for Kinderheilkunde in Berlin and in 1888 published a paper [2] on the subject in the Jahrbuch fur Kinderheilkunde, it took another 60 years for the pathology of aganglionosis to be universally accepted as the cause of this distinct clinical entity bearing Hirschsprung's name.

It soon became apparent that other pseudo-obstructive diseases without aganglionosis but clinically mimicking Hirschsprung's disease (pseudo-Hirschsprung's disease) also existed [3] but only in the past two to three decades the pathological changes (abnormalities in the enteric nerves and muscle) have reliably been identified [4–9].

V.V. Smith, Ph.D., FRCPath (✉)
Paediatric Surgery Unit, Institute of Child Head, University College London, 30 West Avenue, London N31AX, UK
e-mail: v.smith@ich.ucl.ac.uk

The pathology can diffusely affect the entire gastrointestinal tract or only a segment of the bowel. The histological changes are often subtle and can be either congenital (genetic) or acquired and are classified as enteric neuropathies (abnormalities in enteric nervous system) or myopathies (abnormalities in intestinal smooth muscle). Unlike in adults, in children the changes are rarely secondary to a systemic disease but may be seen in muscular dystrophies, cystic fibrosis or mitochondrial cytopathies. In order to identify the subtle changes, a number of different histopathological techniques are required, thus necessitating the preservation of tissue in several different ways.

The optimal diagnostic specimen is a complete circumference of a full-thickness intestinal sample about 4 cm in length taken at a time of a surgical intervention (an exploratory laparotomy or when raising a stoma). The specimen is cut open and a longitudinal block of full-thickness bowel is fixed in formalin and embedded in paraffin-wax for routine histology using haematoxylin and eosin and tinctorial special stains (Masson trichrome, picrosirius, periodic acid Schiff) and immunostains (smooth muscle actin, desmin, CD56, CD117 or c-kit, PGP9.5, S100 and inflammatory markers including HLA-DR). A full-thickness block is snap-frozen for enzyme histochemistry (acetyl cholinesterase and acid phosphatase activities and possible genetic studies) and a thin full-thickness block is fixed in glutaraldehyde for electron microscopy. It is

C. Faure et al. (eds.), *Pediatric Neurogastroenterology: Gastrointestinal Motility and Functional Disorders in Children*, Clinical Gastroenterology,
DOI 10.1007/978-1-60761-709-9_17, © Springer Science+Business Media New York 2013

important that the latter sample is kept whole to facilitate identification of all the layers of the bowel wall.

Care must be taken that the apparent changes seen on routine histology or on electron microscopy are not over-interpreted as pathology, as they may be due to ischaemia and hypoxia during surgery. Equally, the fixation especially for electron microscopy may be suboptimal if too large (thick) pieces of tissue are processed.

In this chapter the histopathology of currently recognised enteric neuropathies and myopathies in children are discussed. The pathology of mesenchymopathies (changes in the population of interstitial cells of Cajal; ICC) and channelopathies are principally considered in Chap. 18.

Enteric Neuropathies (Table 17.1)

Genetic/Congenital Neuropathies

The diagnosis of subtle enteric neuropathies is based on the availability of a sufficient number of myenteric neurons in routine sections of the biopsy/resection analysed. The most obvious abnormality is the absence of enteric neurons (aganglionosis) but disorders with reduced or increased numbers of myenteric neurons are also diagnosed. Rare conditions with intestinal ganglioneuromatosis, neuronal degeneration, neuronal immaturity and abnormalities in the amount of the glial cell component of the myenteric plexus have also been reported. Quantitative analysis is hindered by a lack of normative control data especially in childhood. Subtle abnormalities in the proportions of neurons expressing a particular neurotransmitter cannot be diagnosed on routine sections due to insufficient number of neurons and would require tangential orientation of the plexus in sections or whole mounts and immunohistochemistry but this is expensive of tissue and control data is scarce. Silver staining, which identifies two populations of neurons (argyrophilic and argyrophobic), had been used in the past on tangential sections to identify neural abnormalities [10–12] including an absence of argyrophilic neurons [13]. We now know, however, that argyrophilic neurons in the very young may normally be absent; thus, silver staining is less informative in the young paediatric population [14]. Moreover, the technique of silver staining is capricious and prone to artefacts.

Aganglionosis

Aganglionosis (Hirschsprung's disease) is by far the commonest enteric neuropathy; thus, before embarking on the search for the diagnosis of rarer enteric neuromuscular diseases, Hirschsprung's disease must be excluded on cryostat sections of an adequate suction rectal biopsy containing sufficient submucosa [15]. In aganglionosis no submucosal neurons are found on a haematoxylin and eosin stain and instead there are hypertrophied nerve trunks. An acetylcholinesterase preparation on frozen tissue shows an increase in thick nerve fibres in the muscularis mucosae. In the older baby, thick fibres running transversely as well as vertically in the lamina propria of the mucosa are often found (Fig. 17.1). As a note of caution acetyl cholinesterase enzyme histochemistry is not reliable in samples taken

Table 17.1 Genetic/congenital nerve diseases

Diseases	Genetic defect
Aganglionosis	Multigenic including Ret and/or endothelin signalling and Sox10
Ganglioneuromatosis	*RET M918T* and/or *A883F*
Hypoganglionosis	Not known
Hyperganglionosis	? Enx (Hox11L1)
Glial cells hyperplasia	Not known
Neuronal degeneration	2-bp Δ exon 2 of *FLNA (filamin a)* on chromosome Xq28
Neuronal immaturity	Not known

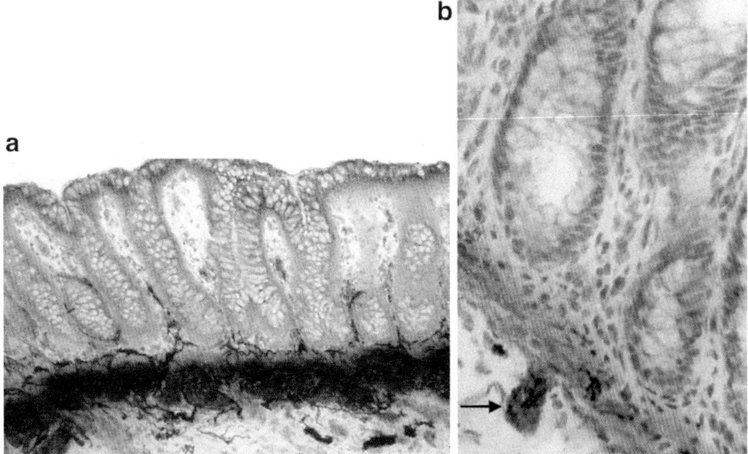

Fig. 17.1 (**a**) Acetyl cholinesterase preparation showing positive thick fibres in the mucularis mucosae and fibres in the lamina propria in Hirschsprung's disease. (**b**) Acetyl cholinesterase activity in normal rectum. A ganglion indicated by *arrow*

proximal to the splenic flexure and the presence of prominent acetyl cholinesterase-positive mucosal nerve fibres in the normal small bowel must not be confused with aganglionosis. In total colonic aganglionosis, an entity first described by Bodian et al. [16] in 1951, the acetyl cholinesterase pattern in the rectal biopsy may be normal and no hypertrophied nerves are seen in the submucosa. The combination of haematoxylin and eosin stain with acetyl cholinesterase enzyme histochemistry is the most reliable way to exclude or confirm the diagnosis [17]. Acetyl cholinesterase activity is best demonstrated by using a method that enhances the colour of the final reaction product as described by Lake et al. 1978 [17]. Some laboratories appear to be reluctant to use frozen tissue and acetyl cholinesterase enzyme histochemistry and have developed methods including immunohistochemistry for calretinin on paraffin sections [18]. The advantage of acetyl cholinesterase histochemistry is that there is an increase in enzyme-reactive nerves in aganglionic bowel whereas with calretinin immunostaining there is an absence or decrease of immunoreactivity. For confirmation of aganglionosis it is far easier to rely on a positive increase in enzyme-reactive nerves rather than the absence of immunoreactive ones.

Ganglioneuromatosis

Intestinal transmural ganglioneuromatosis is a diagnosis not to be missed or taken lightly because it carries serious implications. The distinct appearances can be seen in the submucosa even in a suction rectal biopsy where there is a profound "tumour-like" proliferation of neural tissue (neurons, supporting cells, and nerves) that appear as thickened nerve-like bundles embedded with mature nerve cells (Fig. 17.2). If ganglioneuromatosis is suspected, there is justification to embark in further investigations to exclude multiple endocrine neoplasia type IIB (MEN IIB) requiring germline *M918T* and/or *A883F* mutation analysis of the *RET* proto-oncogene [19].

Children with intestinal ganglioneuromatosis and the above-mentioned molecular diagnosis of MEN IIB inexorably develop medullary thyroid carcinoma [6]. Monitoring the calcitonin concentrations and scanning for adrenal and thyroid masses do not suffice because microscopic medullary thyroid carcinoma can be present without obvious masses on imaging or without raised calcitonin concentrations, even with pentagastrin stimulation. A prophylactic thyroidectomy is recommended, as well as continued surveillance of the adrenal glands for evidence of pheochromocytoma.

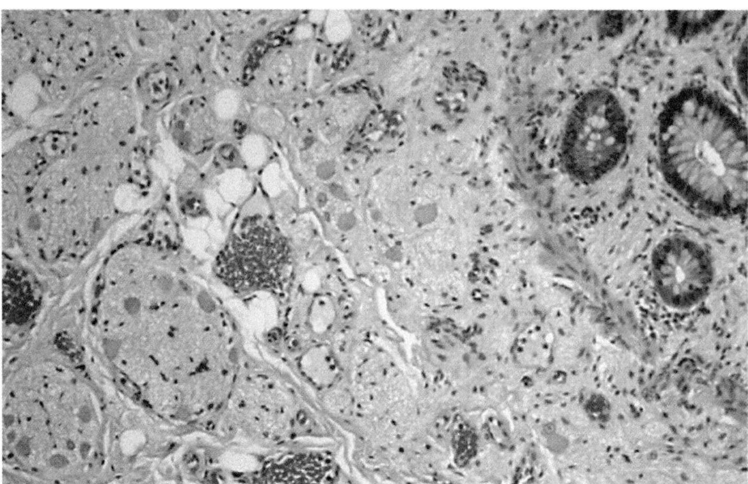

Fig. 17.2 H&E stained section showing ganglioneuromata in the submucosa

Hypoganglionosis

Hypoganglionosis is a disorder in which there is a reduction in myenteric neuronal numbers, hence the specimens suitable for the assessment of hypoganglionosis must be full-thickness intestine. Routine haematoxylin and eosin-stained paraffin sections are suitable for the analysis. In this condition the myenteric ganglia are sparse and small containing grossly reduced numbers of neurons. It can also been seen in the transitional zone of varying length in Hirschsprung's disease proximal to the aganglionic segment, however the transitional zone in addition to hypoganglionosis has thickened nerves trunks. Often the diagnosis can be made semi-quantitatively but for formal assessment of myenteric neuronal density there are normal control data for distal descending colon, terminal ileum and proximal jejunum [20]. Normal density in the colon is 7 ± 2.12 neurons per mm of bowel length examined. In the small bowel the ganglia are more widely spaced and neurons are fewer (4.6 ± 1.51 per mm in ileum, 4 ± 1.07 per mm in jejunum). Counts in a single section are valid provided a sufficient bowel length is analysed. Longitudinally orientated sections are preferred but the counts do not significantly differ even if the orientation is transverse. Bowel lengths less than 10 mm are considered insufficient especially in the small bowel. The normative data are based on haematoxylin and eosin stained paraffin sections of 3 μ(mu)m thickness and the neurons are identified by their amphoteric, granular cytoplasm and open vesicular nuclei with prominent nucleoli but the cytoplasmic appearance alone suffices for a cell to be counted as a neuron. Counts below 2 standard deviations from the control mean are considered abnormal.

Hyperganglionosis

Hyperganglionosis is a disorder in which the myenteric neuronal density is increased. Routine paraffin sections can be used for formal assessment of the neuronal density (see above). Counts above 2 standard deviations from the mean of the control values are considered to be abnormal. Additional features in myenteric hyperganglionosis are seen on acetyl cholinesterase enzyme histochemistry in frozen sections of the bowel. These include ectopic ganglia (Fig. 17.3) in the lamina propria of mucosa and muscularis propria as well as an increase in fine vertical acetyl cholinesterase-positive fibres in the lamina propria of the mucosa. An increase in the number of nerve varicosities may also be seen in the muscularis propria but unlike in aganglionosis in the muscularis mucosae the acetyl cholinesterase pattern is within normal limits.

Glial Cell Hyperplasia

Glial cell hyperplasia was first described in 1990 [21]. In this entity there is a prominent increase in neural elements in the myenteric plexus but it is not accompanied by hyperganglionosis and

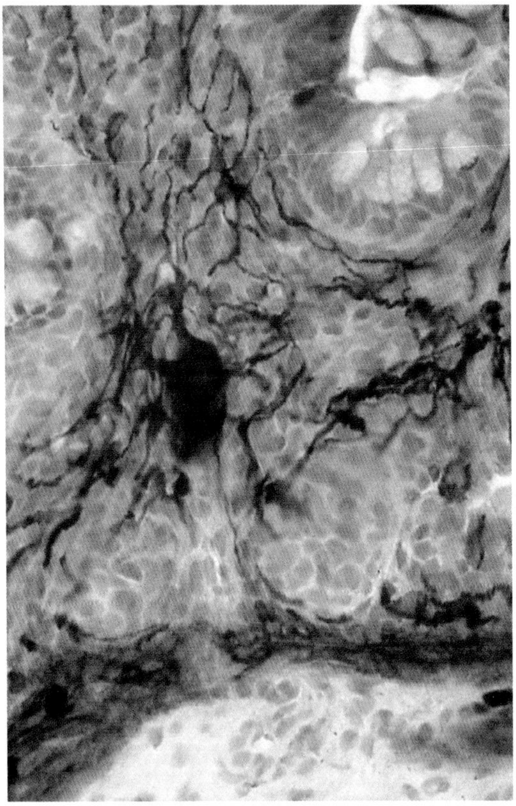

Fig 17.3 Acetyl cholinesterase preparation showing an ectopic ganglion in the lamina propria of the mucosa

may have reduced nerve cell density. The appearances are of an almost continuous myenteric plexus but this is not to be confused with ganglioneuromatosis, which is a distinct histopathological entity (pseudo-tumourous nodular proliferation of glial and neural tissue in which mature nerve cells are embedded—see above). Glial cell hyperplasia can be seen in a distal segment of the colon (personal observation, Smith VV) and distal colonic manometry in these patients is also abnormal (personal observation, Lindley KJ). In one patient with abnormal distal colonic manometry, on histology the abnormal neural tissue was not confined to the myenteric plexus but hyperplastic neural tissue was seen located in the longitudinal muscle coat forming a parallel plexus (Fig. 17.4) to the myenteric plexus as well as traversing from the serosa through the longitudinal muscle coat into the plexus (personal observation, Smith VV).

Neuronal Degeneration

This condition was first described [22] in 1996 in a large kindred in which abnormal myenteric neurons were noted. These were shrunken on routine histology and on ultrastructural examination showed degenerative changes. The inheritance appeared to be X-linked and the linkage was mapped to chromosome Xq28. Later it was shown that there was a two base-pair deletion in exon 2 of the *FILAMIN A* [23].

Neuronal Immaturity

The majority of neonatal neurons are small with a small amount of perikarya (8–15 μ(mu)m in diameter) surrounding the nucleus. With growing age of the child the amount of perikarya increases. In children most neurons measure (20–23 μ(mu) m) and only reach the adult dimensions by the age of 2–5 years when neurons measuring 30–40 μ(mu)m are common. The diagnosis of neuronal immaturity should be considered if inappropriately small neurons are seen in the bowel from an older child [20].

Genetic/Congenital Myopathies (Table 17.2)

Enteric myopathies can result from an abnormal layering of the enteric musculature where there may be a fusion of all the muscle coats resulting in one muscle layer only or there may be additional muscle layers. The former generally affects a segment of the bowel whereas the latter may be segmental or diffuse typically with an additional circular muscle coat [5]. Recently we have also seen two patients with an additional muscle layer on the outside of the longitudinal muscle coat adjacent to the serosa (Personal observation, Smith VV 2009; Fig. 17.5). The diffuse form of an addition circular muscle coat appears to have an X-linked mode of inheritance. Apart from the abnormalities in muscle layering, enteric myopathies may show fibrosis of the muscularis propria with atrophy, drop-out and vacuolation of myocytes (Fig. 17.6). These include a degenerative leiomyopathy with or without evidence of inflammation [24], and thus, some of these may be considered acquired [25].

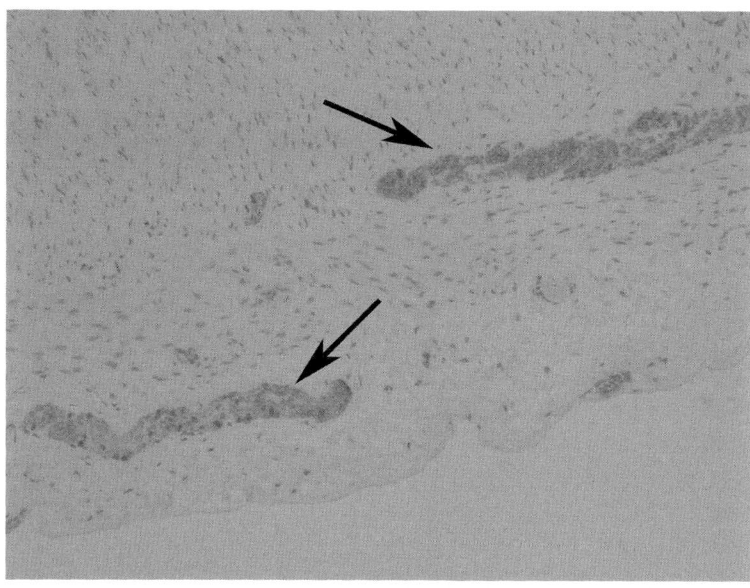

Fig. 17.4 PGP9.5 immunostained section of full-thickness bowel showing “wandering” myenteric plexus (*arrows*)

Table 17.2 Genetic/congenital muscle diseases

Diseases	Observation
Abnormal muscle layering	
Segmental absence of muscle coat	Intrauterine varicella in 2nd trimester
Segmental extra circular muscle coat	Sporadic
Diffuse extra circular muscle coat	X-linked mode of inheritance
Myocyte vacuolation, atrophy and fibrosis	
Myopathy with pink blush and nuclear crowding	? myocyte phenotype changed from contractile to secretory
Myopathy with autophagic activity	? lysosomal activation/defect

Often the changes not only affect the intestine but may also involve the urinary tract in the so-called hollow visceral myopathies within which specific histological phenotypes are seen. In children with vertically acquired human immunodeficiency virus there may be extensive leiomyolysis due to cytomegalovirus enterocolitis [26].

Abnormal Muscle Layering

Segmental Absence of Muscle Layer

This abnormality affects a segment of the bowel showing a fusion of the three enteric muscle coats (muscularis mucosae, circular and longitudinal muscle) to form one single muscle layer with no myenteric plexus or obvious submucosal plexus [5]. The mothers of all the patients with this disorder seen by in our institution have had varicella infection in the second trimester of the pregnancy.

Segmental Extra Muscle Coat

On the inside (lumenal) of the circular muscle coat in this entity there is an extra muscle layer composed of bundles of leiomyocytes with the same orientation as the circular muscle [5]. There also appears to be an additional neural plexus between the additional muscle coat and the muscularis propria. This abnormality affects only the distal bowel and we have not noted it to involve the small intestine. Resection of the abnormal segment restores normal bowel motility.

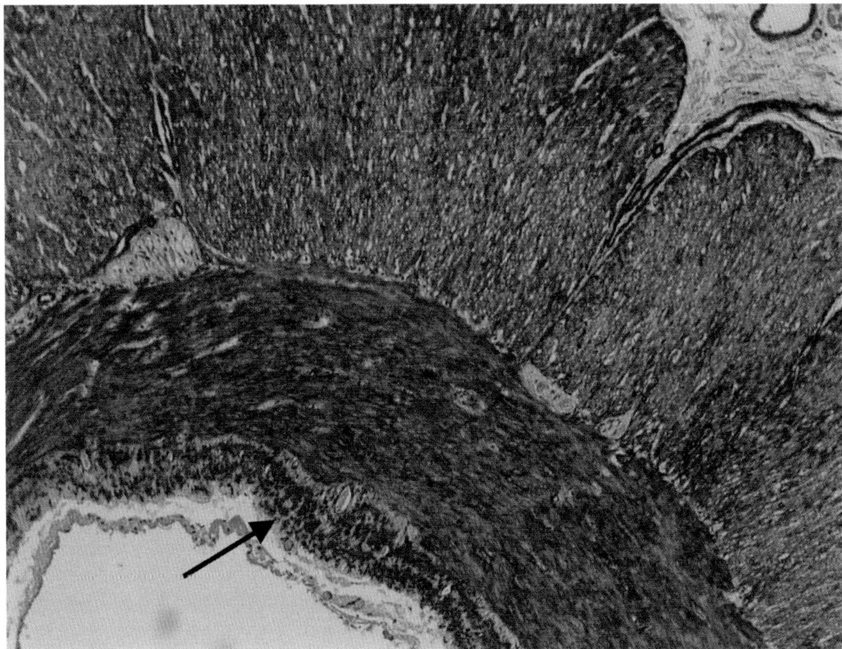

Fig. 17.5 Smooth muscle actin immunostained section showing an additional longitudinal muscle layer (*arrow*)

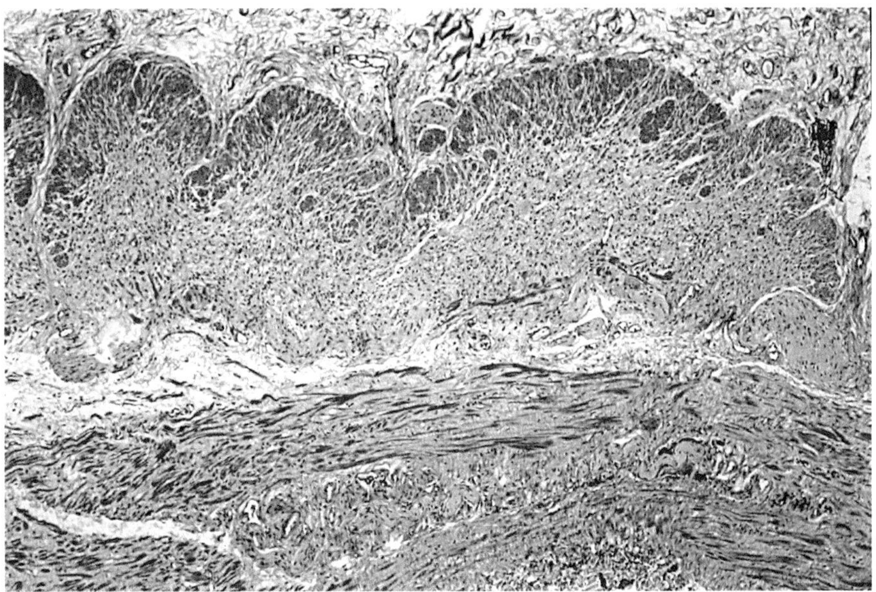

Fig. 17.6 Masson trichrome showing fibrosis, atrophy and drop-out of myocytes in the muscularis propria

Diffuse Extra Muscle Coat

An additional muscle layer found throughout the small and large intestine appears to be the result of a misplaced myenteric plexus bisecting the circular muscle coat (Fig. 17.7) [5]. Clinically it is associated with short bowel, malrotation and megacystis and appears to have an X-linked mode of inheritance.

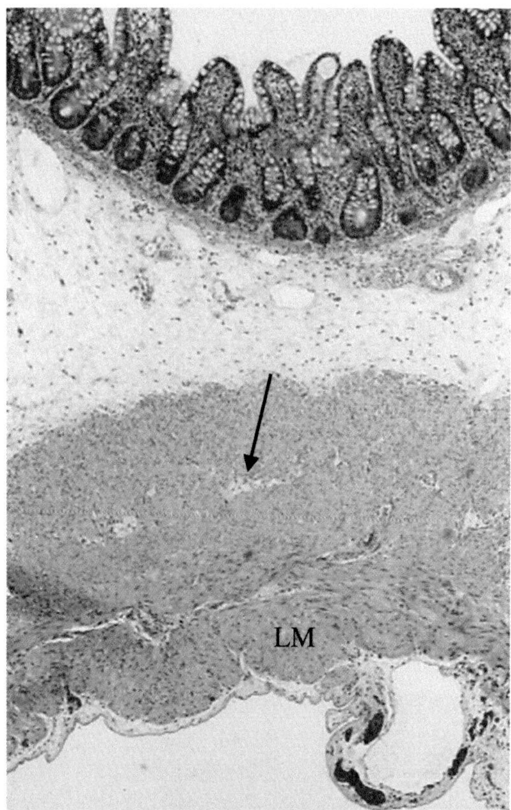

Fig. 17.7 H&E stained section of full-thickness small bowel showing bisected circular muscle by a misplaced myenteric plexus (*arrow*). *LM* longitudinal muscle

Fibrosis, Myocyte Vacuolation and Atrophy

In contrast to enteric neuropathies, which usually affect a segment of the distal bowel, most intestinal myopathies commonly involve the entire gastrointestinal tract and may affect other organs such as the gall bladder and the urinary tract [27] and are often termed hollow visceral myopathies [28]. The most frequently described changes are fibrosis of the muscularis propria, and vacuolation of leiomyocytes together with myocyte atrophy and drop-out. Accumulation of sarcoplasmic glycogen [29] and intramyocyte inclusions [30] has also been described. The latter, although seen in the adults, does not appear to be a feature in paediatric enteric myopathies. These gross changes are easily recognised by light microscopy on a haematoxylin and eosin stain and using connective tissue stains (Masson trichrome and picrosirius) and periodic acid Schiff for glycogen. Lesser degrees of fibrosis, myocyte vacuolation and glycogen accumulation require ultrastructural examination. The use of immunohistochemistry for myocyte contractile proteins and their isoforms is also helpful in explaining the dysmotility [31]. In the paediatric population, the following two specific histological phenotypes are recognised.

Pink Blush and Nuclear Crowding

Haematoxylin and eosin staining throughout the gastrointestinal tract the circular muscle coat shows patchy crowding of myocyte nuclei with areas in which there is a paucity of nuclei [5]. There is a "pink blush" on picrosirius stain corresponding to the areas devoid of nuclei. Electron microscopy reveals that the areas with nuclear paucity are filled with amorphous granular proteinacious material with a few collagen fibre remnants expanding the distance between the leiomyocytes, thus disrupting their electric connectivity (Fig. 17.8). We postulate that the myocytes have changed their phenotype from contractile to secretory producing this granular material. Cases include both sexes and appear sporadic. The urinary tract is also involved showing megacystis/megaureters.

Myopathy with Autophagic Activity

Light microscopy in this phenotype shows profound fibrosis of the muscularis propria with atrophy and loss of leiomyocytes [5]. Enzyme histochemistry for acid phosphatase activity shows reactive lysosomes in the enteric myocytes, which in a normal child should have no acid phosphatase activity. Ultrastructural examination confirms the profound fibrosis with sheets of collagen fibres separating the grossly abnormal and vacuolated myocytes. The vacuoles are dilated lysosomes containing electron dense deg-

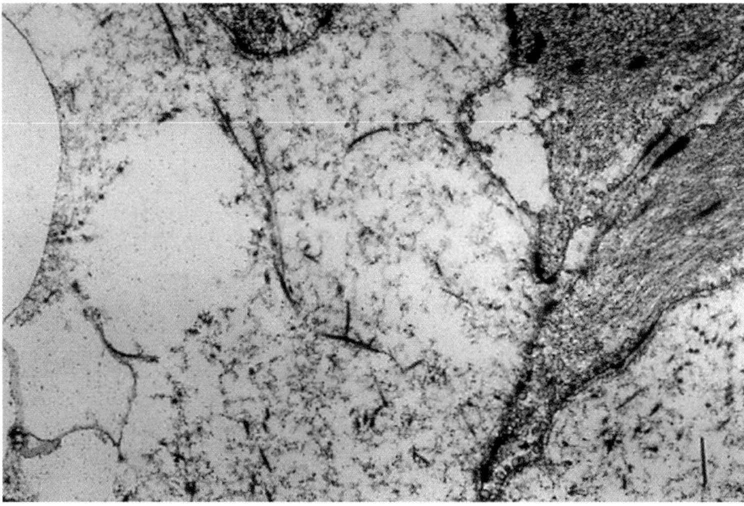

Fig. 17.8 Pink blush and nuclear crowding. Electron micrograph showing separation of myocytes by granular proteinacious material with remnants of collagen fibrils

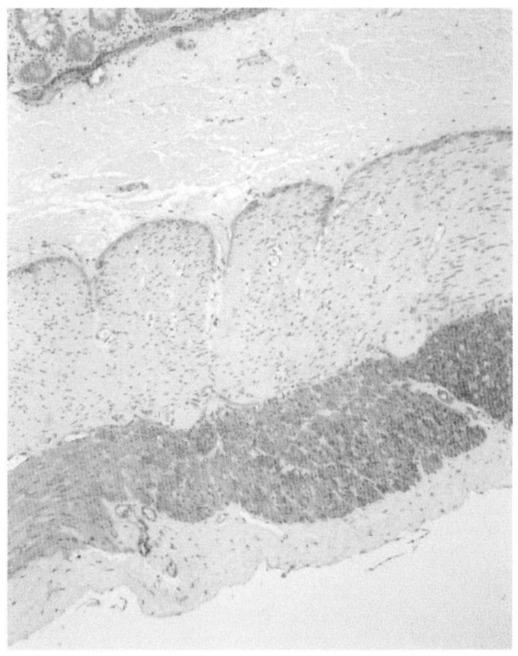

Fig. 17.9 Section of full-thickness bowel showing absent smooth muscle actin activity in bulk of the circular muscle and normal immunoreactivity in other muscle layers including the inner circular muscle

radation products. The abnormality diffusely affects the entire bowel and is associated with megacystis/megaureters. Most patients appear to be sporadic but in one family two siblings (brother and sister) were affected.

Abnormalities in Contractile Proteins

Deficiency of alpha smooth muscle actin (Fig. 17.9) confined to the bulk of the circular muscle, sparing the innermost circular muscle coat (nearest to the lumen), longitudinal muscle and muscularis mucosae was first described in 1992 in an adult patient with life-long intestinal pseudo-obstruction [31]. It was postulated that this deficiency was congenital since the type of myocyte contractility depends on the cocktail of contractile protein isoforms. For instance, actin exists in at least six different isoforms, each of which encoded by a separate gene and expressed in a tissue-specific pattern. There are three alpha isoforms (smooth muscle, skeletal muscle and cardiac muscle) and two gamma isoforms (smooth muscle and cytoplasmic). The beta isoforms are cytoplasmic and are not involved in muscle contraction. The major isoactins in mature intestinal smooth muscle are alpha and gamma smooth muscle actins, the gamma isoform being the largest constituent, although less abundant, the alpha isoform is nevertheless an important component. The proportions of contractile protein isoforms vary in smooth muscle from different tissues [32] and in different stages during development [33] with non-muscle cytoplasmic isoforms predominating in undifferentiated smooth muscle in the

Table 17.3 Diffuse or segmental acquired diseases

Autoimmune ganglionitis
Autoimmune myositis
Eosinophilic ganglionitis
Immune modulation of smooth muscle phenotype by inflammation (eosinophils, mast cells)
Immune modulation of nerves by mucosal eosinophils/ mast cells

early embryo whereas in mature fully differentiated myocytes the muscle specific isoforms (gamma and alpha smooth muscle actin) predominate. These isoforms modulate the type of contraction required; alpha smooth muscle actin for tonic contractions and gamma smooth muscle actin for phasic contractions.

It is also possible that isoprotein proportions may vary in response to various stimuli [34, 35]. Recently it has become evident that insults such as inflammation modulate leiomyocyte contractile protein profile in enteric smooth muscle [7]. Regardless of the mechanism responsible for absent smooth muscle alpha actin immunostaining (congenital vs. acquired) this appearance can contribute to bowel dysmotility.

Diffuse and Segmental Acquired Diseases (Table 17.3)

Autoimmune Ganglionitis

Autoimmune ganglionitis should be suspected if a school-age patient, who had passed meconium within 24 h of birth and had normal bowel habits previously, presents later in life with severe constipation. Although a full-thickness bowel sample is ideal, a biopsy containing sufficient submucosa may give a clue to this entity.

The biopsy shows predominantly T-lymphocytic ganglionitis, initially with intense infiltration involving the ganglia but in time the inflammatory infiltrate is reduced resulting in degeneration and loss of enteric ganglia (Fig. 17.10) [9]. The patient's serum contains IgG-class circulating autoantibodies against enteric nerve cells often indistinguishable from those seen in patients with paraneoplastic disease but no neoplasia is found in these children. The inflammation, unless promptly treated, results in denervation and permanent dysfunction of the entire gastrointestinal tract.

Autoimmune Myositis

In autoimmune myositis the biopsy shows prominent T-lymphocytic infiltration in the muscularis propria, particularly dense around blood vessels and obscuring the myocytes beneath it [7]. If left untreated, the myocytes initially change their contractile protein profile and subsequently degenerate, atrophy and drop-out. In the end-stage disease there is a paucity of enteric myocytes in the muscularis propria, only smooth muscle cells in the capillary walls seem to survive. Anti smooth muscle auto-antibodies are detected on serology.

Eosinophilic Ganglionitis

Enteric ganglia may be affected by an inflammatory infiltrate predominantly composed of eosinophils rather than lymphocytes [8]. The neurons in the ganglia express IL-5 attracting eosinophils into the area and altering neuronal plasticity, function and survival [36] and resulting in a rare, steroid-responsive, acquired form of pseudo-obstruction.

Immune Modulation of Smooth Muscle by Eosinophils and Mast Cells

Predominantly eosinophilic leiomyositis of the muscularis propria is occasionally seen in full-thickness intestinal samples from patients with gut dysmotility. Eosinophil trafficking and activation is said to lead to tissue damage in target organs by releasing eosinophil specific granule proteins (eosinophil derived neurotoxin, eosinophil peroxidase, eosinophil-associated ribonucleases). In addition, eosinophils are regulators of local immune responses. Together with mast cells they are involved in immune modulation and tissues

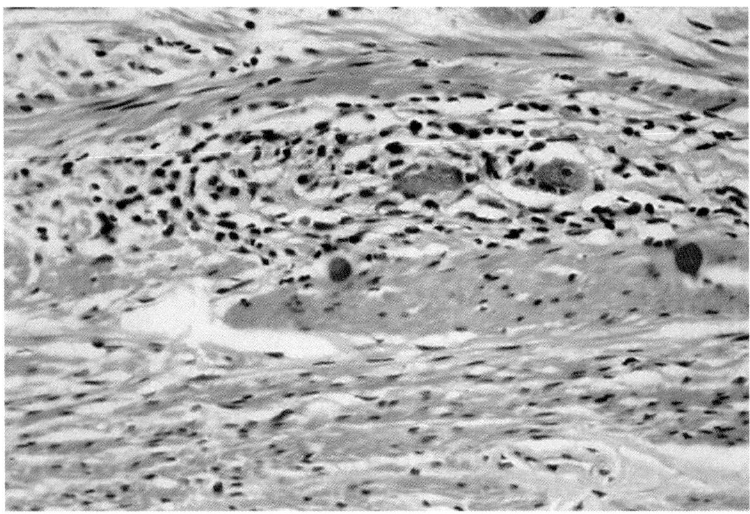

Fig. 17.10 H&E stained section showing lymphocytic myenteric ganglionitis

remodelling and have direct effect on smooth muscle activities [36].

Immune Modulation of Nerves by Mucosal Eosinophils and Mast Cells

Mucosal nerve fibres are in close contact with immunocytes in the lamina propria of the mucosa. In particular eosinophils and mast cells interact with nerves in the mucosa and these interactions are critical for the initiation or disturbance of muscle electrical activity [37]. Activated eosinophils and mast cells release their granules (eosinophil derived neurotoxin, eosinophil peroxidase, eosinophil-associated ribonucleases; and mast cell tryptase and histamine respectively) close to the mucosal nerve fibres activating PAR-2 receptors co-localised with the mucosal nerve fibres and with the loss of myoelectric activity.

Secondary to a Systemic Disease

Unlike in adults, in children enteric neuromuscular diseases secondary to systemic diseases are rare. The pathology of many muscular dystrophies affecting skeletal muscle is well understood and involves dystrophin and dystrophin associated membrane proteins (sarcoglycans, dystroglycans and others). The expression of many of the proteins is shared between skeletal and smooth muscle; thus, the myopathy may not only be confined to skeletal muscle but also affects enteric muscle resulting in bowel dysmotility.

Cystic fibrosis is a multisystem disorder caused as a consequence of defects in the cystic fibrosis membrane regulator (CFTR) protein encoded by *ABBC7* and these mutations are inherently proinflammatory. Meconium ileus and distal ileal obstruction syndrome (DIOS) are seen in patients with cystic fibrosis. In DIOS there is a marked lymphocytic leiomyositis and myenteric ganglionitis, which results in bowel obstruction [38]. The diagnosis of cystic fibrosis should be borne in mind if the intestinal sample shows transmural lymphocytic inflammatory process particularly affecting the muscularis propria and the myenteric plexus. As a consequence there may be myofibroblastic transformation in the bowel wall culminating in disarranged muscle layers (Fig. 17.11).

Mitochondrial cytopathies are regulated by two genomes, mitochondrial DNA and nuclear DNA. In patients with mitochondrial cytopathies such as Kearns-Sayre, MERRF (myoclonic epilepsy and ragged red fibres) and MELAS (myoclonic epilepsy lactic acidosis and stroke-like episodes) with mutations in the mitochondrial DNA and a maternal pattern of inheritance often show abnormal

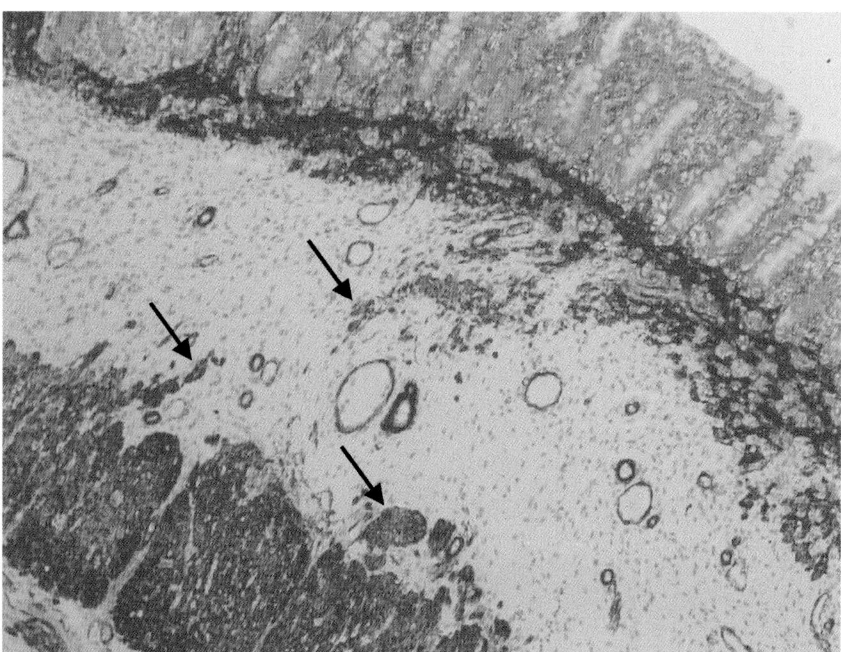

Fig. 17.11 Smooth muscle actin immunostained section of full-thickness bowel showing myofibroblastic transformation (*arrows*)

mitochondria in skeletal myocytes but in enteric smooth muscle cells they are not found even after an intensive search (personal observation, Smith VV). Some mitochondrial cytopathies are clinically associated with gut dysmotility and bear the following acronyms POLIP (polyneuropathy, opthalmoplegia, leukoencephaly and intestinal pseudo-obstruction), OGIMD (oculogastrointestinal muscular dystrophy), MEPOP (mitochondrial encephalomyopathy with sensorymotor polyneuropahy, opthalmoplegia and pseudo-obstruction) and MNGIE (neurogastrointestinal encephalomyopathy) [39]. MNGIE is an autosomal recessive mitochondrial disease with mutations in the nuclear genome and is associated with severe gastrointestinal dysmotility [40]. There are loss-of-function mutations in the nuclear encoded *thymidine phosphorylase* resulting in pathological accumulation of thymidine (deoxythymidine) and uridine (deoxyuridine). The abnormal accumulation of the metabolites creates an imbalance in the mitochondrial nucleotide pool and defects in mitochondrial DNA (depletion, point-mutations and deletions), thus impairing mitochondrial replication and maintenance. Histologically, in one reported case, a thinning of the bowel wall and atrophy and fibrosis of the longitudinal muscle coat has been described [40]. The deltoid muscle had numerous cytochrome oxidase-negative muscle fibres and fibres with increased succinate dehydrogenase activity. Electron microscopy showed abundant mitochondria and cytoplasmic lipid droplets corresponding to vacuolation on light microscopy but these findings are not universal (personal observation, Dr VV Smith). If there is a suspicion of MNGIE, skeletal muscle biopsy may be diagnostic and intestinal tissue is unlikely to be helpful. In addition, thymidine phosphatase activity should be measured in blood white cell preparations, plasma thymidine concentration measured and mutation analysis of the *thymidine phosphorylase* to be undertaken.

The Future

Although in the past couple of decades advances have been made to diagnose enteric neuromuscular diseases, at the present time the methods available to identify the subtle histological changes encountered are basic and require refining [41]. Moreover, difficulties continue to be encountered in securing normal baseline data from children's bowels due to understandable stringent ethical constraints [42].

Following are some of the areas to pursue.

Contractile Protein Isoforms

It is known that the contractile protein cocktail crucially determines the type of smooth muscle contraction. Defects in this process may constitute the basis of some forms of intestinal myopathies in which conventional histology and ultrastructural examination currently fail to demonstrate morphological abnormalities. There is a need to obtain further isoform-specific antibodies to assess the isoform profile of a variety of contractile proteins involved in smooth muscle contraction. Such antibodies could be used to study the ontogeny of isoforms and irregularities in the isoform profile and might identify further patients in whom abnormalities of this type underlie intestinal muscle dysfunction. This could also open the way to more fundamental studies at the genetic and molecular levels.

Muscle Membrane Proteins

Muscle membrane proteins (dystrophin, dystroglycans, sarcoglycans and others) are not only expressed by skeletal muscle but also cardiac and smooth muscle including enteric leiomyocytes. In X-linked dilated cardiomyopathy, which exclusively affects the heart muscle without skeletal muscle involvement, mutations in the *dystrophin* gene are found [43] but the protein levels between different types of muscles vary. Dystrophin levels as low as 30 % suffice to avoid skeletal muscular dystrophy but not cardiac muscle dysfunction. Parallel situations may exist in enteric smooth muscle. A particular level of protein expression may be sufficient to cause leiomyopathy without affecting cardiac or skeletal muscle function, thus warranting further study.

Interstitial Cells of Cajal

ICC are important cells in the control of intestinal motor function by modulating neurotransmission of noncholinergic nonadrenergic (NANC) inhibitory activity [44] but until the mid-1990s they could only be studied by electron microscopy. In 1995 Huizinga et al. demonstrated in the mouse that ICC express c-kit (cd117) and that mice with mutations in *c-kit* lack ICC as well as intestinal pacemaker activity [45]. This observation led to the study of these critically important cells by using immunohistochemistry in intestinal samples from patients with intestinal motility disorders. Many studies have been published with often conflicting results due to the plasticity shown by ICC [46]. There seems to be tremendous potential for meaningful studies on this topic but only after reliable normative data in children have been secured.

CD56 (N-CAM) Immunostaining

CD56-immunostaining is confined to the periphery of the perikarya of enteric neurons, neuronal processes, glial cells and to varicosities in the muscularis propria in post-natal gut. However, in foetal gut (12–23 weeks gestation) enteric muscle in the developing muscularis propria shows positive punctate immunostaining for CD56 (personal observation, VV Smith 1993). We have noted that leiomyocytes in the innermost circular muscle layer may retain CD56-positivity in intestinal samples from some younger patients with intestinal motility disorders (Fig. 17.12). This immunoreactivity was transient in a couple patients disappearing on follow-up sampling. The assumption is that there is a delay in muscle maturation but this is an area that requires a systematic study.

Other areas of potential interest are *channelopathies* and *neurotransmitter receptors,* which have received little attention so far [47]. Histopathology alone, even with electron microscopy as well as enzyme- and immunohistochemisty, does not suffice to identify the subtler changes and there is a need for techniques such as proteomics and

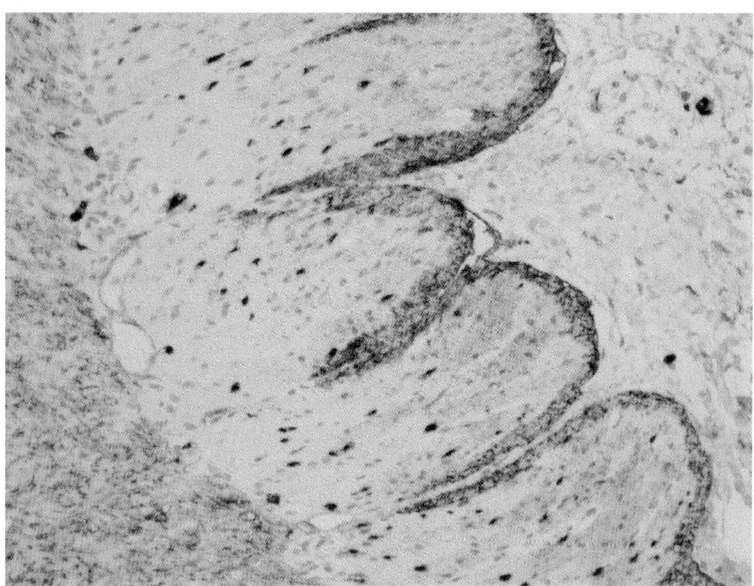

Fig. 17.12 CD56 immunostained section showing abnormal immunoreactivity in the innermost layer of the circular muscle coat (*arrow*)

genomics to identify more abnormalities. The validity of all the aforementioned investigations is underpinned by availability of normative data in childhood, which continues to be a problem in paediatrics.

References

1. Jacobi A. In some important causes of constipation in infants. Am J Obstet. 1886;2:96–113.
2. Hirschsprung H. Stuhltragheit neugeborener in folge von dilatation und hypertrophie des colons. Jahrbuch f Kinderheilkunde. 1888;NF 27:1–4.
3. Ehrenpreis T, Bentley JFR, Nixon HH, Spencer B, Lister J, Duhamel B, Pages R, Katz A. Seminar on pseudo-Hirschsprung'd disease and related disorders. Arch Dis Child. 1966;41:143–54.
4. Heneyke S, Smith VV, Spitz L, Milla PJ. Chronic intestinal pseudo-obstruction: treatment and long term follow-up of 44 patients. Arch Dis Child. 1999;81:21–7.
5. Smith VV, Milla PJ. Histological phenotypes of enteric smooth muscle disease causing functional intestinal obstruction in childhood. Histopathology. 1997;31:112–22.
6. Smith VV, Eng C, Milla PJ. Intestinal ganglioneuromatosis and multiple endocrine neoplasia type 2B: implications for treatment. Gut. 1999;45:143–6.
7. Ruuska TH, Karikoski R, Smith VV, Milla PJ. Acquired myopathic intestinal pseudo-obstruction maybe due to autoimmune enteric leiomyositis. Gastroenterology. 2002;122:1133–9.
8. Schäppi MG, Smith VV, Milla PJ, Lindley KJ. Eosinophilic myenteric ganglionitis is associated with functional intestinal obstruction. Gut. 2003;52:752–5.
9. Smith VV, Gregson N, Foggensteiner L, Neale G, Milla PJ. Acquired intestinal aganglionosis and circulating auto-antibodies without neoplasia or other neural involvement. Gastroenterology. 1997;112:1366–71.
10. Smith B. The myenteric plexus in drug-induced neuropathy. J Neurol Neurosurg Psychiatry. 1968;30:506–10.
11. Smith B. Effect of irritant purgatives on the myenteric plexus in man and the mouse. Gut. 1968;9:139–43.
12. Schuffler MD. Chronic idiopathic intestinal pseudo-obstruction caused by degenerative disorder of the myenteric plexus: the use of Smith's method to define neuropathology. Gastroenterology. 1982;82:476–86.
13. Tanner MS, Smith B, Lloyd JK. Functional intestinal obstruction due deficiency of argyrophilic neurons in the myenteric plexus: familial syndrome presenting with short bowel, malrotation and pyloric hypertrophy. Arch Dis Child. 1976;51:837–41.
14. Smith VV, Milla PJ. Argyrophilia in the developing myenteric plexus. Br J Biomed Sci. 1996;53:278–83.
15. Phillips AD, Smith VV. Intestinal biopsy. In: Kleinman RE, Goulet O-J, Mieli-Vergani G, Sanderson IR, Sherman PM, Schneider BL, editors. Walkers pediatric gastrointestinal disease. 5th ed. Hamilton Ontario Canada: BC Decker Inc.; 2008. p. 1361–73.
16. Bodian M, Carter CO, Ward BC. Hirschsprung's disease. Lancet. 1951;1(6650):302–9.

17. Lake BD, Puri P, Nixon HH, Claireaux AE. Hirschsprung's disease: an appraisal of histochemically demonstrated acetylcholinesterase activity in suction rectal biopsy specimens as an aid to diagnosis. Arch Pathol Lab Med. 1978;102:244–7.
18. Knowles CH, De Giorgio Chairs R, Kapur RP, Bruder E, Farrugia G, Geboes K, Gershon MD, Hutson J, Lindberg G, Martin JE, Meier-Ruge WA, Milla PJ, Smith VV, Vandervinden JM, Veress B, Wedel T. Gastrointestinal neuromuscular pathology (GINMP): guidelines for histological techniques and reporting: Report on behalf of the Gastro 2009 International Working Group. Acta Neuropathol. 2009;118:271–301.
19. Eng C, Marsh DJ, Robinson BG, Chow CW, Patton MA, Southbey MS, Venter DJ, Ponder BAJ, Milla PJ, Smith VV. Germline RET codon 918 mutation in apparently isolated intestinal ganglioneuromatosis. J Clin Endocrinol Metab. 1998;89:4191–4.
20. Smith VV. Intestinal neuronal density in childhood: a baseline for the objective assessment of hypo- and hyperganglionosis. Pediatr Pathol. 1993;13:225–37.
21. Navarro J, Sonsino E, Boige N, Nabarra B, Ferkadji L, Mashako LM, Cezard JP. Visceral neuropathies responsible for chronic intestinal pseudo-obstruction syndrome in pediatric practice: analysis of 26 cases. J Pediatr Gastroenterol Nutr. 1990;11:179–95.
22. Auricchio A, Brancolini V, Casari G, Milla PJ, Smith VV, Devoto M, Ballabio A. The locus for a novel syndromic form of neuronal intestinal pseudo-obstruction maps to Xq28. Am J Hum Genet. 1996;58:743–8.
23. Gargiulo A, Auricchio R, Barone MV, Cotugno G, Reardon W, Milla PJ, Ballabio A, Ciccodicola A, Auricchio A. Filamin A is mutated in X-linked chronic idiopathic intestinal pseudo-obstruction with central nervous system involvement. Am J Hum Genet. 2007;80:751–8.
24. Kaschula ROC, Cywes S, Katz A, Louw JH. Degenerative leiomyopathy with massive megacolon. Myopathic form of chronic idiopathic intestinal pseudo-obstruction occurring in indigenous Africans. Perspect Pediatr Pathol. 1987;11:193–213.
25. Moore SW, Schneider JW, Kaschula RD. Non-familial visceral myopathy: clinical and pathologic features of degenerative leiomyopathy. Pediatr Surg Int. 2002;18:6–12.
26. Smith VV, Williams AJ, Novelli V, Malone M. Extensive enteric leiomyolysis due to Cytomegalovirus enterocolitis in vertically acquired HIV infection in infants. Pediatr Dev Pathol. 2000;3:591–6.
27. Christensen J, Dent J, Malagelada J-R, Wingate DL. Pseudo-obstruction. Gastroenterol Int. 1990;3:107–19.
28. Krishnamurthy S, Schuffler MD. Pathology of neuromuscular disorders of the small intestine and colon. Gastroenterology. 1987;93:610–39.
29. Dieler R, Schroder JM, Skopnik H, Steinau G. Infantile hypertrophic pyloric stenosis: myopathic type. Acta Neuropathol. 1990;80:295–306.
30. Martin JE, Swash M, Kamm MA, Maher K, Cox EL, Gray A. Myopathy of internal anal sphincter with polyglucosan inclusions. J Pathol. 1990;161:221–6.
31. Smith VV, Lake BD, Kamm MA, Nicholls JR. Intestinal pseudo-obstruction with deficient smooth muscle alpha actin. Histopathology. 1992;21:535–42.
32. Fatigati V, Murphy RA. Actin and tropomyosin variants in the smooth muscles. Dependence on tissue type. J Biol Chem. 1984;259:14383–8.
33. Kuroda M. Change of actin isomers during differentiation of smooth muscle. Biochim Biophys Acta. 1985;843:208–13.
34. Li YF, Bowers RL, Haley-Russell D, Moody FG, Weisbrodt NW. Actin and myosin isoforms in gallbladder smooth muscle following cholesterol feeding in prairie dog. Gastroenterology. 1990;99:1460–6.
35. Owens GK, Thompson MM. Developmental changes in isoactin expression in the rat aortic smooth muscle cells in vivo. J Biol Chem. 1986;261:13373–80.
36. Jacobsen EA, Taranova AG, Lee NA, Lee JJ. Eosinophils: singularly destructive effector cells or purveyors of immunoregulation. J Allergy Clin Immunol. 2007;119:1313–20.
37. Schappi MG, Borrelli O, Knafeltz D, Williams S, Smith VV, Milla PJ, Lindley KJ. Mast cell-nerve interactions in children with functional dyspepsia. J Pediatr Gastroenterol Nutr. 2008;47:472–80.
38. Smith VV, Schaeppi MG, Bisset WM, Kiparissi F, Jaffe A, Milla PJ, Lindley KJ. Lymphocytic leiomyositis and myenteric ganglionitis are intrinsic features of cystic fibrosis: studies in distal ileal obstruction syndrome (DIOS) and meconium ileus. J Pediatr Gastroenterol Nutr. 2009;49:42–51.
39. Hirano M, Silvestri G, Blake DM, Lombes A, Minetti C, Bonilla E, Hays AP, Lovelace RE, Butler I, Bertorini TE, et al. Mitochondrial neurogastrointestinal encephalomyopathy (MNGIE): clinical, biochemical, and genetic features of an autosomal recessive mitochondrial disorder. Neurology. 1994;44:721–7.
40. Giordano C, Sebastiani M, Plazzi G, Travaglini C, Sale P, Pinti M, Tancredi A, Liguori R, Montagna P, Bellan M, Valentino ML, Cossarizza A, Hirano M, d'Amati G, Carelli V. Mitochondrial neurogastrointestinal encephalomyopathy: evidence of mitochondrial DNA depletion in the small intestine. Gastroenterology. 2006;130:893–901.
41. Knowles CH, De Giorgio Chairs R, Kapur RP, Bruder E, Farrugia G, Geboes K, Gershon MD, Hutson J, Lindberg G, Martin JE, Meier-Ruge WA, Milla PJ, Smith VV, Vandervinden JM, Veress B, TWedel T. The London classification of gastrointestinal neuromuscular pathology. Gut. 2010;59:882–7.
42. Knowles CH, Veress B, Kapur RP, Wedel T, Farrugia G, Vanderwinden JM, Geboes K, Smith VV, Martin JE, Lindberg G, Milla PJ, de Giorgio R. Quantitation of cellular components of the enteric nervous system in the normal human gastrointestinal tract—report on behalf of the Gastro 2009 International Working

Group. Neurogastroenterol Motil. 2011;23(2):115–24.
43. Neri M, Torelli S, Brown S, Ugo I, Sabatelli P, Merlini L, Spitali P, Rimessi P, Gualandi F, Sewry C, Ferlini A, Muntoni F. Dystrophin levels as low as 30 % are sufficient to avoid muscular dystrophy in the human. Neuromuscul Disord. 2007;17:913–8.
44. Thuneberg L. Interstitial cells of Cajal: intestinal pacemaker cells? Adv Anat Embryol Cell Biol. 1982;71:1–130.
45. Huizinga JD, Thuneberg L, Kluppel M, Malysz J, Mikkelsen HB, Bernstein A. W/kit gene required for interstitial cells of Cajal and for intestinal pacemaker activity. Nature. 1995;373:347–9.
46. Huizinga JD, Zarate N, Farrugia G. Physiology, injury, and recovery of interstitial cells of Cajal: basic and clinical science. Gastroenterology. 2009;137:1548–56.
47. Richardson CE, Morgan JM, Jasani B, Green JT, Rhodes J, Williams GT, Lindstrom J, Wonnacott S, Thomas GA, Smith V. Megacystis-microcolon-intestinal hypoperistalsis syndrome and the absence of the alpha3 nicotinic acetylcholine receptor subunit. Gastroenterology. 2001;121:350–7.

Genetics of Motility Disorder: Gastroesophageal Reflux, Triple A Syndrome, Hirschsprung Disease, and Chronic Intestinal Pseudo-Obstruction

18

Jonathan M. Gisser and Cheryl E. Gariepy

Introduction

The identification of gene mutations associated with a disease often provides important initial insight into its molecular basis and can hold the key to developing an effective therapeutic strategy. After several decades of identifying single gene mutations causing usually rare GI motility disorders, we are beginning to understand the etiology of complex, multigenic motility disorders. In this chapter we review the current genetic understanding of four motility disorders; gastroesophageal reflux disease (GERD), Triple A syndromic achalasia, Hirschsprung disease, and chronic intestinal pseudo obstruction. The molecular and developmental consequences of some of these mutations are described in detail in other chapters.

J.M. Gisser, M.D., M.Sc.
Division of Pediatric Gastroenterology, Hepatology and Nutrition, Pediatrics Department, Center for Molecular and Human Genetics, The Research Institute at Nationwide Children's Hospital, The Ohio State University College of Medicine, Columbus, OH, USA

C.E. Gariepy, M.D. (✉)
Center for Molecular and Human Genetics, Nationwide Children's Research Institute,
700 Children's Drive, WA2015, Columbus, OH 43205, USA
e-mail: cheryl.gariepy@nationwidechildrens.org

Gastroesophageal Reflux Disease

The lower esophageal sphincter is an anatomic and physiologic barrier that limits the backflow of gastric contents into the esophagus while allowing the passage of food into the stomach. In theory, any developmental process affecting the position and function of the lower esophageal sphincter may result in GERD and be genetically influenced. Moreover, a predisposition to complications of lower esophageal sphincter dysfunction may also be genetically influenced. It is therefore likely that the genetic contribution to the symptoms and complications arising from lower esophageal sphincter dysfunction, commonly referred to as GERD, is multifactorial [1]. Pathophysiologic determinants of GERD that may be genetically modulated have been enumerated previously and are listed in Table 18.1 [2]. Since various definitions of GERD are employed in genetic studies and the disease may be genotypically and phenotypically heterogeneous, no clear genetic determinants have yet emerged [1]. To date, evidence for a genetic predisposition to GERD has been inferred from epidemiologic, twin concordance, and genetic linkage studies, with little attention paid to specific host genetic factors. Evidence supporting genetic risk factors in the development of syndromic GERD and complications from GERD also exists, but is beyond the scope of the present discussion.

C. Faure et al. (eds.), *Pediatric Neurogastroenterology: Gastrointestinal Motility and Functional Disorders in Children*, Clinical Gastroenterology,
DOI 10.1007/978-1-60761-709-9_18,

Table 18.1 Pathophysiologic determinants of gastroesophageal reflux disease that could be genetically modulated

Refluxate toxicity
Gastric acid secretion
Duodenogastric reflux
Intrinsic gastric volume and pressure
Gastric compliance
Gastric emptying
Gastric acid volume secretion
Extrinsic pressure on gastric contents
Weight (obesity)
Somatic motor tone (spasticity)
Somatic and crural episodic contractions (cough, wheeze,…)
Gastroesophageal barrier
Lower esophageal sphincter tone
Gastric fundic sensory thresholds (for transient lower esophageal sphincter relaxations)
Crural diaphragm location (relative to sphincter location) and function
Esophageal defenses
Salivary secretion
Peristaltic motor function
Esophageal cytoprotection

[a]Adapted from Orenstein SR, Shalaby TM, Barmada MM, Whitcomb DC. J Pediatr Gastroenterol Nutr. 2002;34(5):506–10. Lippincott Williams & Wilkins, Inc., Philadelphia, publishers

The first studies to infer a genetic component to GERD were case reports describing familial clusters of radiologically confirmed hiatal hernia (reviewed in [3]). In the largest and most detailed of these studies, Carre and colleagues described a kindred of 38 family members across five generations, all of whom were interviewed and subjected to a barium meal. Among this pedigree were 20 individuals with both symptoms of gastroesophageal reflux, and radiologic evidence of hiatal hernia. An autosomal dominant mode of inheritance was suggested [4].

Although familial clusters of hiatal hernia are established, most cases of hiatal hernia are sporadic and most pediatric GERD is not associated with hiatal hernia. Therefore hiatal hernia probably accounts for a small minority of cases of hereditary GERD. Other studies support a familial predisposition to GERD even in the absence of a hiatal hernia. In case control studies, GERD symptoms in relatives of patients with Barrett's metaplasia, and esophageal adenocarcinoma were more prevalent than in spouse controls. A similar increased prevalence among relatives of patients with uncomplicated esophagitis, was not observed in this study, suggesting that only severe GERD is heritable [5]. However, another investigation of patients with abnormal pH studies revealed that relatives of patients with increased esophageal acid exposure were more likely to experience frequent reflux symptoms, even in the absence of GERD complications [6].

Familial clustering of GERD can also arise from shared environmental risk factors rather than genetic factors. In twin studies, conditions that bear a large genetic predisposition are more likely concordant in monozygotic twins than dizygotic twins. Two large-scale studies have investigated the concordance of GERD in mono- and dizygotic twins. In one of these studies, twins belonging to the national Swedish Twin Registry were queried for GERD using a questionnaire. In almost 3,100 twin pairs with GERD, aged 55 years or greater, the concordance was significantly higher among monozygotic twins compared to dizygotic twins, suggesting that heritability accounts for approximately one third of the susceptibility to GERD [7]. A similar study from a twin registry in the United Kingdom corroborated the Swedish study, finding concordance rates of 42% for monozygotic twins versus 26% for dizygotic twins, and concluding that 43% of the predilection to GERD is genetically influenced [8].

In an attempt to detect specific genetic loci associated with GERD, Hu and colleagues performed a genetic linkage analysis of five families in which multiple family members were afflicted with severe pediatric GERD. They found a 9-centiMorgan locus on the long arm of chromosome 13 (13q14; termed GERD1) that segregated with the severe pediatric GERD phenotype in their cohort [9]. A candidate gene in this region is the 5-hydroxytryptamine receptor 2A. However, no coding sequence mutations were identified [9, 10]. The authors proposed that mutations in regulatory or other non-coding regions, null alleles, segmental deletions and duplications, and epigenetic effects in the 13q14 region could still account for the pediatric GERD phenotype in these families [10]. In support of this, a recent case report describes a dysmorphic infant with severe GERD who possesses a 12.8 megabase deletion spanning the GERD1 locus, implicating GERD1 haploinsufficiency in the patient's symptoms [11]. However, independent linkage analyses in different cohorts failed to confirm the association of the 13q14 locus with GERD [12, 13], underscoring the genetic heterogeneity of GERD.

The subjective sensation of GER has been attributed to the exposure of esophageal mucosa to the acidic gastric refluxate causing a mucosal inflammatory response which, in turn, activates afferent sensory nerve pathways. As such, variations in genes that participate in inflammation, wound healing, and sensory neuromodulation could theoretically contribute to the experience of gastroesophageal reflux. With this in mind, three recent studies have focused on genes in these pathways. A study by Chourasia et al. evaluated the relationship of polymorphisms in genes encoding the Interleukin 1B (*IL-1B*) and the interleukin 1 receptor antagonist (*IL-1RN*) to GERD in patients referred to a tertiary center [14]. A single nucleotide polymorphism in the promoter region of the *IL-1B* gene predisposes to increased concentrations of IL-1beta, a potent pro-inflammatory cytokine. In contrast, a polymorphism consisting of two intronic tandem repeats (as opposed to 3–5 repeats) within the *IL-1RN* gene tends to decrease IL-1beta levels and has an anti-inflammatory effect. Hypothesizing that increased gastric inflammation destroys proton-excreting parietal cells, thus lowering esophageal acid exposure, investigators characterized the IL-1 genotypes of 144 patients with confirmed GERD and 368 healthy controls. They found that subjects with genotypes and haplotypes combining to decrease IL-1beta levels had predictably lower gastric mucosal IL-1beta expression, and generally had a higher risk of GERD. These genotypes and haplotypes were also more prevalent in the GERD population [14].

In another genome wide association study, Asling and colleagues collected 36 GERD-affected families and mapped familial GERD to a 35 megabase pair region on chromosome 2q24-q33, confirming this association in a separate cohort. Biopsies from those subjects with abnormal endoscopic or pHmetric findings, or those who had undergone fundoplication, were then subjected to gene expression analysis and the COL3A1 gene (collagen type III alpha I), residing within this locus, was found to be differentially expressed in subjects with GERD compared to controls. As collagen type III contributes to tissue strength, flexibility, and wound response, the authors proposed a mechanism whereby altered collagen type III expression in the esophagus results in a predisposition to esophageal damage in patients with gastroesophageal reflux. Although they immunohistochemically demonstrated increased expression of the collagen III protein in esophageal tissue biopsies, they did not investigate whether this was a cause or a consequence of gastroesophageal reflux. Also, sequencing of the COL3A1 gene in 48 subjects did not identify any causative mutations. The authors propose that disease causing mutations reside in regulatory regions [12].

G-proteins are second messengers involved in the neurotransmission of gastroesophageal sensation. The C825T substitution polymorphism within the gene encoding the G-protein β3 subunit results in enhanced G-protein activation and signal transduction [15], and is associated with functional dyspepsia [16]. On this basis, De Vries and coworkers explored the relationship of the C825T allele with GERD in 363 subjects with either pathologic esophageal acid exposure or a positive symptoms association score for heartburn or regurgitation. Compared to healthy controls, individuals with GERD were more likely to be heterozygous for the C825T. The likelihood of being heterozygous for C825T was highest (adjusted odds ratio 1.5; 95% CI 1.06–2.13) among patients with a positive symptom association score, but no correlation was observed among those with pathologic acid exposure. This suggests that enhanced perception of physiologic acid exposure, and not pathologic acid exposure, underlies the association of C825T heterozygosity and GERD [17].

Each of the above studies propose different heritable host factors in the pathophysiology of

GERD, increasing the likelihood that still other host factors exist. Furthermore, replication and validation of existing studies is required, highlighting the great need for further investigation in this area.

Triple A Syndrome

Triple A syndrome, AAAS is a condition characterized by *a*lacrima, adrenocorticotrophic hormone-resistant *a*drenal insufficiency, and *a*chalasia [18]. Although its name connotes a triad, the syndrome is phenotypically heterogeneous: fewer than three features may be present and additional features not originally identified in the initial report by Allgrove, including progressive autonomic, central, and peripheral nervous system deficits, are associated with the syndrome [19]. The etiology of achalasia in AAAS appears to be distinct from other forms of achalasia [20]. Although it is a rare condition and epidemiologic data are scant, symptoms of swallowing difficulty and achalasia in AAAS usually manifests by the end of the first decade of life and can begin in infancy [21, 22]—in contrast to idiopathic achalasia, where very small minority of patients manifest symptoms before 10 years of age [23]. The diagnosis of achalasia in AAAS relies on the same manometric, radiographic, and endoscopic criteria as for idiopathic achalasia, and the treatment is similar.

Frameshift, point, or missense mutations in the gene *AAAS*, located at 12q13, account for the majority of cases of AAAS [19, 24, 25]. Consanguinity is often present in kindreds of AAAS and the condition segregates in an autosomal recessive pattern. The penetrance of AAAS with bi-allelic mutations in *AAAS* approaches 100%, though expressivity is variable, possibly due to allelic variation or the existence of as yet unidentified modifier genes.

AAAS encodes the ALADIN protein (an acronym for alacrima, achalasia, adrenal insufficiency and neurological disorder) [26, 27]. ALADIN is part of the nuclear pore complex, a large, multiprotein complex spanning the nuclear envelope and forming a selective channel between the cytoplasm and the nucleus [28, 29]. ALADIN is the first nuclear pore protein linked to a human heritable disease. In most cases of AAAS, ALADIN is truncated, resulting in its exclusion from nuclear pore complex and in ectopic cytoplasmic accumulation [30]. This may be due to an inability of the mutant ALADIN protein to anchor to proteins required for nuclear pore complex assembly [31] or to the deletion of a critical nuclear localization signals in the *AAAS* transcript [32]. Although the nucleus and the nuclear pore complex remain morphologically and structurally intact without ALADIN, the nuclear import of selected proteins is interrupted. Proteins involved in DNA repair and the attenuation of oxidative stress fail to localize to the nucleus when ALADIN is absent from the nuclear pore complex [33, 34]. On this basis, it is proposed that defective ALADIN renders cells susceptible to oxidative DNA damage and cell death in a tissue-specific manner [33]. In support of this, fibroblast cultures derived from patients with AAAS possess a higher basal level of reactive oxygen species, a heightened response to oxidative stress and a predilection for premature stress-induced senescence [35]. Given the variety and abundance of macromolecules that depend on a competent nuclear pore complex, it is probable that additional genes and proteins will one day be identified that will further elucidate how the ALADIN defect translates into the observed phenotypes of AAAS.

Hirschsprung Disease

Hirschsprung disease (HSCR) is the developmental absence of enteric ganglion cells from a continuous segment of distal intestine. The enteric ganglia are neural crest-derived and congenital distal aganglionosis is generally attributed to a failure of vagal neural crest cells to complete colonization of the developing intestine between the 5th and 12th week of gestation [36]. A minority of HSCR (30%) is syndromic (associated with other congenital anomalies) with several monogenic syndromes recognized and chromosomal abnormalities found in 12% of cases. Isolated and syndromic HSCR are discussed separately, however, the distinction is not always clear-cut with syndromic phenotypes sometimes not apparent at birth and the implication of several genes in both isolated and syndromic forms of the disease. Approximately 20% of HSCR is familial with a recurrence risk in relatives up to 200 times increased over the general population. HSCR is classified as short-segment disease (S-HSCR) when aganglionosis is distal to the splenic flexure, long-segment (L-HSCR) when aganglionosis begins proximal to the splenic flexure (20% of cases) and total colonic (TC-HSCR) when the entire colon is aganglionic (~5% of cases) [37].

Isolated HSCR

Isolated HSCR is a complex, multigenic disorder with low, sex-dependent penetrance, and variable expression. The incidence of HSCR varies among ethnicities with a range from 1 to 2.8 per 10,000 live births in Hispanics and Asians, respectively [38]. The two major genes implicated in isolated HSCR are the gene encoding the RET (REarranged after Transfection) receptor tyrosine kinase, *RET*, and the gene encoding the endothelin B-receptor, *EDNRB*.

RET is a proto-oncogene that is disease causing in Multiple Endocrine Neoplasia syndrome 2 (MEN2), congenital abnormalities of the kidney and urinary tract [39] and HSCR. A large number of *RET* coding sequence mutations spanning the length of the gene are identified in HSCR. In contrast, MEN2A mutations occur in a cluster of cysteines on exon 10 or exon 11 and the MEN2B mutation is a unique codon substitution, M918T, in the tyrosine kinase domain. HSCR mutations generally reduce biological activity of the receptor whereas MEN2 mutations are activating mutations leading to constitutive dimerization of the receptor in the absence of ligand. However, HSCR and MEN2A occur together in some patients and families, requiring a more complex explanation for the signaling consequences of these mutations [40, 41].

There are two major isoforms of RET produced by alternative splicing of the transcript, RET9 (1,072 amino acids) and RET51 (1,114 amino acids). The evidence is conflicting as to whether both isoforms are equally supportive of enteric nervous system development [42, 43]. The expression of a particular mutation may have significantly different developmental effects depending upon the isoform in which it is expressed. For example, in genetically manipulated mice, a specific mutation in *RET51* produces only distal colon aganglionosis, while the same mutation in *RET9* leads to aganglionosis with parasympathetic, sympathetic, and renal anomalies [43].

Mutations in the coding sequence of *RET* are found in ~50% of familial and 15% of sporadic HSCR. However, most individuals with isolated HSCR carry a non-coding sequence mutation in *RET*. An allele including a single nucleotide change in an enhancer sequence within intron 1 (the "T allele", also known as *rs2435357*) is very common in the USA, European (~24%), and Asian (47% in China) populations and likely plays a pivotal role in HSCR susceptibility despite conferring low penetrance of the phenotype. Coding sequence mutations are more likely to be found in less common forms of the disease (females with familial L-HSCR). The T allele interferes with SOX10 binding to the RET enhancer and is a genetic susceptibility factor in all forms of HSCR (discussed further below) [44]. Interestingly ~5% of the Caucasian population carries a different non-coding sequence polymorphism in *RET* that appears to reduce the risk of HSCR [45].

Glial-Derived Neurotrophic Factor (GDNF) is a ligand that requires the co-receptor GFRα(alpha)1 to activate RET. While targeted disruption of GDNF and GFRα(alpha)1 produces a HSCR-like phenotype in mice, GDNF mutations are a rare cause of HSCR and a GFRα(alpha)1 mutation has only been described in one family with HSCR [46].

EDNRB is a G-protein coupled, heptahelical transmembrane receptor that is activated by the endothelins (EDN1, 2, and 3). While EDNRB accepts all three ligand with equal affinity, developmentally EDN3 is the relevant ligand as targeted disruption in mice of *EDN3* alone (but not *EDN1* or *EDN2*) produces a very similar phenotype as *EDNRB* disruption [47]. Pre-proendothelin is proteolytically activated by Endothelin Converting Enzyme (ECE)1 [48].

Mutations in *EDNRB* and *EDN3* are disease-causing in Waardenburg Syndrome type 4 (WS4, hearing loss and pigment abnormalities with HSCR) and isolated HSCR [49]. While coding sequence *EDN3* mutations are a rare cause of isolated HSCR [50], *EDNRB* coding sequence mutations are found in ~5% of cases with incomplete penetrance of heterozygous mutations [46]. Sanchez-Mejias and colleagues recently reported a single nucleotide polymorphism in an *EDN3* intron significantly overrepresented in HSCR patients and hypothesized that *EDN3* may be a common low-penetrance susceptibility gene for sporadic HSCR, similar to the T allele in *RET* [51]. A heterozygous *ECE1* mutation was identified in a single patient with skip-lesion aganglionosis and other defects (including cardiac defects, craniofacial abnormalities, and autonomic dysfunction, some of which may be related to an absence of active EDN1) [52].

While RET and EDNRB signaling are thought to be independent, genetically there is clear interaction between the two pathways. Mice carrying hypomorphic (causing a partial loss of gene function) non-disease causing mutations of both *RET* and *EDNRB* exhibit aganglionosis and a similar phenomenon is reported in humans [53–55]. *RET* is the major disease causing gene in isolated HSCR, but in most cases alterations in other genes, particularly *EDNRB* and perhaps *EDN3*, modulate clinical expression of the phenotype [44, 56].

Because of the poor genotype–phenotype correlation in isolated HSCR, there is little benefit of mutation screening except for the cancer predisposing MEN2A mutations in *RET* where it is important to identify the syndrome before it becomes symptomatic (see below). Despite this, relative risk figures for isolated HSCR recurrence in siblings exist and depend upon the sex of the known affected individual, the length of aganglionosis in that individual, and the sex of the sibling in question. The lowest recurrence risk is for the female sibling of a male with S-HSCR (1%) and the highest risk is for a male sibling of a female with L-HSCR (33%) [46].

Syndromic HSCR

A wide range of isolated anomalies are reported with HSCR. Cardiac defects (most commonly atrial- or ventricular-septal defects) and renal anomalies are found in ~5% of HSCR patients and should be looked for systematically. For HSCR associated with other congenital anomalies, the prognosis is largely dependent on the severity of the other anomalies. Numerous syndromes are associated with HSCR and the recognition of these syndromes is important for disease prognosis and accurate genetic counseling. Careful evaluation by a clinician familiar with the varied associated syndromes is extremely valuable to the patients and their families. Below we discuss syndromes most commonly associated with HSCR.

HSCR occurs in syndromes with defects in other neural crest-derived tissues, termed neurocristopathies. The neural crest is a transient, multipotent, migratory cell population in the embryo that give rise to diverse tissues of the body, including melanocytes, craniofacial cartilage and bone, cells in the thymus, the cardiac outflow tract, the adrenal medulla, the autonomic nervous system, and the ENS. Multiple endocrine neoplasia (MEN) 2A, 2B, and familial medullary thyroid carcinoma (FMTC) are autosomal dominant cancer predisposition syndromes and neurocristopathies. MEN2A includes medullary thyroid carcinoma (MTC, 70% by age 70), pheochromocytoma (50%), and parathyroid hyperplasia (~25%). MEN2B presents with oral neuroma, marfanoid habitus, and hyperganglionosis (associated with dysmotility) of the gut. It also includes MTC and pheochromocytoma. FMTC and MEN2 are caused by mutations in *RET* and both FMTC and MEN2A are associated with HSCR. The same mutations causing MEN2A and FMTC can cause HSCR suggesting that individuals with

HSCR should be screened for these mutations to allow for early cancer detection [57].

Congenital central hypoventilation syndrome (CCHS) is an autosomal dominant neurocristopathy characterized by an abnormal ventilatory response to hypoxia and hypercapnia due to abnormal autonomic respiratory control. The syndrome can be associated with broader dysfunction of the autonomic nervous system and with neural crest-derived tumors (5–10% of CCHS patients develop neuroblastoma, ganglioblastoma, or ganglioneuroma). CCHS is caused by mutation in *PHOX2B* with a de novo heterozygous in-frame duplication leading to polyalanine expansion being the most common mutation indentified. However, approximately 10% of the parents of CCHS patients will be mosaic for the mutation and may develop late onset central hypoventilation. There is also a clear genotype–phenotype correlation with the risk for tumor development: individuals carrying the most common polyalanine expansion mutation can be reassured, while those carrying a frameshift mutation are at high risk and should be considered for regular screening [58, 59]. Overall, 20% of individuals with CCHS have HSCR with L-HSCR or TCA being most common with a near equal male to female ratio [60]. However, the T allele of RET affects the penetrance of HSCR with the incidence of HSCR climbing to 60% in CCHS patients homozygous for the T allele [61].

The combination of Waardenburg syndrome and HSCR is termed Waardenburg syndrome type 4 (WS4) or the Shah-Waardenburg syndrome. It is called by homozygous mutations of the endothelin-B signaling pathway (*EDNRB* or *EDN3*) or heterozygous *SOX10* mutation. Patients with *SOX10* mutations are also at risk for other neurologic abnormalities including seizures, ataxia, and demyelinating neuropathies. HSCR is also associated with severe congenital deafness in the absence of pigment abnormalities [62].

HSCR also occurs in syndromes that are not neurocristopathies. Trisomy 21 increases the risk of HSCR by 40-fold (0.8% of individuals with trisomy 21 have HSCR) and is by far the most frequent chromosomal abnormality identified in HSCR patients, involving 2–10% of HSCR. HSCR in patients with trisomy 21 shows a more pronounced male predominance and is primarily S-HSCR [63]. Interestingly, the T allele in *RET* intron 1 enhancer discussed above appears to play a role in the expression of HSCR in trisomy 21 as well as sporadic, non-syndromic HSCR. While incidence of the T allele higher in individuals with trisomy 21 HSCR than in individuals with trisomy 21 alone, it is less than that observed in individuals with HSCR alone. This suggests interaction between RET and chromosome 21 genes, perhaps through a reduced HSCR threshold conferred by the extra chromosome 21 [64].

Mowat-Wilson syndrome includes microcephaly, epilepsy, facial dysmorphism, and severe mental retardation. Sixty percent of affected individuals have HSCR. The syndrome is caused by heterozygous de novo inactivating mutations of *ZEB2* [65]. Goldberg-Shprintzen syndrome includes microcephaly, polymicrogyria, facial dysmorphism, cleft palate, iris coloboma, and moderate mental retardation. It is caused by mutation in the gene encoding the kif-1 binding protein (known as *KBP* or *KIAA1279*) [66]. Animal models suggest that this protein is required for axonal outgrowth in the central and peripheral nervous system and for axonal maintenance [67]. The details of how this leads to the HSCR phenotype are yet to be determined.

Bardet-Biedl syndrome (BBS) includes progressive pigmentary retinopathy, hypogonadism, renal abnormalities, mild mental retardation, obesity, and postaxial polydactyly of the hands and feet. HSCR is reported in several cases. It is caused by at least 14 different genes all of which are involved in the function of primary cilia [68]. As with trisomy 21, *PHOX2B* and *EDNRB* mutations, the presence of the T allele of *RET* associated with expression of the aganglionosis phenotype despite independent biochemical signaling pathways [61]. McKusick-Kaufman syndrome is a rare condition allelic to BBS that includes hydrometrocolpos, postaxial polydactyly, and congenital heart defects. HSCR is reported in 10% of cases [69].

Smith-Lemli-Opitz syndrome is characterized by growth retardation, microcephaly, severe metal retardation, dysmorphic facies, hypospadias, and syndactyly of the toes. A high percentage of patients also have HSCR. The syndrome is due to mutation in a gene involved in cholesterol metabolism, 7-dehydro-cholesterol reductase [70, 71]. HSCR occurs with limb anomalies in several other rare syndromes. See Table 18.2 for more on the genetics of isolated and syndromic forms of HSCR.

Table 18.2 Genetics of isolated and syndromic forms of Hirschsprung's disease

Gene	Mutation	Phenotype
A. Isolated Hirschsprung		
RET	Heterozygous loss-of-function of tyrosine kinase receptor (many identified)	Long-segment or total-colonic disease more common
EDNRB	Heterozygous loss-of-function of G protein-coupled receptor	Generally produces short-segment disease
B. Syndromic Hirschsprung		
RET	Heterozygous mutations of cysteines producing constitutive dimerization and activation of the receptor	MEN2A: medullary thyroid carcinoma, pheochromocytoma, parathyroid hyperplasia
Phox2B	Heterozygous loss-of-function mutation of transcription factor Polyalanine expansion most common	Congenital Central Hypoventilation Syndrome: abnormal autonomic respiratory control, frame-shift mutations increase risk of neuroblastoma
EDNRB	Homozygous loss-of-function mutation of G protein-coupled receptor	Waardenburg Syndrome Type 4: pigment abnormalities and deafness
		Waardenburg Syndrome Type 4: pigment abnormalities, deafness. Sox10 mutations also associated with ataxia, neuropathies and seizures
ZEB2	Heterozygous loss-of-function mutation of transcription factor	Mowat-Wilson Syndrome: microcephaly, epilepsy, dysmorphic face, cognitive impairment
KIAA1279	Homozygous loss-of-function in protein involved in microtubule organization	Goldberg-Shprintzen Syndrome: microcephaly, polymicrogyria, dysmorphic face, cleft palate, iris coloboma, mild cognitive impairment
BBS genes	Homozygous loss-of-function in proteins involved in primary cilia	Bardet-Biedl Syndrome: obesity, renal abnormalities, polydactyly, retinitis pigmentosa, hypogonadism, cognitive impairment
DHCR7	Homozgygous loss-of-function of enzyme in cholesterol production pathway	Smith-Lemli-Opitz Syndrome: microcephaly, dysmorphic face, hypotonia, syndactyly, polydactyly, ambiguous genitalia, poor growth
C. Modifying genes		
RET	T allele: single nucleotide substitution in an enhancer sequence	This common allelic variant increases the penetrance of Hirschsprung disease in those with other genetic susceptibilities, like trisomy 21, mutations in EDNRB, Phox2B and BBS genes

Chronic Intestinal Pseudo-Obstruction

Chronic intestinal pseudo-obstruction (CIPO) is a heterogeneous group of rare primary and secondary disorders in which ganglion cells are present throughout the GI tract in a patient with severe failure of intestinal propulsive motility. The anatomic correlates of CIPO are most often absent, subtle, subjective, or non-specific. Most cases are sporadic and non-syndromic, but familial and syndromic forms are reported. CIPO is generally divided into three groups: neuropathic, mesenchymopathic, and myopathic, depending upon whether predominant abnormalities are found in the enteric nervous system, Interstitial Cells of Cajal (ICC), or intestinal smooth muscle, respectively. While a genetic basis is suspected in a large percentage of CIPO, it is established in only a small minority of cases.

Neuropathic

Intestinal Neuronal Dysplasia type B (IND B) is characterized by hyperplasia of the submucosal and mucosal portions of the enteric nervous systems, presents with chronic constipation in the first 6 months of life, and is reported in the proximal gut of some individuals with HSCR [36, 72]. Children with isolated IND B often improve in GI function over time with conservative treatment and do not progress to CIPO [73]. While the diagnosis of IND B remains somewhat controversial, several animal models and its association with HSCR suggest a genetic cause. IND-like hyperplasia of submucosal ganglia occurs in the proximal gut of EDN3-deficient mice [74] and in the small intestine and colon of apparently healthy EDNRB heterozygous rats [75]. Attempts to identify mutations in EDNRB in IND B patients have been unsuccessful [76].

IND A is a rare, fatal syndrome of aplasia or hypoplasia of the enteric sympathetic nerves which presents in the immediate neonatal period with a tonically contracted intestine [77]. The genetics of the disorder are unknown.

Neurofibromatosis 1 (NF1) is a neurocristopathy associated with disordered intestinal motility related to neuroglial proliferation and often tumor formation in the submucosal and myenteric plexus. It is also associated with HSCR. Fifty percent of cases result from de novo mutations and 50% are inherited in an autosomal dominant fashion with highly variable penetrance and phenotypic expression. The NF1 gene encodes neurofibromin which is an upstream regulator of the RAS/RAF/MAPkinase and RAS/RAL intracellular signaling pathways [78]. A GDNF mutation modifies the enteric phenotype of NF1. Individuals carrying both the neurofibromin and GDNF mutation develop NF1 with congenital intestinal dysmotility associated with submucosal plexus hyperplasia [79].

MEN2B is a rare autosomal dominant syndrome characterized by medulary thyroid carcinoma, pheochromocytoma, marfanoid appearance, and ganglioneuromas. The syndrome is most often caused by activating mutation of codon 918 of *RET*. Because 50% of mutations are de novo, a family history is frequently absent. Constipation, often severe, related to intestinal ganglioneuromatosis is present in 40% of patients and may be present at birth [80, 81]. Recognition of this potential cause of severe constipation is clinically important because the intestinal symptoms usually precede endocrine neoplasia. Individuals with MEN2B *RET* mutations develop early onset MTC with metastatic disease reported in infants. Total thyroidectomy during the first month of life is recommended [82].

In addition to being associated with pigment abnormalities and HSCR (WS4), *SOX10* mutations are associated with additional nervous system symptoms, including nystagmus, hypotonia, cerebellar ataxia, and peripheral demyelinating neuropathy [83]. Occasionally the enteric phenotype in individuals with *SOX10* mutations is not HSCR but CIPO with normal appearing ganglia [84].

An X-linked form of CIPO characterized by abnormal argyrophilic "shrunken, degenerating" neurons in the myenteric and submucosal plexus with "nerve fibers in the lamina propria of the colon" associated with pyloric hypertrophy, a short small bowel, and malrotation is reported

[85]. Patients that survive the neonatal period develop severe CNS disease with spasticity and seizures. The syndrome is cause by a deletion in the *FLNA* gene, which encodes a large cytoskeletal protein [86].

Our understanding of CIPO is hampered by a paucity of animal models. Mutations clearly linked to CIPO in humans often cause no disease in mice. For example, mice carrying the MEN2B mutation of RET do not develop intestinal ganglioneuromas [87]. Further, while HOX11L1 knockout mice are a model of CIPO, descriptions of their ENS abnormality are inconsistent. HOX11L1 is expressed in differentiating neurons primarily in the ileocecal region, proximal colon, and gastric cardia where, in a permissive genetic environment, it appears to influence neurotransmitter expression within the ENS: 100% of HOX11L1 knockout mice on one inbred genetic background show signs of intestinal pseudo-obstruction, with most dying in the first month of life and ~30% surviving with distended proximal colons. In contrast, only 15% on a different inbred genetic background developed disease. Strain-specific differences are also noted in the number of enteric neurons that express HOX11L1 [88]. Recently, however, a couple of animal models of myenteric ganglioneuromatosis have been reported. Mice with ENS tissue specific disruption of *PTEN* develop hypertrophy and hyperplasia of the myenteric and submucosal plexus throughout the GI tract with lethal functional obstruction. PTEN deficiency alters intracellular MAPK/ERK signaling and some patients with a ganglioneuromatosis form of CIPO not related to NF1 or MEN2B have decreased expression of PTEN [89]. Decreased immunohistochemical detection of PTEN in the hyperplastic ganglia of individuals with IND B has been reported [90]. Mice that do not express SPRY2, which encodes a fibroblast growth factor pathway antagonist, are another model of myenteric ganglioneuromatosis. These animals have a hyperplastic colonic myenteric plexus (as well as a non-relaxing lower esophageal sphincter), perhaps through increased RET activation. Half of these mice die by 6 weeks of age due to esophageal/intestinal obstruction and the remaining animals are significantly growth restricted [91].

Mesenchymopathic

The ICC are derived from mesenchymal precursor cells and are located adjacent to the myenteric plexus (ICC-MY), along the submucosal boarder of the circular muscle (ICC-SM), within the circular muscle layer in the deep muscular plexus (ICC-DMP), and within muscle bundles of the tunica muscularis (ICC-IM). Various mutations in the gene encoding the receptor tyrosine kinase KIT and its ligand, stem cell factor, produce reductions in some classes of ICC. A reduction in ICC-MY results in mice without intestinal pacemaker activity, a reduction in ICC-IM results in marked reduction in cholinergic excitatory and nitrergic inhibitory input to intestinal smooth muscle. Animal models with genetic reduction in ICC exhibit abnormal intestinal motility patterns without signs of intestinal obstruction, while animals with antibody-mediated ICC reduction in the neonatal period exhibit dysmotility with distension [92, 93]. This likely relates to the severity and subtype of ICC reduction. The absence of ICCs, their abnormal distribution or morphology is suggested to cause CIPO based on several case reports [94].

Myopathic

Myopathic CIPO usually includes a variety of extraintestinal manifestations and myopathies. The Megacystis-Microcolon-Intestinal-Hypoperistalsis Syndrome, MMIHS, is characterized clinically by intestinal and urinary dysfunction and histologically by a reduction in the expression of contractile and cytoskeletal proteins in the intestinal and bladder smooth muscle. The genetic cause of the syndrome remains unknown, although an autosomal recessive pattern of inheritance is observed [95]. Mice with homozygous disruption of the alpha-3/beta-4 neuronal nicotinic acetylcholine receptor genes exhibit a similar phenotype. Both of these genes map to human chromosome 15q24 and a high frequency of polymorphisms in these genes was reported in human patients [96]. MMIHS is also reported in a child with a deletion of a more proximal segment of 15q [97].

A significant fraction of pediatric and adult CIPO patients have mitochondrial defects. These patients almost invariably have or will develop extra-intestinal neurologic or muscle symptoms [98]. A loss-of-function mutation in the thymidine phosphorylase gene (*TYMP*) produces the Mitochondrial Neuro-Gastro-Intestinal Encephalomyopathy (MNGIE) syndrome, a rare autosomal recessive condition beginning in the second decade of life and characterized by CIPO, ptosis, progressive external ophthalmoplegia, peripheral neuropathy, and leukoencephalopathy. Related disorders include MNGIE without leukoencephalopathy that can be caused by mutation in the mitochondrial DNA polymerase gamma gene (*POLG*) leading to mitochondrial depletion, and MELAS (Mitochondrial myopathy, Epilepsy, Lactic acidosis, and Stroke-like episodes) caused by mutation in a mitochondrial transfer RNA [99–102].

References

1. Orenstein SR, Whitcomb DC, Barmada MM. Challenges of examining complex genetic disorders like GERD. J Pediatr Gastroenterol Nutr. 2005;41 Suppl 1:S17–9.
2. Orenstein SR, Shalaby TM, Barmada MM, Whitcomb DC. Genetics of gastroesophageal reflux disease: a review. J Pediatr Gastroenterol Nutr. 2002;34(5):506–10.
3. Trudgill N. Familial factors in the etiology of gastroesophageal reflux disease, Barrett's esophagus, and esophageal adenocarcinoma. Chest Surg Clin N Am. 2002;12(1):15–24.
4. Carre IJ, Johnston BT, Thomas PS, Morrison PJ. Familial hiatal hernia in a large five generation family confirming true autosomal dominant inheritance. Gut. 1999;45(5):649–52.
5. Romero Y, Cameron AJ, Locke III GR, et al. Familial aggregation of gastroesophageal reflux in patients with Barrett's esophagus and esophageal adenocarcinoma. Gastroenterology. 1997;113(5):1449–56.
6. Trudgill NJ, Kapur KC, Riley SA. Familial clustering of reflux symptoms. Am J Gastroenterol. 1999;94(5):1172–8.
7. Cameron AJ, Lagergren J, Henriksson C, Nyren O, Locke III GR, Pedersen NL. Gastroesophageal reflux disease in monozygotic and dizygotic twins. Gastroenterology. 2002;122(1):55–9.
8. Mohammed I, Cherkas LF, Riley SA, Spector TD, Trudgill NJ. Genetic influences in gastro-oesophageal reflux disease: a twin study. Gut. 2003;52(8):1085–9.
9. Hu FZ, Preston RA, Post JC, et al. Mapping of a gene for severe pediatric gastroesophageal reflux to chromosome 13q14. JAMA. 2000;284(3):325–34.
10. Hu FZ, Donfack J, Ahmed A, et al. Fine mapping a gene for pediatric gastroesophageal reflux on human chromosome 13q14. Hum Genet. 2004;114(6):562–72.
11. Champaigne NL, Laird NA, Northup JK, Velagaleti GV. Molecular cytogenetic characterization of an interstitial de novo 13q deletion in a 3-month-old with severe pediatric gastroesophageal reflux. Am J Med Genet A. 2009;149A(4):751–4.
12. Asling B, Jirholt J, Hammond P, et al. Collagen type III alpha I is a gastro-oesophageal reflux disease susceptibility gene and a male risk factor for hiatus hernia. Gut. 2009;58(8):1063–9.
13. Orenstein SR, Shalaby TM, Finch R, et al. Autosomal dominant infantile gastroesophageal reflux disease: exclusion of a 13q14 locus in five well characterized families. Am J Gastroenterol. 2002;97(11):2725–32.
14. Chourasia D, Achyut BR, Tripathi S, Mittal B, Mittal RD, Ghoshal UC. Genotypic and functional roles of IL-1B and IL-1RN on the risk of gastroesophageal reflux disease: the presence of IL-1B-511*T/IL-1RN*1 (T1) haplotype may protect against the disease. Am J Gastroenterol. 2009;104(11):2704–13.
15. Siffert W, Rosskopf D, Siffert G, et al. Association of a human G-protein beta3 subunit variant with hypertension. Nat Genet. 1998;18(1):45–8.
16. Holtmann G, Siffert W, Haag S, et al. G-protein beta 3 subunit 825 CC genotype is associated with unexplained (functional) dyspepsia. Gastroenterology. 2004;126(4):971–9.
17. de Vries DR, ter Linde JJM, van Herwaarden MA, Smout AJPM, Samsom M. Gastroesophageal reflux disease is associated with the C825T polymorphism in the G-protein beta3 subunit gene (GNB3). Am J Gastroenterol. 2009;104(2):281–5.
18. Allgrove J, Clayden GS, Grant DB, Macaulay JC. Familial glucocorticoid deficiency with achalasia of the cardia and deficient tear production. Lancet. 1978;1(8077):1284–6.
19. Sarathi V, Shah NS. Triple-A syndrome. Adv Exp Med Biol. 2010;685:1–8.
20. Di Nardo G, Tullio-Pelet A, Annese V, et al. Idiopathic achalasia is not allelic to alacrima achalasia adrenal insufficiency syndrome at the ALADIN locus. Dig Liver Dis. 2005;37(5):312–5.
21. Brooks B, Kleta R, Stuart C, et al. Genotypic heterogeneity and clinical phenotype in triple A syndrome: a review of the NIH experience 2000–2005. Clin Genet. 2005;68(3):215–21.
22. Milenkovic T, Zdravkovic D, Savic N, et al. Triple A syndrome: 32 years experience of a single centre (1977–2008). Eur J Pediatr. 2010;169(11):1323–8.

23. Marlais M, Fishman JR, Fell JM, Haddad MJ, Rawat DJ. UK incidence of achalasia: an 11-year national epidemiological study. Arch Dis Child. 2010;96(2):192–4.
24. Handschug K, Sperling S, Yoon SJ, Hennig S, Clark AJ, Huebner A. Triple A syndrome is caused by mutations in AAAS, a new WD-repeat protein gene. Hum Mol Genet. 2001;10(3):283–90.
25. Weber A, Wienker TF, Jung M, et al. Linkage of the gene for the triple A syndrome to chromosome 12q13 near the type II keratin gene cluster. Hum Mol Genet. 1996;5(12):2061–6.
26. Huebner A, Kaindl AM, Braun R, Handschug K. New insights into the molecular basis of the triple A syndrome. Endocr Res. 2002;28(4):733–9.
27. Tullio-Pelet A, Salomon R, Hadj-Rabia S, et al. Mutant WD-repeat protein in triple-A syndrome. Nat Genet. 2000;26(3):332–5.
28. Cronshaw JM, Krutchinsky AN, Zhang W, Chait BT, Matunis MJ. Proteomic analysis of the mammalian nuclear pore complex. J Cell Biol. 2002; 158(5):915–27.
29. Huebner A, Kaindl AM, Knobeloch KP, Petzold H, Mann P, Koehler K. The triple A syndrome is due to mutations in ALADIN, a novel member of the nuclear pore complex. Endocr Res. 2004;30(4):891–9.
30. Cronshaw JM, Matunis MJ. The nuclear pore complex protein ALADIN is mislocalized in triple A syndrome. Proc Natl Acad Sci USA. 2003; 100(10):5823–7.
31. Kind B, Koehler K, Lorenz M, Huebner A. The nuclear pore complex protein ALADIN is anchored via NDC1 but not via POM121 and GP210 in the nuclear envelope. Biochem Biophys Res Commun. 2009;390(2):205–10.
32. Kiriyama T, Hirano M, Asai H, Ikeda M, Furiya Y, Ueno S. Restoration of nuclear-import failure caused by triple A syndrome and oxidative stress. Biochem Biophys Res Commun. 2008;374(4):631–4.
33. Hirano M, Furiya Y, Asai H, Yasui A, Ueno S. ALADINI482S causes selective failure of nuclear protein import and hypersensitivity to oxidative stress in triple A syndrome. Proc Natl Acad Sci USA. 2006;103(7):2298–303.
34. Storr HL, Kind B, Parfitt DA, et al. Deficiency of ferritin heavy-chain nuclear import in triple A syndrome implies nuclear oxidative damage as the primary disease mechanism. Mol Endocrinol. 2009;23(12):2086–94.
35. Kind B, Koehler K, Krumbholz M, Landgraf D, Huebner A. Intracellular ROS level is increased in fibroblasts of triple A syndrome patients. J Mol Med (Berl). 2010;88(12):1233–42.
36. Kapur RP. Practical pathology and genetics of Hirschsprung's disease. Semin Pediatr Surg. 2009;18(4):212–23.
37. Imseis E, Gariepy CE. Hirschsprung disease. In: Kleinman RE, Goulet OJ, Mieli-Vergani G, Sanderson IR, Sherman PM, Schneider BL, editors. Pediatric gastrointestinal disease: pathophysiology, diagnosis, and management. 5th ed. Hamilton, Ontario, Canada: BC Decker Inc; 2008. p. 683–93.
38. McCallion A, Chakravarti A. RET and Hirschsprung disease and multiple endocrine neoplasia type 2. In: Epstein CJ, Erickson RP, Wynshaw-Boris A, editors. Inborn errors of development: the molecular basis of clinical disorders of morphogenesis. 2nd ed. New York: Oxford University Press; 2008. p. 512–21.
39. Skinner MA, Safford SD, Reeves JG, Jackson ME, Freemerman AJ. Renal aplasia in humans is associated with RET mutations. Am J Hum Genet. 2008;82(2):344–51.
40. Arighi E, Popsueva A, Degl'Innocenti D, et al. Biological effects of the dual phenotypic Janus mutation of ret cosegregating with both multiple endocrine neoplasia type 2 and Hirschsprung's disease. Mol Endocrinol. 2004;18(4):1004–17.
41. Moore SW, Zaahl M. Familial associations in medullary thyroid carcinoma with Hirschsprung disease: the role of the RET-C620 "Janus" genetic variation. J Pediatr Surg. 2010;45(2):393–6.
42. de Graaff E, Srinivas S, Kilkenny C, et al. Differential activities of the RET tyrosine kinase receptor isoforms during mammalian embryogenesis. Genes Dev. 2001;15(18):2433–44.
43. Jain S, Knoten A, Hoshi M, et al. Organotypic specificity of key RET adaptor-docking sites in the pathogenesis of neurocristopathies and renal malformations in mice. J Clin Invest. 2010;120(3):778–90.
44. Emison ES, Garcia-Barcelo M, Grice EA, et al. Differential contributions of rare and common, coding and noncoding Ret mutations to multifactorial Hirschsprung disease liability. Am J Hum Genet. 2010;87(1):60–74.
45. Griseri P, Lantieri F, Puppo F, et al. A common variant located in the 3′UTR of the RET gene is associated with protection from Hirschsprung disease. Hum Mutat. 2007;28(2):168–76.
46. Amiel J, Sproat-Emison E, Garcia-Barcelo M, et al. Hirschsprung disease, associated syndromes and genetics: a review. J Med Genet. 2008;45(1):1–14.
47. Baynash AG, Hosoda K, Giaid A, et al. Interaction of endothelin-3 with endothelin-B receptor is essential for development of epidermal melanocytes and enteric neurons. Cell. 1994;79(7):1277–85.
48. Yanagisawa H, Yanagisawa M, Kapur RP, et al. Dual genetic pathways of endothelin-mediated intercellular signaling revealed by targeted disruption of endothelin converting enzyme-1 gene. Development. 1998; 125(5):825–36.
49. Verheig JBGM, Hofstra RM. EDNRB, EDN3, and SOX10 and the Shah-Waardenburg Syndrome (WS4). In: Epstein CJ, Erickson RP, Wynshaw-Boris A, editors. Inborn errors of development: the molecular basis of clinical disorders of morphogenesis. 2nd ed. New York: Oxford University Press; 2008. p. 530–6.
50. Bidaud C, Salomon R, Van Camp G, et al. Endothelin-3 gene mutations in isolated and syndromic Hirschsprung disease. Eur J Hum Genet. 1997;5(4):247–51.
51. Sánchez-Mejías A, Fernández RM, López-Alonso M, Antiñolo G, Borrego S. New roles of EDNRB and EDN3 in the pathogenesis of Hirschsprung disease. Genet Med. 2009;12(1):39–43.

52. Hofstra RM, Valdenaire O, Arch E, et al. A loss-of-function mutation in the endothelin-converting enzyme 1 (ECE-1) associated with Hirschsprung disease, cardiac defects, and autonomic dysfunction. Am J Hum Genet. 1999;64(1):304–8.
53. Auricchio A, Griseri P, Carpentieri ML, et al. Double heterozygosity for a RET substitution interfering with splicing and an EDNRB missense mutation in Hirschsprung disease. Am J Hum Genet. 1999;64(4): 1216–21.
54. Puffenberger EG, Hosoda K, Washington SS, et al. A missense mutation of the endothelin-B receptor gene in multigenic Hirschsprung's disease. Cell. 1994;79(7):1257–66.
55. Carrasquillo MM, McCallion AS, Puffenberger EG, Kashuk CS, Nouri N, Chakravarti A. Genome-wide association study and mouse model identify interaction between RET and EDNRB pathways in Hirschsprung disease. Nat Genet. 2002;32(2): 237–44.
56. Emison ES, McCallion AS, Kashuk CS, et al. A common sex-dependent mutation in a RET enhancer underlies Hirschsprung disease risk. Nature. 2005;434(7035):857–63.
57. Moore SW, Zaahl MG. Multiple endocrine neoplasia syndromes, children, Hirschsprung's disease and RET. Pediatr Surg Int. 2008;24(5):521–30.
58. Jennings LJ, Yu M, Rand CM, et al. Variable human phenotype associated with novel deletions of the PHOX2B gene. Pediatr Pulmonol. 2012;47(2): 153–61.
59. Parodi S, Vollono C, Baglietto MP, et al. Congenital central hypoventilation syndrome: genotype-phenotype correlation in parents of affected children carrying a PHOX2B expansion mutation. Clin Genet. 2010;78(3):289–93.
60. Weese-Mayer DE, Rand CM, Berry-Kravis EM, et al. Congenital central hypoventilation syndrome from past to future: model for translational and transitional autonomic medicine. Pediatr Pulmonol. 2009;44(6):521–35.
61. de Pontual L, Zaghloul NA, Thomas S, et al. Epistasis between RET and BBS mutations modulates enteric innervation and causes syndromic Hirschsprung disease. Proc Natl Acad Sci USA. 2009;106(33): 13921–6.
62. Pingault V, Ente D, Dastot-Le Moal F, Goossens M, Marlin S, Bondurand N. Review and update of mutations causing Waardenburg syndrome. Hum Mutat. 2010;31(4):391–406.
63. Freeman SB, Torfs CP, Romitti PA, et al. Congenital gastrointestinal defects in Down syndrome: a report from the Atlanta and National Down Syndrome Projects. Clin Genet. 2009;75(2):180–4.
64. Arnold S, Pelet A, Amiel J, et al. Interaction between a chromosome 10 RET enhancer and chromosome 21 in the Down syndrome-Hirschsprung disease association. Hum Mutat. 2009;30(5):771–5.
65. Saunders CJ, Zhao W, Ardinger HH. Comprehensive ZEB2 gene analysis for Mowat-Wilson syndrome in a North American cohort: a suggested approach to molecular diagnostics. Am J Med Genet A. 2009;149A(11):2527–31.
66. Brooks AS, Bertoli-Avella AM, Burzynski GM, et al. Homozygous nonsense mutations in KIAA1279 are associated with malformations of the central and enteric nervous systems. Am J Hum Genet. 2005;77(1):120–6.
67. Lyons DA, Naylor SG, Mercurio S, Dominguez C, Talbot WS. KBP is essential for axonal structure, outgrowth and maintenance in zebrafish, providing insight into the cellular basis of Goldberg-Shprintzen syndrome. Development. 2008;135(3):599–608.
68. Tobin JL, Di Franco M, Eichers E, et al. Inhibition of neural crest migration underlies craniofacial dysmorphology and Hirschsprung's disease in Bardet-Biedl syndrome. Proc Natl Acad Sci USA. 2008;105(18):6714–9.
69. Sheffield VC, Nishimura D, Stone EM. The molecular genetics of Bardet-Biedl syndrome. Curr Opin Genet Dev. 2001;11(3):317–21.
70. Shefer S, Salen G, Batta AK, et al. Markedly inhibited 7-dehydrocholesterol-delta 7-reductase activity in liver microsomes from Smith-Lemli-Opitz homozygotes. J Clin Invest. 1995;96(4):1779–85.
71. DeBarber AE, Eroglu Y, Merkens LS, Pappu AS, Steiner RD. Smith-Lemli-Opitz syndrome. Expert Rev Mol Med. 2011;13:e24.
72. Meier-Ruge WA, Ammann K, Bruder E, et al. Updated results on intestinal neuronal dysplasia (IND B). Eur J Pediatr Surg. 2004;14(06):384–91.
73. Schimpl G, Uray E, Ratschek M, Höllwarth ME. Constipation and intestinal neuronal dysplasia type B: a clinical follow-up study. J Pediatr Gastroenterol Nutr. 2004;38(3):308–11.
74. Sandgren K, Larsson LT, Ekblad E. Widespread changes in neurotransmitter expression and number of enteric neurons and interstitial cells of Cajal in lethal spotted mice: an explanation for persisting dysmotility after operation for Hirschsprung's disease? Dig Dis Sci. 2002;47(5):1049–64.
75. von Boyen GBT, Krammer H-J, Süss A, Dembowski C, Ehrenreich H, Wedel T. Abnormalities of the enteric nervous system in heterozygous endothelin B receptor deficient (spotting lethal) rats resembling intestinal neuronal dysplasia. Gut. 2002;51(3):414–9.
76. Gath R, Goessling A, Keller KM, et al. Analysis of the RET, GDNF, EDN3, and EDNRB genes in patients with intestinal neuronal dysplasia and Hirschsprung disease. Gut. 2001;48(5):671–5.
77. Fadda B, Maier WA, Meier-Ruge W, Scharli A, Daum R. Neuronal intestinal dysplasia. Critical 10-years' analysis of clinical and biopsy diagnosis. Z Kinderchir. 1983;38(5):305–11.
78. Hanemann CO, Hayward C, Hilton DA. Neurofibromatosis type 1 with involvement of the enteric nerves. J Neurol Neurosurg Psychiatry. 2007;78(10):1163–4.
79. Bahuau M, Pelet A, Vidaud D, et al. GDNF as a candidate modifier in a type 1 neurofibromatosis (NF1) enteric phenotype. J Med Genet. 2001; 38(9):638–43.

80. Evans CA, Nesbitt IM, Walker J, Cohen MC. MEN 2B syndrome should be part of the working diagnosis of constipation of the newborn. Histopathology. 2008;52(5):646–8.
81. King SK, Southwell BR, Hutson JM. An association of multiple endocrine neoplasia 2B, a RET mutation; constipation; and low substance P-nerve fiber density in colonic circular muscle. J Pediatr Surg. 2006;41(2):437–42.
82. Zenaty D, Aigrain Y, Peuchmaur M, et al. Medullary thyroid carcinoma identified within the first year of life in children with hereditary multiple endocrine neoplasia type 2A (codon 634) and 2B. Eur J Endocrinol. 2009;160(5):807–13.
83. Touraine RL, Attié-Bitach T, Manceau E, et al. Neurological phenotype in Waardenburg syndrome type 4 correlates with novel SOX10 truncating mutations and expression in developing brain. Am J Hum Genet. 2000;66(5):1496–503.
84. Pingault V, Girard M, Bondurand N, et al. SOX10 mutations in chronic intestinal pseudo-obstruction suggest a complex physiopathological mechanism. Hum Genet. 2002;111(2):198–206.
85. Auricchio A, Brancolini V, Casari G, et al. The locus for a novel syndromic form of neuronal intestinal pseudoobstruction maps to Xq28. Am J Hum Genet. 1996;58(4):743–8.
86. Gargiulo A, Auricchio R, Barone MV, et al. Filamin A is mutated in X-linked chronic idiopathic intestinal pseudo-obstruction with central nervous system involvement. Am J Hum Genet. 2007;80(4):751–8.
87. Smith-Hicks CL, Sizer KC, Powers JF, Tischler AS, Costantini F. C-cell hyperplasia, pheochromocytoma and sympathoadrenal malformation in a mouse model of multiple endocrine neoplasia type 2B. EMBO J. 2000;19(4):612–22.
88. Parisi MA, Baldessari AE, Iida MH, et al. Genetic background modifies intestinal pseudo-obstruction and the expression of a reporter gene in Hox11L1−/− mice. Gastroenterology. 2003;125(5):1428–40.
89. Puig I, Champeval D, De Santa Barbara P, Jaubert F, Lyonnet S, Larue L. Deletion of Pten in the mouse enteric nervous system induces ganglioneuromatosis and mimics intestinal pseudoobstruction. J Clin Invest. 2009;119(12):3586–96.
90. O'Donnell AM, Puri P. A role for Pten in paediatric intestinal dysmotility disorders. Pediatr Surg Int. 2011;27(5):491–3.
91. Taketomi T, Yoshiga D, Taniguchi K, et al. Loss of mammalian Sprouty2 leads to enteric neuronal hyperplasia and esophageal achalasia. Nat Neurosci. 2005;8(7):855–7.
92. Hennig GW, Spencer NJ, Jokela-Willis S, et al. ICC-MY coordinate smooth muscle electrical and mechanical activity in the murine small intestine. Neurogastroenterol Motil. 2010;22(5):e138–51.
93. Maeda H, Yamagata A, Nishikawa S, et al. Requirement of c-kit for development of intestinal pacemaker system. Development. 1992;116(2):369–75.
94. Feldstein AE, Miller SM, El-Youssef M, et al. Chronic intestinal pseudoobstruction associated with altered interstitial cells of cajal networks. J Pediatr Gastroenterol Nutr. 2003;36(4):492–7.
95. Anneren G, Meurling S, Olsen L. Megacystis-microcolon-intestinal hypoperistalsis syndrome (MMIHS), an autosomal recessive disorder: clinical reports and review of the literature. Am J Med Genet. 1991;41(2):251–4.
96. Lev-Lehman E, Bercovich D, Xu W, Stockton DW, Beaudet AL. Characterization of the human beta4 nAChR gene and polymorphisms in CHRNA3 and CHRNB4. J Hum Genet. 2001;46(7):362–6.
97. Szigeti R, Chumpitazi BP, Finegold MJ, et al. Absent smooth muscle actin immunoreactivity of the small bowel muscularis propria circular layer in association with chromosome 15q11 deletion in Megacystis-Microcolon-Intestinal Hypoperistalsis Syndrome. Pediatr Dev Pathol. 2010;13(4):322–5.
98. Amiot A, Tchikviladzé M, Joly F, et al. Frequency of mitochondrial defects in patients with chronic intestinal pseudo-obstruction. Gastroenterology. 2009;137(1):101–9.
99. de Giorgio R, Volta U, Stanghellini V, et al. Neurogenic chronic intestinal pseudo-obstruction: antineuronal antibody-mediated activation of autophagy via Fas. Gastroenterology. 2008;135(2):601–9.
100. Li V, Hostein J, Romero NB, et al. Chronic intestinal pseudoobstruction with myopathy and ophthalmoplegia. A muscular biochemical study of a mitochondrial disorder. Dig Dis Sci. 1992;37(3):456–63.
101. Cardaioli E, Da Pozzo P, Malfatti E, et al. A second MNGIE patient without typical mitochondrial skeletal muscle involvement. Neurol Sci. 2010;31(4):491–4.
102. Gamez J, Lara MC, Mearin F, et al. A novel thymidine phosphorylase mutation in a Spanish MNGIE patient. J Neurol Sci. 2005;228(1):35–9.

Feeding and Swallowing Disorders

19

Nathalie Rommel and Taher Omari

Introduction

The processes of deglutition and feeding differ although both are complex and interrelated. These terms are used interchangeably and no consensus exists on their definition. The term "deglutition" or "swallowing" refers to the entire act of deglutition from placement of food in the mouth through the pharyngeal phases of the swallow until the material enters the esophagus through the cricopharyngeal juncture while avoiding entry of substances into the airway. Swallowing is a motor event that in order to be successful requires intact and functioning central and peripheral nervous systems and the coordination of actions of multiple muscles of the oral cavity, pharynx and esophagus [1].

The term "feeding" is defined as the overall process whereby the infant or child ingests food. Feeding involves the act of deglutition, but is also influenced by developmental, behavioral and social factors [2]. Therefore, in this chapter the term "feeding problem" is used to address the multi-causal pathology of the child who is not eating. When dealing with infants and children, many clinicians use the term "dysphagia" to describe any type of difficulty with feeding and swallowing or symptom of esophageal dysfunction. In this chapter, however, the term "dysphagia" is used for abnormal oropharyngeal function.

Dysphagia is very common in the pediatric population within a wide range of disorders and hinders the provision of adequate nutrition, affecting growth and development and may lead to significant parental anxiety and family disruption [3, 4]. Epidemiologic data on the prevalence and incidence of feeding and swallowing disorders in pediatric populations are limited. Lindsheid [5] and Burklow [6] summarized studies reporting the estimated prevalence of feeding problems in the pediatric population as ranging from 25 to 45% in typically developing children and 33 to 80% in children with developmental delays. The estimated prevalence of oropharyngeal dysphagia among children with developmental disabilities ranges from 12 to 71% [7, 8]. The incidence of dysphagia is unknown however there is a general agreement that the incidence of swallowing dysfunction is increasing [8–11].

As feeding is a highly integrated, multisystem skill, one or more contributing systems may be dysfunctional. Signs and symptoms frequently cross the traditional boundaries between traditional professional disciplines [12–14]. It is

N. Rommel, M.Sc., Ph.D. (✉)
Department Neurosciences, Experimental Otorhinolaryngology, University of Leuven, Herestraat 49, Leuven 3000, Belgium
e-mail: nathalie.rommel@med.kuleuven.be

T. Omari, Ph.D.
Gastroenterology Unit, Child Youth & Women's Health Service, School of Paediatrics and Reproductive Health University of Adelaide, Adelaide, SA, Australia

C. Faure et al. (eds.), *Pediatric Neurogastroenterology: Gastrointestinal Motility and Functional Disorders in Children*, Clinical Gastroenterology,
DOI 10.1007/978-1-60761-709-9_19, © Springer Science+Business Media New York 2013

nowadays accepted that feeding difficulties in infants and children need to be assessed from multiple perspectives in order to determine the underlying causes. A multidisciplinary approach has been described leading to better identification and treatment of feeding and swallowing disorders [4].

This chapter discusses a variety of oropharyngeal swallowing disorders reported in newborns, infants and children, but does not intend to offer a comprehensive classification of feeding problems in young children. One of the reasons why the relationship between clinical presentation and underlying cause of feeding problems is often unclear relates to the fact that similar signs or symptoms may reflect different etiologies. Because of this lack of a one-to-one correspondence between clinical presentations and underlying causes of dysphagia, careful identification of symptoms, documentation of their pathophysiology and their relation to the mealtimes is crucial in pinpointing the specific cause of feeding disorders.

Oropharyngeal Physiology

Normal swallowing is usually subdivided in three phases: oral, pharyngeal and esophageal. Some descriptions add an initial "oral preparatory phase" which is bolus preparation [15]. While flawless in most individuals, safe and effective swallowing is a very complex process initiated by voluntary actions (oral acceptance and preparation of food and bolus delivery to the pharynx). This in turn initiates the pharyngeal swallow reflex, during which the tongue base propels the bolus backwards, the soft palate seals the nasopharynx, the larynx is elevated, the vocal folds close, the upper esophageal sphincter (UES) relaxes and opens to allow the bolus to pass. The pharyngeal constrictors then clear away any remaining bolus from the pharynx into the esophagus. With increasing age and central nervous system maturation, the oral phase becomes volitional. The pharyngeal phase has both voluntary and involuntary components whereas the esophageal phase is fully involuntary. The entire duration of a swallow sequence is about 1.0–1.5 s in adults as well as in children [16]. Disrupted effectiveness, duration and/or timing of any of these components can result in aspiration.

The UES is the specialized transition zone between the pharynx and the esophagus, which generates an intraluminal high-pressure zone to prevent reflux of material from the esophagus into the pharynx and airways and to prevent entry of air into the digestive tract [17, 18]. Anatomically, the UES is compounded by the inferior pharyngeal constrictor muscle, the cricopharyngeal muscle and the cranial part of the cervical esophagus. The UES also plays a role in allowing passage of esophageal contents during vomiting or belching.

Assessment of Oropharyngeal Dysphagia

The assessment of oropharyngeal dysphagia should consist of two major components: the first one is direct observation of the child's feeding and swallowing skills through clinical oral assessment. The second part is assessing the not-visually obvious motor function of pharynx and esophagus through instrumental testing.

The main goal of the clinical oral assessment is to define the underlying cause and the severity of the feeding and swallowing difficulties. In this problem-solving process, the evaluation of the oral cavity and its functions by observation plays a major role. During the clinical assessment, the oral anatomy, motor skills, reflex activity, responsivity, and swallowing are examined, and the nature of the feeding problem and necessity for further evaluation of pharyngeal swallowing function with instrumental techniques is established. Normal and abnormal oral motor skills have been described extensively in many anatomy text books, as well as in the developmental and rehabilitation literature [19]. In order to feed successfully, a child must adapt to the tactile characteristics of tools (breast, bottle, spoon or cup) and food so that the correct motor responses are performed [20]. Oral motor and sensory based feeding disorders can be differentiated [21] and a structured sensory examination in and around the oral cavity allows the examiner

Table 19.1 Possible signs and symptoms of dysphagia

Signs
Aspiration
Recurrent pneumonia or respiratory infections
Weight loss or slow weight gain or growth
Altered and restricted diet in terms of consistency and volume
Frequent low grade fever
Vomiting
Lengthy feeding times (longer than 30 min)
Dehydration
Food obstruction
Symptoms
Loss of appetite
Coughing and choking during or after meals
Food or liquid spilling from the mouth
Breastfeeding problems
Difficulty breathing or coordinating breathing with eating or drinking
Wet voice (gurgly sound)
Abnormal oral feeding skills
Food refusal (total or during feeding)
Irritability during feeding with increased body tension
Difficult transition from liquids to semisolid and solid food
Lack of attention during feeding
Selective eating
Crying during feeding

to uncover difficulties with the tactile components of feedings. However, it is only possible to observe the reactions to sensations, not the sensations in themselves [17, 22], therefore the term responsivity is more appropriate than sensitivity in the context of dysphagia. The child's ability to respond adequately to tactile input can be assessed during a feeding observation or by a structured sensory examination by grading the sensory input. A sensory baseline on consistency, taste, temperature, tools, area of stimulation and amount needs to be established, defined as the level of tactile input that the child can tolerate without any discomfort. A wide range of tactile responses can be observed and these responses form a continuum of function: aversion, hyperresponsivity, normal tactile responses, absent responses, hyporesponsivity, and absent responses [20]. When tactile responses are severely diminished or absent, a significant sensory impairment should be suspected which can hinder oral feeding. In hyporesponsivity, strong stimulation is required and the responses are slow or partial. A hyperresponse is exaggerated or out of proportion to the strength of the stimulus. While similar to hyperresponses, aversive responses are even stronger and more negative. Both hyperresponses and aversive responses can be part of a general tactile processing problem or be localized to the face and mouth or even more specifically to a certain part of the mouth, most frequently the tongue [23].

During the examination the clinician will also determine whether the parent's reports and perceptions match the observations [24]. Referrals can then be made for further assessment or multidisciplinary management and a targeted treatment plan can be developed. Instrumental assessment has the potential to assess oropharyngeal function objectively if selected and applied properly. The challenging decision is when to refer for instrumental assessment and for what type of testing. The signs and symptoms of dysphagia presented in Table 19.1 are common indicators for further instrumental evaluation of the swallow function.

When supplemental instrumental assessment of the pharyngeal swallow is required, a variety of pharyngeal and UES dysfunctions can be distinguished. The pharyngeal pathology varies from synchronous pharyngeal peristalsis, pharyngeal focal failure, pharyngeal hypocontractility and pharyngeal paralysis. Upper esophageal sphincter patterns range from a normally relaxing UES, to premature contraction to an incomplete or non-relaxing UOS in case of achalasia [25]. How these deglutitive patterns are linked with aspiration risk remains unclear.

Chronic pulmonary aspiration is the most serious complication of swallowing dysfunction causing recurrent pneumonia, progressive lung disease, respiratory disability and even death [26]. Pulmonary aspiration due to swallowing dysfunction (deglutitive aspiration, when the bolus has entered the larynx below the level of the true vocal folds) is a major reason for modification of feeding strategies (oral to tube feeding, avoidance of liquids, etc.) and therefore has a significant impact on quality of life. Deglutitive aspiration can be a cause of recurrent pneumonia, recurrent wheezing, chronic cough, or stridor in infants and children [27].

Many different functional tests are available to rule out aspiration risk and to assess oropharyngeal function during swallowing [17]. Description of every available technique goes beyond the scope of this chapter. Common assessment techniques available for use in the pediatric population include fiberoptic endoscopic evaluation of swallowing (FEES), videofluoroscopy, and pharyngeal-oesophageal manometry. In practice, the use of a particular instrumental technique often depends on the institutional experience, available resources and its commercial availability rather than being based on the performance characteristics of the test. The main argument of using instrumental techniques in addition to clinical examination is to provide a more precise understanding of the biomechanics of the child's swallow which then will lead to a more targeted therapeutic intervention [23]. Specific indicators for videomanometric evaluation are deglutitive aspiration and penetration risk, suspicion of pharyngeal abnormalities or dysfunction, upper esophageal sphincter abnormalities or dysfunction or no therapeutic progress after 2 months after the initial instrumental assessment. Unfortunately, current abilities to diagnose aspiration are limited, as there is evidence that fluoroscopy is poorly predictive of progression to aspiration pneumonia and a normal fluoroscopy cannot entirely rule out feed aspiration [28].

Non-radiological Instrumental Methods: Manometry and Impedance

Manometry can be used to assess pharyngo-esophageal motor function. Pharyngeal weakness or impaired UES relaxation can be relatively easily determined and the technique can be combined with videofluoroscopy. Manometry has been utilized to describe alterations in pressure patterns in relation to age-related changes, neurodegenerative disease, post-surgical dysfunctions, and UES obstruction [29–32]. However, while manometric recordings may identify functional abnormalities that may predispose to aspiration risk, manometry on its own cannot predict circumstances when aspiration is likely. Intraluminal impedance is a technique that can be used to detect failed bolus transport and is easily combined with manometry. The widespread application of impedance measurement to assess the pharyngeal function has been slow to develop because attempts to establish criteria that reliably identify post-swallow residue have been largely unsuccessful [33–35].

Manometric and impedance technologies have evolved in recent years such that catheters with closely spaced pressure-impedance arrays are now more widely available. In the most recent development, high resolution manometry-impedance (or HRMi) recordings have been uniquely combined in the novel technique called Automated Impedance Manometry (AIM) analysis. AIM analysis provides a more objective, non-radiological assessment of pharyngeal function in patients with dysphagia. Unlike videofluoroscopy, this new technique is less resource intensive, easily performed at the bedside and delivers a non-subjective evaluation of swallow parameters (Fig. 19.1). AIM analysis detects swallowing dysfunction via measurement of several swallow function variables and predicts aspiration risk through calculation of a swallow risk index (SRI). The higher the SRI, the more severe the pharyngeal dysfunction and the more likely aspiration will occur [36–38].

Conditions Associated with Feeding Problems

Pediatric dysphagia is associated with multiple etiologies, including anatomic or structural defects and neurologic deficits, either congenital or acquired. Many children have complex medical issues that predispose them to dysphagia and increase their vulnerability to respiratory and growth compromise resulting from the dysphagia. It is important to realize that a previously confirmed diagnosis does not preclude other potential contributing etiologies, for example the diagnosis of esophageal dysmotility

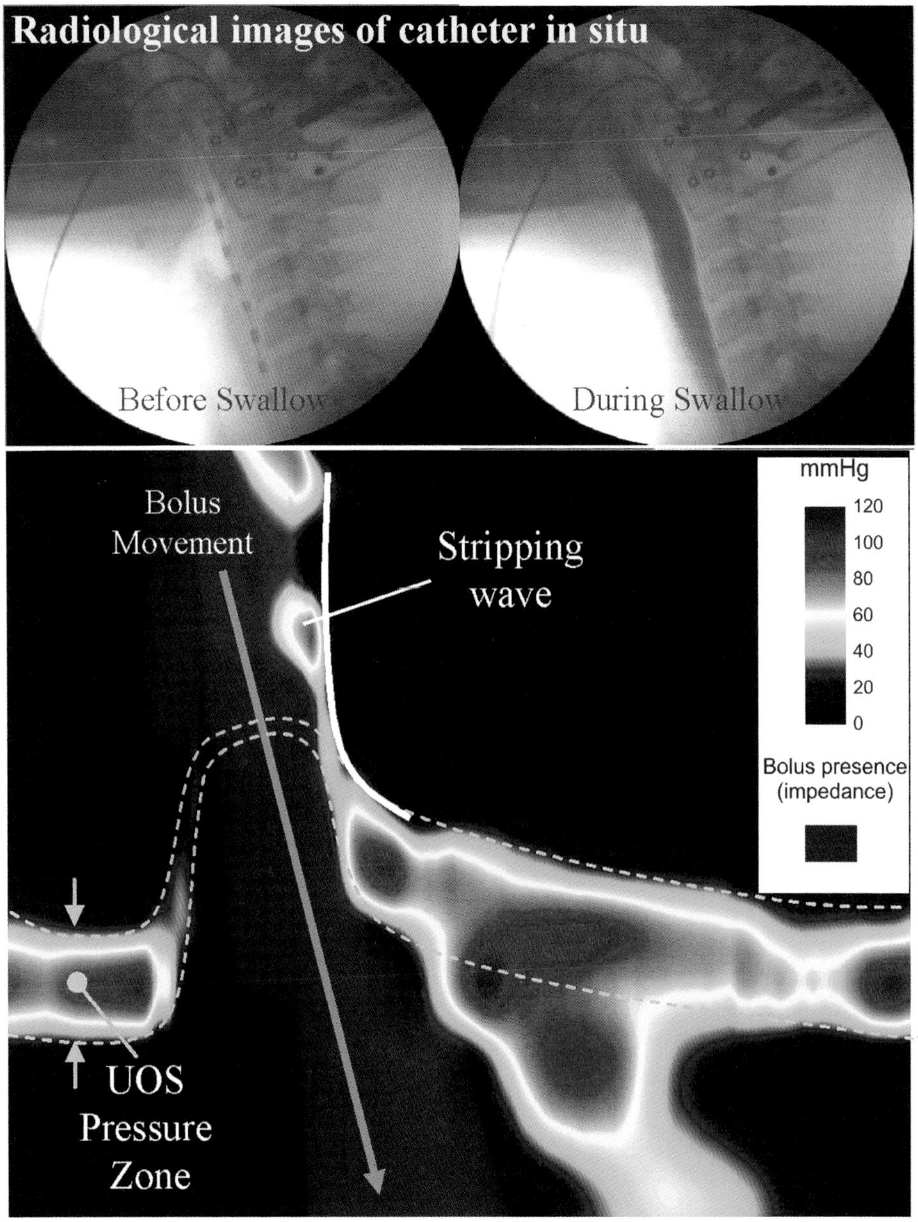

Fig. 19.1 An example of combined manometry and impedance plot of a pharyngeal swallow. This shows the changes in pressure (colors *blue* through *red*) that occur with the pharyngeal stripping wave as well as relaxation and movement of the upper esophageal sphincter (UOS = Upper Oesophageal Sphincter) pressure zone. The conductivity of the bolus swallowed is detected by impedance (*purple shading*). Plot created by M Szczesniak, Dept of Gastroenterology St George Hospital & University of NSW, Sydney Australia

does not exclude the coexistence of oropharyngeal abnormalities. In the following section, we discuss a few of the most common medical conditions associated with feeding and swallowing disorders.

Gastroesophageal Reflux Disease

Gastroesophageal reflux disease (GERD) has been identified as a common underlying condition associated with feeding problems [4, 39]. In infants, GER is recognized as a frequent and usually benign condition which occurs during or after feeding. In the context of feeding problems, GERD is associated with comorbidities such as failure to thrive, feeding difficulties and irritability in relation to feeding. In these circumstances, frequent GER may disrupt or delay normal feeding, or lead to post-feeding irritability, sleep disruption and/or loss of nutrients with overt regurgitation. Unfortunately, such "typical GER-related" symptoms are not specific for GERD and may be due to other causes, such as dietary protein allergy, and the differentiation of symptoms due to GER from symptoms due to other causes remains a significant challenge for most clinicians.

Most common feeding problems associated with GERD are feeding aversion, food refusal and insufficient oral intake. Pain secondary to esophagitis may drive the child to associate pain with feeding and therefore the child may attempt to limit the pain by eliminating eating or by taking small frequent feedings. Snacking may however result in poor oral intake over 24-h period [20].

Neurological Disability

Cerebral palsy (CP) is a common problem, the worldwide incidence being 1.5–3 per 1,000 live births [40]. It is defined as a group of disorders of the development of movement and posture, causing activity limitation, that are attributed to nonprogressive disturbances that occurred in the developing fetal or infant brain. The motor disorders of cerebral palsy are often accompanied by disturbances of sensation, cognition, communication, perception, and/or behavior, and/or by a seizure disorder [41]. CP can be classified in spasticity (79%), dyskinesia (14%), and ataxia (4%) [42].

Children with CP may have feeding problems that affect any or all phases of deglutition. The reports on the prevalence of dysphagia in children with CP vary greatly between 27 and 99% [43–47] depending on the definition of dysphagia used and the population and comorbidities included. Dysphagia has been mostly described in broad CP populations and not specified according to the three main groups. Yet, the differences in muscle tone among these groups cannot be ignored and may cause the type of dysphagia to vary according to the type of CP [46]. Cerebral palsy with hypertonicity may be associated with tongue thrusting, tonic biting and hyperactive gagging. Children with spasticity may present with poor lip closure, tongue thrusting and jaw instability as well thrusting. These inadequate oral motor patterns hinder effective manipulation of food in the oral cavity, appropriate bolus formation and bolus propulsion needed for safe and adequate swallowing. It is important to realize that the child's oral motor skills observed during an oral examination do not necessarily match what is seen at functional mealtimes. Therefore assessment during mealtime process is essential in these children. The child's ability to control movement their tone (hypertonia hypotonia, and/or mixed), their stability, symmetry, degree of independence, and most important head control must be carefully assessed [48] in the child's natural feeding situation.

Children with diplegia and hemiplegia are less likely to have significant dysphagia [45]. Reilly et al. [24] found that tetraplegia was associated with moderate and severe oral-motor dysfunction, and diplegia was more commonly associated with mild oral-motor difficulties. In addition, those children with diplegia were more likely to demonstrate texture-specific problems, whereas children with tetraplegia typically had some level of difficulty with all textures. Potential reasons for the child with spastic quadriplegia to be at an increased risk for dysphagia include the fact that they are dependent feeders and are often unable to communicate [49]. Apart from the type of CP, other factors such as the severity of drooling, postural problems (e.g., scoliosis) the severity of speech disorder, positive history of seizures, episodes of pneumonia [50, 51], presence of GERD [4], developmental retardation [51], and severity of the functional impairment may have an impact on the type of dysphagia. In general, the more severe the functional motor impairment, the more severe the oral motor dysfunction is. Waterman et al. [51] found that the poorer the trunk control, the higher is the risk of dysphagia. Calis et al. [43] reported that the severity of dysphagia was positively related to the Gross Motor Function Classification System Level (GMFCS), but negatively related to the body mass index.

Due to recent advances in instrumental evaluation of dysphagia in children, oropharyngeal patterns of dysphagia are being differentiated in patients with neurological disability. Apart from oral motor disorders such children are often noted to present with pharyngeal hypocontractility or paralysis. Importantly, patients often present with not only pharyngeal but also with oesophageal dysmotility that prevents them from eating orally. Therefore, both pharynx and esophagus should be assessed in terms of motor function in this highly affected group of children.

There are a number of developmental conditions that place children at risk of feeding and swallowing problems. It is well known that children with special needs are at higher risk of acquiring feeding problems [8]. Only a few among such conditions can be discussed in this chapter.

Velo-Cardio-Facial Syndrome

Velo-cardio-facial syndrome (VCFS) is caused by a deletion 22q11.2 and is characterized by mild facial dysmorphia, palatal anomaly, conotruncal cardiac defect, immunodeficiency, and hypocalcaemia [52]. Children with VCFS most often present with feeding difficulties early in life [53, 54] including nasal regurgitation, poor coordination of sucking, swallowing, and breathing and food refusal. Palatal dysfunction may lead to nasal regurgitation during swallowing due to the bolus being forced into the nasal cavity. However, in these children, who are particularly prone to velopharyngeal insufficiency [3, 11], the observed retrograde flow may also be the result of an upper esophageal dysfunction rather than a palatal insufficiency alone [4, 55, 56]. The clinical or radiological observation of retrograde flow and nasal regurgitation should not automatically lead to the diagnosis velopharyngeal insufficiency but require the assessment of the opening profile of the UES.

Autism Spectrum Disorders

Autism Spectrum disorders (ASD) are a group of neurodevelopmental disorders of unknown etiology with onset before 3 years of age and characterized by severe impairment in reciprocal social interaction and communication with a pattern of repetitive or stereotyped behavior [57]. A recent population based study by Ibrahim et al. showed that compared to typically developing children matched for age and gender, children with ASD have an increased incidence of feeding issues, food selectivity and constipation [58]. It was suggested that these problems result from either the behavioral characteristics of children with autism such as ritualistic tendencies, need for routine and thus stereotyped diets or from adverse effects of treatment with psychotropic medications rather than being associated with a primary organic gastrointestinal pathology. Importantly, when children with ASD are compared to typically developing children matched by levels of functioning, children with ASD were only marginally more likely to have more typical feeding problems [59]. Martins et al. showed that the critical difference between both groups lies in the frequency with which children with ASD exhibit the problematic feeding behaviors. They showed that children with ASD are twice as likely to experience feeding problems and that more problems occur at the same time, but they do not necessarily have other feeding problems than those observed in a typical developing child. These findings have important clinical relevance as they indicate that ASD children need more time to overcome difficulties since their behaviors tend to be associated with problems with adapting to change. Feeding therapy therefore should include many steps before the child with ASD should be invited to taste the food, the number depending on the child's capacity to adjust to change. Once oral acceptance is feasible, gradual and repeated taste exposure to small amounts of food may allow the child to accept the food. Their data also suggest that medical care providers should acknowledge that these children are not extremely different from typically developing children in the types of feeding and swallowing problems [59].

Regardless of the prevalence of feeding problems, the most common oral feeding problems observed in children with ASD are selectivity by type and texture. More complex feeding problems such as oropharyngeal dysphagia and food refusal are also often seen, mostly associated with GERD. Constipation as a consequence of poor diet is these children may potentially reinforce the feeding problem by decreasing appetite and thus willingness to try new foods.

Summary

Although many classifications of feeding problems and swallowing difficulties in infants and children are available, it remains important, regardless of the primary medical pathology, to assess the pure biomechanics of swallow physiology in pharynx and esophagus and to do this with assessment techniques which are as objective as possible. Linking clinical signs and symptoms to the objective dysphagic "signature" of the patient is the only way to achieve a proper differential diagnosis of dysphagia and to provide effective treatment.

References

1. Miller A. Deglutition. Physiol Rev. 1982;62:129–84.
2. Milla P. Feeding, tasting and sucking. In: Walker W, Durie P, Hamilton J, Walker-Smith J, Watkins J, editors. Pediatric gastrointestinal disease: pathophysiology, diagnosis, management. Philadelphia, PA: BC Decker; 1991. p. 217–23.
3. Rudolph C, Link D. Feeding disorders in infants and children. Pediatr Clin North Am. 2002;49:97–112.
4. Rommel N, De Meyer AM, Feenstra L, Veereman-Wauters G. The complexity of feeding problems in 700 infants and young children presenting to a tertiary care institution. J Pediatr Gastroenterol Nutr. 2003;37:75–84.
5. Linscheid TR. Behavioral treatments for pediatric feeding disorders. Behav Modif. 2006;30:6–23.
6. Burklow KA, Phelps AN, Schultz JR, et al. Classifying complex pediatric feeding disorders. J Pediatr Gastroenterol Nutr. 1998;27:143–7.
7. Reilly S, Skuse D, Plobete X. Prevelance of feeding problems and oral motor dysfunction in children with cerebral palsy: a community survey. J Pediatr. 1996;129:877–82.
8. Field D, Garland M, Williams K. Correlates of specific childhood feeding problems. J Paediatr Child Health. 2003;39:299–304.
9. Ancel PY, Livinec F, Larroque B, EPIPAGE Study Group, et al. Cerebral palsy among very preterm children in relation to gestational age and neonatal ultrasound abnormalities: the EPIPAGE cohort study. Pediatrics. 2006;117:828–35.
10. Marlow N. Neurocognitive outcome after very preterm birth. Arch Dis Child Fetal Neonatal Ed. 2001;89:F224–8.
11. Hawdon JM, Beauregard N, Slattery J, et al. Identification of neonates at risk of developing feeding problems in infancy. Dev Med Child Neurol. 2000;42:235–9.
12. Bach D, Pouoget S, Belle K. An integrated team approach to the management of patients with oropharyngeal dysphagia. J Allied Health. 1989;18:459–68.
13. Bryan D, Pressman H. Comprehensive team evaluation. In: Rosenthal S, Sheppard J, Lotze M, editors. Dysphagia and the child with developmental disabilities. San Diego: Singular Publishing Group, Inc.; 1995. p. 15–29.
14. Ravich W, Donner M, Kashima H, Buchholz D, Marsh B, Hendrix T, Kramer S, Jones B, Bosma J, Siebens A, Linden P. The swallowing center: concepts and procedures. Gastrointest Radiol. 1985;10:255–61.
15. Logemann J. Evaluation and treatment of swallowing disorders. Austin, TX: Pro Ed; 1983. p. 1–249.
16. Arvedson J, Lefton-Greif M. Anatomy, physiology and development of deglutition. In: Arvedson J, Lefton-Greif M, editors. Pediatric videofluoroscopic swallow studies. San Antonio, TX: Communication Skill Builders; 1998. p. 13–30.
17. Arvedson J. Assessment of pediatric dysphagia and feeding disorders: clinical and instrumental approaches. Dev Disabil Res Rev. 2008;14(2):118–27.
18. Singh S, Hamdy S. The upper oesophageal sphincter. Neurogastroenterol Motil. 2005;17 Suppl 1:3–12.
19. Morris S. Pre-speech assessment scale: a rating scale for the development of the pre-speech behaviors from birth through two years. Clifton, NJ: JA Preston; 1982.
20. Wolf L, Glass R. Clinical feeding evaluation. In: Wolf L, Glass R, editors. Feeding and swallowing in infants and children: pathophysiology, diagnosis and treatment. San Diego: Therapy Skill Builders; 1992. p. 85–147.
21. Palmer M, Heyman M. Assessment and treatment of sensory versus motor-based feeding problems in very young children. Infants Young Child. 1993;6:67–73.
22. Arvedson J. Oral-motor and feeding assessment. In: Arvedson J, Brodsky L, editors. Pediatric swallowing and feeding: assessment and management. San Diego: Singular; 1993. p. 249–92.
23. Rommel N. Assessment techniques for babies and children. In: Murdoch B, Chicero J, editors. Dysphagia: foundation theory and practice. London: Wiley Publishers Ltd; 2006. p. 466–86.

24. Reilly S, Wisbeach A, Carr L. Assessing feeding in children with neurological problems. In: Southall A, Schwartz A, editors. Feeding problems in children. Oxford: Radcliffe Medical Press; 2000. p. 153–71.
25. Rommel N, Omari T. Abnormal pharyngo-esophageal function in infants and young children: diagnosis with high-resolution manometry. J Pediatr Gastroenterol Nutr. 2011;52:S29–30.
26. Boesch RP, Daines C, Willging JP, Kaul A, Cohen AP, Wood RE, et al. Advances in the diagnosis and management of chronic pulmonary aspiration in children. Eur Respir J. 2006;28:847–61.
27. Sheikh S, Allen E, Shell R, Hruschak J, Iram D, Castile R, et al. Chronic aspiration without gastroesophageal reflux as a cause of chronic respiratory symptoms in neurologically normal infants. Chest. 2001;120:1190–5.
28. Croghan JE, Burke EM, Caplan S, et al. Pilot study of 12 month outcomes of nursing home patients with aspiration on videofluoroscopy. Dysphagia. 1994;9:141–6.
29. Shaker R, Ren J, Podvrsan B, Dodds WJ, Hogan WJ, Kern M, Hoffmann R, Hintz J. Effect of aging and bolus variables on pharyngeal and upper esophageal sphincter motor function. Am J Physiol Gastrointest Liver Physiol. 1993;264:G427–32.
30. Yokoyama M, Mitomi N, Tetsuka K, Tayama N, Niimi S. Role of laryngeal movement and effect of aging on swallowing pressure in the pharynx and upper esophageal sphincter. Laryngoscope. 2000;110:434–9.
31. Cook IJ, Blumbergs P, Cash K, Jamieson GG, Shearman DJ. Structural abnormalities of the cricopharyngeus muscle in patients with pharyngeal (Zenker's) diverticulum. J Gastroenterol Hepatol. 1992;7:556–62.
32. Dantas RO, Cook IJ, Dodds WJ, Kern MK, Lang IM, Brasseur JG. Biomechanics of cricopharyngeal bars. Gastroenterology. 1990;99:1269–74.
33. Omari TI, Rommel N, Szczesniak MM, et al. Assessment of intraluminal impedance for the detection of pharyngeal bolus flow during swallowing in healthy adults. Am J Physiol Gastrointest Liver Physiol. 2006;290:G183–8.
34. Szczesniak MM, Rommel N, Dinning PG, et al. Optimal criteria for detecting bolus passage across the pharyngo-oesophageal segment during the normal swallow using intraluminal impedance recording. Neurogastroenterol Motil. 2008;20:440–7.
35. Szczesniak MM, Rommel N, Dinning PG, et al. Intraluminal impedance detects failure of pharyngeal bolus clearance during swallowing: a validation study in adults with dysphagia. Neurogastroenterol Motil. 2009;21:244–52.
36. Omari TI, Dejaeger E, Vanbeckevoort D, et al. A method to objectively assess swallow function in adults with suspected aspiration. Gastroenterology. 2011;140:1454–63.
37. Omari T, Dejaeger E, Van Beckevoort D, et al. A novel method for the non-radiological assessment of ineffective swallowing. Am J Gastroenterol. 2011;106:1796.
38. Omari T, Papathanasopoulos A, Dejaeger E, et al. Reproducibility and agreement of pharyngeal automated impedance manometry with videofluoroscopy. Clin Gastroenterol Hepatol. 2011;9(10):862–7.
39. Schwarz SM, Corredor J, Fisher-Medina J, Cohen J, Rabinowitz S. Diagnosis and treatment of feeding disorders in children with developmental disabilities. Pediatrics. 2001;108:671–6.
40. Prevalence and characteristics of children with cerebral palsy in Europe. Dev Med Child Neurol. 2002;44:633–40.
41. Bax M, Goldstein M, Rosenbaum P, et al. Proposed definition and classification of cerebral palsy. Dev Med Child Neurol. 2005;47:571–6.
42. Bax M, Tydeman C, Flodmark O. Clinical and MRI correlates of cerebral palsy: the European Cerebral Palsy Study. JAMA. 2006;296:1602–8.
43. Calis EA, Veugelers R, Sheppard JJ, Tibboel D, Evenhuis HM, Penning C. Dysphagia in children with severe generalized cerebral palsy and intellectual disability. Dev Med Child Neurol. 2008;50:625–30.
44. Gisel EG, Applegate-Ferrante T, Benson JE, Bosma JF. Effect of oral sensorimotor treatment on measures of growth, eating efficiency and aspiration in the dysphagic child with cerebral palsy. Dev Med Child Neurol. 1995;37:528–43.
45. Motion S, Northstone K, Emond A, Stucke S, Golding J. Early feeding problems in children with cerebral palsy: weight and neurodevelopmental outcomes. Dev Med Child Neurol. 2002;44:40–3.
46. Sullivan PB, Lambert B, Rose M, Ford-Adams M, Johnson A, Griffiths P. Prevalence and severity of feeding and nutritional problems in children with neurological impairment: Oxford Feeding Study. Dev Med Child Neurol. 2000;42:674–80.
47. Ozdemirkiran T, Secil Y, Tarlaci S, Ertekin C. An EMG screening method (dysphagia limit) for evaluation of neurogenic dysphagia in childhood above 5 years old. Int J Pediatr Otorhinolaryngol. 2007;71:403–7.
48. Strudwick S. Oral motor impairment and swallowing dysfunction: assessment and management. In: Sullivan PB, editor. Feeding and nutrition in children with neurodevelopmental disability. London: Mac Keith press; 2009. p. 35–56.
49. Casas MJ, Kenny DJ, McPherson KA. Swallowing/ventilation interactions during oral swallow in normal children and children with cerebral palsy. Dysphagia. 1994;9:40–6.
50. Senner JE, Logemann J, Zecker S, Gaebler-Spira D. Drooling, saliva production, and swallowing in cerebral palsy. Dev Med Child Neurol. 2004;46:801–6.
51. Waterman ET, Koltai PJ, Downey JC, Cacace AT. Swallowing disorders in a population of children with cerebral palsy. Int J Pediatr Otorhinolaryngol. 1992;24:63–71.
52. McDonald-McGinn D, Kirschner R, Goldmuntz E, et al. The Philadelphia story: the 22q11.2 deletion: report on 250 patients. Genet Couns. 1999;10:11–24.

53. Rommel N, Vantrappen G, Devriendt K, et al. Retrospective analysis of feeding and speech disorders in 50 patients with velo-cardio-facial syndrome. Genet Couns. 1999;10:71–8.
54. Eicher P, Donald-McGinn DM, Fox C, et al. Dysphagia in children with a 22q11.2 deletion: unusual pattern found on modified barium swallow. J Pediatr. 2000;137:158–64.
55. Vantrappen G, Rommel N, Cremers C, et al. The velo-cardio-facial syndrome: the otorhinolaryngeal manifestations and implications. Int J Pediatr Otorhinolaryngol. 1998;45:133–41.
56. Rommel N, Davidson G, Cain T, Hebbard G, Omari T. Videomanometric evaluation of pharyngo-oesophageal dysmotility in children with velocardiofacial syndrome. J Pediatr Gastroenterol Nutr. 2008;46:87–91.
57. American Psychiatric Association. Diagnostic and statistical manual of mental disorders. 4th ed. Washington DC: American Psychiatric Association; 1994.
58. Ibrahim S, Voigt R, Katusic S, et al. Incidence of gastrointestinal symptoms in children with autism: a population-based study. Pediatrics. 2009;124:680–6.
59. Martins Y, Young RL, Robson D. Feeding and eating behaviors in children with autism and typically developing children. J Autism Dev Disord. 2008;38:1878–87.

20 Esophageal Motor Disorders: Achalasia, Diffuse Esophageal Spasm, Nonspecific Motor Disorders, Eosinophilic Esophagitis

Hayat Mousa and Ann Aspirot

General Background Physiology

The esophagus is a collapsible organ in the digestive tract with the main function of transporting contents from the mouth to the stomach. The muscle layer is composed of circular, longitudinal, striated, and smooth muscle to assist peristalsis. Its three primary parts are the upper esophageal sphincter (UES), esophageal body (EB), and lower esophageal sphincter (LES). The UES is made of three muscles and cricoid cartilage which prevent inspired air from entering the digestive tract as well as esophageal contents from refluxing into the hypopharynx [1, 2]. Anterior to the EB are the larynx and trachea; the EB descends along the front of the vertebral column [3]. During swallows it collapses, distending to the anterior–posterior 2 cm and laterally to 3 cm. Primary peristalsis is initiated by either wet or dry swallows and facilitates esophageal clearance [4]. Secondary peristalsis occurs in response to refluxed materials or esophageal distention and contributes to the esophageal clearance [5]. Central and neural circuitry must coordinate in order for peristalsis to continue through the esophagus. The LES, comprising the gastroesophageal junction, works to prevent gastroesophageal reflux (GER) episodes, though allowing gaseous reflux contents.

Manometry is the primary assessment method for esophageal motor activity, specifically contractions [6]. It measures UES and LES pressures, esophageal body contraction amplitude, and peristaltic sequences [7, 8]. Manometry is a diagnostic tool recommended for use only after endoscopy and fluoroscopy have ruled out organic pathology [9]. Typically a manometry catheter is inserted from the pharynx to the stomach. The catheter has sensors which detect pressure and muscle contractions as the patient swallows, although it can be difficult to perform in the presence of pharyngeal or upper esophageal obstructions, severe coagulopathy cardiac conditions causing intolerance to vagal stimulation, and patient noncompliance [6, 7, 10]. Accurate diagnosis is obtained with proper instrumentation, standard technique and evaluation. Interpretation of the manometric tracings can be altered by the patient activity, body position, age, and gender [8, 11, 12]. More

H. Mousa, M.D. (✉)
Division of Gastroenterology, Nationwide Children Hospital, J West 1985, Columbus, OH, 43205, USA
e-mail: hayat.mousa@nationwidechildrens.org

A. Aspirot, M.D.
Pediatric Surgery Division, Department of Surgery, Sainte-Justine University Health Center, University of Montreal, Montreal, QC, Canada

C. Faure et al. (eds.), *Pediatric Neurogastroenterology: Gastrointestinal Motility and Functional Disorders in Children*, Clinical Gastroenterology,
DOI 10.1007/978-1-60761-709-9_20, © Springer Science+Business Media New York 2013

details about the different methods used to measure esophageal manometry are addressed in chapter 8.

Evaluation of Esophageal Bolus Transit and Clearance

There are several options to evaluate bolus transit and clearance:

Cineradiography

Cineradiology or video fluorography (VFG), is a method examining different phases of swallowing to identify motor abnormalities [13]. In this test, the patient digests, or is injected with, various concentrations of barium while altering body position to evaluate esophageal mucosa, motility, and structures [14–16]. The swallows are followed by several radiographs which detect esophageal clearance. Abnormal peristalsis identified in at least two swallows defines abnormal motility [15]. VFG is generally used as a screening tool with high sensitivity, though affected by number of swallows and body positions [16, 17].

Esophageal Transit Scintigraphy

Scintigraphy focuses on esophageal emptying, evaluates bolus transit in segments, and identifies reflux episodes [18]. In this test, the patient ingests a radio-labeled bolus and several images are taken to inspect bolus transit and clearance [19]. The study measures the level of radioactivity as it relates to clearance. Use of liquidized bolus is more standardized than semisolid bolus. Also, patients usually usually lie in the supine position to eliminate gravity as a source of error [18]. Scintigraphy is more sensitive than VFG, though the necessary equipment is not as widely available. More details about esophageal transit scintigraphy are addressed in Chap. 14.

Esophageal Impedance and pH Monitoring

Another method involves esophageal impedance and pH monitoring. When combined, these techniques can assess bolus transit, clearance, and chemical content of the bolus or refluxate. Similar to manometry, a catheter with several sensors is utilized for assessment. Several liquid and viscous swallows are required. Impedance demonstrates 97% concordance with fluoroscopy, though only fluoroscopy can study swallows with a solid bolus [20]. Among its many advantages, impedance can be (repeatedly) employed on pregnant women and children because it does not involve radiation; it also relates to esophageal mucosal integrity [21]. However, swallowed air can make brief changes in impedance unrelated to bolus transit.

Esophageal Function Testing

Esophageal function testing (EFT) is a union of manometry and multichannel intraluminal impedance monitoring. EFT gathers information on bolus transit patterns, swallow associated events, nonobstructive dysphagia, chest pain, and general motility disorders [22, 23]. It is also a helpful evaluation tool before antireflux surgery. Again, catheters are used for evaluation and several types are available depending on how many channels, sensors, pressure transducers, are needed [24]. In one exam, EFT provides information previously gathered in separate exams from manometry and fluoroscopy, even though it is typically used after both of those methods produce negative results [22]. By evaluating the transit time, EFT classifies esophageal dysmotility into two categories: either abnormal manometry with abnormal transit or abnormal manometry with normal transit. Abnormal manometry with abnormal transit includes conditions such as achalasia, scleroderma, ineffective esophageal motility, and distal esophageal spasm. Abnormal manometry with normal transit includes conditions such as nutcracker esophagus, hypertensive LES, hypotensive LES, and poor relaxing LES.

Esophageal Dysmotility

Prevalence of Esophageal Dysmotility in Children and Adolescents

As reported previously by Glassman et al., up to 25% of children and adolescents who present with chest pain, dysphagia, and vomiting have abnormal esophageal motility study [25]. The most common patterns of esophageal dysmotility in symptomatic children with dysphagia, chest pain, and vomiting are diffuse esophageal spasm (33%), achalasia (19%), hypotensive lower esophageal sphincter (14%), aperistaltic distal esophagus (14%), nutcracker esophagus (10%), and hypertensive lower esophageal sphincter in (10%) [25].

Clinical Presentation of Esophageal Dysmotility

Dysphagia

Swallowing is an important developmental process for human life. It requires the coordination between the mouth, pharynx, and esophagus for successful completion. Esophageal dysphagia or difficulty swallowing can be the result of behavioral, developmental, neurological, respiratory, GER, and inflammatory diseases [26, 27]. It is observed in 25–45% of developing children and even more in those with developmental disorders [28]. Dysphagia can occur with solid foods and/or liquids. Exclusively experiencing solid food dysphagia is more characteristic of a mechanical rather than a neurological disorder, whereas solid and/or liquid dysphagia is characteristic of neuromuscular disorder [27]. A child may indicate dysphagia by demonstrating little interest in food or eating, displaying straining or extension of muscles during feedings, taking extensive time to complete feeding, spilling food or liquid out of the mouth, emesis, coughing or gagging during feeding, struggling with breathing/stridor when feeding, and failing to thrive [26]. Patients undergo barium esophagogram or upper GI endoscopy to evaluate UES function, or manometry to assess motility when esophageal dysphagia is suspected [26, 27]. In infants, parents may additionally be provided a questionnaire and/or a physician may observe the child while feeding.

Chest Pain

Noncardiac chest pain can be indicative of esophageal dysmotility in infants and children. Because the heart and esophagus have similar neural pain pathways, it can be difficult to determine cardiac and noncardiac chest pain [29]. Compared to other sources to noncardiac chest pain (i.e., musculoskeletal pain and asthma), studies indicate that gastrointestinal diseases represent less than 10–15% of cases [30]. Glassman et al. reviewed the cases of 83 children aged 1–20 years with chest pain and vomiting or dysphagia for prevalence of esophageal motility disorders. Of the 83, 47 had normal esophageal manometry and endoscopy [25]. The remaining 36 patients had evidence of esophageal disease, indicated by either abnormal endoscopy, abnormal manometry, or both. Among the 21 patients with abnormal manometry, diffuse esophageal spasm was the most common diagnosis followed by achalasia, hypotensive LES, aperistalsis, nutcracker esophagus, and hypertensive LES. Most of these patients (16 of 21) were symptomatic of their disease. Berezin et al. performed a similar study of 51 children, aged 8–20 years, of which 27 were found to have idiopathic chest pain [29]. Twenty-one of those patients were diagnosed with esophagitis or diffuse esophageal spasm using manometry and histology; though only five had abnormal motility. Additionally, Glassman et al. found that with treatment chest pain was more easily resolved than esophageal symptoms.

Foreign Body Impaction

Children ingest materials that become impacted in the esophagus, usually in the upper esophagus, and obstruct esophageal transit; by comparison ingested items rarely enter the tracheobronchial tree [31, 32]. Children primarily ingest nonfood items such as coins and small toys, whereas adults tend to have impacted meat and bones [32]. Children with meat impactions should be evaluated for either anatomic esophageal malformation, motility/functional disorders or eosinophilic esophagitis [31].

Classification: The Chicago Classification 2009

High-resolution esophageal pressure topography (HROPT) is a novel technical development in the study of motility. Traditionally, manometry was used to examine esophageal motility but did not report pressures within the organ; this was a task reserved for pressure topography. HROPT provides the benefits of manometry and pressure topography in one technique. The Chicago Classification is a schema used to categorize results of HROPT used in clinical evaluations. It is based on a study of 400 patients and 75 controls by Kahrilas et al. [33]. In summary, HROPT classifies nonspecific esophageal motility disorders, diffuse esophageal spasm, nutcracker esophagus subtypes, vigorous achalasia, and functional obstruction. Among its advantages, HROPT is easily interpreted and standardized, saves time, provides high-quality data, and allows for more specific diagnoses.

Esophageal Motility Disorders

Esophageal Achalasia

Esophageal achalasia is a primary motor disorder presenting with dysphagia secondary to functional obstruction due to the dysfunction of the body of the esophagus and the lower esophageal sphincter. It is characterized by the absence of peristalsis and incomplete relaxation of the lower esophageal sphincter.

Epidemiology and Incidence

Achalasia is an infrequent adult disease with an incidence of 1.63/100,000 and a prevalence of 10.8/100,000, based on a recent population-based study [34]. Because of the relative rarity of childhood and adolescent achalasia, much of the literature on achalasia is based on the adult population, with information by pediatric gastroenterologists noted only in case series and retrospective studies. An incidence of less than 0.1/100,000 has been found in children in England and Wales [35]. Most of the cases are diagnosed between 7 and 15 years. Infants are rarely affected (6%), but symptoms are described to be present during the first year of life in 18% [36]. Infantile achalasia is reported as case reports in the literature [37]. Diagnosis may not be as rigorous in young children as it is in adults [35], many published cases were not confirmed by esophageal manometry, the gold standard diagnostic tool.

Pathophysiology

Acquired degeneration of the Auerbach's myenteric plexus is the primary mechanism of achalasia. Loss of nitrergic inhibitory enteric neurons occurring prior to loss of cholinergic neurons results in an imbalance between excitatory and inhibitory input leading to ineffective esophageal peristalsis and incomplete lower esophageal sphincter relaxation [38]. Nitric oxide (NO) is the predominant inhibitory neurotransmitter but others have been described such as vasopeptide intestinal peptide (VIP). Studies on resected specimen have demonstrated decreased number of myenteric ganglia, lymphocytic infiltrate, and collagen deposition within ganglia. Some specimens had normal number of myenteric ganglion cells, but myenteric fibrosis was observed. Preservation of cholinergic excitatory neurons could explain the occurrence of vigorous achalasia which has been hypothesized to be an earlier form of the disease [39]. These findings suggest a progressive immune mediated destruction of neuronal cells. The pathologic findings could be different in childhood achalasia where less neuronal inflammation was found [40].

Etiology

Achalasia can be primary (idiopathic) or secondary. The etiology of primary achalasia remains unknown. Numerous hypotheses have been proposed including infection, hereditary, and autoimmunity. Chagas disease is the prototype of secondary achalasia that is caused by the parasite *Trypanosma cruzi*. The disease is common in South and Central America. Whether the disease is similar to idiopathic achalasia remains controversial [41]. Because of the associated inflammatory infiltration mainly composed of lymphocytes, viruses such as measles, HSV-1, and VZV have been suspected as a cause of idiopathic achalasia. A cause–effect relationship between viruses and achalasia has yet to be identified. Studies have associated achalasia with trisomy 21 [42], Hirschsprung's disease [43], Allgrove's syndrome, and familial dysautonomia, which suggest a genetic link. However, familial history is the exception in achalasic patients even in the pediatric age [36]. Allgrove's or 4 "A" syndrome, which presents with achalasia, alacrima, autonomic disturbance, and corticotrophin (ACTH) insensitivity, is the only condition associated with achalasia that has been linked to a specific chromosomal anomaly which is the AAAS gene on chromosome 12q13 [44–46]. Because of the rarity of achalasia in childhood, it is important to refer younger patients to Genetics and screen for adrenal insufficiency. The third broad hypothesis is autoimmunity that could precipitate an immune reaction directed to the esophageal myenteric ganglia. Studies are contradictory in demonstrating a link between antineuronal antibodies and achalasia [38, 47].

Clinical Presentation

Achalasia presents with progressive dysphagia (first for liquids and eventually for solid food), chest pain, and regurgitation of undigested food, not mixed with gastric secretions [48]. Nurko and Rosen [49] summarized the clinical symptoms in 528 pediatric patients from 23 series. The most common symptoms are vomiting (80%) and dysphagia (75%). Weight loss is reported in 64% and failure to thrive in 31%. Chest pain and odynophagia are sometimes present (45%), but less common in younger children. Diagnosis is often delayed in children because of multiple factors including lower incidence of achalasia, incapacity to verbalize complaints, and unspecific symptoms, such as food refusal and failure to thrive. Parents will sometimes report that their child is a slow eater. Children additionally present nocturnal symptoms such as choking and regurgitated food on the pillow (21%). Respiratory symptoms occur in 44% which is more frequent than in the adult population. In children, regurgitation, respiratory problems, and failure to thrive are frequently attributed to gastroesophageal reflux (GER) which is much more predominant than achalasia in this population. Extraesophageal complications of achalasia include recurrent pulmonary aspirations and tracheal compression by the megaesophagus. Sudden death has also been reported.

Differential Diagnosis

Apart from GER, differential diagnosis includes mechanical obstruction by foreign body, intrinsic esophageal pathology (esophageal stenosis, leiomyomas), and extrinsic compression of the esophagus (foregut duplication, mediastinal tuberculosis). Malignant neoplasms are more frequently seen in the adult population but need to be included in the differential diagnosis even in children. Chagas disease is always a possibility in patients coming from endemic regions. Achalasia has also been mistaken as eating disorders [50], emphasizing the importance of a thorough evaluation of the upper gastrointestinal tract anatomy and function in patients suspected of having primary anorexia nervosa.

Diagnosis

Diagnosis is often delayed because of the poor specificity of symptoms and the overlap with other more frequent pathologies such as gastroesophageal reflux disease. The specific workup includes radiographic studies, upper endoscopy, and esophageal manometry to confirm the diagnosis of achalasia.

Radiography

Plain chest radiograph may show an air-fluid level in the lower chest, a widened mediastinum, and an absent gastric bubble [51]. Contrast esophagogram will demonstrate the stagnation of contrast in the distal esophagus and possibly absent or tertiary peristalsis. The typical dilated esophagus tapering smoothly at its distal end ("bird's beak") is not necessary to make the diagnosis, but is highly suggestive of the disease. Using manometry as the gold standard, Parkman found a positive predictive value of 96%, a sensitivity of 100% and a specificity of 98% [52]. However, the correlation of severity as assessed by esophagogram and patient's symptoms is poor, which can also lead to a delayed diagnosis [53]. Barium esophagogram is also useful to monitor the success of treatment.

Endoscopy

Upper endoscopy may show retained food in a dilated esophagus. The gastroesophageal junction may appear tight (difficult to distend with air insufflation) but it is usually possible to reach the stomach. The main goal of upper endoscopy is to rule out mechanical obstruction at the gastroesophageal junction (pseudoachalasia) [54]. If pseudoachalasia is suspected, further investigation with ultrasound, endoscopic ultrasonography, and other imaging studies will help to differentiate between the numerous neoplastic and non-neoplastic causes of pseudoachalasia [55].

Manometry

The diagnosis of achalasia is confirmed by esophageal manometry. Absence of peristalsis in the esophageal body is the sine qua non criteria to diagnose esophageal achalasia [48]. Frequently, the lower esophageal sphincter relaxation is incomplete (residual pressure above 8 mmHg) [56, 57]. Hypertensive lower esophageal sphincter (resting pressure above 45 mmHg) is sometimes seen as well as an increased esophagogastric gradient. Recently, high-resolution esophageal manometry has been used more frequently and has permitted a better understanding of the motility abnormalities found in achalasia. Based on topographic plot characteristics, Pandolfino [58] has proposed a classification of achalasia in three subtypes:

- Type I: Classic achalasia: Mean integrated LES relaxation pressure (IRP) ≥15 mmHg, absent peristalsis, no or minimal distal esophageal pressurization.
- Type II: Achalasia with esophageal compression: Mean IRP ≥15 mmHg, absent peristalsis, with panesophageal pressurization to greater than 30 mmHg in ≥20% of swallows (Fig. 20.1.)
- Type III: Spastic achalasia. Mean IRP ≥15 mmHg, absent peristalsis and spasm (contractile front >8 cm^{-1}) in ≥20% of swallows with or without compartmentalized pressurization (Fig. 20.2).

These subtypes have different prognosis implication with type II having the best response to any therapy (pneumatic dilation, Heller myotomy, botulinum toxin) while type III have the worst response to all treatments. This information can be brought in the discussion with the patients and parents and also may guide the clinician in the therapeutic decision.

Treatment

Achalasia affects permanently the esophageal motility. Treatments for achalasia, similar to other esophageal disorders, focus on relieving symptoms [59]. The three primary types of treatment are pharmacologic, endoscopic, and surgical. The therapy of choice in children is still debated [60]. Proper treatment of achalasia is important to prevent progression toward dilated mega-esophagus where esophagectomy may become inevitable. Barium esophagogram can help monitor success of the treatment plan (Table 20.1).

Pharmacologic treatments include nitrates, calcium channel blockers, and phosphodiesterase inhibitors. Although significant decrease of lower esophageal sphincter pressure has been observed by manometry, symptom improvement occurred in 53–87% of patients [61]. In some cases, these medications are used temporarily while determining a more effective means of treatment. Pharmacologic interventions are also the treatment of choice for patients who are not candidates for or do not wish to receive more aggressive therapy. These medications have frequent side effects (headache, hypotension). Experience in children is limited to calcium channel blockers and nitrates and consists mainly of case reports [62–64]. Isosorbide dinitrate patch (long acting nitrate) has been used in an 8-year-old [63] with

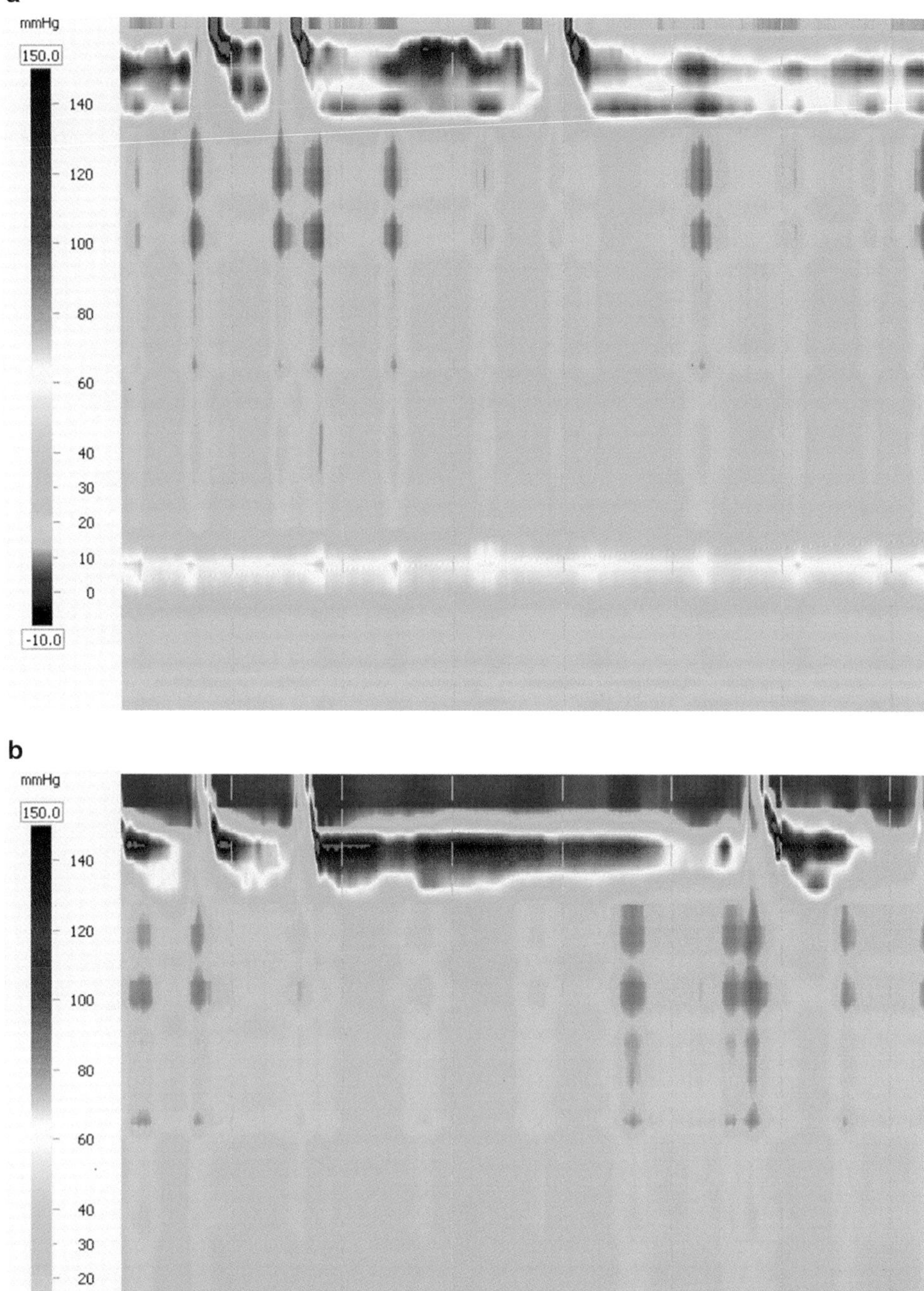

Fig. 20.1 Type II esophageal achalasia (with compression)

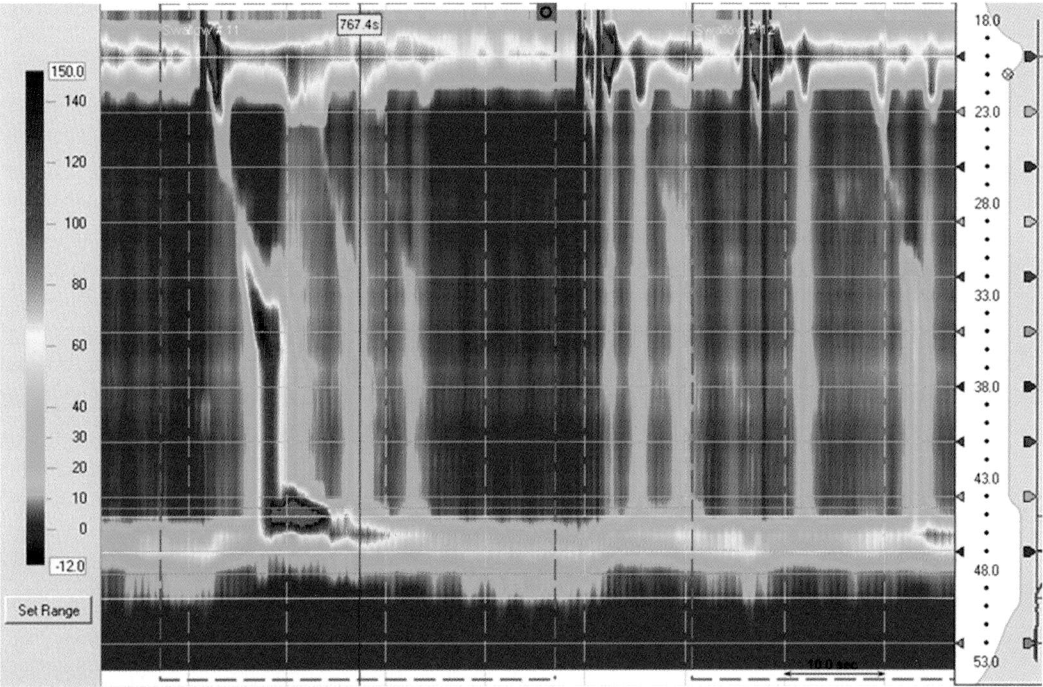

Fig. 20.2 Type III esophageal achalasia (spastic)

good short-term success. Nifedipine (10 mg) before meal was used in four adolescents with good clinical response and a decrease of LES pressure on manometry but there was recurrence of symptoms when the medication was stopped [62]. Long-term pharmacologic therapy is not actually recommended. Short use can be useful while waiting for definitive therapy (establishing weight gain, awaiting school vacation).

Endoscopic therapies include botulinum toxin injection into the LES, pneumatic dilation, and stenting. The use of intrasphincteric botulinum toxin was first reported by Pasricha et al. [65]. This potent neurotoxin blocks the release of acetylcholine at the neuromuscular junction leading to decreased lower esophageal sphincter pressure. A double-blind placebo-controlled trial demonstrated a good initial response in adults [66]. Long-term results showed that it is necessary to repeat the injection and the response decreases with repeated injections [67]. Experience in children is once again limited to retrospective case series [68–71], but shows similar results of good initial clinical response and high rate of recurrence. The data are however insufficient to conclude to the same certitude as in the adult population. Botulinum toxin injection can also be used as a diagnostic tool in patients with early and unclear diagnosis [72]. However, submucosal fibrosis resulting from intrasphincteric injections may complicate the subsequent surgical myotomy [73]. Esophageal dilation is the oldest treatment modality [48]. Balloon dilation is preferred over rigid bougienage because it is thought to permit a controlled tearing of the muscle fibers, even though it was not proven in animal studies [74]. It is less invasive than surgical treatment and is considered the most effective nonsurgical treatment of achalasia in adults [75, 76], and the first-line treatment in some pediatric centers [60]. The main complication is esophageal perforation which was reported in 1.6% of patients [75, 76]. Long-term efficacy of pneumatic dilation ranges from 40 to 60% [77–79]. Pediatric results are variable and difficult to compare because of the nonstandardization of the technique [49]. Pneumatic dilation can also serves as a rescue therapy after an incomplete

Table 20.1 Analysis of selected esophageal motility disorder treatment methods

Method of treatment	Associated disorders	Advantages	Disadvantages	Success
Acid suppression	DES, NE, NEMDs, SSc	Relieves GERD symptoms	May only treat GERD symptoms	Low success in children
Antibiotics	Caustic ingestion, CIIP, SSc			
Botox injection	Achalasia	Suitable for long-term use	May contribute to fibrosis at injection site	
Elemental diet	Caustic ingestion, EoE, DES, NE, SSc	Quick resolution of symptoms	Formulas not palatable Lower quality of life Cost/insurance coverage	Compliance difficult for children
Elimination diet	EoE, CIIP	Still allows for some food intake by mouth	Requires careful review of all food choices for allergens Does not always indicate specific food allergen at fault	Must continue elimination for long-term resolution
Esophageal dilation	Achalasia, caustic ingestion, DES, EoE, NE	Highly effective when strictures are also present	Chest pain Esophageal perforations	Common treatment in adults
Other surgical procedures	Achalasia, caustic ingestion, DES, HD, NE		Complications may further complicate disease	Usually successful with rare complications
Systemic or topical corticosteroids	EoE, SSc	Direct administration to eosinophilia (topical) Variety of administration (swallowed or inhaled)	Low bioavailability May not fully penetrate eosinophilia (topical)	Satisfactory symptom resolution High rate of symptom relapse upon discontinuation

myotomy [51]. Temporary self-expanding metallic stent is a new therapeutic option that has been used in patients as young as 12 years old but more studies and long-term experience is needed before recommending it [80].

Surgical treatment usually consists of a longitudinal division of the muscle fibers of the lower esophageal sphincter and proximal stomach coupled or not with an antireflux procedure. The name of Heller myotomy comes from the first description of this procedure by Ernest Heller in 1913 [59]. Laparoscopic Heller myotomy is now the most commonly performed surgical treatment of achalasia because it reduces the morbidity compared to the open approach. It has been shown to be as effective as open approaches [81] and superior to thoracoscopic approach [82, 83]. Clinical response after myotomy ranges from 83 to 100% [84] and the benefits persists in 67 to 85% in long-term (more than 10 years) studies [85, 86]. Randomized controlled trials compared favorably laparoscopic Heller myotomy to pneumatic dilation [87, 88]. Clinical deterioration over time has been associated with GER [89] which has led to randomized controlled studies comparing Heller myotomy with and without fundoplication [90]. Recently, it has been suggested that a more aggressive balloon dilatation results in comparable results to myotomy [91, 92]. Based on long-term success rates of 47–82% at 10 years, laparoscopic Heller myotomy with partial fundoplication is considered by many the surgical procedure of choice [75, 93, 94]. However, a study has reported that up to 30% of myotomized patients will require re-treatment within the first 12 years [95]. Pandolfino has reported different response to therapy according to the type of achalasia. According to his classification, type I (classic) achalasia responds best to Heller myotomy, type II (with compression) responds to any therapy, and type III (spastic) has a poor response to any therapy [58].

Laparoscopic Heller myotomy has also been found safe and effective in children [96]. Rates of good to excellent results of 90.9% have been reported [97–99]. As in the adult literature [100], the same surgical controversies exist which include extension of the myotomy [101], addition of fundoplication [102], and type of fundoplication if performed. Complications after Heller myotomy include esophageal perforation, phrenic nerve paralysis, hemorrhage, herniation of stomach. Long-term complications are persistent dysphagia and GER. The intra-operative use of endoscopy [103] and esophageal manometry [104] have been suggested to decrease the rate of incomplete myotomy. It is important to emphasize that while myotomy should improve the bolus transit by reducing the LES pressure, ineffective peristalsis can still remain an issue (Fig. 20.3) [105].

An approach to the child with persistent dysphagia after myotomy has been proposed since it is a frequent and debilitating problem [106]. Differential diagnosis of this problem include esophageal dysmotility, incomplete myotomy, fibrosis at the distal end of the myotomy, obstructive fundoplication, esophageal stricture and preoperative error in diagnosis [107–109]. A thorough evaluation is the basis of management, starting with a good clinical history. Contrast esophagogram and esophageal manometry complete the initial work up. Depending on the findings, endoscopy with pneumatic dilation may be indicated as the first therapeutic step. Surgical treatment is reserved for persistent significant obstruction of the distal esophagus [106].

Outcome

Regardless of the elected therapy, patients must continue with regular follow-up to prevent progression toward a more serious disease. A rare, yet critical complication of achalasia is squamous cell carcinoma in the esophagus. It is thought to result from stasis and uncontrolled bacterial growth [110]. Based on a review of the literature, Dunaway has reported a mean prevalence of 3% which represents of 50-fold increased risk over the general population [111]. Chronic gastroesophageal reflux resulting from the successful treatment of achalasia is also a risk factor for the development of adenocarcinoma [112, 113]. More recently, a prospective cohort study of 448 achalasia patients reported esophageal cancer in 3.3% with an annual incidence of 0.34 and, despite structured endoscopic surveillance, most

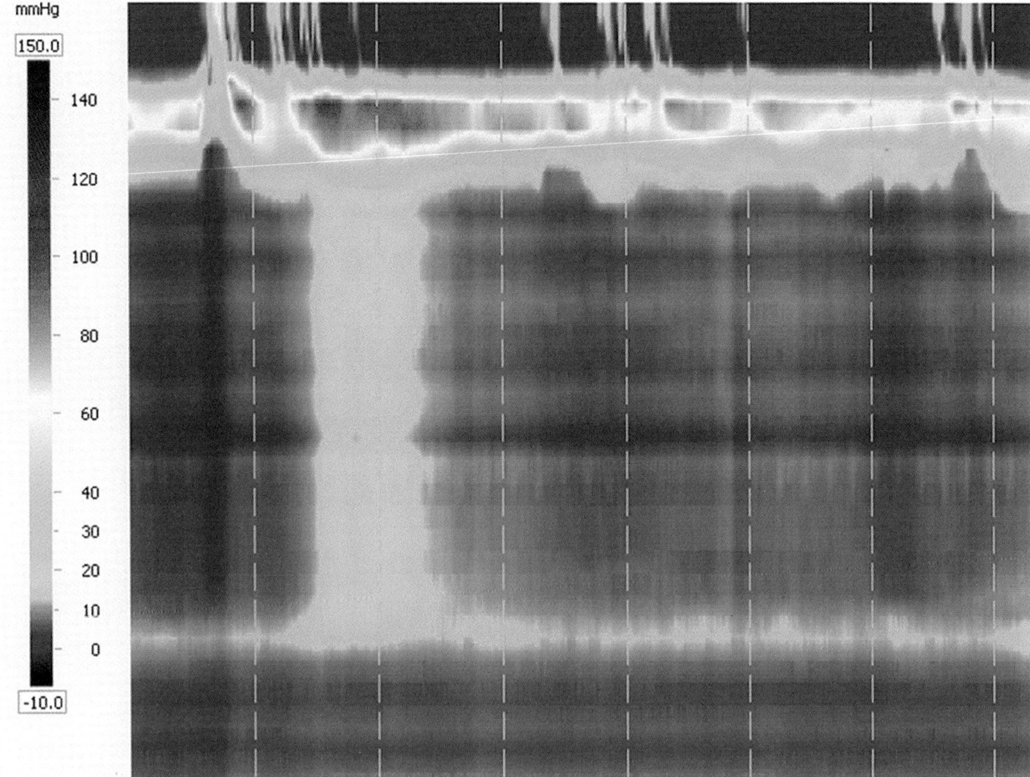

Fig. 20.3 Postoperative esophageal manometry after Heller myotomy

neoplastic lesions were detected at an advanced stage [114]. However, the overall life expectancy of patients with achalasia does not appear to be significantly decreased [115] and up to now, no cases of esophageal carcinoma have been reported in patients who had achalasia diagnosed as children [49]. Routine diagnostic tests are not recommended but patients developing recurrence or development of new symptoms should be investigated thoroughly.

Diffuse Esophageal Spasm and Nutcracker Esophagus

The incidence in children is not known and the literature is scarce, limited to case reports and small case series [25, 116]. In a retrospective study of 83 children with chest pain investigated by esophageal manometry and endoscopy, Glassman identified 4 patients with DES.

Diffuse esophageal spasm (DES) and nutcracker esophagus (NE), also known as hypertensive peristalsis, are benign and very rare, representing less than 10% of abnormal adult manometry diagnoses [117–119]. The etiology and pathogenesis of both conditions remain unknown [117]. Both DES and NE share symptoms of intermittent dysphagia and chest pain, with or without swallowing [16, 117, 120, 121]. Symptoms are usually experienced while eating or drinking [117, 120]. DES tends to present comorbidly in infants and children [122]. Infants may additionally present with apnea and brachycardia and younger children with aspiration pneumonia; symptoms of older children most resemble those observed in adults [123]. Because symptoms are intermittent, it is easy to distinguish these two conditions from more progressive diseases (i.e., achalasia and esophageal cancer) [120].

There is controversy regarding the diagnosis and treatment of DES and NE. Both can be diagnosed using manometry; however, only clinical symptoms are helpful to diagnose DES [120, 121]. pH monitoring can determine whether gastroesophageal reflux disease (GERD) is present which identifies need for anti-GERD therapies in treatment [124]. Barium esophagograms are often normal in DES and NE patients [120]. Possible treatment options for DES and NE include pharmaceutical interventions, surgery, and anti-GERD therapies [120]. Nitrates, calcium channel blockers, and botulinum toxin, all decrease LES pressure; though esophageal function is further complicated when the LES becomes too relaxed due to medications [124–126]. Anxiolytics may be used in DES patients diagnosed with anxiety or depression [120, 121]. The use of visceral analgesics (tricyclic antidepressants, serotonin reuptake inhibitors (SSRIs)) improved global symptoms scores in individuals with esophageal contraction abnormalities and DES. There is no evidence on the effect of visceral analgesics on NE. *Medical and surgical* approaches are intended to alleviate pain and decrease severity of symptoms [120]. Patients may undergo pneumatic dilation to relieve symptoms but the procedure is not consistently effective because the balloon can be difficult to place. Surgery is usually reserved for those patients with dysphagia and hypertensive sphincter. Selecting a treatment option should be used based on bolus transit and manometry findings [9].

Eosinophilic Esophagitis

Eosinophilic Esophagitis (EoE) is a condition in which the esophagus becomes inflamed due to infiltration by eosinophils. Detection of ≥15–21 eosinophils/HPF in squamous epithelium is postulated as qualifying criterion for EoE diagnosis though some controversy remains [127–131]. Eosinophilic infiltration is common in the GI tract in cases of eosinophilic gastroenteritis, allergic colitis, IBD, and GER [132, 133]. EoE is now appreciated as a condition separate from GERD and reflux esophagitis [128]. The exact incidence and prevalence of EoE remains unknown. Dohil et al. suggest a prevalence of 30 in 100,000 people [134]. It is postulated that 10% of children with GER, unresponsive to acid suppression therapies have EoE [128]. Overall, prevalence tends to be higher in individuals with a history of dysphagia and pre-diagnosed/existing cases of GERD, reflux esophagitis, and food impaction [130].

Etiopathogenesis of EoE remains unknown, though researchers suggest infiltration is related to food allergen hypersensitivity in non-idiopathic cases of EoE [128]. GERD, aperistalsis, dysphagia, and poor esophageal clearance are described as complications of EoE [128, 133, 135].

Mechanisms responsible for esophageal dysmotility associated with EoE are somewhat uncertain. Eosinophils contain substances that cause inflammation and may damage surrounding tissue when released [136]. A suggested trigger of inflammation in epithelial cells of the esophagus is eotaxin-3, an eosinophil chemoattractant [133]. This inflammation subsequently penetrates other cell layers. For instance, it may lead to inflammation of the epithelium which furthers dysmotility [130, 133]. Axonal necrosis is thought to result from eosinophilic degranulation creating damaged nerve tissue and consequently weak esophageal contractions. Increased eosinophil cationic protein (ECP) is shown to result from the co-culture of eosinophils and fibroblasts; ECP encourages abnormal fibroblast contractions [133, 136].

The following are symptoms of EoE in adults: dysphagia, food impaction and retrosternal pain with or without swallowing [129, 132, 133, 137]. Pediatric patients may additionally experience vomiting, abdominal pain, failure to thrive, food aversion, feeding difficulties, and other symptoms imitating GERD [128, 137, 138]. Normal frequency of reflux episodes, an allergic history, and poor response to acid suppression are also characteristic of EoE patients [128]. Due to symptom overlap between EoE and GERD, diagnosis must be confirmed by endoscopy [139, 140].

The diverse array of EoE symptoms speak to the variety of treatment options available to EoE patients: diet management, fluticasone inhalants,

Table 20.2 Summary of EoE treatment methods

Method of treatment	Advantages	Disadvantages	Success
Elimination diet	Still allows for some food intake by mouth	Requires careful review of all food choices for allergens	Must continue elimination for long-term resolution
		Does not always indicate specific food allergen at fault	
Elemental diet	Quick resolution of symptoms	Formulas not palatable	Compliance difficult for children
		Lower quality of life	
		Cost/insurance coverage	
Acid suppression	Can distinguish between EoE and GERD	May only treat GERD symptoms	Low success in children
Topical corticosteroids	Direct administration to areas with eosinophilia	May not fully penetrate eosinophilia	High rate of symptom relapse
Systemic corticosteroids	Variety of administration (swallowed or inhaled)	Low bioavailability	Satisfactory symptom resolution
Esophageal dilation	Highly effective when strictures are also present	Chest pain	Common treatment in adults
		Esophageal perforations	

acid suppression, topical and systemic corticosteroids, and esophageal dilation [138]. Esophageal dilation is a surgical treatment option more common in adults with strictures, but is also used for pediatric EoE [138, 141]. The primary, yet rare risks associated with esophageal dilation are wall disruption and perforation [138]. Patients may prefer this method of treatment after seeing no improvement with dietary or other medical intervention (Table 20.2).

Collagen Vascular Disorders

Among collagen vascular disorders, scleroderma is the most severe and commonly manifests in the gastrointestinal tract. Other collagen vascular disorders with esophageal manifestations are systemic lupus erythematosus (SLE), mixed connective tissue diseases (MCTDs), Sjörgen syndrome, and rheumatoid arthritis. Scleroderma consists of the hardening of tissues resulting from an autoimmune response. Systemic scleroderma (SSc) is characterized by collagen deposition in body tissue, especially the esophagus. SSc affects esophageal tissue and motility in 75–90% of adult cases [142, 143]; pediatric studies indicate lower prevalence [144, 145]. In a multi-center study, Foeldvari et al. reported 65% (88/135) of pediatric SSc patients presented GI tract involvement [146]. Of those 135 cases, under 50% ($n=63$) involved the esophagus [146].

A study of SSc revealed that childhood-onset is sometimes preceded by trauma in the area of deposition; a unique phenomenon compared to adult cases of scleroderma [145]. In the presence of SSc, esophageal manometry reveals an incompetent LES and low-amplitude smooth muscle contractions of the esophagus [142]. The retrograde movement of gastric contents, related to low LES pressure, exposes the esophagus to acidity, which can further compromise peristalsis. Frequent contact between acidic gastric contents and esophageal mucosa degrades tissue quality; esophagitis, bleeding, and strictures are other known complications. However, studies have noted that many who experience esophageal dysmotility secondary to SSc are sometimes asymptomatic [142, 147]. Aside from manometry, barium esophagram, 24-h ambulatory pH, and endoscopy are also used to diagnose the extent of esophageal disturbance secondary to SSc [142]. Autoimmune markers such as the anti-endonuclear antigens anti-ScL-70 and anti-centromere antibodies may be present.

Common symptoms of SSc with esophageal involvement are dysphagia, chest pain, weight loss, food impaction, and early satiety [142, 148]. Weber et al. reported reflux events in over 60% of pediatric patients with SSc [147]. Overall mortality for SSc with esophageal involvement is very rare; death is usually a consequence of multi-system involvement [145, 146]. Treatment of SSc primarily involves immunosuppressants (prednisone, methotrexate, mycophenolate mofetil, tumor necrosis factor-alpha, cyclophosphamide) [145, 149]. However, there is no specific treatment for SSc esophageal involvement. Gunawardena and McHugh suggest proton pump inhibitors, bulking agents, nutritional supplements, and antibiotics as additional treatment options [148, 150].

Chronic Idiopathic Intestinal Pseudo-Obstruction

Chronic idiopathic intestinal pseudo-obstruction (CIIP) is a rare primary disorder that involves the entire gastrointestinal tract. Esophageal involvement is very common [151, 152]. Non-idiopathic intestinal pseudo-obstruction is usually secondary to systemic, metabolic, genetic or mitochondrial etiologies. CIIP is often diagnosed during infancy and childhood and symptoms are usually both severe and frequent at onset. Patients with esophageal involvement present clinical symptoms of GER, dysphagia, nausea and vomiting, and weight loss [153]. Dysphagia, however, is usually a chief complaint when CIIP is secondary to another disorder.

Abnormal manometry findings include uncoordinated or low-amplitude contractions with swallowing [152, 154]; these findings are more common than aperistalsis. Decreased LES pressure is also a common finding. Pharmacologic treatment of CIIP is similar to that of other esophageal motility disorders, involving antiemetics, prokinetics, and antispasmodics.

Hirschsprung's Disease

Lack or poor formation of the enteric nervous system defines Hirschsprung's Disease (HD). Though primarily a disease of the small and large bowel, HD is occasionally associated with abnormal esophageal motility indicated by poor peristaltic wave propagation [155, 156]. Staiano et al. examined esophageal involvement in children with HD, in comparison to those with idiopathic megacolon and healthy controls with no esophageal or colonic diseases. Abnormalities in the amplitude and frequency of distal esophageal body contractions were significantly higher in HD patients than other groups [157]. The severity of HD in this group was unrelated to esophageal involvement.

Caustic Ingestion

Caustic ingestion of harmful substances is a common accident among young children, especially in developing countries. Common signs and symptoms include salivation, oropharyngeal burns, vomiting, bleeding, epigastric and retrosternal pain, and malignant transformation [158, 159]. A recent study examined the extent of esophageal damage in 94 toddlers (mean age 38 months) who experienced caustic ingestion [159]. Over 80% of cases had second to third degree esophageal burns which were highly associated with the development of esophageal strictures. Strictures occurred in 46 cases overall (49%) and were associated with development of dysphagia, contributing to poor nutrient intake, and dysmotility.

Esophageal manometry has revealed hypoperistalsis, usually with normal UES and LES function, in cases of caustic ingestion [160, 161].

Ineffective Esophageal Motility

Spechler and Castell defined ineffective esophageal motility (IEM) as having low or normal esophageal sphincter pressure, normal LES relaxation, and greater than 30% low-amplitude waves characterized by the following: wave amplitude <30 mmHg, peristalsis that does not travel the length of the esophagus, simultaneous contractions <30 mmHg, or aperistalsis [162]. Currently there is little data regarding IEM in the pediatric population. Literature suggests IEM as a predictor for GERD in adults, though the nature of the association is controversial. It has not yet been determined whether IEM is a rare primary disorder or merely secondary to increased acid exposure. IEM hypocontractions and incomplete peristalsis of the esophagus may be diagnosed using manometry and/or high-frequency intraluminal ultrasound (HFIUS). Pioneered by Mittal [163], HFIUS provides real-time images of esophageal function which has proven especially beneficial during manometry. Using HFIUS, Kim et al. sought to examine esophageal muscle thickness in patients diagnosed with IEM [164]. Of 283 eligible patients, 46 (16%) had IEM, with just over half of those cases associated with GERD ($n=26$). The non-GERD IEM group had greater LES muscle thickness than the GERD group, supporting an association, but not causal relationship between the two. HFIUS, coupled with manometry, will likely become an increasingly utilized examination and diagnostic tool for gastroenterologists as more data is collected on IEM [162, 165].

Nonspecific Esophageal Motility Disorders

Nonspecific esophageal motility disorders (NEMDs) capture those cases with abnormal manometry, but without characteristics of an established disorder [118, 120, 166]. Criteria for NEMDs are ≥30% of wet swallows with nontransmitted or low-amplitude contractions or at least one of the following contraction abnormalities: triple-peaked contraction, retrograde contraction, prolonged duration peristaltic waves (>6 s), or isolated incomplete LES relaxation (>8 mmHg) [166]. Low-amplitude contractions are thought to be the most common manometric finding [167]. NEMDs differ from achalasia in that with swallows there are intermittent normal and abnormal peristaltic waves; while complete lack of peristalsis is characteristic of achalasia. Additionally, NEMDs involve low-amplitude waves, whereas DES typically involves high-amplitude pressure waves. Despite these notably distinct symptoms, it is suggested that NEMDs may be an early disease state of achalasia and DES [167]. Naftali et al. reported a minority of patients who progressed from NEMD to achalasia or DES diagnosed during a repeat manometry test.

Common symptoms are dysphagia, vomiting, chest and epigastric pain, and food impactions [118, 120, 124]. NEMDs are rarer than other primary esophageal motility disorders, such as achalasia and DES. In a cohort of 154 children with upper GI symptoms, 30 were not diagnosed with GER. Of those 30 patients, 43% ($n=13/30$) were found to have NEMDs, representing 8% of the entire cohort [168]. In addition to normal esophageal pH, many of those diagnosed demonstrated normal endoscopic appearance and esophageal histology; thus clinical findings (i.e., food impaction) are of great significance with regard to NEMDs [168]. Palliative treatment interventions for NEMDs usually involve antispasmodic agents, prokinetics, antacids (when GER is present), and/or PPIs [118, 120]. Improvement with these methods is variable; some patients may even improve without pharmacologic intervention [168].

References

1. Kahrilas PJ, et al. Upper esophageal spincter function during deglutition. Gastroenterology. 1988;95(1):52–62.
2. Sivarao DV, Goyal RK. Functional anatomy and physiology of the upper esophageal sphincter. Am J Med. 2000;108(Suppl 4a):27S–37.
3. Kuo B, Urma D. Esophagus—anatomy and development. In: Goyal RK, Shaker R, editors. Goyal and Shaker's GI Motility Online. New York: Nature Publishing Group; 2006.
4. Miller MJ, Kiatchoosakun P. Relationship between respiratory control and feeding in the developing infant. Semin Neonatol. 2004;9(3):221–7.
5. Holloway RH. Esophageal body motor response to reflux events: secondary peristalsis. Am J Med. 2000;108(Suppl 4a):20S–6.
6. Passaretti S, et al. Standards for oseophageal manometry. A position statement from the gruppo italinao di studio motilita apparato digerente (gismad). Dig Liver Dis. 2000;32(1):46–56.
7. Katz P, Menin R, Gideon R. Utility and standards in esophageal manometry. J Clin Gastroenterol. 2008;42(5):620–6.
8. Chitkara DK, Fortunado C, Nurko S. Prolonged monitoring of esophageal motor function in healthy children. J Pediatr Gastroenterol Nutr. 2004;38(2):192–7.
9. Tutuian R, et al. Symptom and function heterogenicity among patients with distal esophageal spam: studies using combined impedance-manometry. Am J Gastroenterol. 2006;101:464–9.
10. Gideon R. Manometry: technical issues. Gastrointest Endosc Clin N Am. 2005;15(2):243–55.
11. Bremner RM, et al. Normal esophageal body function: a study using ambulatory esophageal monometry. Am J Gastroenterol. 1998;93:183–7.

12. Pursnani K, et al. Comparison of lower oesophageal sphincter pressure measurement using circumferential vs unidirectional transducers. Neurogastroenterol Motil. 1997;9(3):177–80.
13. Russo S, et al. Videofluorography swallow study of patients with systemic sclerosis. Gastrointest Radiol. 2009;114:948–59.
14. Fordham LA. Imaging of the esophagus in children. Radiol Clin North Am. 2005;43(2):283–302.
15. Levine MS, Rubesine SE, Laufer I. Barium esophagography: a study for all seasons. Clin Gastroenterol Hepatol. 2008;6(1):11–25.
16. Summerton SL. Radiographic evaluation of esophageal function. Gastrointest Endosc Clin N Am. 2005;15(2):231–42.
17. Schima W, et al. Esophageal motor disorders: videofluoroscopic and manometric evaluation-prospective study in 88 symptomatic patients. Radiology. 1992;185:487–91.
18. Mariani G, et al. Radionucleotide gastroesophageal motor studies. J Nucl Med. 2004;15(2):231–42.
19. Iascone C, et al. Use of radiographic esophageal transit in the assessment of patients with symptoms of reflux and non-specific esophageal motor disorders. Dis Esophagus. 2004;17(3):218–22.
20. Imam H, et al. Bolus transit patterns in healthy subjects: a study using simultaneous impedance monitoring, videoesophagram, and esophageal manometry. Am J Physiol Gastrointest Liver Physiol. 2005;288(5):G1000–6.
21. Brednoord AJ, et al. Technology review: esophageal impedance monitoring. Am J Gastroenterol. 2007;102(1):187–94.
22. Bredneoord AJ, Smout AJ. Esophageal motility testing: impedance-based transit measurement and high-resolution manomotry. Gastroenterol Clin North Am. 2008;37(4):775–91.
23. Tutuian R, Castell DO. Esophageal function testing: role of combined multichannel intraluminal impedance and manometry. Gastrointest Endosc Clin N Am. 2005;4:265–75.
24. Savarino E, Tutuian R. Combined multichannel intraluminal impedance and manometry testing. Dig Liver Dis. 2008;40(3):167–73.
25. Glassman MS, et al. Spectrum of esophageal disorders in children with chest pain. Dig Dis Sci. 1992;37(5):663–6.
26. Prasse JE, Kikano GE. An overview of pediatric dysphagia. Clin Pediatr. 2009;48(3):247–51.
27. Lawal A, Shaker R. Esophageal dysphagia. Phys Med Rehabil Clin N Am. 2008;19:729–45.
28. Lefton-Greif MA. Pediatric dysphagia. Phys Med Rehabil Clin N Am. 2008;19(4):837–51.
29. Berezin S, et al. Chest pain of gastrointestinal origin. Arch Dis Child. 1988;63:1457–60.
30. Eslick GD. Classification, natural history, epidemiology, and risk factors of noncardiac chest pain. Dis Mon. 2008;54(9):593–603.
31. Webb WA. Management of foreign bodies of the upper gastrointestinal tract: update. Gastrointest Endosc. 1995;41(1):39–51.
32. Macpherson RI, et al. Esophageal foreign bodies in children: diagnosis, treatment, and complications. Am J Roentgenol. 1996;166:919–24.
33. Ghosh SK, et al. Oesophageal peristaltic transition zone defects: real but few and far between. Neurogastroenterol Motil. 2008;20(12):1283–90.
34. Sadowski DC, et al. Achalasia: incidence, prevalence and survival. A population-based study. Neurogastroenterol Motil. 2010;22(9):256–61.
35. Mayberry JF, Mayell MJ. Epidemiological study of achalasia in children. Gut. 1988;29(1):90–3.
36. Myers NA, Jolley SG, Taylor R. Achalasia of the cardia in children: a worldwide survey. J Pediatr Surg. 1994;29(10):1375–9.
37. Asch MJ, et al. Esophageal achalasia: diagnosis and cardiomyotomy in a newborn infant. J Pediatr Surg. 1974;9(6):911–2.
38. Kraichely RE, Farrugia G. Achalasia: physiology and etiopathogenesis. Dis Esophagus. 2006;19(4):213–23.
39. Goldblum JR, Rice TW, Richter JE. Histopathologic features in esophagomyotomy specimens from patients with achalasia. Gastroenterology. 1996;111(3):648–54.
40. Bohl J, et al. Childhood achalasia: a separate entity? Z Gastroenterol. 2007;45(12):1273–80.
41. Herbella FA, Oliveira DR, Del Grande JC. Are idiopathic and Chagasic achalasia two different diseases? Dig Dis Sci. 2004;49(3):353–60.
42. Wallace RA. Clinical audit of gastrointestinal conditions occurring among adults with Down syndrome attending a specialist clinic. J Intellect Dev Disabil. 2007;32(1):45–50.
43. Kelly JL, et al. Coexistent Hirschsprung's disease and esophageal achalasia in male siblings. J Pediatr Surg. 1997;32(12):1809–11.
44. Kimber J, et al. Allgrove or 4 "A" syndrome: an autosomal recessive syndrome causing multisystem neurological disease. J Neurol Neurosurg Psychiatry. 2003;74(5):654–7.
45. Brooks AS, et al. Homozygous nonsense mutations in KIAA1279 are associated with malformations of the central and enteric nervous systems. Am J Hum Genet. 2005;77(1):120–6.
46. Khelif K, et al. Achalasia of the cardia in Allgrove's (triple A) syndrome: histopathologic study of 10 cases. Am J Surg Pathol. 2003;27(5):667–72.
47. Moses PL, et al. Antineuronal antibodies in idiopathic achalasia and gastro-oesophageal reflux disease. Gut. 2003;52(5):629–36.
48. Pohl D, Tutuian R. Achalasia: an overview of diagnosis and treatment. J Gastrointestin Liver Dis. 2007;16(3):297–303.
49. Rosen R, Nurko S. Other motor disorders. In: Walker WA, editor. Pediatric gastrointestinal disease. Hamilton: BC Decker Inc; 2004. p. 424–62.
50. Dabritz J, et al. Achalasia mistaken as eating disorders: report of two children and review of the literature. Eur J Gastroenterol Hepatol. 2010;22(7):775–8.

51. Berquist WE, et al. Achalasia: diagnosis, management, and clinical course in 16 children. Pediatrics. 1983;71(5):798–805.
52. Parkman HP, et al. Optimal evaluation of patients with nonobstructive esophageal dysphagia. Manometry, scintigraphy, or videoesophagography? Dig Dis Sci. 1996;41(7):1355–68.
53. Blam ME, et al. Achalasia: a disease of varied and subtle symptoms that do not correlate with radiographic findings. Am J Gastroenterol. 2002;97(8):1916–23.
54. Eckardt AJ, Eckardt VF. Current clinical approach to achalasia. World J Gastroenterol. 2009;15(32):3969–75.
55. Liu W, et al. The pathogenesis of pseudoachalasia: a clinicopathologic study of 13 cases of a rare entity. Am J Surg Pathol. 2002;26(6):784–8.
56. Castell JA, Gideon MR, Castell DO. Esophageal manometry. In: Schuster MM, editor. Atlas of gastrointestinal motilily in health and disease. Hamilton: BC Decker; 2002. p. 69–85.
57. Pandolfino JE, Kahrilas PJ. AGA technical review on the clinical use of esophageal manometry. Gastroenterology. 2005;128(1):209–24.
58. Pandolfino JE, Kwiatek MA, Nealis T. Achalasia: a new clinically relevant classification by high resolution manometry. Gastroenterology. 2008;135:1526–33.
59. Williams VA, Peters JH. Achalasia of the esophagus: a surgical disease. J Am Coll Surg. 2009;208(1):151–62.
60. Jung C, et al. Treatments for pediatric achalasia: Heller myotomy or pneumatic dilatation? Gastroenterol Clin Biol. 2010;34(3):202–8.
61. Vaezi MF, Richter JE. Current therapies for achalasia: comparison and efficacy. J Clin Gastroenterol. 1998;27(1):21–35.
62. Maksimak M, Perlmutter DH, Winter HS. The use of nifedipine for the treatment of achalasia in children. J Pediatr Gastroenterol Nutr. 1986;5(6):883–6.
63. Efrati Y, et al. Radionuclide esophageal emptying and long-acting nitrates (Nitroderm) in childhood achalasia. J Pediatr Gastroenterol Nutr. 1996;23(3):312–5.
64. Smith H, et al. The use of nifedipine for treatment of achalasia in children. J Pediatr Gastroenterol Nutr. 1988;7(1):146.
65. Pasricha PJ, et al. Treatment of achalasia with intrasphincteric injection of botulinum toxin. A pilot trial. Ann Intern Med. 1994;121(8):590–1.
66. Pasricha PJ, et al. Intrasphincteric botulinum toxin for the treatment of achalasia. N Engl J Med. 1995;332(12):774–8.
67. Pasricha PJ, et al. Botulinum toxin for achalasia: long-term outcome and predictors of response. Gastroenterology. 1996;110(5):1410–5.
68. Khoshoo V, LaGarde DC, Udall Jr JN. Intrasphincteric injection of Botulinum toxin for treating achalasia in children. J Pediatr Gastroenterol Nutr. 1997;24(4):439–41.
69. Walton JM, Tougas G. Botulinum toxin use in pediatric esophageal achalasia: a case report. J Pediatr Surg. 1997;32(6):916–7.
70. Hurwitz M, et al. Evaluation of the use of botulinum toxin in children with achalasia. J Pediatr Gastroenterol Nutr. 2000;30(5):509–14.
71. Ip KS, et al. Botulinum toxin for achalasia in children. J Gastroenterol Hepatol. 2000;15(10):1100–4.
72. Katzka DA, Castell DO. Use of botulinum toxin as a diagnostic/therapeutic trial to help clarify an indication for definitive therapy in patients with achalasia. Am J Gastroenterol. 1999;94(3):637–42.
73. Smith CD, et al. Endoscopic therapy for achalasia before Heller myotomy results in worse outcomes than Heller myotomy alone. Ann Surg. 2006;243(5):579–84. discussion 584–6.
74. Vantrappen G, Janssens J. To dilate or to operate? That is the question. Gut. 1983;24(11):1013–9.
75. Campos GM, et al. Endoscopic and surgical treatments for achalasia: a systematic review and meta-analysis. Ann Surg. 2009;249(1):45–57.
76. Kadakia SC, Wong RK. Pneumatic balloon dilation for esophageal achalasia. Gastrointest Endosc Clin N Am. 2001;11(2):325–46. vii.
77. West RL, et al. Long term results of pneumatic dilation in achalasia followed for more than 5 years. Am J Gastroenterol. 2002;97(6):1346–51.
78. Chan KC, et al. Short-term and long-term results of endoscopic balloon dilation for achalasia: 12 years' experience. Endoscopy. 2004;36(8):690–4.
79. Karamanolis G, et al. Long-term outcome of pneumatic dilation in the treatment of achalasia. Am J Gastroenterol. 2005;100(2):270–4.
80. Zhao JG, et al. Long-term safety and outcome of a temporary self-expanding metallic stent for achalasia: a prospective study with a 13-year single-center experience. Eur Radiol. 2009;19(8):1973–80.
81. Ali A, Pellegrini CA. Laparoscopic myotomy: technique and efficacy in treating achalasia. Gastrointest Endosc Clin N Am. 2001;11(2):347–58. vii.
82. Patti MG, et al. Comparison of thoracoscopic and laparoscopic Heller myotomy for achalasia. J Gastrointest Surg. 1998;2(6):561–6.
83. Stewart KC, et al. Thoracoscopic versus laparoscopic modified Heller Myotomy for achalasia: efficacy and safety in 87 patients. J Am Coll Surg. 1999;189(2):164–9. discussion 169–70.
84. Spechler SJ. AGA technical review on treatment of patients with dysphagia caused by benign disorders of the distal esophagus. Gastroenterology. 1999;117(1):233–54.
85. Malthaner RA, et al. Long-term results in surgically managed esophageal achalasia. Ann Thorac Surg. 1994;58(5):1343–6. discussion 1346–7.
86. Jara FM, et al. Long-term results of esophagomyotomy for achalasia of esophagus. Arch Surg. 1979;114(8):935–6.
87. Csendes A, et al. Late results of a prospective randomised study comparing forceful dilatation and oesophagomyotomy in patients with achalasia. Gut. 1989;30(3):299–304.
88. Kostic S, et al. Pneumatic dilatation or laparoscopic cardiomyotomy in the management of newly diag-

nosed idiopathic achalasia. Results of a randomized controlled trial. World J Surg. 2007;31(3):470–8.
89. Csendes A, et al. Very late results of esophagomyotomy for patients with achalasia: clinical, endoscopic, histologic, manometric, and acid reflux studies in 67 patients for a mean follow-up of 190 months. Ann Surg. 2006;243(2):196–203.
90. Richards WO, et al. Heller myotomy versus Heller myotomy with Dor fundoplication for achalasia: a prospective randomized double-blind clinical trial. Ann Surg. 2004;240(3):405–12. discussion 412–5.
91. Zerbib F, et al. Repeated pneumatic dilations as long-term maintenance therapy for esophageal achalasia. Am J Gastroenterol. 2006;101(4):692–7.
92. Vela MF, et al. The long-term efficacy of pneumatic dilatation and Heller myotomy for the treatment of achalasia. Clin Gastroenterol Hepatol. 2006;4(5):580–7.
93. Zaninotto G, et al. Four hundred laparoscopic myotomies for esophageal achalasia: a single centre experience. Ann Surg. 2008;248(6):986–93.
94. Jeansonne LO, et al. Ten-year follow-up of laparoscopic Heller myotomy for achalasia shows durability. Surg Endosc. 2007;21(9):1498–502.
95. Lopushinsky SR, Urbach DR. Pneumatic dilatation and surgical myotomy for achalasia. JAMA. 2006;296(18):2227–33.
96. Askegard-Giesmann JR, et al. Minimally invasive Heller's myotomy in children: safe and effective. J Pediatr Surg. 2009;44(5):909–11.
97. Mehra M, et al. Laparoscopic and thoracoscopic esophagomyotomy for children with achalasia. J Pediatr Gastroenterol Nutr. 2001;33(4):466–71.
98. Rothenberg SS, et al. Evaluation of minimally invasive approaches to achalasia in children. J Pediatr Surg. 2001;36(5):808–10.
99. Patti MG, et al. Laparoscopic Heller myotomy and Dor fundoplication for esophageal achalasia in children. J Pediatr Surg. 2001;36(8):1248–51.
100. Litle VR. Laparoscopic Heller myotomy for achalasia: a review of the controversies. Ann Thorac Surg. 2008;85(2):S743–6.
101. Tannuri AC, et al. Laparoscopic extended cardiomyotomy in children: an effective procedure for the treatment of esophageal achalasia. J Pediatr Surg. 2010;45(7):1463–6.
102. Corda L, et al. Laparoscopic oesophageal cardiomyotomy without fundoplication in children with achalasia: a 10-year experience: a retrospective review of the results of laparoscopic oesophageal cardiomyotomy without an anti-reflux procedure in children with achalasia. Surg Endosc. 2010;24(1):40–4.
103. Adikibi BT, et al. Intraoperative upper GI endoscopy ensures an adequate laparoscopic Heller's myotomy. J Laparoendosc Adv Surg Tech A. 2009;19(5):687–9.
104. Jafri M, et al. Intraoperative manometry during laparoscopic Heller myotomy improves outcome in pediatric achalasia. J Pediatr Surg. 2008;43(1):66–70. discussion 70.
105. Tovar JA, et al. Esophageal function in achalasia: preoperative and postoperative manometric studies. J Pediatr Surg. 1998;33(6):834–8.
106. Pensabene L, Nurko S. Approach to the child who has persistent dysphagia after surgical treatment for esophageal achalasia. J Pediatr Gastroenterol Nutr. 2008;47(1):92–7.
107. Zaninotto G, et al. Etiology, diagnosis, and treatment of failures after laparoscopic Heller myotomy for achalasia. Ann Surg. 2002;235(2):186–92.
108. Zaninotto G, et al. Treatment of esophageal achalasia with laparoscopic Heller myotomy and Dor partial anterior fundoplication: prospective evaluation of 100 consecutive patients. J Gastrointest Surg. 2000;4(3):282–9.
109. Zaninotto G, et al. Minimally invasive surgery for esophageal achalasia. J Laparoendosc Adv Surg Tech A. 2001;11(6):351–9.
110. Sandler RS, et al. The risk of esophageal cancer in patients with achalasia. A population-based study. JAMA. 1995;274(17):1359–62.
111. Dunaway PM, Wong RK. Risk and surveillance intervals for squamous cell carcinoma in achalasia. Gastrointest Endosc Clin N Am. 2001;11(2):425–34. ix.
112. Zendehdel K, et al. Risk of esophageal adenocarcinoma in achalasia patients, a retrospective cohort study in Sweden. Am J Gastroenterol. 2011;106(1):57–61.
113. Brucher BL, et al. Achalasia and esophageal cancer: incidence, prevalence, and prognosis. World J Surg. 2001;25(6):745–9.
114. Leeuwenburgh I, et al. Long-term esophageal cancer risk in patients with primary achalasia: a prospective study. Am J Gastroenterol. 2010;105(10):2144–9.
115. Eckardt VF, Hoischen T, Bernhard G. Life expectancy, complications, and causes of death in patients with achalasia: results of a 33-year follow-up investigation. Eur J Gastroenterol Hepatol. 2008;20(10):956–60.
116. Fontan JP, et al. Esophageal spasm associated with apnea and bradycardia in an infant. Pediatrics. 1984;73(1):52–5.
117. Sperandio M, et al. Diffuse esophageal spasm: not diffuse but distal esophageal spasm (des). Dig Dis Sci. 2003;48(7):1380–4.
118. Smout AJ. Advances in esophageal motor disorder. Curr Opin Gastroenterol. 2008;24:285–9.
119. Tutuian R, Castell DO. Review article: oesophageal spasm-diagnosis and management. Aliment Pharmacol Ther. 2006;23(10):1393–402.
120. Adler DG, Romero Y. Primary esophageal motility disorders. Mayo Clin Proc. 2001;76(2):195–200.
121. Grubel C, et al. Diffuse esophageal spasm. Am J Gastroenterol. 2008;103:450–7.
122. Rosen J, et al. Diffuse esophageal spasm in children (abstract). J Pediatr Gastroenterol Nutr. 2005;41(4):561.
123. Hussain SZ, Di Lorenzo C. Motility disorders. Diagnosis and treatment for the pediatric patient. Pediatr Clin North Am. 2002;49(1):27–51.

124. Herbella FAM, et al. Primary versus secondary esophageal motility disorders: diagnosis and implications for treatment. J Laparoendosc Adv Surg Tech A. 2009;19(2):195–8.
125. Allen ML, DiMarino AJ. Manometric diagnosis of diffuse esophageal spasm. Dig Dis Sci. 1996;41(7):1346–9.
126. Lacy BE, Weiser K. Esophageal motility disorders: medical therapy. J Clin Gastroenterol. 2008;2(5):652–8.
127. Putnam PE. Eosinophilic esophagitis in children: clinical manifestations. Gastroenterol Clin North Am. 2008;37:369–81.
128. Markowitz JE, Liacouras CA. Eosinophilic esophagitis. Gastroenterol Clin North Am. 2003;32(2003):949–66.
129. Nurko S, Rosen R, Furuta GT. Esophageal dysmotility in children with esoinophilic esophagitis: a study using prolonged esophageal manometery. Am J Gastroenterol. 2009;104:3050–7.
130. Rothenberg ME. Biology and treatment of eosinophilic esophagitis. Gastroenterology. 2009;137:1238–49.
131. Orenstein SR, et al. The spectrum of pediatric eosinophilic esophagitis beyond infancy: a clinical series of 30 children. Am J Gastroenterol. 2000;95:1422–30.
132. Xu X, et al. Mast cells and eosinophils have a potential profibrogenic role in Crohn Disease. Scand J Gastroenterol. 2004;39:440–7.
133. Nurko S, Rosen R. Esophageal dysmotility in patients who have eosinophilic esophagitis. Gastrointest Endosc Clin N Am. 2008;18(1):73–89. ix.
134. Dohil R, et al. Oral viscuous budesonide is effective in children with eosinophilic esophagits in a randomized, placedbo-controlled trail. Gastroenterology. 2010;139:418–29.
135. Hejazi RA, et al. Disturbances of esophageal motility in esoinophilic esophagitis: a case series. Dysphagia. 2010;25:231–7.
136. Zagai U, et al. The effect of eosinophils on collagen gel contraction and implications for tissue remodeling. Clin Exp Immunol. 2004;135:427–33.
137. Straumann A. The natural history and complications fo esoinophilic esophagits. Gastrointest Endosc Clin N Am. 2008;18(1):99–118.
138. Shah A, Hirano I. Treatment of esosinophilic esophagitis: drugs, diet, or dilation? Curr Gastroenterol Rep. 2007;9(3):181–8.
139. Putnam PE. Evaluation of the child who has eosinophilic esophagitis. Immunol Allergy Clin North Am. 2009;29:1–10.
140. Liacouras CA. Eosinophilic esophagitis. Curr Opin Pediatr. 2004;16(5):560–6.
141. Aceves SS, Furuta GT, Spechler SJ. Integrated approach to treatment of children and adults with eosinophilic esophagitis. Gastrointest Endosc Clin N Am. 2008;18:195–217.
142. Ntoumazios SK, et al. Esophageal involvement in scleroderma: gastroesophageal reflux, the common problem. Semin Arthritis Rheum. 2006;36:173–81.
143. Duraj V, et al. Esophageal damages in systemic scleroderma (abstract). Med Arch. 2007;61(1):47–8.
144. Vancheeswaran R, et al. Childhood-onset secleroderma: is it different from adult-onset disease? Arthritis Rheum. 1996;39(6):1041–9.
145. Denton CP, Derrett-Smith EC. Juvenile-onset systemic sclerosis: children are not small adults. Rheumatology. 2008;48:96–7.
146. Foeldvari I, et al. Favourable outcome in 135 children with juvenile systemic sclerosis: results of a multinational survey. Rheumatology. 2000;39:556–9.
147. Weber P, et al. Twenty-four hour intraesophageal pH monitoring in children and adolescents with scleroderma and mixed connective tissue disease (abstract). J Rheumatol. 2000;27(11):2692–5.
148. Gunawardena H, McHugh N. Features and recommended treatment of systemic sclerosis. Prescriber. 2008;19(18):56–65.
149. Hedrich CM, et al. Presentations and treatment of childhood scleroderma: Localized scleroderma, eosinophilic fasciitis, systemic sclerosis, and graft-versus-host disease. Clin Pediatr (Phila). 2011;50(7):604–14.
150. Domsic R, Fasanella K, Bielefeldt K. Gastrointestinal manifestations of systemic sclerosis. Dig Dis Sci. 2008;53:1163–74.
151. Antonucci A, et al. Chronic intestinal pseudo-obstruction. World J Gastroenterol. 2008;14(19):2953–61.
152. Boige N, et al. Manometrical evaluation in visceral neuropathies in children. J Pediatr Gastroenterol Nutr. 1994;19(1):71–7.
153. Panganamamula KV, Parkman HP. Chronic pseudo-obstruction. Curr Treat Options Gastroenterol. 2005;8:3–11.
154. Byrne WJ, et al. Chronic idiopathic intestinal pseudo-obstruction syndrome in children—clinical characteristics and prognosis. J Pediatr. 1977;90(4):585–9.
155. de Lorijn F, Boechxstaens GE, Benninga MA. Symptomatology, pathophysiology, diagnostic work-up, and treatment of Hirschsprung disease in infancy and childhood. Curr Gastroenterol Rep. 2007;9:245–53.
156. Faure C, et al. Duodenal and esophageal manometry in total colonic aganglionosis. J Pediatr Gastroenterol Nutr. 1994;18(2):193–9.
157. Staiano A, et al. Esophageal motility in children with Hirschsprung's disease. Am J Dis Child. 1991;145(3):310–3.
158. Karagiozoglou-Lampoudi T, et al. Conservative management of caustic substance ingestion in a pediatric department setting, short-term and long-term outcome. Dis Esophagus. 2010;2(42):86–91.
159. Sanchez-Ramirez CA, et al. Caustic ingestion and oesophageal damage in children: clinical spectrum and feeding practices. J Pediatr Child Health. 2011;47(6):378–80.

160. Dantas RO, Mamede RC. Esophageal motility in patients with esophageal caustic injury. Am J Gastroenterol. 1996;91(6):1157–61.
161. Genc A, Mutaf O. Esophageal motility changes in acute and late periods of caustic esophageal burns and their relation to prognosis in children. J Pediatr Surg. 2002;37(11):1526–8.
162. Spechler SJ, Castell D. Classification of oesophageal motility abnormalities. Gut. 2001;49:145–51.
163. Mittal KR. Motor and sensory function of the esophagus: revelations through ultrasound imaging. J Clin Gastroenterol. 2005;39 Suppl 2:S42–8.
164. Kim JH, et al. Is all ineffective esophageal motility the same? A clinical and high-frequency intraluminal US study. Gastrointest Endosc. 2008;68:422–31.
165. Botoman VA. How effective are we at understanding ineffective esophageal motility? Gastrointest Endosc. 2008;68(3):432–3.
166. Leite LP, et al. Ineffective esophageal motility (IEM): the primary finding in patients with nonspecific esophageal motility disorder. Dig Dis Sci. 1997;42(9):1859–65.
167. Naftali T, et al. Nonspecific esophageal motility disorders may be an early stage of a specific disorder, particularly achalasia. Dis Esophagus. 2009;22:611–5.
168. Rosario JA, et al. Nonspecific esophageal motility disorders in children without gastroesophageal reflux. J Pediatr Gastroenterol Nutr. 1999;28(5):480–5.

Gastric Motor Disorders: Gastroparesis and Dumping Syndrome

21

Miguel Saps and Ashish Chogle

Introduction

Normal gastrointestinal function relies on the coordinated action of motor, sensory, digestive, secretory and excretory function. Coordinated motility is essential for the orderly digestion, absorption, and elimination of waste. Adequate gastrointestinal motility requires integration of the autonomic nervous system (intrinsic and extrinsic sympathetic and parasympathetic nerves), neurotransmitters, and enteric smooth muscle cells. Sensory extrinsic neurons respond to various stimuli, including the presence of food in the gastrointestinal tract by triggering complex reflex mechanisms with final effectors in the smooth muscle cells in the gut wall, blood vessels, and glandular cells. Alterations at any level of these complex processes may result in altered motility.

M. Saps, M.D.
Pediatric Gastorenterology, Hepatology and Nutrition Division, Pediatrics Department, Children's Memorial Hospital, Northwestern University, Chicago, IL, USA

A. Chogle, M.D., M.P.H. (✉)
Division of Gastroenterology, Hepatology and Nutrition, Children's Memorial Hospital, 2300 Children's Plaza, Box 65, Chicago, IL 60614-3363, USA
e-mail: achogle@childrensmemorial.org

Gastroparesis

Gastroparesis is a gastric motor disorder characterized by delayed emptying of gastric contents into the duodenum in the absence of mechanical obstruction. The pathogenesis and pathophysiology of gastroparesis are often complex and poorly understood. Multiple processes affecting the extrinsic motor neurons, enteric motor neurons, interstitial cells of Cajal, and smooth-muscle cells may lead to altered physiological mechanisms resulting in gastroparesis. Pathophysiological mechanisms vary and include exaggerated relaxation of the fundus, poor antral contractility, uncoordinated antro-pyloro-duodenal function and persistent pylorospasm. The pathophysiological mechanisms and etiological agents involved in development of gastroparesis are sometimes identified but it is not infrequent that despite thorough diagnostic studies the etiologic causes and pathophysiological mechanisms of gastroparesis remain unknown. Gastroparesis may present with a variety of symptoms including early satiety, bloating, abdominal discomfort or pain, anorexia, halitosis, nausea, and vomiting of "old" undigested food and weight loss but can also be paucisymptomatic or asymptomatic. Diagnosis is based on the clinical presentation, exclusion of other causes of persistent vomiting, and the objective demonstration of delayed gastric emptying (Fig. 21.1). Etiological factors (Table 21.1) associated with gastroparesis vary with the child's age.

C. Faure et al. (eds.), *Pediatric Neurogastroenterology: Gastrointestinal Motility and Functional Disorders in Children*, Clinical Gastroenterology,
DOI 10.1007/978-1-60761-709-9_21, © Springer Science+Business Media New York 2013

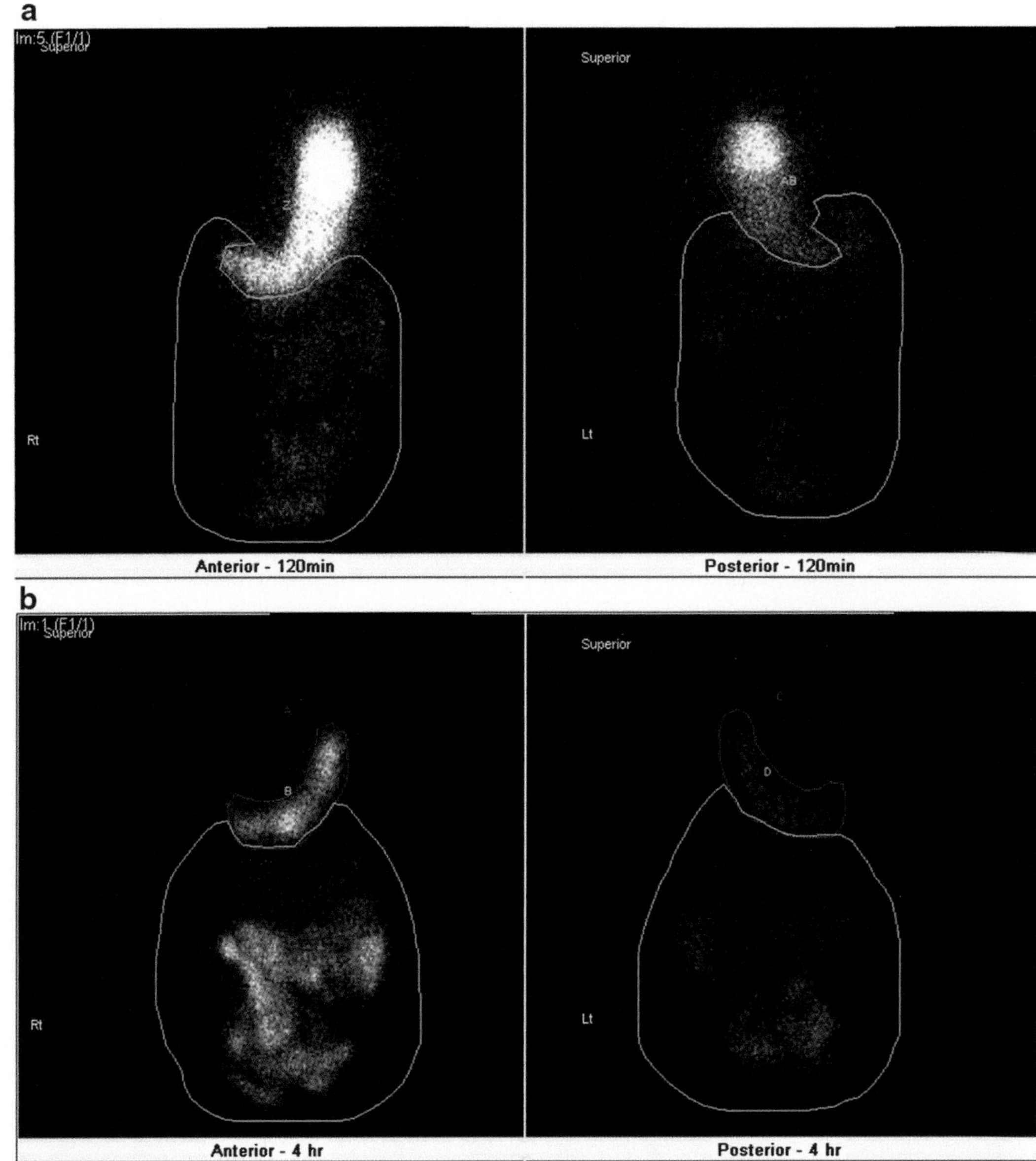

Fig. 21.1 Gastric emptying scan showing delayed gastric emptying with greater than 60% and 10% Tc 99 m sulfur colloid activity in the stomach at 2 and 4 h respectively

Immaturity

Gastric electrical and motor activity matures with gestational age [1, 2]. Extreme preterm birth is associated with immature gastric function. Premature neonates may present transient manifestations of intestinal ileus that mimic intestinal pseudo-obstruction. A case series reported abdominal distension, dilated loops of bowel throughout the abdomen without evidence of obstruction and failure to pass stools in seven infants with an average gestational age of 30 weeks that recovered after several weeks [3]. Mature patterns of motor contractile activity are only achieved in late stages of gestation. Normal gastric electrical rhythm and mature patterns of gastric liquid emptying have been shown in infants of 32 weeks of gestational age [1]. Normal

Table 21.1 Etiology of gastroparesis in children

Idiopathic
Post-infectious
Rotavirus
EBV
CMV
Norwalk virus
Parvo-virus like agents
Mycoplasma
Borellia
Postsurgical
Thoracic and abdominal surgeries
Vagotomy
Partial gastrectomy
Metabolic
Diabetes mellitus type I
Hypothyroidism
Hyperthyroidism
Hyperparathyroidism
Addison's disease
Hypopituitarism
Chronic renal failure
Amyloidosis
Immune/inflammatory
Cow milk protein allergy
Eosinophilic gastroenteropathy
Celiac disease
Crohn's disease
Autoimmune dysautonomia
Drug induced
Anticholinergics
Opioids
Tricyclic antidepressants
Proton-pump inhibitors
H2 receptors antagonists
Antacids
Diphenhydramine
Sucralfate
Octreotide
Beta-adrenergic agonists
Calcium channel blockers
Levodopa
Other
GERD
Hirschsprung's disease
Neuronal intestinal dysplasia
Peripheral neuropathies
Mitochondrial disorders
CNS or other chronic illnesses
Caustic ingestions
Radiation
Portal hypertension
Marijuana consumption

gastric motility is fully developed by 34 weeks of gestational age [4]. Gastric electrical activity progressively acquires the adult pattern in the first decade of life [5]. Small enteral feedings lead to a rapid increase in motility, digestion, and absorptive capacity of the immature gastrointestinal tract [6]. Early life experiences including environmental and nociceptive factors affecting the digestive tract and airway may delay postnatal gastro-enteric motor maturation.

Post-Infectious

Post-infectious gastroparesis is common in children [7]. Multiple pathologic agents including rotavirus, EBV, CMV, Norwalk virus, parvo-virus like agents, mycoplasma, and Lyme disease have been associated with gastroparesis in children [7–9]. Symptoms usually present days or months following an acute intercurrent illness. Consultation is often late and the etiologic agents are rarely isolated. Post-viral gastroparesis in children is transient and tends to resolve spontaneously over several months. Follow-up studies of children diagnosed with post-infectious gastroparesis have shown resolution of symptoms in 6 months to 2 years in all cases [7, 9].

Peripheral Neuropathies

Peripheral neuropathies may involve different nerve groups. A subgroup of these patients manifests with a more prominent and selective involvement of the autonomic nervous system. Some of these patients can have an identifiable cause such as diabetes, amyloidosis, or inherited autonomic neuropathy while others have no identifiable cause and are considered as having an *idiopathic autonomic neuropathy*.

Diabetes Mellitus

Diabetes as a cause of gastroparesis is commonly reported in adults but rarely investigated in children. The pathophysiology of diabetic gastroparesis is multifactorial and includes hyperglycemia, electrolyte imbalances, vagal parasympathetic dysfunction, loss of neuronal nitric oxide expression and enteric neurons, gastric smooth muscle abnormalities, and disruption of interstitial cells of Cajal [10–14]. Antral hypomotility is the most common motor abnormality in children with IDDM [15–18]. Gastric electrical dysrhythmias, gastrointestinal symptoms and delayed gastric emptying have been demonstrated in diabetic children few years after diagnosis [15, 17]. A study in children with IDDM and gastrointestinal complaints has shown that autonomic neuropathy was not an etiological factor of gastrointestinal symptoms in this group of children [19]. Glycemic control and delayed gastric emptying are closely related. Gastroparesis can contribute to worsening glycemic control due to the slow and erratic gastric emptying while blood glucose levels measured 180 min after meals have been correlated with prolonged gastric emptying time [15]. The study has also shown a significant increase in gastric electrical dysrhythmias in diabetic children compared with healthy controls. Gastrointestinal symptoms, delayed gastric emptying have been reported in children within 1–7 years of onset of IDDM [17]. A study on 40 consecutive children diagnosed with insulin-dependent diabetes mellitus (IDDM) 5 years prior to the study has shown delayed gastric emptying time in 2/3 of children [15]. Children with IDDM have lower serum motilin concentrations compared with healthy control [19]. A study in children with IDDM has shown improvement in gastrointestinal symptoms, gastric emptying function, and better glycemic control with the use of erythromycin [17].

Autoimmune Neuropathy

Autoimmune gastrointestinal dysmotility is a limited form of autoimmune dysautonomia. It usually presents with subacute onset of autonomic dysfunction, unexplained nausea and vomiting and confirmed gastroparesis sometimes associated with a previous illness (possibly infectious) [20]. Most of these cases are now considered within the spectrum of *autoimmune autonomic neuropathy* and specifically as *autoimmune autonomic ganglionopathy*. The spectrum of autoimmune autonomic disorders is broad and patients can have presence of one or more autoantibodies and localized or generalized gastrointestinal dysmotility and dysautonomic manifestations. Patients typically present with gastroparesis, constipation, abnormal pupillary light response, anhidrosis, marked dry eyes and dry mouth (sicca complex), neurogenic bladder, and orthostatic hypotension that usually reach peak autonomic failure within 3 months [21]. More commonly, autoantibodies related gastrointestinal dysmotility disorders are limited to specific areas and may manifest as isolated foregut dysmotility such as achalasia, esophageal dysmotility or pyloric stenosis. Symptoms may include dysphagia, odynophagia, early satiety, postprandial epigastric discomfort, nausea, vomiting, unexplained weight loss with malnutrition, abdominal pain, and intractable constipation or diarrhea. High titers of antibodies specific for the neuronal ganglionic nicotinic acetylcholine receptor (nAChR) are frequently found in patients with severe forms of *autoimmune autonomic ganglionopathy* [22]. A decrease in antibody titers is frequently associated with improved autonomic function. Gastrointestinal dysmotilities associated with dysautonomia have been reported in patients with anti-neuronal nuclear autoantibody, type 1 (ANNA-1, "anti-Hu") and other neuronal voltage-gated cation channel antibodies (voltage-gated calcium channels (VGCCs), voltage-gated potassium channels (VGKCs), glutamic acid decarboxylase (GAD)) [23, 24]. Autoimmune gastrointestinal dysmotility disorders may sometimes be part of paraneoplastic syndromes. No cases of autoimmune autonomic neuropathy have been published in children, however cation channel antibodies have been found in some unpublished cases in adolescents with gastrointestinal dysmotility. Autoimmune gastrointestinal dysmotility can also be associated other autoantibodies and autoimmune disorders (diabetes, lupus, Raynaud, hypothyroidism, and pernicious anemia). Approximately half of the patients in one study had coexistence of plasma membrane cation channel autoantibodies with antibody markers of organ-specific autoimmunity (skeletal muscle striational, GAD65, thyroid or gastric parietal cell specificities) [23].

Hirschsprung's Disease

A study on adults with a history of *Hirschsprung's disease*, neuronal intestinal dysplasia or hypoganglionosis found abnormal esophageal, gastric and gut motility in 2 of 12 cases studied [25]. A study on 21 children who underwent GI transit time study and a scintigraphic gastric emptying test several years after surgery showed delayed gastric emptying in 57% of patients and prolonged total gastrointestinal time in patients with a history of Hirschsprung's disease compared with healthy controls suggesting that gastrointestinal dysmotility persists long after surgical correction [26, 27].

Central Nervous System Disorders

Children with *central nervous system disorders* and other chronic illnesses have been shown to have a high incidence of gastric dysrhythmias and gastroparesis with abnormal antroduodenal motility [28–30]. Foregut dysmotility including esophageal dysmotility, and delayed gastric emptying is frequent in children with central nervous system disorders [31].

Gastroparesis may occur as part of a mitochondrial disorder. Studies have identified accumulation of mitochondrial A3243G mutation in the stomach in a group of patients with gastric dysmotility and gastric symptoms and a leukocytic point mutation of mitochondrial DNA at nucleotide position 3243 [32]. Mitochondrial encephalomyopathy with lactic acidosis and stroke-like episodes (MELAS) is characterized by the involvement of skeletal muscle and central nervous system and occasional urinary or gastrointestinal symptoms. An A-to-G point mutation at position 3243 of mitochondrial DNA was found in patients with MELAS [33].

Myopathies

Autoimmune disorders of the connective tissue such as polymyositis and dermatomyositis are characterized by inflammation and degeneration of muscle. Both inflammatory myopathies are frequently associated with delayed gastric and esophageal emptying secondary to malfunction of the smooth muscle of the upper gastrointestinal tract. Gastric and esophageal dysfunctions correlate with the severity of the peripheral skeletal muscle weakness [34].

Postsurgical

Gastroparesis often develops after upper abdominal and thoracic surgeries and is frequently associated with injury of the vagal nerve. Increases in intragastric volumes, impaired proximal gastric responses to meals and to balloon insufflation, and heightened perception of gastric distention also have been observed after vagotomy [35]. The exact mechanisms responsible for *postsurgical gastroparesis* remain unclear but are likely to be multifactorial. Abnormalities of antral peristalsis and fundic tone are demonstrable in patients with postsurgical gastroparesis. In one study, eight of nine patients with gastroparesis had no fasting motor activity, whereas asymptomatic postoperative controls exhibited normal migrating motor complex activity [36]. Intestinal manipulation leading to mast cells degranulation and altered bowel motility has been proposed as an important pathophysiological mechanism of postoperative dysmotility. A randomized placebo controlled study showed that the administration of mast cell stabilizers such as ketotifen prior to the surgery prevented the inflammatory response, and the development of postoperative gastroparesis [37]. Symptoms of postsurgical gastroparesis secondary to vagal injury gradually improve with time possibly due to the ability of the enteric nervous system to adapt to the loss of vagal input or occurrence of vagal reinnervation [38].

Immune and Inflammatory

Food Allergy

Electrographic studies have shown severe gastric dysrhythmias in infants with *cow's milk protein allergy* [28]. Measurement of gastric half-emptying time by electrical impedance tomography has shown delayed gastric emptying in children sensitized to cow's milk. Gastroesophageal reflux and cow's milk allergy frequently coexist in infants. Delayed gastric emptying and gastric cardiac distension associated with cow's milk protein allergy may elicit transient relaxations of the lower esophageal sphincter (tLESR) through vagally mediated reflexes worsening gastroesophageal reflux symptoms.

A study on a murine model of eosinophilic gastrointestinal inflammation has shown eosinophilic infiltration in close proximity to damaged enteric nerves [39]. Similar findings were described in humans. Electrogastrographic changes, mast cell degranulation in proximity to the gastric nerve fibers were found in patients exhibiting a positive food challenge [40]. Although the mechanism remains unclear, it has been proposed that the release of the major basic protein by eosinophils may induce muscarinic receptor dysfunction, alteration of smooth muscle contraction leading to gastric dysmotility and delayed gastric emptying [41].

Celiac Disease and Inflammatory Bowel Diseases

Celiac disease is frequently associated with gastrointestinal dysmotility. Patients will celiac disease often present delayed esophageal, gastric and small intestinal transit time and accelerated colonic transit [42]. A study comparing antro-duodeno-jejunal motility of untreated celiac disease patients, celiac patients on a gluten-free diet and healthy controls showed upper gut motor abnormalities in 80% of untreated celiac patients [43]. Gastric emptying rate of solids is delayed in patients with untreated celiac disease while prolonged gluten withdrawal normalizes gastric emptying time in all celiac disease patients [44]. A case series of five patients with clinically inactive inflammatory bowel disease and persistent symptoms of nausea, vomiting and weight loss in the absence of strictures have shown evidence of upper gut dysmotility. A study on gastric emptying in adult patients with nonobstructive *Crohn's disease*, revealed slow gastric emptying in a subgroup of symptomatic patients who complained of bloating, early satiety, and abdominal distention [45].

Gastroesophageal Reflux and Functional Dyspepsia

Studies have shown that delayed gastric emptying may play a role in the pathophysiology of gastroesophageal reflux in a subgroup of children. Gastric emptying rate in children older than 6 years, suffering from gastroesophageal reflux was shown to be significantly delayed as compared to normal children older than 6 years. No delay was observed in children younger than 3 years [46]. Thus gastroparesis could be a contributory factor in the pathophysiology of gastroesophageal reflux in older children. Gastric motor disorders and characteristic motility patterns may be present in functional gastrointestinal disorders such as functional dyspepsia and rumination. An in-depth discussion of these disorders can be found in other sections of this book.

Other

Gastroparesis is a recognized complication of other *endocrine disorders* such as hypothyroidism, hyperthyroidism, hyperparathyroidism, Addison's disease and hypopituitarism. Fifty percent of critically ill patients exhibit severe gastroparesis [41, 47]. In these patients, gastroparesis can be explained by the elevation of fasting and nutrient stimulated CCK and PYY and suppression of fasting ghrelin [48, 49].

Caustic ingestion was also shown to lead to delayed liquid gastric emptying even in the absence of symptoms [50]. Various *drugs* including anticholinergics, opioids, tricyclic antidepressants, proton-pump inhibitors, H2 receptors antagonists, diphenhydramine, antacids, sucralfate, octreotide, beta-adrenergic agonists, calcium channel blockers, and levodopa among others may delay gastric emptying [51–53]. Even after thorough diagnostic studies the etiologic causes and pathophysiological mechanisms of gastroparesis frequently remain unknown.

Marijuana consumption slows down motility and delays gastric emptying. Cannabinoid receptors are expressed in the enteric nervous system. Cannabinoid signaling modulates synaptic activity in the nervous system. Activation of CB1 receptors on myenteric neurons results in presynaptic depression inhibiting neuronal activity, synaptic transmission, and axonal mitochondrial transport [54, 55].

Treatment

Treatment of gastroparesis include dietary and lifestyle modifications, prokinetics agents, intrapyloric injection of botulinum toxin, and gastric electrical stimulation, an intervention that although does not consistently improve emptying has been shown to help alleviate symptoms and improve quality of life. Diagnostic testing and specific treatment modalities of gastric motility disorders are covered in other chapters of this book.

Dumping Syndrome

Dumping syndrome is characterized by the onset of gastrointestinal and vasomotor symptoms following the ingestion of a meal. The underlying gastrointestinal motor abnormality in dumping syndrome is acceleration of gastric emptying leading to fluid shifts and changes in glucose homeostasis. Early symptoms comprise both gastrointestinal and vasomotor symptoms. Gastrointestinal symptoms include abdominal pain, diarrhea, borborygmi, nausea and bloating. Vasomotor symptoms consist of fatigue, a desire to lie down after meals, facial flushing, palpitations, perspiration tachycardia, hypotension and syncope. The rapid emptying of hyperosmolar contents into the small intestine results in a fluid shift from the intravascular compartment into the intestinal lumen, leading to small bowel distention. This initiates release of various humoral and neural mediators and increased intestinal contractility [56]. The administration of intravenous fluids does not prevent clinical manifestations of early dumping syndrome [57]. Late dumping occurs 1–2 h after a meal and is characterized predominantly by systemic vascular symptoms, including hypoglycemia, perspiration, palpitations, hunger, fatigue, confusion, aggression, tremor, and syncope. Physical examination may reveal orthostatic changes, including a fall in blood pressure and increased heart rate. The rapid delivery of gastric contents to the small bowel leads to the rapid absorption of glucose into the circulation and hyperglycemia, which subsequently stimulates the rapid release of insulin followed by reactive hypoglycemia [56]. Uncontrolled severe dumping can result in the fear of food or eating and subsequent weight loss. Clinical manifestations of one or both of these phases may be present in each patient. It is estimated that manifestations of early phases of dumping occur in 75% of all affected patients [58]. Dumping syndrome may be seen after surgical procedures such as esophagectomy, gastrectomy, vagotomy with pyloroplasty, bariatric surgery, and fundoplication. It has been reported to occur in up to 30% of children undergoing anti-reflux surgery [59]. In a recent study, 35% adult patients with cyclic vomiting syndrome, 13% with diabetes mellitus and 10% with irritable bowel syndrome were found to have dumping syndrome [60]. A provocative test for assessing dumping syndrome can be used to confirm clinical suspicion. This test is a modification of the oral glucose tolerance test and involves the ingestion of 50 g or 75 g glucose in solution after an overnight fast. Immediately before and up to 180 min after ingestion of this solution, the blood glucose concentration, hematocrit, pulse rate, and blood pressure are measured at 30 min intervals. The provocative test is considered positive if late (120–180 min) hypoglycemia occurs, or if an early (30 min) increase in hematocrit of more than 3% occurs. The best predictor of dumping syndrome seems to be a rise in the pulse rate of more than 10 beats per minute after 30 min [61]. Assessments of gastric emptying might show that this process occurs rapidly in patients with dumping syndrome—especially for liquid nutrients—but this test does not seem to have good diagnostic sensitivity or specificity, probably because rapid emptying occurs early after meal ingestion, a phase that is not analyzed closely or separately in many protocols of gastric emptying testing [61, 62].

Treatment of dumping syndrome includes lifestyle modifications and dietary measures. Dietary recommendations include eating smaller portions by dividing the recommended daily energy intake between six meals, increasing the viscosity of food by adding uncooked cornstarch, guar gum, or pectin to the meals and delaying liquid intake up to 30 min after the meal [63]. Readily absorbable carbohydrates should be minimized in the diet to prevent late dumping. Patients are advised to lie down for at least 30 min after meals to decrease gastric emptying and prevent symptoms of hypovolemia. Use of acarbose is recommended in patients with manifestations of late dumping, as it interferes with carbohydrate absorption in the small intestine and has been shown to improve glucose tolerance and reduce hypoglycemia [64]. Acarbose inhibits the α-glycosidase-mediated production of monosaccharides from carbohydrates in the epithelial brush border cells of the small intestine. Acarbose, given three times daily at 50–100 mg doses to patients with dumping syndrome, showed an improvement in glucose tolerance, a decreased release of gastrointestinal hormones and a reduction in the incidence of hypoglycemia [64–67]. Octreotide has been reported to be beneficial in patients with dumping syndrome who fail to respond to dietary measures. Octreotide delays gastric emptying and small bowel transit, inhibits the release of gastrointestinal hormones, delays monosaccharide absorption, decreases insulin secretion, and prevents hemodynamic changes [68, 69]. Surgical re-intervention or continuous enteral feeding may be considered in refractory cases.

References

1. Cucchiara S, et al. Gestational maturation of electrical activity of the stomach. Dig Dis Sci. 1999;44(10):2008–13.
2. Riezzo G, et al. Gastric electrical activity and gastric emptying in term and preterm newborns. Neurogastroenterol Motil. 2000;12(3):223–9.
3. Lamireau T, et al. Transient intestinal pseudo-obstruction syndrome in premature infants. Arch Fr Pediatr. 1993;50(4):301–6.
4. Riezzo G, et al. Maturation of gastric electrical activity, gastric emptying and intestinal permeability in preterm newborns during the first month of life. Ital J Pediatr. 2009;35(1):6.
5. Cheng W, Tam PK. Gastric electrical activity normalises in the first decade of life. Eur J Pediatr Surg. 2000;10(5):295–9.
6. Owens L, Burrin DG, Berseth CL. Minimal enteral feeding induces maturation of intestinal motor function but not mucosal growth in neonatal dogs. J Nutr. 2002;132(9):2717–22.
7. Sigurdsson L, et al. Postviral gastroparesis: presentation, treatment, and outcome. J Pediatr. 1997;131(5):751–4.
8. Huang S, et al. Mycoplasma infections and different human carcinomas. World J Gastroenterol. 2001;7(2):266–9.
9. Naftali T, et al. Post-infectious gastroparesis: clinical and electrogastrographic aspects. J Gastroenterol Hepatol. 2007;22(9):1423–8.
10. Horvath VJ, Vittal H, Ordog T. Reduced insulin and IGF-I signaling, not hyperglycemia, underlies the diabetes-associated depletion of interstitial cells of Cajal in the murine stomach. Diabetes. 2005;54(5):1528–33.
11. James AN, et al. Regional gastric contractility alterations in a diabetic gastroparesis mouse model: effects of cholinergic and serotoninergic stimulation. Am J Physiol Gastrointest Liver Physiol. 2004;287(3):G612–9.
12. Keshavarzian A, Iber FL, Vaeth J. Gastric emptying in patients with insulin-requiring diabetes mellitus. Am J Gastroenterol. 1987;82(1):29–35.
13. Shah V, et al. Nitric oxide in gastrointestinal health and disease. Gastroenterology. 2004;126(3):903–13.
14. Takahashi T, et al. Impaired intracellular signal transduction in gastric smooth muscle of diabetic BB/W rats. Am J Physiol. 1996;270(3 Pt 1):G411–7.
15. Cucchiara S, et al. Gastric emptying delay and gastric electrical derangement in IDDM. Diabetes Care. 1998;21(3):438–43.
16. Franzese A, et al. Domperidone is more effective than cisapride in children with diabetic gastroparesis. Aliment Pharmacol Ther. 2002;16(5):951–7.
17. Reid B, et al. Diabetic gastroparesis due to postprandial antral hypomotility in childhood. Pediatrics. 1992;90(1 Pt 1):43–6.
18. White NH, et al. Reversal of neuropathic and gastrointestinal complications related to diabetes mellitus in adolescents with improved metabolic control. J Pediatr. 1981;99(1):41–5.
19. Vazeou A, et al. Autonomic neuropathy and gastrointestinal motility disorders in children and adolescents with type 1 diabetes mellitus. J Pediatr Gastroenterol Nutr. 2004;38(1):61–5.

20. Lobrano A, et al. Postinfectious gastroparesis related to autonomic failure: a case report. Neurogastroenterol Motil. 2006;18(2):162–7.
21. Klein CM, et al. The spectrum of autoimmune autonomic neuropathies. Ann Neurol. 2003;53(6):752–8.
22. Vernino S, et al. Autoantibodies to ganglionic acetylcholine receptors in autoimmune autonomic neuropathies. N Engl J Med. 2000;343(12):847–55.
23. Dhamija R, et al. Serologic profiles aiding the diagnosis of autoimmune gastrointestinal dysmotility. Clin Gastroenterol Hepatol. 2008;6(9):988–92.
24. Tornblom H, et al. Autoantibodies in patients with gut motility disorders and enteric neuropathy. Scand J Gastroenterol. 2007;42(11):1289–93.
25. Tomita R, et al. Upper gut motility of Hirschsprung's disease and its allied disorders in adults. Hepatogastroenterology. 2003;50(54):1959–62.
26. Miele E, et al. Persistence of abnormal gastrointestinal motility after operation for Hirschsprung's disease. Am J Gastroenterol. 2000;95(5):1226–30.
27. Staiano A, et al. Autonomic dysfunction in children with Hirschsprung's disease. Dig Dis Sci. 1999;44(5):960–5.
28. Ravelli AM, Milla PJ. Vomiting and gastroesophageal motor activity in children with disorders of the central nervous system. J Pediatr Gastroenterol Nutr. 1998;26(1):56–63.
29. Werlin SL. Antroduodenal motility in neurologically handicapped children with feeding intolerance. BMC Gastroenterol. 2004;4:19.
30. Zangen T, et al. Gastrointestinal motility and sensory abnormalities may contribute to food refusal in medically fragile toddlers. J Pediatr Gastroenterol Nutr. 2003;37(3):287–93.
31. Sullivan PB. Gastrointestinal disorders in children with neurodevelopmental disabilities. Dev Disabil Res Rev. 2008;14(2):128–36.
32. Fujii A, et al. Gastric dysmotility associated with accumulation of mitochondrial A3243G mutation in the stomach. Intern Med. 2004;43(12):1126–30.
33. Inoue K, et al. High degree of mitochondrial 3243 mutation in gastric biopsy specimen in a patient with MELAS and diabetes complicated by marked gastrointestinal abnormalities. Diabetes Care. 2003;26(7):2219.
34. Horowitz M, et al. Abnormalities of gastric and esophageal emptying in polymyositis and dermatomyositis. Gastroenterology. 1986;90(2):434–9.
35. Azpiroz F, Malagelada JR. Gastric tone measured by an electronic barostat in health and postsurgical gastroparesis. Gastroenterology. 1987;92(4):934–43.
36. Malagelada JR, et al. Gastric motor abnormalities in diabetic and postvagotomy gastroparesis: effect of metoclopramide and bethanechol. Gastroenterology. 1980;78(2):286–93.
37. The FO, et al. The role of mast cell stabilization in treatment of postoperative ileus: a pilot study. Am J Gastroenterol. 2009;104(9):2257–66.
38. Shafi MA, Pasricha PJ. Post-surgical and obstructive gastroparesis. Curr Gastroenterol Rep. 2007;9(4):280–5.
39. Hogan SP, et al. A pathological function for eotaxin and eosinophils in eosinophilic gastrointestinal inflammation. Nat Immunol. 2001;2(4):353–60.
40. Schappi MG, et al. Mast cell-nerve interactions in children with functional dyspepsia. J Pediatr Gastroenterol Nutr. 2008;47(4):472–80.
41. Tarling MM, et al. A model of gastric emptying using paracetamol absorption in intensive care patients. Intensive Care Med. 1997;23(3):256–60.
42. Tursi A. Gastrointestinal motility disturbances in celiac disease. J Clin Gastroenterol. 2004;38(8):642–5.
43. Bassotti G, et al. Antroduodenojejunal motor activity in untreated and treated celiac disease patients. J Gastroenterol Hepatol. 2008;23(7 Pt 2):e23–8.
44. Rocco A, et al. Tissue ghrelin level and gastric emptying rate in adult patients with celiac disease. Neurogastroenterol Motil. 2008;20(8):884–90.
45. Annese V, et al. Gastric emptying of solids in patients with nonobstructive Crohn's disease is sometimes delayed. J Clin Gastroenterol. 1995;21(4):279–82.
46. Di Lorenzo C, et al. Gastric emptying with gastro-oesophageal reflux. Arch Dis Child. 1987;62(5):449–53.
47. Heyland DK, et al. Impaired gastric emptying in mechanically ventilated, critically ill patients. Intensive Care Med. 1996;22(12):1339–44.
48. Nematy M, et al. Changes in appetite related gut hormones in intensive care unit patients: a pilot cohort study. Crit Care. 2006;10(1):R10.
49. Nguyen NQ, et al. Fasting and nutrient-stimulated plasma peptide-YY levels are elevated in critical illness and associated with feed intolerance: an observational, controlled study. Crit Care. 2006;10(6):R175.
50. Mittal BR, et al. Delayed gastric emptying in patients with caustic ingestion. Nucl Med Commun. 2008;29(9):782–5.
51. Maes BD, et al. Influence of octreotide on the gastric emptying of solids and liquids in normal healthy subjects. Aliment Pharmacol Ther. 1995;9(1):11–8.
52. Marano AR, et al. Effect of sucralfate and an aluminum hydroxide gel on gastric emptying of solids and liquids. Clin Pharmacol Ther. 1985;37(6):629–32.
53. Tougas G, et al. Omeprazole delays gastric emptying in healthy volunteers: an effect prevented by tegaserod. Aliment Pharmacol Ther. 2005;22(1):59–65.
54. Boesmans W, et al. Cannabinoid receptor 1 signalling dampens activity and mitochondrial transport in networks of enteric neurones. Neurogastroenterol Motil. 2009;21(9):958–e77.
55. Galligan JJ. Cannabinoid signalling in the enteric nervous system. Neurogastroenterol Motil. 2009;21(9):899–902.
56. Ukleja A. Dumping syndrome: pathophysiology and treatment. Nutr Clin Pract. 2005;20(5):517–25.
57. Johnson LP, Sloop RD, Jesseph JE. Etiologic significance of the early symptomatic phase in the dumping syndrome. Ann Surg. 1962;156:173–9.

58. Connor F. Gastrointestinal complications of fundoplication. Curr Gastroenterol Rep. 2005;7(3):219–26.
59. Samuk I, et al. Dumping syndrome following Nissen fundoplication, diagnosis, and treatment. J Pediatr Gastroenterol Nutr. 1996;23(3):235–40.
60. Hejazi RA, Patil H, McCallum RW. Dumping syndrome: establishing criteria for diagnosis and identifying new etiologies. Dig Dis Sci. 2010;55(1):117–23.
61. van der Kleij FG, et al. Diagnostic value of dumping provocation in patients after gastric surgery. Scand J Gastroenterol. 1996;31(12):1162–6.
62. Vecht J, Masclee AA, Lamers CB. The dumping syndrome. Current insights into pathophysiology, diagnosis and treatment. Scand J Gastroenterol. 1997;223(Suppl):21–7.
63. Borovoy J, Furuta L, Nurko S. Benefit of uncooked cornstarch in the management of children with dumping syndrome fed exclusively by gastrostomy. Am J Gastroenterol. 1998;93(5):814–8.
64. Gerard J, Luyckx AS, Lefebvre PJ. Acarbose in reactive hypoglycemia: a double-blind study. Int J Clin Pharmacol Ther Toxicol. 1984;22(1):25–31.
65. Hasegawa T, et al. Long-term effect of alpha-glucosidase inhibitor on late dumping syndrome. J Gastroenterol Hepatol. 1998;13(12):1201–6.
66. Lyons TJ, et al. Effect of acarbose on biochemical responses and clinical symptoms in dumping syndrome. Digestion. 1985;31(2–3):89–96.
67. McLoughlin JC, Buchanan KD, Alam MJ. A glycoside-hydrolase inhibitor in treatment of dumping syndrome. Lancet. 1979;2(8143):603–5.
68. Bredenoord AJ, et al. Gastric accommodation and emptying in evaluation of patients with upper gastrointestinal symptoms. Clin Gastroenterol Hepatol. 2003;1(4):264–72.
69. Thumshirn M, et al. Gastric mechanosensory and lower esophageal sphincter function in rumination syndrome. Am J Physiol. 1998;275(2 Pt 1):G314–21.

Chronic Intestinal Pseudo-Obstruction

22

Paul E. Hyman and Nikhil Thapar

Chronic intestinal pseudo-obstruction (CIPO), far from a single entity, represents a heterogenous group of disorders affecting gut neuromuscular function. Such conditions are rare and vary in cause, severity, course, and response to therapy [1–6]. Most are severe, disabling and characterized by repetitive episodes or continuous symptoms and signs of bowel obstruction, including radiographic documentation of dilated bowel with air-fluid levels, in the absence of a fixed, lumen-occluding lesion [7]. At the present time, CIPO remains largely a clinical diagnosis based on phenotype, rather than pathology or manometry. The most common signs are abdominal distention and failure to thrive, and the most common symptoms are vomiting, constipation or diarrhea and abdominal pain. Heterogeneity in pseudo-obstruction includes, but is not limited to, a wide spectrum of abnormal gastric, small intestinal, and colonic myoelectrical activity and contractions as well as histologic abnormalities in nerve and muscle. The genetics for most CIPO conditions is poorly characterized. Although these diseases have distinctive pathophysiologic characteristics, they are considered together because of their clinical and therapeutic similarities (See Table 22.1 for list of heterogeneity).

Etiology

CIPO may occur as a primary disease or as a secondary manifestation of a large number of other conditions that transiently (e.g., hypothyroidism, phenothiazine overdose) or permanently (e.g., scleroderma, amyloidosis) alter bowel motility (Table 22.2) [8–40].

Most congenital forms of neuropathic and myopathic CIPO are both rare and sporadic. There is no family history of pseudo-obstruction, no associated syndrome, and no evidence of other predisposing factors such as toxins, infections, ischemia, or autoimmune disease. Such conditions are likely to represent new mutations. More rarely, CIPO appears to show familial inheritance and a number of genes have been implicated. This is discussed in detail elsewhere in the book. Briefly, there are reports of autosomal-dominant [41, 42] and -recessive [43–46] neuropathic, and dominant [47, 48] and recessive [49, 50] myopathic patterns of inheritance. In the autosomal-dominant diseases, expressivity and penetrance are

P.E. Hyman, M.D. (✉)
Gastroenterology Division, Children's Hospital, Louisiana State University, 200 Henry Clay Ave, New Orleans, LA 70118, USA
e-mail: paulhyman@aol.com

N. Thapar, B.Sc.(hon), B.M.(hon), M.R.C.P., M.R.C.P.C.H., Ph.D.
Gastroenterology Unit, University College London, Institute of Child Health, Division of Neurogastroenterology and Motility, London, UK

Department of Paediatric Gastroenterology, Great Ormond Street Hospital for Children, London, UK

C. Faure et al. (eds.), *Pediatric Neurogastroenterology: Gastrointestinal Motility and Functional Disorders in Children*, Clinical Gastroenterology,
DOI 10.1007/978-1-60761-709-9_22, © Springer Science+Business Media New York 2013

Table 22.1 Features of chronic intestinal pseudo-obstruction in pediatric patients

Onset
Congenital
Acquired
Acute
Gradual
Presentation
Megacystis—microcolon intestinal hypoperistalsis syndrome
Acute neonatal bowel obstruction, with or without megacystitis
Chronic vomiting and failure to thrive
Chronic abdominal distention and failure to thrive
Cause
Sporadic
Familial
Toxic
Ischemic
Viral
Inflammatory
Autoimmune
Area of involvement
Entire gastrointestinal tract
Segment of gastrointestinal tract
Megaduodenum
Small bowel
Colon
Pathology
Myopathy
Neuropathy
Lymphocytic or eosinophilic ganglionitis
Absent neurons
Immature neurons
Degenerating neurons
Absent cells of Cajal
Intestinal neuronal dysplasia
No microscopic abnormality

variable; some of those affected die in childhood, but those less affected are able to reproduce. An X-linked recessive form of neuropathic pseudo-obstruction has been mapped to its locus, Xq28 [51]. A recessive form of CIPO is described in mitochondrial neurogastrointestinal encephalopathy (MNGIE) [52]. When counseling families, a thorough family history is essential, and screening tests of relatives should be considered to seek milder phenotypic expression.

CIPO may result from exposure to toxins during critical developmental periods in utero. A few children with fetal alcohol syndrome [52] and a few exposed to narcotics in utero have neuropathic forms of CIPO. Presumably, any substance

Table 22.2 Causes of secondary acute, subacute, and chronic intestinal pseudo-obstruction in children

Toxic
Ketamine
Carbamazepine
Clonidine
Atropine and other anticholinergics
Theophyllin
Fludarabin
Vinblastin and other vinca alkaloids
Neuroleptics
Antidepressants
Phenothiazine
Opiates
Calcium channel blockers
Fetal alcohol syndrome [8]
Metabolic
Electrolyte imbalance (hypo K^+, hyper Mg^{2+}, hypo Ca^{2+}) [9]
Hypothyroidism
Hypoparathyroidism
Carnitine deficiency [10]
Vitamin E deficiency ("brown-bowel syndrome") [11, 12]
Infectious
Viral: CMV [13], EBV [14, 15], Herpes Zoster [16], Rotavirus [17]
Trypanosoma cruzei (young adults)
Lyme disease [18]
Immune
Celiac disease
Systemic sclerosis [19]
Lupus (myopathy) [20]
Autoimmune leiomyositis [21, 22]
Autoimmune enteric ganglionitis (with anti-enteric neurons antibodies, anti-PCNA antibodies) [23, 24]
Guillain-Barré syndrome [25]
Tumoral
Neural crest cell tumor: neuroblastoma, ganglioneuroblastoma [26]
Pheochromocytoma [27]
Thymoma (with anti-acetylcholine receptor antibodies) [28]
Striated myopathy
Myotonic dystrophy [29, 30]
Duchenne muscular dystrophy [31]
Desmin myopathy [32]
Mitochondrial myopathy [33, 34]
Central or peripheral generalized neuropathy
Degenerative process: diabetes, amyloidosis (not reported in children)
Mitochondrial neurogastrointestinal encephalopathy (MNGIE) [35]
Familial dysautonomia [36]
Acquired cholinergic dysautonomia or acquired pandysautonomia [37]

(continued)

Table 22.2 (continued)

Miscellaneous
Angioedema [38]
Postradiation enteropathy [39]
Kawasaki [40]

that alters neuronal migration or maturation might affect the development of the enteric plexuses and cause CIPO.

Children with chromosomal abnormalities or syndromes may suffer from pseudo-obstruction. Children with Down syndrome have a higher incidence of Hirschsprung's disease than the general population and may have abnormal esophageal motility [53] and neuronal dysplasia in the myenteric plexus. Rare children with Down syndrome have a myenteric plexus neuropathy so generalized and so severe that they present with pseudo-obstruction. Children with neurofibromatosis, multiple endocrine neoplasia type IIB, and other chromosome aberrations and autonomic neuropathies may suffer from neuropathic constipation. Children with Duchenne's muscular dystrophy sometimes develop pseudo-obstruction, especially in the terminal stages of life [54]. Esophageal manometry and gastric emptying are abnormal in Duchenne's dystrophy, suggesting that the myopathy includes gastrointestinal smooth muscle even in asymptomatic children [31]. Acquired pseudo-obstruction may be a rare complication of infection from cytomegalovirus [13] or Epstein-Barr virus [14]. Most recently, JC virus (JCV) a polyomavirus that can infect brain glial cells to cause severe illness has been shown to be present in the myenteric plexuses of adult patients with CIPO. JCV in enteroglial cells suggested a pathological role for this virus in enteric neuropathy [55]. This is yet to be shown in pediatric CIPO. Immunocompromised children and immunosuppressed transplant recipients seem at higher risk than the general population for acquired myenteric plexus neuropathy. Acquired CIPO might result from myenteric plexus neuritis from persistent viral infection or an autoimmune inflammatory response. Mucosal inflammation causes abnormal motility. With celiac disease [56], Crohn's disease, and the chronic enterocolitis associated with Hirschsprung's disease some patients develop dilated bowel and symptoms due, not to anatomic obstruction, but to a neuromuscular disorder presumably related to the effects of inflammatory mediators on mucosal afferent sensory nerves or motor nerves in the enteric plexuses. Other causes of CIPO associated with inflammation include myenteric neuritis associated with antineuronal antibodies [23] and intestinal myositis [22, 57].

Pathology (See Chap. 17)

There may be histologic abnormalities in the muscle or nerve or, rarely, both [58]. More recently there have also been descriptions of CIPO due to mesenchymopathies or deficiencies in interstitial cells of Cajal [59]. Assessment of such pathology in motility disorders is not standardized and therefore mesenchymopathy as a distinct entity remains unclear [24]. Histology is normal in about 10% of cases that are studied appropriately, although there is great variability in available expertise and protocols. Moreover, it is often difficult to determine what changes are primary, and what changes in nerve cell dropout and muscle fibrosis are caused by chronic distension and consequent ischemia. Recent initiatives are attempting to address this variability [60–62]. In cases of normal gross neuromuscular histopathology there may be an abnormality in neuronal diversity (subtype dropout) or some biochemical aspect of stimulus-contraction coupling.

When laparotomy is imminent for a child with pseudo-obstruction, there must be timely communication between the surgeon and the pathologist. Although a laparotomy is not generally undertaken for biopsy alone, increasing expertise with laparoscopy has facilitated it's use for the assessment of histopathology where confirmation is required prior to definitive surgery or to inform prognosis. When surgery is indicated (e.g., for colectomy, cholecystectomy, or creation of an ileostomy) a plan should be made to obtain a full-thickness bowel biopsy specimen at least 2 cm in diameter. As discussed in Chap. 17 the tissues should be processed for routine and specialized histopathology studies including H&E, tinctorial stains, immunohistochemistry (IHC) and also for enzyme histochemistry and electron microscopy.

Muscle disease may be inflammatory but more often is not. In light microscopy of both familial and sporadic forms of hollow visceral myopathy, the muscularis appears thin. The external longitudinal muscle layer is more involved than the internal circular muscle, and there may be extensive fibrosis in the muscle tissue. By electron microscopy there are vacuolar degeneration and disordered myofilaments.

Neuropathic disease used to be examined with silver stains of the myenteric plexus [63, 64] and routine histologic techniques but the former has largely been superceded by IHC. The presence of neurons in the submucous plexus of a suction biopsy specimen eliminates Hirschsprung's disease as a diagnostic possibility but is inadequate for the evaluation of other neuropathies. There may be maturational arrest of the myenteric plexus. This hypoganglionosis is characterized by fewer neurons, which may be smaller than normal. Apart from abnormal development phenotypes other pathologies include neuronal degeneration, inflammation, and inclusion bodies. Maturational arrest can be a primary congenital disorder or can occur secondary to ischemia or infection. Changes can be patchy or generalized.

Intestinal neuronal dysplasia [65], or hyperganglionosis, is a histologic diagnosis defined by these findings: (1) hyperplasia of the parasympathetic neurons and fibers of the myenteric (and sometimes submucous) plexus, characterized by increases in the number and size of ganglia, thickened nerves, and increases in neuron cell bodies; (2) increased acetyl cholinesterase-positive nerve fibers in the lamina propria; (3) increased acetylcholine esterase-positive nerve fibers around submucosal blood vessels; (4) heterotopic neuron cell bodies in the lamina propria, muscle, and serosal layers. The first two criteria are obligatory.

Children with intestinal neuronal dysplasia are a heterogeneous group. Children with primary pseudo-obstruction due to neuronal dysplasia may have disease that is limited to the colon or disseminated. Other children may have neuronal dysplasia associated with prematurity, protein allergy, chromosome abnormalities, MEN IIB, and neurofibromatosis; however, intestinal neuronal dysplasia is an occasional incidental finding in bowel specimens examined for reasons unrelated to motility. Intestinal neuronal dysplasia correlates poorly with motility-related symptoms [66]. Thus, a pathologic diagnosis of intestinal neuronal dysplasia neither predicts clinical outcome nor influences management.

Clinical Features

Presentation

More than half the affected children develop symptoms at or shortly after birth. A few cases are diagnosed in utero, by ultrasound findings of polyhydramnios and megacystis and marked abdominal distention. Intestinal malrotation is found in both neuropathic and myopathic congenital forms of pseudo-obstruction. Of children who present at birth, about 40% have an intestinal malrotation. In the most severely affected infants symptoms of acute bowel obstruction appear within the first hours of life. Less severely affected infants present months later with symptoms of vomiting, diarrhea, and failure to thrive. A few patients have megacystis at birth and insidious onset of gastrointestinal symptoms over the first few years. More than three quarters of the children develop symptoms by the end of the first year of life, and the remainder present sporadically through the first two decades.

Although there is individual variation in the number and intensity of signs and symptoms, it may be useful to note the relative frequencies in this population (Table 22.3). Abdominal distention and vomiting are the most common features, complaints of about three quarters of the patients. Constipation, episodic or intermittent abdominal pain, and poor weight gain are features in about 60% of cases. Diarrhea is a complaint in one third. Urinary tract smooth muscle is affected in those with both hollow visceral neuropathy and hollow visceral myopathy, about one fifth of all

Table 22.3 Clinical symptoms in children with chronic intestinal pseudo-obstruction

Study	Abdominal distension	Vomiting	Constipation	Failure to thrive	Abdominal pain	Diarrhea	Dysphagia
Faure et al. [1] $n=105$	100	94	70	64	46	29	9
Vargas et al. [2] $n=87$	73	50	51	23	NA	21	2
Granata et al. [3] $n=59$	59	31	27	NA	NA	26	NA
Schuffler et al. [4, 5] $n=30$	23	19	20	15	NA	16	NA
Heneyke et al. [6] $n=44$	31	40	31	NA	NA	–	NA
Total $n=325$	286 (88%)	234 (72%)	199 (61%)	102 (31%)	–	92 (28%)	11 (3%)

NA not available

pseudo-obstruction patients. Often these children are severely affected at birth and are described by the phenotype *megacystis-microcolon intestinal hypoperistalsis syndrome* [2].

The majority of children's clinical course is characterized by relative remissions and exacerbations. Factors that precipitate deteriorations include intercurrent infections, general anesthesia, psychological stress, and poor nutritional status.

The radiographic signs are those of intestinal obstruction, with air-fluid levels, dilated stomach, small intestine, and colon, or microcolon in those studied because of obstruction at birth [6]. There may be prolonged stasis of contrast material placed into the affected bowel, so it is prudent to use a nontoxic, isotonic, water-soluble medium to prevent barium from solidifying. Children who feel well still show radiographic evidence of bowel obstruction. The greater problem arises when children develop an acute deterioration. Radiographs demonstrate the same patterns of bowel obstruction that are seen when the child feels well. In children who previously had surgery, it can be difficult to discriminate between physical obstruction related to adhesions and an episodic increase in CIPO symptoms.

Table 22.4 Differential diagnosis of CIP in children

Aerophagia
Gastroparesis
Functional constipation
Cyclic vomiting syndrome
Chronic abdominal pain with psychological dysfunction (pain-associated disability syndrome)
Bacterial overgrowth of various origins (lactase deficiency, disaccharidase deficiency, intestinal duplication)
Aerodigestive fistula
Pediatric illness falsification (Munchausen-by-proxy syndrome, fabricated or induced illness imposed on a child)

Diagnosis

An incorrect CIPO label can result from misdiagnosis of infant and toddler victims of pediatric illness falsification, known in the United Kingdom as Fabricated or Induced Illness, formerly known as Münchausen's syndrome by proxy [67]. Well-meaning clinicians inadvertently cocreate disease as they respond to a caretaker's symptom fabrications by performing tests and procedures, including parenteral nutrition support, repeated surgery, and even small bowel transplantation [68]. Adolescents with disabling abdominal pain arising from psychiatric diseases such as pain disorder, posttraumatic stress disorder, and Asperger's syndrome may also confuse gastroenterologists [69]. A differential diagnosis for CIPO is provided in Table 22.4.

Diagnostic testing provides information about the nature and severity of the pathophysiology. Manometric studies are more sensitive than radiographic tests to evaluate the strength and coordination of contraction and relaxation in the esophagus, gastric antrum, small intestine, colon, and anorectal area.

In affected children scintigraphy demonstrates delayed gastric emptying of solids or liquids and reflux of intestinal contents back into the stomach. Dilated loops of bowel predispose to bacterial overgrowth, so breath hydrogen testing may reveal elevations in fasting breath hydrogen and a rapid increase in breath hydrogen with a carbohydrate meal.

Esophageal manometry is abnormal in about half those affected by CIPO. In children with myopathy, contractions are low amplitude but coordinated in the distal two-thirds of the esophagus. Lower esophageal sphincter pressure is low, and sphincter relaxation is complete. When the esophagus is affected by neuropathy, contraction amplitude in the esophageal body may be high, normal, low, or absent. There may be simultaneous, spontaneous, or repetitive contractions [70, 71]. Relaxation of the lower esophageal sphincter may be incomplete or absent.

Antroduodenal manometry findings are always abnormal with intestinal pseudo-obstruction involving the upper gastrointestinal tract; however, manometry is often also abnormal in partial or complete small bowel obstruction. Although the manometric patterns of true obstruction differ from those of CIPO in adults [72, 73], such a distinction is not always clear. Contrast radiography and, as a last resort, exploratory laparotomy are best for differentiating true obstruction from pseudo-obstruction. Antroduodenal manometry should not be used as a test to differentiate true bowel obstruction from pseudo-obstruction. Manometry may help to determine the physiologic correlates for the symptoms, to assess drug responses, and for prognosis [70, 74–76]. Intestinal myopathy causes low-amplitude coordinated contractions, and neuropathy causes uncoordinated contractions [77]. Pain with each high-amplitude antral contraction suggests gastric hyperalgesia. Interpretation of antroduodenal manometry requires recognition of normal and abnormal features (Table 22.5).

The abnormalities in pseudo-obstruction are commonly discrete and easily interpreted by eye (see Chap. 9). They contrast markedly with normal features of antroduodenal manometry.

In most cases the manometric abnormality correlates with clinical severity of the disease. For example, children with total aganglionosis have contractions of normal amplitude that are never organized into migrating motor complexes (MMCs), fed patterns, or even bursts or clusters of contractions but are simply a monotonous pattern of random events. Children with such a pattern are dependent on total parenteral nutrition (TPN). More than 80% of children with MMCs are nourished enterally, but more than 80% of children without MMCs require partial or total parenteral nutrition [75].

Table 22.5 Antroduodenal manometric features from studies of 300 children

Normal features
Migrating motor complex (MMC) (fasting)
Postprandial (phase 2-like) pattern
Abnormal features in duodenum
Absent MMC phase 3
Sustained tonic contractions
Retrograde propagation of phase 3
Giant single-propagating contractions
Absent phase 2 with increased phase 3 frequency
Persistently low-amplitude or absent contractions
Prolonged nonpropagating clusters
Postprandial abnormalities
Antral hypomotility after a solid nutrient meal
Absent or decreased motility
Failure to induce a fed pattern (MMC persists)

[a]Each of these features is recognized by visual inspection of the recording. From Tomomasa T, DiLorenzo C, Morikawa A, et al. Analysis of fasting antroduodenal manometry in children. Dig Dis Sci. 1996;41:195–203.

Normal antroduodenal manometry and absence of dilated bowel in a patient with CIPO symptoms shifts the emphasis from medical to psychological illness [78]. It is often difficult for families to consider and engage in psychological intervention, especially when the decision is based on a "lack of medical findings." Thus it is important to interpret the antroduodenal manometry as a positive prognostic indicator, *especially* when the results are normal.

Colon manometry is abnormal in colonic pseudo-obstruction [79]. The normal features of colon manometry in children include (1) high-amplitude propagating contractions (phasic contractions stronger than 60 mmHg amplitude) propagating over at least 30 cm; (2) a gastrocolic response (the increase in motility that follows a meal); and (3) an absence of discrete abnormalities.

With neuropathic disease contractions are normal or reduced in amplitude, but there are no high-amplitude propagating contractions or gastrocolic response. With myopathy there are usually no colonic contractions (see Chap. 10).

There are several pitfalls with intestinal and colonic manometry. In dilated bowel no contractions are recorded and manometry is not diagnostic. Recordings filled with respiratory and movement artifacts from agitated, angry, crying patients are uninterpretable. Acute pseudo-obstruction is usually associated with ileus, so that an absence of contractions may not reflect the underlying abnormality. Manometry is most likely to be helpful when performed in a cooperative patient at a time when the patient is feeling well. Anorectal manometry is usually normal in CIPO. There is an absence of the rectoinhibitory reflex only in Hirschsprung's disease and in some patients with intestinal neuronal dysplasia. In a few specialized centers, electrogastrography is a noninvasive screening test for evaluation of children thought to have CIPO [80]. Skin electrodes are placed over the stomach, just as surface electrodes are placed over the heart to perform electrocardiography. The electrical slow-wave rhythms of the gastric body and antrum are recorded. Gastric slow waves normally occur at a rate of 3 per minute. Gastric neuropathies are characterized by decreases (bradygastria) or increases (tachygastria) in slow-wave frequency. Gastric myopathies are characterized by reduced power, a measure of signal amplitude.

Treatment

Nutrition Support

The goal of nutrition support is to achieve normal growth and development with the fewest possible complications and the greatest patient comfort. In children with CIPO, motility improves as nutritional deficiencies resolve and worsens as malnutrition recurs.

Roughly a third of affected children require prolonged periods of partial or total parenteral nutrition (TPN). One third require total or partial tube feedings, and the rest eat by mouth. In those with intestinal neuropathies about 30% need TPN. In those with enteric myopathies over 70% need TPN. TPN is the least desirable means of achieving nutritional sufficiency because of the potential for life-threatening complications. In the absence of enteral nutrients, the gastrointestinal tract does not grow or mature normally. In the absence of the postprandial rise in trophic and stimulant gastrointestinal hormones, bile stasis and liver disease develop [81]. TPN-associated cholelithiasis [82] and progressive liver disease are important causes of morbidity and mortality in children with pseudo-obstruction. The minimal volume, composition, and route of enteral support required to reverse or prevent the progression of gastrointestinal complications have not been determined. It seems likely that a complex liquid formula containing protein and fat, given by mouth or gastrostomy tube, and contributing 10–25% of the child's total calorie requirement would be sufficient to stimulate postprandial increases in splanchnic blood flow and plasma concentrations of gastrin and other trophic factors. Every effort should be extended to maximize enteral nutritional support in parenteral nutrition-dependent children.

Continuous feeding via gastrostomy or jejunostomy may be effective when bolus feedings fail. Most children with visceral myopathy and a few with neuropathy have an atonic stomach and almost no gastric emptying. In these children, a feeding jejunostomy may be helpful for the administration of medications and for drip feedings [83]. Care must be taken to place a jejunostomy into an undistended bowel loop.

Drugs

Drugs to stimulate intestinal contractions are helpful in a minority of children with CIPO. Bethanechol, neostigmine, metoclopramide, and domperidone have not been useful. Perhaps the best documented benefit of pharmacoptherapy for CIPO has come from serotonergic drugs. The combined 5HT4 agonist and 5HT3 antagonist cisapride's mechanism of action is to bind to serotonin receptors on the motor nerves of the myenteric plexus, facilitating release of acetylcholine and stimulating gastrointestinal smooth muscle contraction. It appeared most likely to improve symptoms in children with MMCs and without dilated bowel [84] and acted by increasing the number and strength of contractions in the duodenum of children with CIPO. It did not initiate the MMC in patients without it or inhibit discrete abnormalities. Cisapride was withdrawn from the commercial marketplace in much of the world in the early 2000s because of concerns related to rare fatal cardiac arrhythmias. In the USA today cisapride is available at no cost to individual patients after successful application to the Federal Drug Administration for an Investigational New Drug application, and approval by a local Human Subjects Committee. The pure 5HT4 agonist tegaserod held similar promise for CIPO, but was also withdrawn for cardiovascular concerns similar to those about cisapride. Newer serotonergic agents are being tested but their effect in CIPO is not yet studied.

Erythromycin, a motilin receptor agonist, appears to facilitate gastric emptying in those with neuropathic gastroparesis by stimulating high-amplitude 3-min antral contractions, relaxing the pylorus, and inducing antral phase 3 episodes in doses of 1–3 mg/kg intravenously [85] or 3–5 mg/kg orally. Erythromycin does not appear to be effective for more generalized motility disorders [85], is ineffective for stimulating colonic contractility [86].

Octreotide, a somatostatin analogue, given subcutaneously, induces small intestinal phase 3-like clustered contractions and suppresses phase 2 [87]. However, the clusters may not propagate, or may propagate in either direction and intestinal transit and nutrient absorption are optimal during phase 2. Augmentin, a combination of amoxacillin and clavulinate, increases contractions in the small bowel [88]. Augmentin may be useful in selected CIPO cases to increase the contractions and treat bacterial overgrowth.

Antibiotics are used for bacterial overgrowth. Bacterial overgrowth is associated with steatorrhea, fat-soluble vitamin malabsorption, and malabsorption of the intrinsic factor—vitamin B_{12} complex. It is possible that bacterial overgrowth contributes to bacteremia and frequent episodes of central venous catheter-related sepsis and to TPN-associated liver disease. Bacterial overgrowth, mucosal injury, malabsorption, fluid secretion, and gas production may contribute to chronic intestinal dilatation, which may further impair motility. Chronic antibiotic use may result in the emergence of resistant strains of bacteria or overgrowth with fungi. Thus, treating bacterial overgrowth must be considered on an individual basis.

Excessive gastrostomy drainage may result from retrograde flow of intestinal contents into the stomach or from gastric acid hypersecretion. Gastric secretory function or gastric pH should be tested before beginning antisecretory drugs. Histamine H_2-receptor antagonists may be used to suppress gastric acid hypersecretion. Tolerance develops after a few months of intravenous use [89], so the drug should be given orally when possible. When a drug is added to TPN, gastric pH should be assessed at regular intervals to monitor drug efficacy. Induction of achlorhydria is inadvisable because it promotes bacterial overgrowth in the stomach.

Constipation is treated initially with oral polyethylene glycol solutions, suppositories, or enemas. Oral lavage solutions often cause abdominal distention because of delayed small bowel transit in children with pseudo-obstruction. For constipation and small bowel disease, cecostomy or appendicostomy may simplify management by bypassing the small bowel [90]. If colon manometry shows no colon contractions, the most efficient course is ileostomy and colon resection. An ileostomy takes the resistance of the anal sphincter out of the system, and facilitates flow of chyme from the higher pressures from gastric contractions to the absence of pressure at the stoma.

Acute pain due to episodes of pseudo-obstruction is best treated by decompressing distended bowel. Opioids are rarely needed if the bowel is promptly decompressed. It is appropriate to consider nonsteroidal anti-inflammatory agents (e.g., ketorolac) and epidural anesthetics as alternatives to, or in combination with, systemic opioids.

Chronic pain can be a problem in children with congenital pseudo-obstruction and is common in adolescents who have autoimmune or inflammatory disease and progressive loss of intestinal function. Pain consists of a nociceptive component and an affective component. Patients with chronic pain benefit from a multidisciplinary approach including not only attention to gastrointestinal disease but also mental health assessment and treatment for the affective pain component. Collaboration with pain management specialists is beneficial for optimizing the care of pseudo-obstruction patients who complain of chronic pain. Multiple modalities for pain relief are useful: cognitive behavioral therapy, massage, relaxation, hypnosis, psychotherapy, yoga, and drugs all have shown positive effects. Drugs that reduce afferent signaling, improving chronic visceral pain, include the tricyclic antidepressants, clonidine, and gabapentin [91]. Opioid use is inadvisable, because opioids disorganize intestinal motility, tolerance to opioids develops rapidly, and opioid withdrawal can simulate the visceral pain of acute pseudo-obstruction.

Sympathetic plexus neurolysis, by interrupting sympathetic efferent (and inhibitory) activity on upper digestive tract, improved symptoms in CIPO patients [92–94].

Surgery

One of the management challenges in pseudo-obstruction is the evaluation and reevaluation of newborns and children with episodic acute obstructive symptoms. Although most acute episodes represent pseudo-obstruction, it is important to intervene with surgery when the episode is a true bowel obstruction, appendicitis, or another surgical condition. Many children with episodes of acute pseudo-obstruction undergo repeated exploratory laparotomies. It is important to avoid unnecessary abdominal surgery in children with pseudo-obstruction for several reasons: (1) They often suffer from prolonged postoperative ileus: (2) Adhesions create a diagnostic problem each time there is a new obstructive episode: (3) Adhesions following laparotomy may distort normal tissue planes and make future surgery riskier in terms of bleeding and organ perforation. After several laparotomies turn up no evidence of mechanical obstruction, the surgeon may choose a more conservative management plan for subsequent episodes, including pain management, nutritional support, and abdominal decompression.

Gastrostomy was the only procedure that reduced the number of hospitalizations in adults with pseudo-obstruction [95], and the experience with children seems to be similar [96]. Gastrostomy provides a quick and comfortable means of evacuating gastric contents and relieves pain and nausea related to gastric and bowel distention. Continued "venting" may decompress more distal regions of small bowel, precluding nasogastric intubation and pain medication. Gastrostomy is used for enteral feeding and enteral administration of medication. Gastrostomy placement should be considered for those receiving parenteral nutrition and for children who will need tube feedings longer than 2 months. In many patients, endoscopic gastrostomy placement is ideal. In those with contraindications to endoscopic placement, surgical placement is appropriate. Care must be taken to place the ostomy in a suitable position, above the gastric antrum in the midbody.

Fundoplication is rarely indicated for pseudo-obstruction. After fundoplication, symptoms change from vomiting to repeated retching [97]. In children with pseudo-obstruction, vomiting is reduced by venting the gastrostomy. Acid reflux is controlled with antisecretory medication.

Results of pyloroplasty or Roux-en-*Y* gastrojejunostomy to improve gastric emptying in pseudo-obstruction have been poor; gastric emptying remains delayed. Altering the anatomy rarely improves the function of the dilated fundus and body. Small bowel resections or tapering operations may provide relief for months or even years; however, when the lesion is present in other areas of bowel those areas gradually dilate and symptoms recur.

Ileostomy can decompress dilated distal small bowel and provide further benefit by removing from the circuit the high-pressure zones at the end of the bowel namely the colon and the anal sphincter. Transit of luminal contents is always from a high-pressure zone to a lower-pressure one. In pseudo-obstruction patients with gastric antral contractions but no effective small bowel contractions, bowel transit improves with the creation of an ileostomy because of the absence of resistance to flow at the ostomy site.

Colectomy is sometimes necessary in severe congenital pseudo-obstruction to decompress an abdomen so distended that respiration is impaired. In general, colon diversions are inadvisable because of a high incidence of diversion colitis [98]. Diversion colitis can cause abdominal pain, tenesmus, hematochezia and may worsen motility of the proximal intestine as chemical by-products of inflammation circulate to vulnerable tissues.

Subtotal colectomy with ileoproctostomy cures rare children with neuropathic pseudo-obstruction confined to the colon. Typically these children are able to eat normally and grow, but they are unable to defecate spontaneously. They differ from children with functional constipation in that their stools are never huge or hard, there is no retentive posturing, the history of constipation begins at birth, and there are often extrarectal fecal masses. Colon pathology may show neuronal dysplasia, maturational arrest, or no diagnostic abnormality, but colon manometry is always abnormal, without high-amplitude propagating contractions or a postprandial rise in motility index. Before colectomy for constipation, antroduodenal manometry may be necessary to determine whether the upper gastrointestinal tract is involved. Abnormal antroduodenal manometry is a relative contraindication to colectomy because upper gastrointestinal symptoms appear after colon resection [99]. Before surgery, a psychological evaluation may help to assess the possibility of psychiatric disease and somatization masquerading as colon disease and to prepare the patient for the procedures.

A cecostomy using a small "button" ostomy appliance for regular infusion of colonic lavage solution has not been effective for severe colonic pseudo-obstruction. The abdomen distends, but the colon does not empty.

There is increasing experience with the pacemakers in gut motility disorders although the experience is limited to gastroparesis, not CIPO [100].

Failed medical management may signal a need for total bowel resection. Rarely, a mucosal secretory disorder complicates the management of pseudo-obstruction. Several liters of intestinal secretions drain from enteric orifices each day. When secretions cannot be controlled with loperamide, anticholinergics, antibiotics, steroids, or somatostatin analogue, it may be necessary to resect the entire bowel to avoid life-threatening electrolyte abnormalities and nutritional disturbances caused by the large volume losses. Total bowel resection may reduce episodes of bacterial transmigration across dilated bowel to eliminate repeated life-threatening central venous catheter infections [101]. Total bowel resection should be considered alone or in combination with small bowel transplantation. Small bowel or combined liver–bowel transplants have the potential to cure children with pseudo-obstruction. Transplant results in CIPO children are similar to results in children undergoing transplantation for short bowel syndrome or intractable diarrhea [102]. (See also Chap. 46.)

Outcomes

The prognosis of children with CIPO remains guarded, with risk of mortality as high as 30% in the first year of life. Complications of parenteral nutrition are the cause of death in a majority of children [103, 104]. Thus, TPN is life saving, but measures to avoid TPN and, once started, to discontinue TPN are appropriate. Children with lower socioeconomic status tend to be on TPN longer than children from high socioeconomic status, suggesting that those with better health care access are aggressively moved away from parenteral nutrition [103]. The quality of life for surviving children with pseudo-obstruction and their families is reduced compared to others with chronic disease [103]. The factors responsible for reduced quality of life in CIP were chronic pain and the caretaker's time commitment for participating in their child's medical care [103]. Adverse prognostic factors include early onset disease, enteric myopathies, associated malrotation, and absent phase 3 of the migrating motor complex on small intestinal manometry. A few children with congenital neuropathic CIPO improve with time. Several factors may be responsible. First, caloric needs are greatest in the first year, and decrease in subsequent years. Thus, the infant who can digest 50% of his or her caloric needs in the first year, may have no change in motility, but digest 100% of his or her lessening caloric needs in subsequent years. Second, motility may improve spontaneously. The mechanisms for improvement in this small group are unexplained.

References

1. Faure C, Goulet O, Ategbo S, et al. Chronic intestinal pseudoobstruction syndrome: clinical analysis, outcome, and prognosis in 105 children. French-Speaking Group of Pediatric Gastroenterology. Dig Dis Sci. 1999;44:953–9.
2. Granata C, Puri P. Megacystis-microcolon-hypoperistalsis syndrome. J Pediatr Gastroenterol Nutr. 1997;25:12–9.
3. Heneyke S, Smith VV, Spitz L, et al. Chronic intestinal pseudo-obstruction: treatment and long term follow up of 44 patients. Arch Dis Child. 1999;81 :21–7.
4. Krishnamurthy S, Heng Y, Schuffler MD. Chronic intestinal pseudo-obstruction in infants and children caused by diverse abnormalities of the myenteric plexus. Gastroenterology. 1993;104:1398–408.
5. Schuffler MD. Visceral myopathy of the gastrointestinal and genitourinary tracts in infants. Gastroenterology. 1988;94:892–8.
6. Vargas JH, Sachs P, Ament ME. Chronic intestinal pseudo-obstruction syndrome in pediatrics: results of a national survey by members of the North American Society of Pediatric Gastroenterology and Nutrition. J Pediatr Gastroenterol Nutr. 1988;7:323–32.
7. Connor FL, Di Lorenzo C. Chronic intestinal pseudo-obstruction: assessment and management. Gastroenterology. 2006;130(2 Suppl 1):S29–36.
8. Uc A, Vasiliauskas E, Piccoli D, et al. Chronic intestinal pseudo-obstruction associated with fetal alcohol syndrome. Dig Dis Sci. 1997;42:1163–7.
9. Golzarian J, Scott Jr HW, Richards WO. Hypermagnesemia-induced paralytic ileus. Dig Dis Sci. 1994;39:1138–42.
10. Weaver LT, Rosenthal SR, Gladstone W, et al. Carnitine deficiency: a possible cause of gastrointestinal dysmotility. Acta Paediatr. 1992;81:79–81.
11. Horn T, Svendsen LB, Nielsen R. Brown-bowel syndrome. Review of the literature and presentation of cases. Scand J Gastroenterol. 1990;25:66–72.
12. Ward HC, Leake J, Milla PJ, et al. Brown bowel syndrome: a late complication of intestinal atresia. J Pediatr Surg. 1992;27:1593–5.
13. Sonsino E, Movy R, Foucaud P, et al. Intestinal pseudo-obstruction related to cytomegalovirus infection of the myenteric plexus. N Engl J Med. 1984;311:196–7.
14. Besnard M, Faure C, Fromont-Hankard G, et al. Intestinal pseudo-obstruction and acute pandysautonomia associated with Epstein-Barr virus infection. Am J Gastroenterol. 2000;95:280–4.
15. Vassallo M, Camilleri M, Caron BL, et al. Gastrointestinal motor dysfunction in acquired selective cholinergic dysautonomia associated with infectious mononucleosis. Gastroenterology. 1991;100:252–8.
16. Debinski HS, Ahmed S, Milla PJ, et al. Electrogastrography in chronic intestinal pseudoobstruction. Dig Dis Sci. 1996;41:1292–7.
17. Sigurdsson L, Flores A, Putnam PE, et al. Postviral gastroparesis: presentation, treatment, and outcome. J Pediatr Gastroenterol Nutr. 1997;131:751–4.
18. Chatila R, Kapadia CR. Intestinal pseudoobstruction in acute Lyme disease: a case report. Am J Gastroenterol. 1998;93:1179–80.
19. Ortiz-Alvarez O, Cabral D, Prendiville JS, et al. Intestinal pseudo-obstruction as an initial presentation of systemic sclerosis in two children. Br J Rheumatol. 1997;36:280–4.
20. Perlemuter G, Chaussade S, Wechsler B, et al. Chronic intestinal pseudo-obstruction in systemic lupus erythematosus. Gut. 1998;43:117–22.
21. Ginies JL, Francois H, Joseph MG, et al. A curable cause of chronic idiopathic intestinal pseudo-obstruction in children: idiopathic myositis of the small intestine. J Pediatr Gastroenterol Nutr. 1996;23:426–9.
22. Ruuska TH, Karikoski R, Smith VV, et al. Acquired myopathic intestinal pseudo-obstruction may be due to autoimmune enteric leiomyositis. Gastroenterology. 2002;122:1133–9.
23. De Giorgio R, Barbara G, Stanghellini V, et al. Clinical and morphofunctional features of idiopathic myenteric ganglionitis underlying severe intestinal motor dysfunction: a study of three cases. Am J Gastroenterol. 2002;97:2454–9.
24. Smith VV, Gregson N, Foggensteinor L, et al. Acquired intestinal aganglionosis and circulating autoantibodies without neoplastic or other neuronal involvement. Gastroenterology. 1997;112:1366–71.
25. Burns TM, Lawn ND, Low PA, et al. Adynamic ileus in severe Guillain-Barre syndrome. Muscle Nerve. 2001;24:963–5.

26. Gohil A, Croffie JM, Fitzgerald JF, et al. Reversible intestinal pseudoobstruction associated with neural crest tumors. J Pediatr Gastroenterol Nutr. 2001;33:86–8.
27. Salazar A, Naik A, Rolston DD. Intestinal pseudoobstruction as a presenting feature of a pheochromocytoma. J Clin Gastroenterol. 2001;33:253–4.
28. Anderson NE, Hutchinson DO, Nicholson GJ, et al. Intestinal pseudo-obstruction, myasthenia gravis, and thymoma. Neurology. 1996;47:985–7.
29. Bodensteiner JB, Grunow JE. Gastroparesis in neonatal myotonic dystrophy. Muscle Nerve. 1984;7:486–7.
30. Bruinenberg JF, Rieu PN, Gabreels FM, et al. Intestinal pseudo-obstruction syndrome in a child with myotonic dystrophy. Acta Paediatr. 1996;85:121–3.
31. Leon SH, Schuffler MD, Kettler M, et al. Chronic intestinal pseudoobstruction as a complication of Duchenne's muscular dystrophy. Gastroenterology. 1986;90:455–9.
32. Dalakas MC, Park KY, Semino-Mora C, et al. Desmin myopathy, a skeletal myopathy with cardiomyopathy caused by mutations in the desmin gene. N Engl J Med. 2000;342:770–80.
33. Chinnery PF, Jones S, Sviland L, et al. Mitochondrial enteropathy: the primary pathology may not be within the gastrointestinal tract. Gut. 2001;48:121–4.
34. Haftel LT, Lev D, Barash V, et al. Familial mitochondrial intestinal pseudo-obstruction and neurogenic bladder. J Child Neurol. 2000;15:386–9.
35. Nishino I, Spinazzola A, Papadimitriou A, et al. Mitochondrial neurogastrointestinal encephalomyopathy: an autosomal recessive disorder due to thymidine phosphorylase mutations. Ann Neurol. 2000;47:792–800.
36. Axelrod FB, Gouge TH, Ginsburg HB, et al. Fundoplication and gastrostomy in familial dysautonomia. J Pediatr Gastroenterol Nutr. 1991;118:388–94.
37. Inamdar S, Easton LB, Lester G. Acquired postganglionic cholinergic dysautonomia: case report and review of the literature. Pediatrics. 1982;70:976–8.
38. Eck SL, Morse JH, Janssen DA, et al. Angioedema presenting as chronic gastrointestinal symptoms. Am J Gastroenterol. 1993;88:436–9.
39. Perino LE, Schuffler MD, Mehta SJ, et al. Radiation-induced intestinal pseudoobstruction. Gastroenterology. 1986;91:994–8.
40. Fang SB, Lee HC, Huang FY, et al. Intestinal pseudo-obstruction followed by major clinical features of Kawasaki disease: report of one case. Acta Paediatr Taiwan. 2001;42:111–4.
41. Mayer EA, Schuffler MD, Rotter JI, et al. Familial visceral neuropathy with autosomal dominant transmission. Gastroenterology. 1986;91:1528–35.
42. Roy AD, Bharucha H, Nevin NC, et al. Idiopathic intestinal pseudo-obstruction: a familial visceral neuropathy. Clin Genet. 1980;18:291–7.
43. Faulk DL, Anuras S, Gardner D. A familial visceral myopathy. Ann Intern Med. 1987;89:600–6.
44. Haltia M, Somer H, Palo J, et al. Neuronal intranuclear inclusion disease in identical twins. Ann Neurol. 1984;15:316–21.
45. Patel H, Norman MG, Perry TL, et al. Multiple system atrophy with neuronal intranuclear hyaline inclusions. Report of a case and review of the literature. J Neurol Sci. 1985;67:57–65.
46. Schuffler MD, Bird TD, Sumi SM, et al. A familial neuronal disease presenting as intestinal pseudo-obstruction. Gastroenterology. 1978;75:889–98.
47. Schuffler MD, Lowe MC, Bill AH. Studies of idiopathic intestinal pseudo-obstruction. I. Hereditary hollow visceral myopathy: clinical and pathological studies. Gastroenterology. 1977;73:327–8.
48. Schuffler MD, Pope CE. Studies of idiopathic intestinal pseudo-obstruction. II. Hereditary hollow visceral myopathy: family studies. Gastroenterology. 1977;73:339–44.
49. Anuras S, Mitros FA, Nowak TV, et al. A familial visceral myopathy with external ophthalmoplegia and autosomal recessive transmission. Gastroenterology. 1983;84:346–53.
50. Ionasescu V, Thompson SH, Ionasescu R, et al. Inherited ophthalmoplegia with intestinal pseudo-obstruction. J Neurol Sci. 1983;59:215–28.
51. Auricchio A, Brancolini V, Casari G, et al. The locus for a novel syndromatic form of neuronal intestinal pseudo-obstruction maps to Xq28. Am J Hum Genet. 1996;58:743–8.
52. Van Goethem G, Schwartz M, Löfgren A, et al. Novel POLG mutations in progressive external ophthalmoplegia mimicking mitochondrial neurogastrointestinal encephalomyopathy. Eur J Hum Genet. 2003;11:547–9.
53. Miele E, Tozzi A, Staiano A, et al. Persistence of abnormal gastrointestinal motility after operation for Hirschsprung's disease. Am J Gastroenterol. 2000;95(5):1226–30.
54. Staiano A, Corraziari E, Andriotti MR, et al. Upper gastrointestinal tract motility in children with progressive muscular dystrophy. J Pediatr Gastroenterol Nutr. 1992;121:720–4.
55. Selgrad M, De Giorgio R, Fini L, et al. JC virus infects the enteric glia of patients with chronic idiopathic intestinal pseudo-obstruction. Gut. 2009;58:25–32.
56. Cucchiara S, Bassotti G, Castellucci G, et al. Upper gastrointestinal motor abnormalities in children with celiac disease. J Pediatr Gastroenterol Nutr. 1995;21:435–42.
57. Ginies JL, Francois H, Joseph MG, et al. A curable cause of chronic idiopathic intestinal pseudo-obstruction in children: idiopathic myositis of the small intestine. J Pediatr Gastroenterol Nutr. 1996;23:426–9.
58. Krishnamurthy S, Schuffler MD. Pathology of neuromuscular disorders of the small intestine and colon. Gastroenterology. 1987;93:610–39.
59. Streutker CJ, Huizinga JD, Campbell F, et al. Loss of CD117 (c-kit)- and CD34-positive ICC and

associated CD34-positive fibroblasts defines a subpopulation of chronic intestinal pseudo-obstruction. Am J Surg Pathol. 2003;27(2):228–35.
60. Knowles CH, De Giorgio R, Kapur RP, et al. Gastrointestinal neuromuscular pathology: guidelines for histological techniques and reporting on behalf of the Gastro 2009 International Working Group. Acta Neuropathol. 2009;118:271–301.
61. Knowles CH, De Giorgio R, Kapur RP, et al. The London Classification of gastrointestinal neuromuscular pathology: report on behalf of the Gastro 2009 International Working Group. Gut. 2010;59:882–7.
62. Knowles CH, Farrugia G. Gastrointestinal neuromuscular pathology in chronic constipation. Best Pract Res Clin Gastroenterol. 2011;25(1):43–57.
63. Schuffler MD, Jonak Z. Chronic idiopathic intestinal pseudo-obstruction caused by a degenerative disorder of the myenteric plexus: the use of Smith's method to define the neuropathology. Gastroenterology. 1982;82:476–86.
64. Smith B. The neuropathology of the alimentary tract. London: Edward Arnold; 1972.
65. Schofield ED, Yunis EJ. Intestinal neuronal dysplasia. J Pediatr Gastroenterol Nutr. 1991;12:182–9.
66. Cord-Udy CL, Smith VV, Ahmed S, et al. An evaluation of the role of suction rectal biopsy in the diagnosis of intestinal neuronal dysplasia. J Pediatr Gastroenterol Nutr. 1997;24:1–6.
67. Hyman PE, Bursch B, Zeltzer L. Discriminating chronic intestinal pseudo-obstruction from pediatric condition falsification in toddlers. Child Maltreat. 2002;7(2):132–7.
68. Kosmach B, Tarbell S, Reyes J, et al. "Munchausen by proxy" syndrome in a small bowel transplant recipient. Transplant Proc. 1996;28:2790–1.
69. Hyman PE, Bursch B, Sood M, et al. Visceral pain-associated disability syndrome: a descriptive analysis. J Pediatr Gastroenterol Nutr. 2002;35:663–8.
70. Boige N, Faure C, Cargill G, Mashako LM, Cordeiro-Ferreira G, Viarme F, Cezard JP, Navarro J. Manometrical evaluation in visceral neuropathies in children. J Pediatr Gastroenterol Nutr. 1994;19:71–7.
71. Schuffler MD, Pope II CE. Esophageal motor dysfunction in idiopathic intestinal pseudoobstruction. Gastroenterology. 1976;70:677–82.
72. Camilleri M. Jejunal manometry in distal subacute mechanical obstruction: significance of prolonged simultaneous contractions. Gut. 1989;30:468–75.
73. Summers RW, Anuras S, Green J. Jejunal manometry patterns in health, partial intestinal obstruction, and pseudo-obstruction. Gastroenterology. 1983;85:1301–6.
74. Fell JME, Smith VV, Milla PJ. Infantile chronic idiopathic intestinal pseudo-obstruction: the role of small intestinal manometry as a diagnostic tool and prognostic indicator. Gut. 1996;39:306–11.
75. Hyman PE, DiLorenzo C, McAdams L, et al. Predicting the clinical response to cisapride in children with chronic intestinal pseudo-obstruction. Am J Gastroenterol. 1993;88:832–6.
76. Tomomasa T, DiLorenzo C, Morikawa A, et al. Analysis of fasting antroduodenal manometry in children. Dig Dis Sci. 1996;41:195–203.
77. Tomomasa T, Itoh Z, Koizumi T, Kitamura T, Suzuki N, Matsuyama S, Kuroume T. Manometric study on the intestinal motility in a case of megacystis-microcolon-intestinal hypoperistalsis syndrome. J Pediatr Gastroenterol Nutr. 1985;4:307–10.
78. Cucchiara S, Borrelli O, Salvia G, Iula VD, Fecarotta S, Gaudiello G, Boccia G, Annese V. A normal gastrointestinal motility excludes chronic intestinal pseudoobstruction in children. Dig Dis Sci. 2000;45:258–64.
79. Di Lorenzo C, Flores AF, Reddy SN, et al. Colonic manometry in children with chronic intestinal pseudo-obstruction. Gut. 1993;34:803–7.
80. Devane SP, Ravelli AM, Bisset WM, et al. Gastric antral dysrhythmias in children with chronic idiopathic intestinal pseudo-obstruction. Gut. 1992;33:1477–81.
81. Dahms BB, Halpin Jr TC. Serial liver biopsies in parenteral nutrition-associated cholestasis of early infancy. Gastroenterology. 1981;81:136–44.
82. Roslyn JJ, Berquist WE, Pitt HA, et al. Increased risk of gallstones in children receiving total parenteral nutrition. Pediatrics. 1993;71:784–9.
83. Di Lorenzo C, Flores A, Hyman PE. Intestinal motility and jejunal feeding in children with chronic intestinal pseudo-obstruction. Gastroenterology. 1995;108:1379–85.
84. Di Lorenzo C, Reddy SN, Villanueva-Meyer J, et al. Cisapride in children with chronic intestinal pseudo-obstruction: an acute, double-blind crossover placebo controlled trial. Gastroenterology. 1991;101:1564–70.
85. Di Lorenzo C, Flores AF, Tomomasa T, et al. Effect of erythromycin on antroduodenal motility in children with chronic functional gastrointestinal symptoms. Dig Dis Sci. 1994;39:1399–404.
86. Dranove J, Horn D, Reddy SN, et al. Effect of intravenous erythromycin on the colonic motility of children and young adults during colonic manometry. J Pediatr Surg. 2010;45:777–83.
87. Di Lorenzo C, Lucanto C, Flores AF, et al. Effect of octreotide on gastrointestinal motility in children with functional gastrointestinal symptoms. J Pediatr Gastroenterol Nutr. 1998;27(5):508–12.
88. Gomez R, Fernandez S, Aspiroz A, et al. Effect of amoxicillin-clavulanate on gastrointestinal motility in children. J Pediatr Gastroenterol Nutr. 2012;54(6):780–4.
89. Hyman PE, Garvey TQ, Abrams CE. Tolerance to intravenous ranitidine. J Pediatr Gastroenterol Nutr. 1987;110:794–6.
90. Youssef NN, Barksdale Jr E, Griffiths JM, et al. Management of intractable constipation with antegrade enemas in neurologically intact children. J Pediatr Gastroenterol Nutr. 2002;34:402–5.

91. Rosner H, Rubin L, Kestenbaum A. Gabapentin adjunctive therapy in neuropathic pain states. Clin J Pain. 1996;12:56–8.
92. Teitelbaum JE, Berde CB, Nurko S, Buonomo C, Perez-Atayde AR, Fox VL. Diagnosis and management of MNGIE syndrome in children: case report and review of the literature. J Pediatr Gastroenterol Nutr. 2002;35:377–83.
93. Devulder J, De Laat M, Rolly G. Stellate ganglion block alleviates pseudo-obstruction symptoms followed by episodes of hypermetropia: case report. Reg Anesth. 1997;22:284–6.
94. Khelif K, Scaillon M, Govaerts MJM, Vanderwinden JM, De Laet MH. Bilateral thoracoscopic splanchnicectomy in chronic intestinal pseudo-obstruction: report of two paediatric cases. Gut. 2006;55:293–4.
95. Pitt HA, Mann LL, Berquist WE, et al. Chronic intestinal pseudo-obstruction: management with total parenteral nutrition and a venting enterostomy. Arch Surg. 1985;120:614–8.
96. Michaud L, Guimber D, Carpentier B, Sfeir R, Lambilliotte A, Mazingue F, Gottrand F, Turck D. Gastrostomy as a decompression technique in children with chronic gastrointestinal obstruction. J Pediatr Gastroenterol Nutr. 2001;32:82–5.
97. Di Lorenzo C, Flores A, Hyman PE. Intestinal motility in symptomatic children with fundoplication. J Pediatr Gastroenterol Nutr. 1991;12:169–73.
98. Ordein J, DiLorenzo C, Flores A, et al. Diversion colitis in children with pseudo-obstruction. Am J Gastroenterol. 1992;87:88–90.
99. Sigurdsson L, Reyes J, Kocoshis SA, et al. Intestinal transplantation in children with chronic intestinal pseudo-obstruction. Gut. 1999;45:570–4.
100. Lin Z, Sarosiek I, Forster J, et al. Two-channel gastric pacing in patients with diabetic gastroparesis. Neurogastroenterol Motil. 2011;23(10):912–e396.
101. Mughal MM, Irving MH. Treatment of end stage chronic intestinal pseudo-obstruction by subtotal enterectomy and home parenteral nutrition. Gut. 1988;29(11):1613–7.
102. Nayyar N, Mazariegos G, Ranganathan S, et al. Pediatric small bowel transplantation. Semin Pediatr Surg. 2010;19(1):68–77.
103. Mousa H, Hyman PE, Cocjin J, et al. Long term outcome of congenital intestinal pseudo-obstruction. Dig Dis Sci. 2002;47:2298–305.
104. Schwankovsky L, Mousa H, Rowhani A, et al. Quality of life outcomes in congenital chronic intestinal pseudo-obstruction. Dig Dis Sci. 2002;47:1965–8.

Hirschsprung Disease

23

Robert O. Heuckeroth

There are many excellent articles on Hirschsprung disease (HSCR) that provide detailed information about the clinical presentation, epidemiology, genetics, diagnosis, and associated medical problems [1–9]. This chapter summarizes and simplifies the complex HSCR literature. Percentages in the text and tables are estimates, since widely divergent numbers are presented in different manuscripts.

The enteric nervous system (ENS) is an integrated network of neurons and glia that controls most aspects of intestinal function. This includes intestinal motility, response to luminal and intramural stimuli, regulation of epithelial activity and control of blood flow. To perform these tasks, neurons are distributed along the entire length of the bowel in a well-ordered and finely regulated manner. When the ENS is absent or defective in any region of the bowel, profound problems with intestinal function occur causing significant morbidity and in some cases death.

Introduction

Hirschsprung disease, the most well understood intestinal motility disorder, is characterized by the complete absence of enteric neurons (i.e., aganglionosis) in the myenteric and submucosal plexus of the distal bowel. In the absence of ganglion cells, the bowel tonically contracts causing a functional intestinal obstruction. Many, but not all, clinical manifestations of HSCR result from the tonic contraction of aganglionic bowel.

Nomenclature describing the extent of aganglionosis in HSCR is not consistent. However, most affected individuals have "short segment" disease where aganglionosis is restricted to the rectosigmoid region of the colon [7, 8, 10]. "Long-segment" HSCR aganglionosis extends proximal to the sigmoid colon and is usually distinguished from "total colonic" aganglionosis. In a small percentage of cases, aganglionosis extends into the small bowel leading to very serious life-long disability often requiring total parenteral nutrition (Table 23.1) [7, 8]. Although some authors have suggested that clinical presentation varies with the length of aganglionosis [4], others claim that clinical symptoms are not related to the extent of disease [1]. From a practical standpoint, it is best to assume that the extent of aganglionosis and the severity and character of symptoms are unrelated.

Clinical Presentation

HSCR is debilitating and can be fatal. Clinical presentation is highly variable and diagnosis requires a high index of suspicion (Table 23.2). Recognizing HSCR is important since surgical management dramatically reduces disease morbidity and mortality.

R.O. Heuckeroth, M.D., Ph.D. (✉)
Department of Pediatrics, Division of Gastroenterology, Hepatology, and Nutrition, Washington University School of Medicine, 660 South Euclid Avenue, Campus Box 8208, St. Louis, MO 63110, USA
e-mail: heuckeroth@kids.wustl.edu

C. Faure et al. (eds.), *Pediatric Neurogastroenterology: Gastrointestinal Motility and Functional Disorders in Children*, Clinical Gastroenterology,
DOI 10.1007/978-1-60761-709-9_23,

Table 23.1 Extent of aganglionosis

Short segment	74–89%
Long segment	12–22%
Total colon	4–13%
Small bowel	3–5%

Adapted from Haricharan and Georgeson [8]

Table 23.2 Presenting symptoms in HSCR

Symptom	Comment
Abdominal distension	Very Common in HSCR or anatomic bowel obstruction
Bilious emesis	Common and suggests HSCR or anatomic defects
Constipation	Common in older children with HSCR but also in healthy toddlers and infants
Diarrhea	Foul smelling, bloody or "explosive" diarrhea suggests enterocolitis (HAEC)
Delayed Meconium	Common in HSCR, but many infants with HSCR do not have delayed passage of meconium
Bowel perforation	Should raise concern for HSCR

In the current era, most people with HSCR are diagnosed by 6 months of age [11–13], but it is not unusual to diagnose HSCR in older children and HSCR has been diagnosed in adults up to 73 years of age [14]. HSCR needs to be considered in anyone with severe chronic constipation that began in early infancy, especially if suppositories or enemas are needed for stool passage. However, because constipation is common, affecting up to 35% of all children [15, 16], and HSCR is rare (1/5,000 people), recognizing distinct features that suggest HSCR is important for diagnosis. Furthermore, constipation is only one feature of HSCR. Typical presentations for HSCR include:

1. **Neonatal intestinal obstruction**
   Infants present with marked abdominal distension and bilious emesis. Distension may be severe enough to cause respiratory compromise. Obstruction may occur on the first day of life, but children may also initially have apparently normal bowel movements or "mild constipation" and then present acutely with abdominal distension and vomiting at an older age. Because HSCR requires a high index of suspicion for diagnosis, some infants are hospitalized repeatedly for episodes of presumed "gastroenteritis" that were actually a manifestation of HSCR associated intestinal obstruction. A key clinical distinction is that gastroenteritis may cause severe vomiting, but does not typically cause as much abdominal distension as HSCR. Vomiting associated with infectious enteritis is also usually followed by diarrhea, whereas intestinal obstruction should be accompanied by reduced stool passage. A distended abdomen occurs in 57–93% of infants with Hirschsprung disease and bilious emesis occurs in 19–37% [1, 8, 17–19].
2. **Neonatal bowel perforation**
   HSCR presents with bowel perforation about 5% of the time [20, 21] and HSCR causes about 10% of all neonatal bowel perforations [22]. Symptoms may not be specific and include poor feeding, emesis, abdominal distension, constipation, diarrhea, and lethargy. In two series with 55 cases reported [20, 21] only one child was more than 2 months old. The majority of the perforations were in the cecum or ascending colon and 15% were in the appendix. Many of the children with bowel perforation had long-segment disease (34% total colonic aganglionosis, with an additional 23% having aganglionosis proximal to the splenic flexure). Since long-segment HSCR is less common than short segment disease (see Table 23.1), proximal colon perforation in a young infant should dramatically raise concern for long-segment HSCR. In 55% of reported cases, the perforation was proximal to the transition zone and occurred in ganglion cell containing bowel. In 13% the perforation was at the transition zone. In 30%, however, the perforation occurred in aganglionic bowel distal to the transition zone.
3. **Delayed passage of meconium**
   Delayed passage of meconium should suggest the diagnosis of HSCR, but defining HSCR risk in infants with delayed passage of meconium is challenging because the timing of meconium passage reported for healthy infants is variable. In a study of 979 infants older than 34 weeks gestational age in the United States, 97% passed meconium by 24 h of life, and 99.8% passed meconium by 36 h of life [23]. Breast feeding or bottle feeding did not influence the timing of the first bowel movement and multivariate analysis

demonstrated that only prematurity was a significant predictor of delayed passage of meconium. A similar study in Turkey [24] also demonstrated that 724/743 (97%) passed meconium by 24 h after birth and 740/743 (99.6%) passed meconium by the time that they were 48 h old. However, a smaller study in the Netherlands, reported only 56/71 (79%) of term infants passed meconium by 24 h after birth [25] and in a study of 267 healthy infants in Nigeria, only 92% passed their first bowel movement by 48 h after birth [26]. In the Nigerian study, 5% of the infants were preterm, but even if the preterm infants are excluded, the data suggest that at most 97% of the healthy full term infants studied passed their first bowel movement by the time they were 48 h old. Excluding premature infants from the analysis is important since prematurity predisposes to delayed passage of meconium. A study of 611 infants reported that only 57% of infants less than 29 weeks EGA, 66% of infants between 29 and 32 weeks EGA, and 80% of infants between 32 and 37 weeks EGA [27] passed meconium by the end of their "second calendar day" and 1% of premature infants did not pass meconium until after day of life 9. In children with Hirschsprung disease, delayed passage of meconium is much more common than in healthy infants. Nonetheless, up to 50% of children with HSCR pass meconium by 48 h after birth [17, 28, 29], so passage of meconium within 48 h of birth does not exclude a diagnosis of HSCR.

4. **Chronic severe constipation**
   HSCR causes constipation, but constipation unrelated to HSCR is very common and HSCR is rare, so constipation alone usually does not indicate HSCR. "Severe" constipation and constipation beginning within the first few months of life does increase concern for HSCR and the likelihood of disease. For example, in one study, rectal biopsy was performed on all children over a year of age who were referred to a specialty center for consultation and who had constipation refractory to more than 6 months of medical management. 19 out of 395 biopsies demonstrated HSCR (5%), a 250-fold increased risk compared to the population prevalence of HSCR (1/5,000) [30]. Constipation in isolation also appears to be an uncommon presentation of HSCR in infants. In particular, the wide range of normal bowel movement frequency in healthy infants makes it difficult to use constipation as the only indication to evaluate for HSCR. In a study of 911 healthy children in Turkey (Tunc 2008) between 2 and 12 months of age, mean stool frequency was once a day, but at 2 months of age stool frequency varied from once a week to eight times per day.
5. **Abdominal distension relieved by rectal stimulation or enema**
   In children with HSCR, rectal exam or other forms of rectal stimulation may cause a sudden "explosive" release of intraluminal contents and relieve abdominal distension. This is uncommon in other conditions and should raise concern about HSCR. Rectal exam is, however, not otherwise useful in identifying children with HSCR. In particular, "anal tone" is not a reliable indicator of disease.
6. **Enterocolitis**
   Defining when children have enterocolitis presents its own challenges (see below for symptoms), but enterocolitis is a dangerous and common presentation for HSCR. When enterocolitis occurs, children with HSCR have diarrhea instead of constipation.

Who Should be Biopsied to Evaluate for Hirschsprung Disease?

Rectal biopsy is the "gold standard" diagnostic test for HSCR (see below). Unless another diagnosis is evident, children with the following clinical presentations *should undergo* rectal biopsy to evaluate for Hirschsprung disease:

1. Neonates with significant abdominal distension, especially in combination with bilious vomiting or delayed passage of meconium.
2. Neonates with bowel perforation.

Also *consider* rectal biopsy for Hirschsprung disease in children with:

1. Neonatal bloody diarrhea. Given the low incidence of infectious enteritis in breast fed or formula fed neonates, bloody diarrhea in neonates is concerning for HSCR associated enterocolitis (see below).

2. Healthy appearing full term infants with delayed passage of meconium even in the absence of other symptoms. Since Hirschsprung disease occurs in 1:5,000 infants, but delayed passage of meconium for more than 48 h after birth probably happens in at least 1:1,000 healthy infants, most children (i.e., >80%) who have delayed passage of meconium for 48 h will not have HSCR, but the risk of HSCR is probably 5–20%. Given the risks associated with untreated HSCR, I usually recommend biopsy in this setting. Assuming that 97% of healthy full term infants pass meconium by 24 h of life, only about 1:150 children with passage of meconium >24 h after birth, but <48 h after birth will have HSCR. The value of rectal biopsy in this setting is more questionable, unless other symptoms of HSCR are present.
3. Young children with constipation refractory to oral medication. Constipation beginning after a year of age is rarely due to HSCR. Constipation that improves dramatically with oral medication is also unlikely to be due to HSCR. Remember too that the common form of functional constipation that occurs in toddlers may be challenging to treat, so it can be challenging to know if toddlers are truly "refractory to oral medication."

Red Flags (conditions that should raise suspicion for HSCR):

1. Constipation with episodes of abdominal distension or vomiting. Constipation does not cause vomiting, but many disorders cause both vomiting and reduced bowel movement frequency including HSCR.
2. Growth failure. This is a common feature of untreated HSCR.
3. Trisomy 21. HSCR occurs in 1:100 children with Down syndrome so HSCR should be more readily suspected in children with trisomy 21.
4. The presence of additional anomalies also increases the likelihood of HSCR, but remember that most children with HSCR do not have other medical problems.

Given the diverse presenting symptoms of HSCR, it remains difficult to decide who to evaluate. The more "classic" features of HSCR present, the more likely the child has HSCR. Given the high morbidity and mortality in untreated HSCR, evaluation for HSCR should be performed in many children who do not end up having this disease to avoid missing this potentially life threatening medical problem.

Diagnostic Strategies

HSCR by definition means that affected individuals do not have ganglion cells in the distal bowel. Rectal biopsy is therefore required to make the diagnosis and is considered the "gold standard" approach [31]. A number of other strategies for diagnosing HSCR are used, but each has problems.

1. **Rectal suction biopsy**
   This is a simple procedure taking only a few minutes using an instrument designed to take small pieces of the rectal mucosa (e.g., Noblett or rbi2 instrument) to reduce the risk of bowel perforation or hemorrhage [32]. Because there are no sensory nerve endings that respond to cutting in the area of the rectum where the biopsies are obtained, sedation and pain medicines are not required, but sedation is sometimes used in older children. Biopsies should be obtained at 2–3 cm from the dentate line (i.e., the transition between rectal and squamous mucosa) because there is a physiological submucosal aganglionosis in the terminal rectum. From a practical standpoint, however, some authors advocate obtaining biopsies at multiple levels (e.g., 1, 2, and 3 cm from the dentate line) because precise positioning of the biopsy can be difficult. Biopsy tissues obtained are sectioned, stained and examined by a pathologist to identify ganglion cells. There is some controversy about the optimal staining method, but hematoxylin and eosin and acetylcholinesterase are commonly used techniques [31, 32]. A meta-analysis analyzing data from 993 patients indicated that the mean sensitivity of rectal suction biopsy for HSCR is 93%, and the mean specificity is 98% [33]. A more recent manuscript documents 935 cases of HSCR diagnosed by rectal mucosal biopsy (a total of 19,365 biopsies in 6,615 children) with no false positive or false negative diagnoses (i.e., 100% sensitivity and specificity) [34]. Serious

bleeding and bowel perforation are uncommon with rectal suction biopsy, but can occur. One series of 1,340 biopsies [35] reported three bowel perforations (0.2%), one death (0.07%), and three rectal hemorrhage (0.2%) requiring blood transfusion. More recent studies also document low but non-zero rates of serious bleeding or bowel perforation (no complications in 297 children [36]; no complications in 88 infants [37]; and 2 episodes of bleeding requiring transfusion (0.7%) plus one episode of rectal perforation and sepsis (0.035%) in 272 children [38]). The most common problem with rectal suction biopsies, however, is that they are so small that they are "inadequate" 6–26% of the time requiring repeat biopsy to make a diagnosis [36, 38, 39].

2. **Anorectal manometry**
   This method tests for the rectoanal inhibition reflex using a small balloon attached to a tube inserted into the rectum [33]. This reflex is absent in children with HSCR. Sensitivity and specificity of anorectal manometry are 91 and 94% respectively, but this test is not required to diagnose HSCR [33]. Furthermore, the equipment needed to do this test is expensive, patient cooperation is needed, and significant experience is needed to evaluate results in infants less than a year of age, so the test is not widely available.
3. **Contrast enema**
   This is a radiology test where images are obtained as contrast is infused into the colon via the anal canal to look for evidence of the distal bowel contraction that occurs in areas of aganglionosis. The change in bowel caliber between contracted distal aganglionic bowel and more dilated ganglion cell containing bowel is called the "transition zone" and suggests HSCR. Although contrast enema may have value in planning the surgical approach to HSCR, the radiographic and anatomic transition from aganglionic to ganglion cell containing bowel may not be in the same location. It should also be noted that in total colonic HSCR there is no colon transition zone. Furthermore, the sensitivity (70%) and specificity (50–80%) are considerably lower using contrast enema for HSCR diagnosis than other methods [19, 33]. The role of contrast enema in HSCR diagnosis therefore remains a matter of debate.
4. **Full thickness rectal biopsy**
   Deeper biopsies can be performed by a surgeon under general anesthesia if the diagnosis remains uncertain after rectal suction biopsy.

Epidemiology/Genetics Overview

HSCR is a multigenic disorder that affects approximately 1/5,000 infants. At least 10 specific gene defects are associated with HSCR. For short segment disease there is an approximately 4:1 male to female ratio, but for total colonic aganglionosis, the male to female ratio is near 2:1. HSCR has been reported throughout the world in many ethnic groups. There are geographic and racial differences described in HSCR incidence, but these data are difficult to evaluate. Most reports have not been replicated over extended time periods and the difficulty in HSCR diagnosis increases uncertainty in interpreting regional data. Furthermore, it is often not possible to determine from large-scale epidemiological studies the number of affected individuals who share mutations by common descent, so data may be skewed by families with multiple affected members, such as has been described in some Mennonite communities [40]. HSCR incidence per 10,000 live births in California were reported as 1.0, 1.5, 2.1, and 2.8 for Hispanics, Caucasian-Americans, African-Americans and Asians respectively [41]. HSCR incidence was reported as 1.4 per 10,000 in Denmark, 1.8–2.1 per 10,000 in Japan [7], and 2.3 per 10,000 in British Columbia [42]. Considerably higher rates of HSCR are reported in some small geographic areas or ethnic groups. For example, HSCR incidence is 2.9 per 10,000 in Tasmania [43], 5.6 per 10,000 for native Alaskans [44], 7.3 per 10,000 in Pohnpei State in the Federated States of Micronesia [45], and 5.6 per 10,000 in Oman [46]. In Oman, rates of consanguinity are reported to be high (75% first or second cousins). Founder effects within populations, nutritional factors, or environmental toxins may also account for these differences in HSCR incidence.

Recurrence risk for siblings of children with HSCR is dramatically elevated compared to the general population, but HSCR is a non-Mendelian disease and risk varies from 1:3 to 1:100

[6, 47], depending on the sex of the proband and the extent of aganglionosis. Because female sex protects against HSCR and because long-segment disease implies more serious genetic risk than short segment disease, male siblings of females with long-segment HSCR have a 33% chance of HSCR, while new sisters have only a 9% risk. Siblings of males with long-segment HSCR have a recurrence risk of 17 and 13% in new brothers and sisters respectively. For a male proband with short segment HSCR the risk of recurrence is 5% in male siblings, but only 1% in female siblings. For a female proband with short segment disease, recurrence risk is 5 and 3% for new male and female siblings respectively. These complex epidemiologic and recurrence risk data are a direct reflection of the genetic underpinnings of HSCR. While these "average" data are helpful in discussions with families, far better estimates of HSCR recurrence risk could theoretically be obtained using modern molecular genetic techniques.

Associated Medical Problems

HSCR is an isolated anomaly in ~70% of affected individuals, but ~30% of children with HSCR have additional birth defects, including the ~12% of children with HSCR who have chromosomal anomalies [9, 29, 42, 48–50]. A very wide range of additional defects have been reported in children with HSCR. The most common defects are congenital heart disease, sensory neural problems, kidney and urinary tract, and skeletal anomalies. Many different chromosomal defects have been described in people with HSCR, but trisomy 21 is by far the most common. There are also >30 genetic syndromes associated with HSCR (reviewed in Amiel 2008). A few HSCR associated syndromes are summarized in Table 23.3.

Surgical Management

Although Harald Hirschsprung first described children with the disease that now bears his name in 1886 [51], the pathophysiology of HSCR and management strategies remained unknown until the first successful surgical approach was described in 1948 [52]. There are many modifications of the original pull-through surgery, but the most common procedures today are the Swenson, Duhamel, and Soave endorectal techniques with modification of surgical approaches for total colonic HSCR [1, 2, 53]. For each of these procedures, intraoperative biopsies are obtained to determine the extent of aganglionosis. The Swenson procedure involves complete resection of the aganglionic bowel with reanastomosis of ganglion cell containing bowel to a 1–2 cm rectal cuff. In the Duhamel modification, ganglion cell containing bowel is brought through the retrorectal space and anastomosed to a segment of aganglionic rectum using a side-to-side anastomosis. In the Soave procedure as modified by Boley, the rectal mucosa and submucosa are removed, the ganglion cell containing bowel is pulled through a muscular cuff of distal aganglionic bowel, and then attached within 1 cm of the anal verge. There are innumerable studies of surgical outcome, but few large-scale systematic comparisons are available [54], so it remains unclear that one procedure is better than another. Over the past decade there have been three major changes in surgical management. These include laparoscopic surgery, transanal surgery, and increased use of one-step surgical procedures [8, 55–58]. A recent analysis of transanal versus transabdominal surgery suggests that the children who had transanal endorectal pull-through procedures for HSCR had fewer complications and lower rates of enterocolitis [13].

Cost for Initial Management

For children with HSCR, initial hospitalization costs average $100,000 and the hospital stay averages almost a month [59]. Taking into account HSCR incidence and birth rates, estimated costs for initial care of children with HSCR in the United States is at least $86 million/year. This cost estimate does not include the expense of lost work time or other expenses families encounter while caring for an ill child. Estimates also do not

Table 23.3 Selected HSCR associated syndromes

Syndrome name	Genetic defect	Comments
MEN2A = Multiple Endocrine Neoplasia 2A	RET mutation in codons 609, 611, 618, or 620	~2% of children with HSCR may have MEN2A RET mutations; 20–30% of families with Ret 609, 611, 618, or 620 mutations have members with both FMTC and HSCR
FMTC = Familial medullary thyroid carcinoma		
Down Syndrome	Trisomy 21	1% of children with trisomy 21 have HSCR; 2–10% of children with HSCR have Down's
WS4 = Waardenburg Syndrome	WS4A = EDNRB	9% of children with HSCR have WS4
	WS4C = SOX10	Syndrome includes HSCR, deafness and pigmentary abnormalities
CCHS = Congenital central hypoventilation syndrome	PHOX2B	20% of children with CCHS have HSCR; 0.5–1.5% of children with HSCR have CCHS
MWS = Mowat-Wilson Syndrome	ZFHX1B	60% of children with MWS have HSCR; 6% of children with HSCR have MWS; Syndrome includes HSCR, intellectual disability, epilepsy, dysmorphic facial features, brain and heart defects
Goldberg-Sphrintzen Megacolon Syndrome	KIAA1279	Syndrome includes HSCR, intellectual disability, dysmorphic facial features, brain and heart defects

include the cost of ongoing care after the initial hospitalization, which in some cases may be significant, especially in children with enterocolitis. For children with aganglionosis extending into the small bowel, long term parenteral nutrition also adds dramatically to cost and disease morbidity. Finding new ways to treat or prevent HSCR therefore remains desirable.

Enterocolitis

Hirschsprung disease associated enterocolitis (HAEC) is common, can occur at any time before or after surgery, and is the most frequent cause of death in infants and children with HSCR. Death from HAEC occurs because HSCR predisposes to bacterial translocation into the bloodstream that leads to sepsis. Nonetheless, recognizing HAEC is difficult and until recently there was no standard clinical definition for HAEC. In 2009 a consensus of expert surgeons and gastroenterologists developed a systematic scoring system to identify children with HSCR [60]. Components of the score include "explosive" diarrhea, foul smelling diarrhea, or bloody diarrhea. Additional components include abdominal distension, explosive discharge of gas and stool with rectal exam, reduced peripheral perfusion, lethargy and fever. Radiographic findings include multiple air fluid levels, distended loops of bowel, sawtooth and irregular mucosal lining, pneumatosis and rectosigmoid cutoff sign with the absence of distal air. Laboratory findings include leukocytosis and a left shift. Many of these features are also listed as presenting symptoms for HSCR because HAEC is common in children with HSCR, especially before surgery.

The reason that children with HSCR develop HAEC is not clear, but enterocolitis does not occur in children with "severe" functional constipation. Possible predisposing factors for HAEC in children with HSCR include residual partial bowel obstruction, defects in epithelial integrity, or abnormalities in the immune system [61]. Partial obstruction may result from stricture or from intestinal dysmotility causing increased intraluminal pressure and possibly changes in gut flora. Epithelial dysfunction may occur because enteric neurons and glia support normal bowel epithelial cell function and mucin production [62–67]. Problems with intestinal immunity may occur because the ENS directly regulates the intestinal immune system [68–70]. Furthermore, some of the genes defective in children with HSCR have roles in development of the immune system.

For example, RET is important for Peyer's patch formation [71], while EDNRB is important for normal spleen development [72]. Given the diverse genetic underpinnings of HSCR, there may be more than one mechanism for HAEC.

Optimal methods to treat or prevent HAEC are not yet known. Current treatment includes bowel rest, nasogastric tube drainage, intravenous fluids, decompression of dilated bowel via rectal dilation and/or rectal irrigation with normal saline, and the use of broad spectrum antibiotics [61]. Routine rectal irrigation [73] and the long-term use of metronidazole in children at high risk of enterocolitis may also reduce the frequency of HAEC episodes. Because HAEC is potentially fatal, it is critical that families understand symptoms of enterocolitis and that plans are in place for prompt treatment should these symptoms arise.

Long Term Outcome

Untreated HSCR is a deadly disease, but outcome with modern surgical methods and improved medical management strategies is dramatically better than in the past. Nonoperative management leads to very high mortality rates (e.g., >50–80%), and reports from the 1970s describe mortality rates of 25–35% [1, 74] even with surgical treatment. HSCR death rates today remain about 2–6%, in large part attributable to enterocolitis [7, 10, 29, 75, 76]. Enterocolitis occurs commonly both before and after surgery for HSCR (25–45% of children) [13, 59, 77, 78]. Long-term outcome even years after surgery also remains less than ideal with only 45–89% having normal bowel function. Many individuals continue to have fecal soiling (4–29%), constipation (3–22%), or permanent stomas (7–10%) [79–81]. Normal bowel function is even less common in children with Down syndrome (34%). Bowel function appears to improve as children get older with "normal" continence in 58% at 5–10 years after surgery, 68% at 10–15 years after surgery, and 89% at 15–20 years after surgery in one study [79]. In this analysis 7% had marked limitation in their social life 5–10 years after surgery, although this problem improved as children became older.

Lessons from Mouse Models

There are many mouse models with distal bowel or total intestinal aganglionosis that mimic human HSCR [82–87]. This includes mice with mutations in *Ret, Sox10, Ednrb, Edn3, Ece1, Phox2b, β(Beta)1 integrin, Ihh,* and *Pax3.* Mutations in several additional genes affect ENS structure or function but do not cause distal bowel aganglionosis including *Nrtn, Gfra2, Gdnf, Shh, Nt3, Trkc, Sprty2, Dcc,* and *Hlx1*. These model organisms support the human genetic data that identified mutations causing HSCR and also provide additional insight into disease pathogenesis. Mouse models are particularly valuable because they provide direct evidence that specific genetic defects cause specific anomalies. There are a several simple lessons from these model organisms that are relevant to human clinical disease. First, the ENS is often abnormal in the proximal bowel of mice with distal bowel aganglionosis [88], suggesting that many of the ongoing problems in children with HSCR occur because the "normal" proximal bowel is not really normal. Furthermore, areas in the distal bowel that contain ganglion cells may be profoundly hypoganglionic, a problem that is not apparent with the limited biopsies that are obtained during surgery for children with HSCR. Finally in some mouse models, ENS anatomy is nearly normal, but function is profoundly abnormal [89] emphasizing that even sophisticated pathological methods may not provide the information needed to optimize intestinal function. There are human correlates to these observations in mice including the observation that motility problems of the stomach, small bowel and esophagus are common in humans with HSCR [90–94].

The Future of Hirschsprung Disease

Outcomes for children with HSCR today are quite good, but many challenges remain. The primary problems and opportunities include:

1. There have been major advances in our understanding of the genetic underpinnings

of HSCR, but these findings are not yet routinely incorporated into clinical practice. Furthermore, there is no consensus about what type of molecular genetic testing, if any, should be performed on children with HSCR. One reasonable argument is that all children with HSCR should be tested for RET mutations that cause MEN2A, but this is still not common practice. As genetic testing becomes less expensive and the capacity to test for many mutations simultaneously increases, it may become practical to perform more comprehensive analysis that would provide information about the risk of other medical problems. It is important that we develop user friendly methods to understand the type of complex genetic data that are relevant for children with HSCR.

2. Enterocolitis remains a common cause of morbidity and the most common cause of mortality in children with HSCR. We need to have a more complete understanding of factors that predispose to HAEC and new ways to prevent this problem. More research is needed to understand the impact of the ENS on mucosal integrity and on immune system function. We also need more information about whether specific HSCR predisposing mutations increase the risk of HAEC. Most importantly we ought to know if there are factors that can be modified to reduce HAEC frequency or severity. Are there changes in surgical approach that would help? Would probiotics be useful? Are there additional medications that could reduce HAEC rates? Would a more systematic analysis of pathology at the time of surgery help? These questions must be investigated in more detail.
3. We need improved methods to evaluate and visualize the ENS. Recent intriguing experiments suggest that advanced acousto-optic spectral imaging techniques might be useful during surgery [95], but these methods require further development and testing. The ability to visualize the ENS without biopsy could potentially make surgery faster and provide better data about the location of the anatomic transition zone. These data might improve surgical outcomes and reduce post-surgical HAEC rates by enhancing the surgeon's ability to evaluate the density of bowel innervation intra-operatively. They could also reduce the cost of surgery.
4. We need to determine if there are ways to reduce HSCR occurrence rates or to reduce the extent of aganglionosis in affected individuals. New data from our laboratory suggest that many environmental factors, including maternal vitamin A levels, may impact the likelihood that children develop HSCR [96]. Reports of monozygotic twins discordant for HSCR also suggest that HSCR is not a purely genetic disease [29, 49, 97, 98]. Large-scale epidemiological studies coupled with work in model systems should be pursued to identify maternal drugs, health conditions, or nutritional problems that could be modified to prevent HSCR.
5. We need to find new ways to replace or repair the ENS when it is damaged or when development is defective. New very exciting studies of ENS stem cells provide hope for the future, but many obstacles need to be overcome for stem cell replacement therapy to become a practical treatment strategy [99–103]. Specifically, we need to know how to differentiate stem cells into specific types of neurons or glia, to implant those cells close to where they are needed, and to encourage stem cells to establish a functional enteric neuron network.

Summary

Over the past century dramatic advances have been made in Hirschsprung disease diagnosis, surgical management, developmental biology and genetics. Ongoing studies provide new hope that we will be able to reduce HSCR incidence, prevent HAEC, replace missing enteric neurons using stem cells, image the ENS intra-operatively, improve surgical techniques, and incorporate genetics into clinical practice.

References

1. Sieber WK. Hirschsprung's disease. Curr Probl Surg. 1978;15(6):1–76.
2. Skinner MA. Hirschsprung's disease. Curr Probl Surg. 1996;33(5):389–460.
3. Dasgupta R, Langer JC. Hirschsprung disease. Curr Probl Surg. 2004;41(12):942–88.
4. Martucciello G. Hirschsprung's disease, one of the most difficult diagnoses in pediatric surgery: a review of the problems from clinical practice to the bench. Eur J Pediatr Surg. 2008;18(3):140–9.
5. Coran AG, Teitelbaum DH. Recent advances in the management of Hirschsprung's disease. Am J Surg. 2000;180(5):382–7.
6. Amiel J, Sproat-Emison E, Garcia-Barcelo M, et al. Hirschsprung disease, associated syndromes and genetics: a review. J Med Genet. 2008;45(1):1–14.
7. Suita S, Taguchi T, Iciri S, Nakatsuji T. Hirschsprung's disease in Japan: analysis of 3852 patients based on a nationwide survey in 30 years. J Pediatr Surg. 2005;40(1):197–201. discussion 201–192.
8. Haricharan RN, Georgeson KE. Hirschsprung disease. Semin Pediatr Surg. 2008;17(4):266–75.
9. Godbole K. Many faces of Hirschsprung's disease. Indian Pediatr. 2004;41(11):1115–23.
10. Ikeda K, Goto S. Diagnosis and treatment of Hirschsprung's disease in Japan. An analysis of 1628 patients. Ann Surg. 1984;199(4):400–5.
11. Singh SJ, Croaker GD, Manglick P, et al. Hirschsprung's disease: the Australian Paediatric Surveillance Unit's experience. Pediatr Surg Int. 2003;19(4):247–50.
12. Klein MD, Coran AG, Wesley JR, Drongowski RA. Hirschsprung's disease in the newborn. J Pediatr Surg. 1984;19(4):370–4.
13. Kim AC, Langer JC, Pastor AC, et al. Endorectal pull-through for Hirschsprung's disease-a multicenter, long-term comparison of results: transanal vs transabdominal approach. J Pediatr Surg. 2010;45(6):1213–20.
14. Chen F, Winston 3rd JH, Jain SK, Frankel WL. Hirschsprung's disease in a young adult: report of a case and review of the literature. Ann Diagn Pathol. 2006;10(6):347–51.
15. Wald ER, Di Lorenzo C, Cipriani L, Colborn DK, Burgers R, Wald A. Bowel habits and toilet training in a diverse population of children. J Pediatr Gastroenterol Nutr. 2009;48(3):294–8.
16. van den Berg MM, Benninga MA, Di Lorenzo C. Epidemiology of childhood constipation: a systematic review. Am J Gastroenterol. 2006;101(10):2401–9.
17. Hackam DJ, Reblock KK, Redlinger RE, Barksdale Jr EM. Diagnosis and outcome of Hirschsprung's disease: does age really matter? Pediatr Surg Int. 2004;20(5):319–22.
18. Teitelbaum DH, Cilley RE, Sherman NJ, et al. A decade of experience with the primary pull-through for hirschsprung disease in the newborn period: a multicenter analysis of outcomes. Ann Surg. 2000; 232(3):372–80.
19. Diamond IR, Casadiego G, Traubici J, Langer JC, Wales PW. The contrast enema for Hirschsprung disease: predictors of a false-positive result. J Pediatr Surg. 2007;42(5):792–5.
20. Surana R, Quinn FMJ, Puri P. Neonatal intestinal perforation in Hirschsprung's disease. Pediatr Surg Int. 1994;9:501–2.
21. Newman B, Nussbaum A, Kirkpatrick Jr JA. Bowel perforation in Hirschsprung's disease. AJR Am J Roentgenol. 1987;148(6):1195–7.
22. Bell MJ. Perforation of the gastrointestinal tract and peritonitis in the neonate. Surg Gynecol Obstet. 1985;160(1):20–6.
23. Metaj M, Laroia N, Lawrence RA, Ryan RM. Comparison of breast- and formula-fed normal newborns in time to first stool and urine. J Perinatol. 2003;23(8):624–8.
24. Tunc VT, Camurdan AD, Ilhan MN, Sahin F, Beyazova U. Factors associated with defecation patterns in 0-24-month-old children. Eur J Pediatr. 2008;167(12):1357–62.
25. Bekkali N, Hamers SL, Schipperus MR, et al. Duration of meconium passage in preterm and term infants. Arch Dis Child Fetal Neonatal Ed. 2008; 93(5):F376–9.
26. Ameh N, Ameh EA. Timing of passage of first meconium and stooling pattern in normal Nigerian newborns. Ann Trop Paediatr. 2009;29(2): 129–33.
27. Weaver LT, Lucas A. Development of bowel habit in preterm infants. Arch Dis Child. 1993;68(3 Spec No):317–20.
28. Reding R, de Ville de Goyet J, Gosseye S, et al. Hirschsprung's disease: a 20-year experience. J Pediatr Surg. 1997;32(8):1221–5.
29. Jung PM. Hirschsprung's disease: one surgeon's experience in one institution. J Pediatr Surg. 1995; 30(5):646–51.
30. Rahman N, Chouhan J, Gould S, et al. Rectal biopsy for Hirschsprung's disease–are we performing too many? Eur J Pediatr Surg. 2010;20(2):95–7.
31. Martucciello G, Pini Prato A, Puri P, et al. Controversies concerning diagnostic guidelines for anomalies of the enteric nervous system: a report from the fourth International Symposium on Hirschsprung's disease and related neurocristopathies. J Pediatr Surg. 2005;40(10):1527–31.
32. Kapur RP. Practical pathology and genetics of Hirschsprung's disease. Semin Pediatr Surg. 2009; 18(4):212–23.
33. de Lorijn F, Kremer LC, Reitsma JB, Benninga MA. Diagnostic tests in Hirschsprung disease: a systematic review. J Pediatr Gastroenterol Nutr. 2006;42(5):496–505.
34. Buder E, Meier-Ruge WA. Twenty years diagnostic competence center for Hirschsprung disease in Basel. Chirurg. 2010;81(6):572–6.
35. Rees BI, Azmy A, Nigam M, Lake BD. Complications of rectal suction biopsy. J Pediatr Surg. 1983; 18(3):273–5.

36. Santos MM, Tannuri U, Coelho MC. Study of acetylcholinesterase activity in rectal suction biopsy for diagnosis of intestinal dysganglionoses: 17-year experience of a single center. Pediatr Surg Int. 2008;24(6):715–9.
37. Hall NJ, Kufeji D, Keshtgar A. Out with the old and in with the new: a comparison of rectal suction biopsies with traditional and modern biopsy forceps. J Pediatr Surg. 2009;44(2):395–8.
38. Alizai NK, Batcup G, Dixon MF, Stringer MD. Rectal biopsy for Hirschsprung's disease: what is the optimum method? Pediatr Surg Int. 1998;13(2–3): 121–4.
39. Kobayashi H, Li Z, Yamataka A, Lane GJ, Miyano T. Rectal biopsy: what is the optimal procedure? Pediatr Surg Int. 2002;18(8):753–6.
40. Puffenberger EG, Kauffman ER, Bolk S, et al. Identity-by-descent and association mapping of a recessive gene for Hirschsprung disease on human chromosome 13q22. Hum Mol Genet. 1994;3(8): 1217–25.
41. Torfs CP (1998) An epidemiological study of Hirschsprung disease in a multiracial California population. The Third International Meetings: Hirschsprung disease and related neurocristopathies. Evian, France
42. Spouge D, Baird PA. Hirschsprung disease in a large birth cohort. Teratology. 1985;32(2):171–7.
43. Koh CE, Yong TL, Fenton EJ. Hirschsprung's disease: a regional experience. ANZ J Surg. 2008;78(11): 1023–7.
44. Schoellhorn J, Collins S. False positive reporting of Hirschsprung's disease in Alaska: an evaluation of Hirschsprung's disease surveillance, birth years 1996–2007. Birth Defects Res A Clin Mol Teratol. 2009;85(11):914–9.
45. Meza-Valencia BE, de Lorimier AJ, Person DA. Hirschsprung disease in the U.S. associated Pacific Islands: more common than expected. Hawaii Med J. 2005;64(4):96–8. 100–101.
46. Rajab A, Freeman NV, Patton MA. Hirschsprung's disease in Oman. J Pediatr Surg. 1997;32(5):724–7.
47. Badner JA, Sieber WK, Garver KL, Chakravarti A. A genetic study of Hirschsprung disease. Am J Hum Genet. 1990;46(3):568–80.
48. Pini Prato A, Musso M, Ceccherini I, et al. Hirschsprung disease and congenital anomalies of the kidney and urinary tract (CAKUT): a novel syndromic association. Medicine (Baltimore). 2009; 88(2):83–90.
49. Sarioglu A, Tanyel FC, Buyukpamukcu N, Hicsonmez A. Hirschsprung-associated congenital anomalies. Eur J Pediatr Surg. 1997;7(6):331–7.
50. Abbag FI. Congenital heart diseases and other major anomalies in patients with Down syndrome. Saudi Med J. 2006;27(2):219–22.
51. Skaba R. Historic milestones of Hirschsprung's disease (commemorating the 90th anniversary of Professor Harald Hirschsprung's death). J Pediatr Surg. 2007;42(1):249–51.
52. Swenson O, Bill Jr AH. Resection of rectum and rectosigmoid with preservation of the sphincter for benign spastic lesions producing megacolon; an experimental study. Surgery. 1948;24(2):212–20.
53. Marquez TT, Acton RD, Hess DJ, Duval S, Saltzman DA. Comprehensive review of procedures for total colonic aganglionosis. J Pediatr Surg. 2009;44(1):257–65. discussion 265.
54. Langer JC. Response to Dr Swenson's article: Hirschsprung's disease—a complicated therapeutic problem: some thoughts and solutions based on data and personal experience over 56 years. J Pediatric Surg. 2004;39(10):1449–53.
55. Teitelbaum DH, Coran AG. Primary pull-through for Hirschsprung's disease. Semin Neonatol. 2003;8(3): 233–41.
56. Rangel SJ, de Blaauw I. Advances in pediatric colorectal surgical techniques. Semin Pediatr Surg. 2010;19(2):86–95.
57. De La Torre L, Langer JC. Transanal endorectal pull-through for Hirschsprung disease: technique, controversies, pearls, pitfalls, and an organized approach to the management of postoperative obstructive symptoms. Semin Pediatr Surg. 2010;19(2):96–106.
58. Georgeson KE, Robertson DJ. Laparoscopic-assisted approaches for the definitive surgery for Hirschsprung's disease. Semin Pediatr Surg. 2004;13(4):256–62.
59. Shinall Jr MC, Koehler E, Shyr Y, Lovvorn 3rd HN. Comparing cost and complications of primary and staged surgical repair of neonatally diagnosed Hirschsprung's disease. J Pediatr Surg. 2008;43(12): 2220–5.
60. Pastor AC, Osman F, Teitelbaum DH, Caty MG, Langer JC. Development of a standardized definition for Hirschsprung's-associated enterocolitis: a Delphi analysis. J Pediatr Surg. 2009;44(1):251–6.
61. Vieten D, Spicer R. Enterocolitis complicating Hirschsprung's disease. Semin Pediatr Surg. 2004; 13(4):263–72.
62. Bush TG, Savidge TC, Freeman TC, et al. Fulminant jejuno-ileitis following ablation of enteric glia in adult transgenic mice. Cell. 1998;93(2):189–201.
63. Bjerknes M, Cheng H. Modulation of specific intestinal epithelial progenitors by enteric neurons. Proc Natl Acad Sci USA. 2001;98(22):12497–502.
64. Van Landeghem L, Mahe MM, Teusan R, et al. Regulation of intestinal epithelial cells transcriptome by enteric glial cells: impact on intestinal epithelial barrier functions. BMC Genomics. 2009;10:507.
65. Savidge TC, Newman P, Pothoulakis C, et al. Enteric glia regulate intestinal barrier function and inflammation via release of S-nitrosoglutathione. Gastroenterology. 2007;132(4):1344–58.
66. Murphy F, Puri P. New insights into the pathogenesis of Hirschsprung's associated enterocolitis. Pediatr Surg Int. 2005;21(10):773–9.
67. Mattar AF, Coran AG, Teitelbaum DH. MUC-2 mucin production in Hirschsprung's disease: possible association with enterocolitis development. J Pediatr Surg. 2003;38(3):417–21. discussion 417–421.

68. Ruhl A. Glial cells in the gut. Neurogastroenterol Motil. 2005;17(6):777–90.
69. Neunlist M, Van Landeghem L, Bourreille A, Savidge T. Neuro-glial crosstalk in inflammatory bowel disease. J Intern Med. 2008;263(6):577–83.
70. Genton L, Kudsk KA. Interactions between the enteric nervous system and the immune system: role of neuropeptides and nutrition. Am J Surg. 2003; 186(3):253–8.
71. Veiga-Fernandes H, Coles MC, Foster KE, et al. Tyrosine kinase receptor RET is a key regulator of Peyer's patch organogenesis. Nature. 2007;446(7135): 547–51.
72. Cheng Z, Wang X, Dhall D, et al. Splenic lymphopenia in the endothelin receptor B-null mouse: implications for Hirschsprung associated enterocolitis. Pediatr Surg Int. 2011;27(2):145–50.
73. Marty TL, Seo T, Sullivan JJ, Matlak ME, Black RE, Johnson DG. Rectal irrigations for the prevention of postoperative enterocolitis in Hirschsprung's disease. J Pediatr Surg. 1995;30(5):652–4.
74. Momoh JT. Hirschsprung's disease: problems of diagnosis and treatment. Ann Trop Paediatr. 1982; 2(1):31–5.
75. Rescorla FJ, Morrison AM, Engles D, West KW, Grosfeld JL. Hirschsprung's disease. Evaluation of mortality and long-term function in 260 cases. Arch Surg. 1992;127(8):934–41. discussion 941–932.
76. Sherman JO, Snyder ME, Weitzman JJ, et al. A 40-year multinational retrospective study of 880 Swenson procedures. J Pediatr Surg. 1989;24(8):833–8.
77. Menezes M, Puri P. Long-term outcome of patients with enterocolitis complicating Hirschsprung's disease. Pediatr Surg Int. 2006;22(4):316–8.
78. Haricharan RN, Seo JM, Kelly DR, et al. Older age at diagnosis of Hirschsprung disease decreases risk of postoperative enterocolitis, but resection of additional ganglionated bowel does not. J Pediatr Surg. 2008;43(6):1115–23.
79. Niramis R, Watanatittan S, Anuntkosol M, et al. Quality of life of patients with Hirschsprung's disease at 5–20 years post pull-through operations. Eur J Pediatr Surg. 2008;18(1):38–43.
80. Menezes M, Corbally M, Puri P. Long-term results of bowel function after treatment for Hirschsprung's disease: a 29-year review. Pediatr Surg Int. 2006; 22(12):987–90.
81. Gunnarsdottir A, Sandblom G, Arnbjornsson E, Larsson LT. Quality of life in adults operated on for Hirschsprung disease in childhood. J Pediatr Gastroenterol Nutr. 2010;51(2):160–6.
82. Heanue TA, Pachnis V. Enteric nervous system development and Hirschsprung's disease: advances in genetic and stem cell studies. Nat Rev Neurosci. 2007;8(6):466–79.
83. Newgreen D, Young HM. Enteric nervous system: development and developmental disturbances–part 1. Pediatr Dev Pathol. 2002;5(3):224–47.
84. Newgreen D, Young HM. Enteric nervous system: development and developmental disturbances–part 2. Pediatr Dev Pathol. 2002;5(4):329–49.
85. Gariepy CE. Intestinal motility disorders and development of the enteric nervous system. Pediatr Res. 2001;49(5):605–13.
86. Gershon MD. Lessons from genetically engineered animal models. II. Disorders of enteric neuronal development: insights from transgenic mice. Am J Physiol. 1999;277(2 Pt 1):G262–7.
87. Burzynski G, Shepherd IT, Enomoto H. Genetic model system studies of the development of the enteric nervous system, gut motility and Hirschsprung's disease. Neurogastroenterol Motil. 2009;21(2):113–27.
88. Jain S, Naughton CK, Yang M, et al. Mice expressing a dominant-negative Ret mutation phenocopy human Hirschsprung disease and delineate a direct role of Ret in spermatogenesis. Development. 2004;131(21):5503–13.
89. Gianino S, Grider JR, Cresswell J, Enomoto H, Heuckeroth RO. GDNF availability determines enteric neuron number by controlling precursor proliferation. Development. 2003;130(10):2187–98.
90. Medhus AW, Bjornland K, Emblem R, Husebye E. Motility of the oesophagus and small bowel in adults treated for Hirschsprung's disease during early childhood. Neurogastroenterol Motil. 2010; 22(2):154–60. e149.
91. Medhus AW, Bjornland K, Emblem R, Husebye E. Liquid and solid gastric emptying in adults treated for Hirschsprung's disease during early childhood. Scand J Gastroenterol. 2007;42(1):34–40.
92. Miele E, Tozzi A, Staiano A, Toraldo C, Esposito C, Clouse RE. Persistence of abnormal gastrointestinal motility after operation for Hirschsprung's disease. Am J Gastroenterol. 2000;95(5):1226–30.
93. Faure C, Ategbo S, Ferreira GC, et al. Duodenal and esophageal manometry in total colonic aganglionosis. J Pediatr Gastroenterol Nutr. 1994;18(2):193–9.
94. Staiano A, Corazziari E, Andreotti MR, Clouse RE. Esophageal motility in children with Hirschsprung's disease. Am J Dis Child. 1991;145(3):310–3.
95. Frykman PK, Lindsley EH, Gaon M, Farkas DL. Spectral imaging for precise surgical intervention in Hirschsprung's disease. J Biophotonics. 2008; 1(2):97–103.
96. Fu M, Sato Y, Lyons-Warren A, et al. Vitamin A facilitates enteric nervous system precursor migration by reducing Pten accumulation. Development. 2010;137(4):631–40.
97. Hannon RJ, Boston VE. Discordant Hirschsprung's disease in monozygotic twins: a clue to pathogenesis? J Pediatr Surg. 1988;23(11):1034–5.
98. Siplovich L, Carmi R, Bar-Ziv J, Karplus M, Mares AJ. Discordant Hirschsprung's disease in monozygotic twins. J Pediatr Surg. 1983;18(5):639–40.
99. Hotta R, Natarajan D, Thapar N. Potential of cell therapy to treat pediatric motility disorders. Semin Pediatr Surg. 2009;18(4):263–73.
100. Druckenbrod NR, Epstein ML. Age-dependent changes in the gut environment restrict the invasion of the hindgut by enteric neural progenitors. Development. 2009;136(18):3195–203.

101. Lindley RM, Hawcutt DB, Connell MG, Edgar DH, Kenny SE. Properties of secondary and tertiary human enteric nervous system neurospheres. J Pediatr Surg. 2009;44(6):1249–55. discussion 1255–1246.
102. Metzger M, Caldwell C, Barlow AJ, Burns AJ, Thapar N. Enteric nervous system stem cells derived from human gut mucosa for the treatment of aganglionic gut disorders. Gastroenterology. 2009;136(7): 2214–25. e2211–2213.
103. Thapar N. New frontiers in the treatment of Hirschsprung disease. J Pediatr Gastroenterol Nutr. 2009;48 Suppl 2:S92–4.

24 Motility Problems in Developmental Disorders: Cerebral Palsy, Down Syndrome, William Syndrome, Familial Dysautonomia, and Mitochondrial Disorders

Annamaria Staiano and Massimo Martinelli

Cerebral Palsy

Cerebral palsy (CP) refers to a group of chronic, nonprogressive disorders of movement, posture, and tone due to central nervous system damage before cerebral development is complete. The prevalence of CP is approximately 2 per 1,000 live births. The different types of CP vary from series to series, with the spastic type being the most frequent, while periventricular leukomalacia and/or cortical/cerebral atrophy represents the main neuropathological correlates [1]. The survival of children with severe neurological disorders, such as cerebral palsy, has created a major challenge for medical care. Gastrointestinal motor dysfunction, such as gastroesophageal reflux disease (GERD), dysphagia, vomiting, and chronic constipation, is known to occur frequently in children with different degrees of CNS damage. The degree of GI dysmotility seems to correlate with the degree of brain damage [2]. Swallowing disorders are common in patients affected by CP. In the study by Del Giudice and colleagues, the authors found that 30 of the 35 patients with CP presenting with dysphagia had swallowing disorders. The great majority of patients showed dysfunction of the oral phase of swallowing with abnormal formation of the alimentary bolus due to either uncoordinated movements of the tongue or it being contracted and rigid. Alternatively, they had a normal bolus but huge defects in its propulsion toward the oropharynx, due to the lack of finely coordinated movements of the tongue against the palate. Swallowing disorders have significant implications for development, nutrition, respiratory health, and GI function of this group of patients [3]. The development of dysphagia is associated with a progressive reduction of food intake and represents the main pathogenic factor for malnutrition [4]. At the same time, swallowing disorders can often cause recurrent episodes of pulmonary aspiration. For all these reasons, it is essential to diagnose these conditions as early as possible. Videofluoroscopic swallow studies are considered to be a valuable diagnostic tool for children with CP, given their ability to assess both pharyngeal motility and airway protection during swallowing. There is growing evidence that the method of feeding is an important variable in outcomes of children with more severe CP. In those patients with dysphagia, undernutrition, and associated respiratory diseases, the adoption of gastrostomy tube feeding is recommended [5–7]. The American Academy of Cerebral Palsy and Developmental Medicine considers gastrostomy feeding as a valuable alternative nutritional source in this group of children [6]. GERD is very common in patients with a severe neurologic impairment. The incidence is reported to be between 70 and 90%, depending on the different investigations used including esophageal

A. Staiano, M.D. (✉) • M. Martinelli, M.D.
Pediatric Gastoenterology Division, Pediatrics Department, University of Naples "Federico II", Via Pansini No 5, Naples 80131, Italy
e-mail: staiano@unina.it

C. Faure et al. (eds.), *Pediatric Neurogastroenterology: Gastrointestinal Motility and Functional Disorders in Children*, Clinical Gastroenterology,
DOI 10.1007/978-1-60761-709-9_24, © Springer Science+Business Media New York 2013

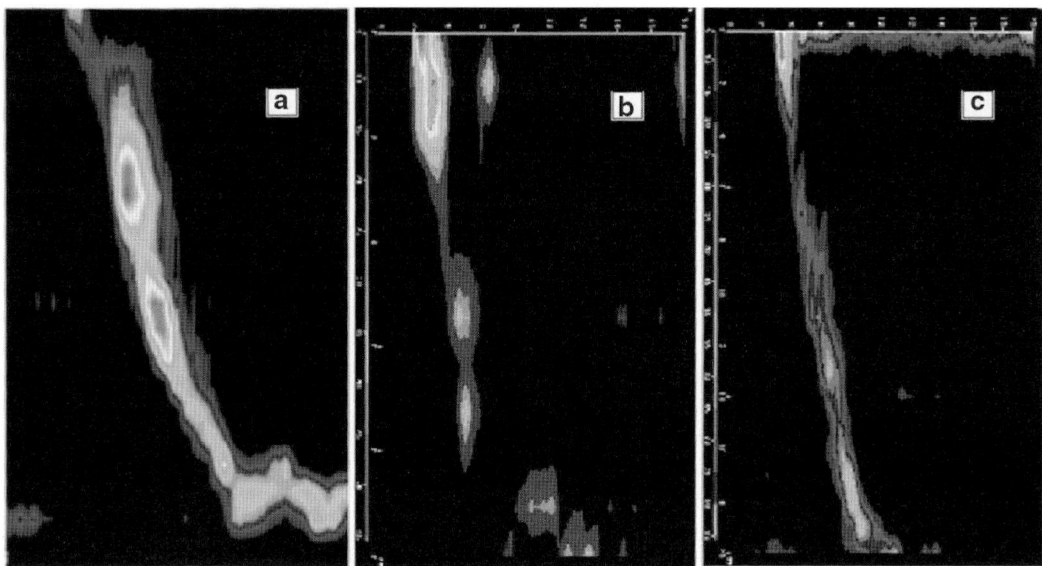

Fig. 24.1 Examples of high-resolution esophageal manometry tracings in a control subject (**a**) and in two patients (**b** and **c**) affected by cerebral palsy. Note in (**a**) a normal esophageal tracing, whereas in (**b**) hypotensive lower esophageal sphincter and low-amplitude contraction. In (**c**), marked hypomotility of the smooth muscle region is visible.

pH studies and/or upper GI endoscopy [3, 8]. The pathogenesis of GERD in children with CP seems to relate mainly to the impaired motility of the esophagus. Our group demonstrated that most of the neurological patients affected by GERD showed prolonged gastric emptying and abnormal esophageal motility. The main abnormalities consisted of significantly low amplitudes of the lower esophageal sphincter (LES) and esophageal contraction waves and an increased number of simultaneous waves, compared to control children (Fig. 24.1) [3]. These findings, part of a more generalized dysmotility of the GI tract, together with the other conditions often present in these children, such as spasticity, prolonged adoption of supine position, scoliosis, seizures, and reduced amounts of swallowed saliva consequent to the drooling, increase the predisposition to the development of GERD and may be responsible for the high failure rate of both medical and surgical treatments in this category of patients. The correct therapeutical approach to GERD in CP patients is still controversial. According to the recent ESPGHAN–NASPGHAN guidelines on gastroesophageal reflux, antisecretory therapy should be optimized. Long-term treatment with PPIs is often effective for symptom control and maintenance of remission. Baclofen is recommended to control vomiting [9]. An alternative medical approach is represented by the use of an elemental diet. We described a lower incidence of GERD in neurologically impaired children with refractory esophagitis treated with amino acid-based formula [10]. However, conventional medical management is less effective in neurologically impaired children. At the same time, surgical intervention is associated with high operative risk given the poor physical condition of the patients. The benefit/risk ratio of antireflux surgery in patients with persistent symptoms despite optimized medical therapy is not clear. Nissen fundoplication has been associated with several complications in neurologically impaired children. In addition, postoperative morbidity rates are up to 50%, reoperation rates up to 20%, and mortality substantial [11, 12]. Recently, the advent of laparoscopic Nissen fundoplication has become the procedure of choice. Esposito and colleagues reported a 30% rate of postoperative complications and 6% rate of reoperation [13].

Constipation represents another frequent and often undiagnosed problem in patients with CP. The prevalence of the chronic constipation varies from 25 to 75% of patients with CP [3]. Chronic constipation is the result of prolonged colonic transit, which is secondary to the underlying gut dysmotility. Colonic transit time seems to be delayed predominantly in the left colon and rectum [14]. It has been suggested that disruption of the neural modulation of colonic motility may play a predominant role in the development of constipation in neurologic disease. This could explain why prokinetic drugs have little impact on the delayed colonic transit seen in children with brain damage. The low fiber and fluid intake as well as the frequent delay in diagnosis certainly contribute to the development and the reinforcement of constipation in neurologically impaired children. Our group demonstrated the efficacy of dietary fiber glucomannan in improving bowel frequency in children with severe brain damage, despite no measurable effects on delayed transit [15].

Down Syndrome

About 77% of neonates affected by Down syndrome (DS) present with or develop associated GI abnormalities [16]. Cleves et al., in a recent cohort study, showed, besides congenital heart defects, an elevated relative risk for GI malformations (OR 67.07) in infants with DS [17]. The most frequent GI malformation associated with DS is Hirschsprung disease; however, esophageal atresia, tracheoesophageal fistula, duodenal atresia or stenosis, and imperforate anus were all described. Some of the most common functional GI symptoms reported by DS patients are dysphagia for liquids and solids, vomiting/GER, and heartburn, as well as other esophageal dysmotility symptoms [18]. Children affected by DS are at high risk of GERD [19] and its serious complications such as oropharyngeal aspiration and pneumonia. As for other conditions with neurological impairment such as CP, treatment of GERD in DS patients should associate optimized antisecretory therapy to behavioral measures including feeding and positional changes. Despite optimized medical therapy, some DS patients with GERD, especially patients with respiratory complications of GERD, need antireflux surgery [20]. It has been observed however that neurological impairment and GI disease necessitating surgery have been independently associated with poorer development outcome [21]. With regard to esophageal motor disorders, different cases of association between achalasia and DS have been described in the literature, and although achalasia remains a rare entity, it should be considered in any DS patient who presents with dysphagia [22]. Among the most common motor disorders in DS children and adults, unexplained chronic constipation is included [23]. In children with chronic constipation, it is important to exclude Hirschsprung disease (HSCR), observed in approximately 1 on 200–300 DS patients [24]. About 30% of HSCR patients have a recognized chromosomal abnormality, a recognized syndrome, or additional congenital anomalies, the most frequent of which is DS [25]. Moore et al., studying a population of 408 HSCR patients, reported a prevalence of 3.2% of DS with an 85% association with other anomalies [26]. The well-described correlation between DS and HSCR indicates a possible role for chromosome 21 in the etiology of HD. Nevertheless, the existence of trisomy 21 although seemingly increasing the risk of developing HSCR does not invariably lead to its occurrence. In the literature several studies investigating the role of chromosome 21 as a potential candidate area for a modifying gene in HSCR exist [27], but in the last few years, the possible role of genes mapping outside chromosome 21 (such as SOD1, ITGB2, protein s-100 beta) is emerging. Also well studied has been the relationship between the major susceptibility genes associated with HSCR (RET and EDNRB) and the DS. Arnold et al. [28] demonstrated that the RET enhancer polymorphism RET 19.7 at chromosome 10q11.2 is associated with HSCR in DS individuals. Interestingly, the RET19.7 T allele frequency is significantly different between individuals with DS alone (0.26 ± 0.04), HSCR alone (0.61 ± 0.04), and HSCR and DS (0.41 ± 0.04), demonstrating an association and interaction between RET and chromosome 21 gene dosage. Similarly a novel EDNRB variant was identified in DS patients with HSCR [29]. Moreover, there appears to be a significantly higher overall incidence of preoperative enterocolitis and postoperative enterocolitis in DS with HSCR [30].

Williams Syndrome

Williams syndrome (WS), also known as Williams–Beuren syndrome, is due to a homozygous deletion of a contiguous gene on the long arm of chromosome 7 (7q11.23) [31]. The estimated prevalence of WS is 1 in 7,500 live births [32]. Most individuals with WS (99%) have a 1.5 megabase deletion in 7q11.23 encompassing the elastin gene (ELN) and 25–35 other genes, all of which are detectable by fluorescent in situ hybridization (FISH) [33]. Clinical features of WS include distinctive facial anomalies; congenital heart defects, in particular supravalvular aortic stenosis; slight to severe mental retardation; herniae; growth deficiency; and infantile hypercalcemia [34]. Gastrointestinal symptoms such as chronic abdominal pain, feeding problems, constipation, and gastroesophageal reflux disease are seen relatively frequently in children with WS [35]. Hypercalcemia may contribute to irritability, vomiting, constipation, and muscle cramps; it is more common in infancy but may recur in adults [36].

Familial Dysautonomia

Familial dysautonomia, also known as Riley–Day syndrome, is an autosomal recessive disorder, which occurs predominantly in the Ashkenazi Jewish population and has an incidence of about 1 in 1,370 individuals. It is associated with a complex neurological disorder that affects the sensory system and the autonomous nervous system functions [37]. Although FD is caused by one gene and the penetrance is always complete, there is a great deal of variation in expression. The sensory dysfunction is characterized by alterations of small fiber neuronal populations such that FD patients have impaired sensations of temperature, pain, and vibration. The autonomic dysfunction affects multiple systems and it is characterized by cyclic manifestations of a typical "dysautonomic crisis"; these crises represent systemic reactions to physiologic and psychological stress: gastrointestinal perturbations such as vomiting are the predominant part of the constellation of symptoms seen during an episode; other symptoms include hypertension, tachycardia, diaphoresis, personality changes, blotching of the skin, piloerection, functional ileus, and dilatation of pupils [38]. Malfunction of the gastrointestinal tract is the main clinical manifestation of FD with oropharyngeal incoordination being one of the earliest symptoms. Discoordinated swallow is found in about the 60% of patients with FD, and it is often responsible for the development of severe feeding alteration, malnutrition, and recurrent aspiration, which can lead to chronic lung disease. Cineradiographic swallowing studies may document the level of functional ability [39, 40]. According to Axelrod et al., up to 80% of children will require gastrostomy prior to the age of 1 year [37]. However, the prominent GI gastrointestinal symptom is the propensity to vomit. Vomiting can occur cyclically as a part of dysautonomic crises or daily in response to stress or arousal. The efficacy of diazepam in reducing vomiting during autonomic crises suggests that the crisis is caused by a central phenomenon, probably developed from autonomic seizures [41]. Gastroesophageal reflux is another common problem. Sundaram and colleagues found a prevalence of 95% of GERD in a sample study of 174 FD patients [42]. A major contributor to the development of GERD is represented by dysfunction and increased relaxation of the lower esophageal sphincter. The LES is controlled by postganglionic parasympathetic fibers within the vagus nerve and preganglionic sympathetic fibers. The parasympathetic circuits are able to control both the relaxation and the contraction of LES, while the sympathetic system evokes exclusively the contraction. The pathogenesis of GERD is correlated to the reported degeneration of sympathetic nervous system and the consequent prevalence of parasympathetic firing. Medical management including H2 antagonists should be tried; however, if symptoms persist and events such as hematemesis occur, surgical intervention is recommended.

Mitochondrial Disorders

Mitochondrial disorders (MD) refer to a clinically heterogeneous group of disorders that arise as a result of dysfunction of the mitochondrial respiratory chain. They can be caused by either inherited or spontaneous mutations of nuclear (nDNA) or mitochondrial DNA (mtDNA) which lead to altered functions of the proteins or RNA molecules that normally reside in mitochondria. Defects in nDNA can be inherited from either parent, while defects in the genes of the mtDNA are maternally inherited. Mitochondria are present in virtually all cell types of human body and their damage primarily affects the main energy-dependent tissues such as brain, heart, liver, skeletal muscles, kidney, and the endocrine and respiratory systems [43]. Mitochondrial disorders primarily affect children, but adult onset is becoming more common. More than 100 mtDNA abnormalities associated with MD have been described in the literature, with some resulting in profound disability and premature death [44, 45]. GI symptoms are reported in 15% of MD patients occurring usually in childhood, before the onset of more classical symptoms of MD [46].

Mitochondrial Disorders Presenting with Motility Problems

The major MD presenting with GI symptoms are mitochondrial neurogastrointestinal encephalomyopathy (MNGIE) (peripheral neuropathy, ophthalmoparesis, leukoencephalopathy, muscle wasting, cachexia) in which GI symptoms (especially from chronic intestinal pseudo-obstruction and diarrhea) are present in 45–67% of patients [47–49]; Leigh syndrome (subacute necrotizing encephalomyelopathy resulting in hypotonia, bulbar paresis, abnormal eye movements, lack of coordination of extremities, and regressive psychomotor development) [50]; Kearns–Sayre syndrome (chronic progressive external ophthalmoplegia, atypical pigmentary retinopathy, ataxia, and heart block); and MELAS syndrome (mitochondrial encephalopathy, lactic acidosis, and stroke-like episodes) [51]. Other MD are characterized by nonspecific GI symptoms and present with dysphagia, gastroesophageal delayed gastric emptying, feeding difficulties, gastroesophageal reflux (GER) and/or vomiting, diarrhea, failure to thrive, and abdominal pain. Different mtDNA mutations have been associated with GI disorders in MD. Recently Horvath et al. found a new heteroplasmic mutation in the anticodon stem of mitochondrial tRNA of a girl presenting with clinical symptoms of MNGIE-like GI dysmotility and cachexia [52]. In MELAS it is common to find an A3243G mutation in transfer RNA (tRNA) Leu (UUR) [53]. Mutations in the nuclear gene encoding SURF1, a mitochondrial protein involved in cytochrome c oxidase assembly, have been noted in many patients with Leigh syndrome [54]. GI symptoms are predominantly localized in the upper GI tract. Chitkara et al. reported six children with MD who presented upper GI symptoms such as vomiting, food aversion, GER, poor suck, and feeding intolerance [46]. Fifteen percent of patients with Kearns–Sayre, an MD characterized by deletions in cytochrome c oxidase deficiency, present swallowing difficulties and dysphagia [55]. Shaker et al. described the manometric characteristics of a cervical dysphagia in a patient with Kearns–Sayre observing absence of pharyngeal peristalsis, abnormally low upper esophageal sphincter resting pressure, and absence of proximal esophageal peristalsis [56]. Vomiting and dysphagia have been described in patients with Leigh syndrome [57]. Dysphagia seems to be due to primary esophageal dysmotility, neurogenic causes, or a combination of these two factors. Dysmotility disorders like delayed gastric emptying and intestinal pseudo-obstruction have been shown in child [46, 58] and adult patients with MD [59]. Gastroparesis has been associated with various diseases and may occur as part of a MD [60]. There is no consensus regarding management of patients with gastroparesis who do not respond to simple antiemetic or prokinetic therapy. Tatekawa et al. proposed a new surgical technique in a refractory gastroparesis 12-year-old girl with pyruvate dehydrogenase complex deficiency [60]. Intestinal pseudo-obstruction is an increasingly recognized clinical feature of MD, mainly in MNGIE and less frequently in MELAS, and may represent an important cause of chronic intestinal failure. The pathogenesis of intestinal pseudo-obstruction in MD is still unclear. Giordano et al. showed in two studies performed in one and four patients suffering from MNGIE, respectively, smooth muscle cell atrophy, mitochondrial proliferation, and mtDNA depletion in the muscularis propria of the small intestine [61, 62]. Their pathogenetic hypothesis was that in MNGIE patients the baseline low abundance of mtDNA molecules may predispose smooth muscle cells of the external layer of muscularis propria to the toxic effects of circulating dThd and dUrd.

References

1. Kuban KC, Leviton A. Cerebral palsy. N Engl J Med. 1994;330:188–95.
2. Staiano A, Cucchiara S, Del Giudice E, Andreotti MR, Minella R. Disorders of oesophageal motility in children with psychomotor retardation and gastro-oesophageal reflux. Eur J Pediatr. 1991;150:638–41.
3. Del Giudice E, Staiano A, Capano G, et al. Gastrointestinal manifestations in children with cerebral palsy. Brain Dev. 1999;21:307–11.
4. Campanozzi A, Capano G, Miele E, et al. Impact of malnutrition on gastrointestinal disorders and gross motor abilities in children with cerebral palsy. Brain Dev. 2007;29:25–9.
5. Schwarz SM, Corredor J, Fisher-Medina J, Cohen J, Rabinowitz S. Diagnosis and treatment of feeding disorders in children with developmental disabilities. Pediatrics. 2001;108:671–6.
6. Samson-Fang L, Butler C, O'Donnell M. AACPDM. Effects of gastrostomy feeding in children with cerebral palsy: an AACPDM evidence report. Dev Med Child Neurol. 2003;45:415–26.
7. Sullivan PB, Juszczak E, Bachlet AM, et al. Gastrostomy tube feeding in children with cerebral palsy: a prospective, longitudinal study. Dev Med Child Neurol. 2005;47:77–85.
8. Wesley JR, Coran AG, Sarahan TM, Klein MD, White SJ. The need for evaluation of gastroesophageal reflux in brain-damaged children referred for feeding gastrostomy. J Pediatr Surg. 1981;16:866–71.
9. Vandenplas Y, Rudolph CD, Di Lorenzo C, et al. North American Society for Pediatric Gastroenterology Hepatology and Nutrition, European Society for Pediatric Gastroenterology Hepatology and Nutrition. Pediatric gastroesophageal reflux clinical practice guidelines: joint recommendations of the North American Society for Pediatric Gastroenterology, Hepatology, and Nutrition (NASPGHAN) and the European Society for Pediatric Gastroenterology, Hepatology, and Nutrition (ESPGHAN). J Pediatr Gastroenterol Nutr. 2009;49:498–547.
10. Miele E, Staiano A, Tozzi A, Auricchio R, Paparo F, Troncone R. Clinical response to amino acid-based formula in neurologically impaired children with refractory esophagitis. J Pediatr Gastroenterol Nutr. 2002;35:314–9.
11. Richards CA, Andrews PL, Spitz L, Milla PJ. Nissen fundoplication may induce gastric myoelectrical disturbance in children. J Pediatr Surg. 1998;33:1801–5.
12. Richards CA, Carr D, Spitz L, Milla PJ, Andrews PL. Nissen-type fundoplication and its effects on the emetic reflex and gastric motility in the ferret. Neurogastroenterol Motil. 2000;12:65–74.
13. Esposito C, Van Der Zee DC, Settimi A, Doldo P, Staiano A, Bax NM. Risks and benefits of surgical management of gastroesophageal reflux in neurologically impaired children. Surg Endosc. 2003;17:708–10.
14. Staiano A, Del Giudice E. Colonic transit and anorectal manometry in children with severe brain damage. Pediatrics. 1994;94(2 Pt 1):169–73.
15. Staiano A, Simeone D, Del Giudice E, Miele E, Tozzi A, Toraldo C. Effect of the dietary fiber glucomannan on chronic constipation in neurologically impaired children. J Pediatr. 2000;136:41–5.
16. Spahis JK, Wilson GN. Down syndrome: perinatal complications and counseling experiences in 216 patients. Am J Med Genet. 1999;89:96–9.
17. Cleves MA, Hobbs CA, Cleves PA, Tilford JM, Bird TM, Robbins JM. Congenital defects among liveborn infants with Down syndrome. Birth Defects Res A Clin Mol Teratol. 2007;79:657–63.
18. Zarate N, Mearin F, Hidalgo A, Malagelada J. Prospective evaluation of esophageal motor dysfunction in Down's syndrome. Am J Gastroenterol. 2001;96:1718–24.
19. Buchin PJ, Levy JS, Schullinger JN. Down syndrome and the gastro-intestinal tract. J Clin Gastroenterol. 1986;8:111–4.
20. Vernon-Roberts A, Sullivan PB. Fundoplication versus post-operative medication for gastro-oesophageal reflux in children with neurological impairment undergoing gastrostomy. Cochrane Database Syst Rev. 2007.
21. van Trotsenburg AS, Heymans HS, Tijssen JG, de Vijlder JJ, Vulsma T. Comorbidity, hospitalization, and medication use and their influence on mental and motor development of young infants with Down syndrome. Pediatrics. 2006;118:1633–9.
22. Okawada M, Okazaki T, Yamataka A, Lane GJ, Miyano T. Down's syndrome and esophageal achalasia: a rare but important clinical entity. Pediatr Surg Int. 2005;21:997–1000.
23. Wallace RA. Clinical audit of gastrointestinal conditions occurring among adults with Down syndrome attending a specialist clinic. J Intellect Dev Disabil. 2007;32:45–50.
24. Quinn FM, Surana R, Puri P. The influence of trisomy 21 on outcome in children with Hirschsprung's disease. J Pediatr Surg. 1994;29:781–3.

25. Chakravarti A, Lyonnet S. Hirschsprung disease. In: Scrivner CR, Beaudet AR, Sly W, Valle D, editors. The metabolic and molecular bases of inherited disease. 8th ed. New York: McGraw-Hill; 2001. p. 6231–55.
26. Moore SW. The contribution of associated congenital anomalies in understanding Hirschsprung's disease. Pediatr Surg Int. 2006;22:305–15.
27. Puffenberger E, Kauffman E, Bolk S, et al. Identity-bydescent and association mapping of a recessive gene for Hirschsprung disease on human chromosome 13q22. Hum Mol Genet. 1994;3:1217–25.
28. Arnold S, Pelet A, Amiel J, et al. Interaction between a chromosome 10 RET enhancer and chromosome 21 in the Down syndrome–Hirschsprung disease association. Hum Mutat. 2009;30:771–5.
29. Zaahl MG, du Plessis L, Warnich L, Kotze MJ, Moore SW. Significance of novel endothelin-B receptor gene polymorphisms in Hirschsprung's disease: predominance of a novel variant (561C/T) in patients with co-existing Down's syndrome. Mol Cell Probes. 2003;17:49–54.
30. Morabito A, Lall A, Gull S, Mohee A, Bianchi A. The impact of Down's syndrome on the immediate and long-term outcomes of children with Hirschsprung's disease. Pediatr Surg Int. 2006;22:179–81.
31. Merla G, Ucla C, Guipponi M, Reymond A. identification of additional transcripts in the Williams-Beuren syndrome critical region. Hum Genet. 2002;110:429–38.
32. Stromme P, Bjornstad PG, Ramstad K. Prevalence estimation of Williams syndrome. J Child Neurol. 2002;17:269–71.
33. Lowery MC, Morris CA, Ewart A, Brothman LJ, Zhu XL, Leonard CO, et al. Strong correlation of elastin deletions, detected by FISH, with Williams syndrome: evaluation of 235 patients. Am J Hum Genet. 1995;57:49–53.
34. Greenberg F. Williams syndrome professional symposium. Am J Med Genet Suppl. 1990;6:85–8.
35. Morris CA, Demsey SA, Leonard CO, Dilts C, Blackburn BL. Natural history of Williams syndrome: physical characteristics. J Pediatr. 1988;113:318–26.
36. Morris CA, Pober V, Wang P, et al. Medical guidelines for Williams syndrome. Williams Syndrome Association Website. 1999.
37. Axelrod FB. Familial dysautonomia. Muscle Nerve. 2004;29:352–63.
38. Axelrod FB, Maayan C. Familial dysautonomia. In: Burg FD, Ingelfinger JR, Wald ER, Polin RA, editors. Gellis and Kagen's current pediatric therapy. 16th ed. Philadelphia, PA: WB Saunders; 2007.
39. Krausz Y, Maayan C, Faber J, Marciano R, Mogle P, Wynchank S. Scintigraphic evaluation of esophageal transit and gastric emptying in familial dysautonomia. Eur J Radiol. 1994;18:52–6.
40. Margulies SI, Brunt PW, Donner MW, Silbiger ML. Familial dysautonomia. A cineradiographic study of the swallowing mechanism. Radiology. 1968;90:107–11.
41. Axelrod FB, Zupanc M, Hilz MJ, Kramer EL. Ictal SPECT during autonomic crisis in familial dysautonomia. Neurology. 2000;55:122–5.
42. Sundaram V, Axelrod FB. Gastroesophageal reflux in familial dysautonomia: correlation with crisis frequency and sensory dysfunction. J Pediatr Gastroenterol Nutr. 2005;40:429–33.
43. Johns D. Mitochondrial DNA and disease. N Engl J Med. 1995;333:638–44.
44. Wallace D, Lott M, Torroni A, Brown M. Report on the committee on human mitochondrial DNA. Genome Priority Reports. 1993;1:727–57.
45. Servidei S. Mitochondrial encephalomyopathies: gene mutation. Neuromusc Disorders. 1997;7:XIII–XVIII.
46. Chitkara DK, Nurko S, Shoffner JM, Buie T, Flores A. Abnormalities in gastrointestinal motility are associated with diseases of oxidative phosphorylation in children. Am J Gastroenterol. 2003;98:871–7.
47. Gillis LA, Sokol RJ. Gastrointestinal manifestations of mitochondrial disease. Gastroenterol Clin North Am. 2003;32:789–817.
48. Nishino I, Spinazzola A, Papadimitriou A, Hammans S, Steiner I, Hahn CD, Connolly AM, Verloes A, Guimaraes J, Maillard I, Hamano H, Donati MA, Semrad CE, Russell JA, Andreu AL, Hadjigeorgiou GM, Vu TH, Tadesse S, Nygaard TG, Nonaka I, Hirano I, Bonilla E, Rowland LP, DiMauro S, Hirano M. Mitochondrial neurogastrointestinal encephalomyopathy: an autosomal recessive disorder due to thymidine phosphorylase mutations. Ann Neurol. 2000;47:792–800.
49. Nishino I, Spinazzola A, Hirano M. Thymidine phosphorylase gene mutations in MNGIE, a human mitochondrial disorder. Science. 1999;283:689–92.
50. Miyabayashi S, Narisawa K, Iinuma K. Cytochrome C oxidase deficiency in two siblings with Leigh encephalomyelopathy. Brain Dev. 1984;6:362–72.
51. Johns DR. Seminars in medicine of the Beth Israel Hospital, Boston. Mitochondrial DNA and disease. N Engl J Med. 1995;333:638–44.
52. Horvath R, Bender A, Abicht A, et al. Heteroplasmic mutation in the anticodon-stem of mitochondrial tRNAVal causing MNGIE-like gastrointestinal dysmotility and cachexia. J Neurol. 2009;256:810–5.
53. Chinnery PF, Jones S, Sviland L. Mitochondrial enteropathy: the primary pathology may not be within the gastrointestinal tract. Gut. 2001;48:121–4.
54. Zhu Z, Yao J, Johns T, et al. SURF1, encoding a factor involved in the biogenesis of cytochrome c oxidase, is mutated in Leigh syndrome. Nat Genet. 1998;20:337–43.
55. Bril V, Rewcastle NB, Humphrey J. Oculoskeletal myopathy with abnormal mitochondria. Can J Neurol Sci. 1984;11:390–4.
56. Shaker R, Kupla JI, Kidder TM, Arndorfer RC, Hofmann C. Manometric characteristics of cervical dysphagia in a patient with the Kearns-Sayre syndrome. Gastroenterology. 1992;103:1328–31.
57. Naviaux RK. The spectrum of mitochondrial disease. In: Hirsch D, editor. Mitochondrial and metabolic disorders—a primary care physician's guide. Oradell, NJ: Psy-Ed Corp; 1997. p. 3–10.
58. Amiot A, Tchikviladzé M, Joly F, et al. Frequency of mitochondrial defects in patients with chronic

intestinal pseudo-obstruction. Gastroenterology. 2009;137:101–9
59. Amiot A, Tchikviladzé M, Joly F, et al. Frequency of mitochondrial defects in patients with chronic intestinal pseudo-obstruction. Gastroenterology. 2009; 137:101–9.
60. Tatekawa Y, Komuro H. A technical surgery for refractory gastroparesis in a patient with a mitochondrial disorder. Pediatr Surg Int. 2010;26:655–8.
61. Giordano C, Sebastiani M, Plazzi G, et al. Mitochondrial neurogastrointestinal encephalomyopathy: evidence of mitochondrial DNA depletion in the small intestine. Gastroenterology. 2006;130:893–901.
62. Giordano C, Sebastiani M, De Giorgio R, et al. Gastrointestinal dysmotility in mitochondrial neurogastrointestinal encephalomyopathy is caused by mitochondrial DNA depletion. Am J Pathol. 2008;173:1120–8.

Part IV

Motility Disorders after Surgery and Developmental Anomalies of the Enteric Neuromuscular System Secondary to Anatomical Malformations

Esophageal Atresia

25

Julie Castilloux and Christophe Faure

Esophageal atresia (EA) with or without tracheoesophageal fistula (TEF) is a common congenital anomaly, with an incidence of 1:3,500. Since the first successful surgery in 1941, anesthetic, surgical, and neonatal care have improved tremendously, and our interest is now geared toward preventing short- and long-term morbidity in these children [1]. Besides pulmonary and orthopedic complications [2], motor disorders of the esophagus leading to gastroesophageal reflux (GER) [3–8], chronic dysphagia [5, 9, 10], and esophageal stricture [3–5, 8, 11, 12] remain the most frequent long term problems. Later, complications potentially related to chronic acid and pepsin exposure of the esophageal mucosa, such as Barrett's esophagus [12] and esophageal carcinoma [8] have also been reported.

J. Castilloux, M.D. (✉)
Division of Pediatric Gastroenterology, Pediatric Department, Centre Hospitalier Universitaire Laval, 2705 boul Laurier, Quebec City, QC G1V 4G2, Canada
e-mail: julie.castilloux@mail.chuq.qc.ca

C. Faure, M.D.
Division of Pediatric Gastroenterology, Department of Pediatrics, Sainte-Justine, University Health Center, Université de Montréal, 3175 Côte Sainte-Catherine, Montréal, H3T1C5 QC, Canada

Clinical Symptoms

Gastroesophageal Reflux

GER, as assessed by pH monitoring, affects the majority of children [1, 3–5] and adults [10, 12] with EA with an incidence of 22–58% and may be very severe leading to esophagitis and worsening of the pulmonary condition [10]. Using impedance testing in 24 children with EA, Fröhlich et al. demonstrated an abnormal bolus index in 67% of the patients. Weakly acid reflux showed a higher tendency to be related to symptoms than did acid reflux [13]. However, the low baseline impedance, secondary to the poor esophageal function and/or stasis of liquid especially in the lower esophagus, appears to impair the capacity of MII-pH to accurately capture the changes associated with reflux in these patients [14]. EA patients are at high risk of developing severe GER for several reasons: esophageal dysmotility, modification of the His angle, iatrogenic hiatal hernia, smaller portion of the intrathoracic part of esophagus, vagal nerve surgical injury, and anomalies of gastric motility [15–17]. Romeo et al. reported that 36% of patients with EA have delayed gastric emptying on scintigraphy and 45% abnormal gastric peristalsis on manometry [18]. Because esophagitis is known to provoke esophageal hypomotility, many authors suggest that, at least in the first year of life, all patients need antacid protection and should undergo endoscopic surveillance [8, 19].

C. Faure et al. (eds.), *Pediatric Neurogastroenterology: Gastrointestinal Motility and Functional Disorders in Children*, Clinical Gastroenterology,
DOI 10.1007/978-1-60761-709-9_25, © Springer Science+Business Media New York 2013

Dysphagia

Frequent symptoms of esophageal dysfunction such as dysphagia, episodes of foreign body impaction, heartburn, and vomiting are often detected during purposeful interrogation [20, 21]. Studies in children [3, 5, 10] and in adults [12, 20, 22] have reported that dysphagia is very common occurring in 45–85% of patients [5, 8, 15, 20, 21]. It might be caused by an anastomotic stricture or rarely by eosinophilic esophagitis [23] but is most frequently related to esophageal dysmotility. It can be associated with increased risk of esophageal foreign body impaction and feeding difficulties [1, 8, 12, 15]. A step-by-step investigation may consist of a barium swallow to exclude a stricture, an upper endoscopy to exclude peptic or eosinophilic esophagitis, then an esophageal manometry, and a possible trial of a prokinetic.

Dumping Syndrome

Dumping syndrome is often unrecognized, and its diagnosis delayed. In children with EA, it is most often encountered after a fundoplication or in patients with microgastria [24]. It has also been reported in EA patients with no other precipitating factors [25]. Whether gastric motility disorder may be primitive or secondary to vagus nerve injury is unknown.

Esophageal Motility in Patients with EA

Esophageal dysmotility is practically universal in all patients with EA. It involves mostly peristalsis and may exist even when symptoms are absent [26].

Upper Esophageal Sphincter

The upper esophageal sphincter (UES) function has been reported to be normal by most authors [15, 16, 26], but incomplete relaxation has been described in newborns [27]. When evaluated by videomanometry, an inadequate coordination between pharyngeal contraction and UES relaxation was found [28].

Esophageal Body

Esophageal body dysfunction is present in nearly all patients with EA. It is found in children [13, 15, 16, 21, 26–31] and persists all life long as demonstrated by adult studies [12, 16, 20, 32]. Manometric studies have so far been conducted with standard techniques and found a lack of coordination of peristalsis or no peristaltic waves in the entire esophagus or limited to a segment [10, 15, 20, 26, 28, 29]. Amplitudes are usually low. Simultaneous contractions of low or normal amplitude, similar to achalasia, have been reported [12, 15]. Tovar et al. used a combined 24-h manometry and pH-metry and found a virtual absence of propulsive waves leading to a uniform pattern of long nocturnal episodes of GER in those with a failing sphincteric barrier [21]. Using conventional manometric technique in 101 adults, Sistonen et al. demonstrated non-propagating peristalsis with weak and simultaneous esophageal pressure waves in 80% of patients, with ineffective distal esophageal peristalsis in all [12]. Manometrical abnormalities were significantly worse in those with epithelial metaplasia [12]. Using high-resolution manometry (HREM), a recent study was conducted on 39 patients (34 with type C EA and 5 with type A) with a median age of 8 years. HREM results were abnormal in all patients. Three different esophageal motility patterns were derived from HREM tracing analysis: aperistalsis, pressurization, and distal peristalsis (Fig. 25.1). Five patients were asymptomatic and were found in each group. GERD-related symptoms predominated in the aperistalsis group, and dysphagia was more prevalent in the distal peristalsis group [33].

Lower Esophageal Sphincter

In most studies, lower esophageal sphincter (LES) function is generally similar to controls except for occasional reduced pressure and

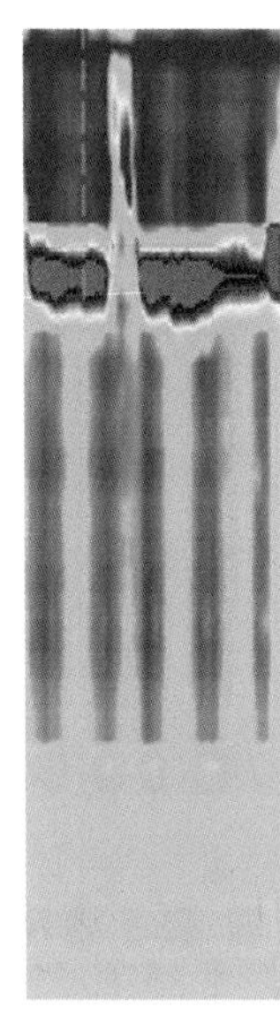
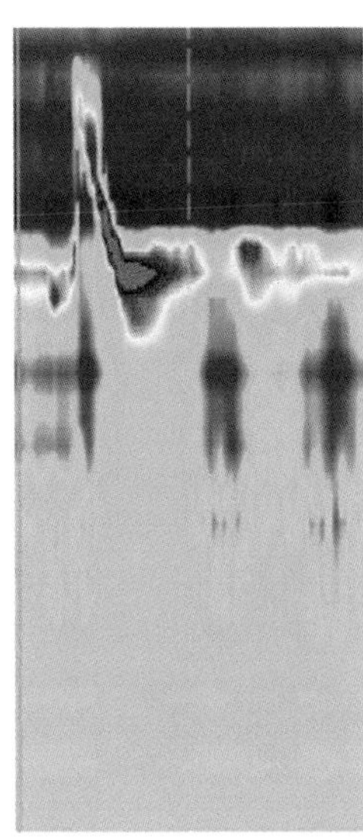
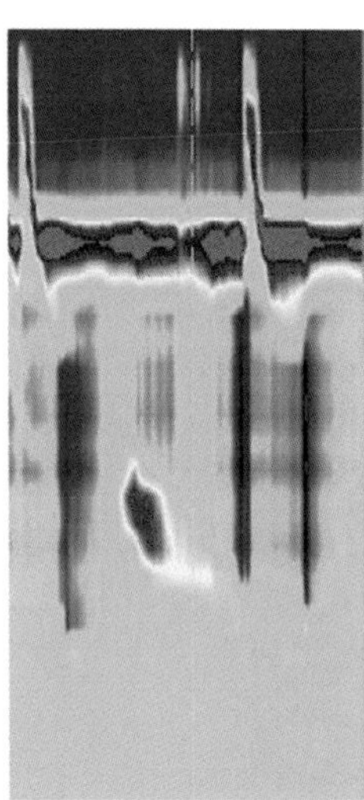

Fig. 25.1 High-resolution esophageal manometry tracings recorded in patients with esophageal atresia. Three patterns are recognized: aperistalsis pattern (A), pressurization pattern (B), and distal (weak) peristalsis pattern (C)

incomplete relaxation [10, 16, 20, 27, 29]. Dutta et al. found that the LES pressure correlated with the severity of GER [26].

Etiology of the Esophageal Dysmotility

The etiology of the esophageal motility disorder remains unclear and controversial. It may be caused by (1) intrinsic factors related to abnormal development of the esophageal smooth muscle and intrinsic innervation and vagus nerve or (2) operative maneuvers. Data indicating a key role of congenital malformation are gaining strength.

Primary Motility Disorder of the Esophagus

Prior to surgery, esophageal manometry conducted in 20 newborn with EA showed motor abnormalities in the proximal (pouch) and distal esophagus [27]. Similarly, abnormal esophageal motility patterns with aperistalsis have been described in adults with tracheoesophageal fistula without atresia before surgical repair [34, 35]. Pathological data support the role of abnormal intrinsic and vagal innervation of the esophagus. Detailed pathological analysis of esophageal myenteric plexuses in dead EA newborn reported profound abnormalities in the Auerbach plexus (plexus hypoplasia, abnormal interganglionic network) [36]. Other studies found hypoplasia of esophageal innervation or smooth muscle [37] in the upper pouch [38] or in the fistula [37, 39]. Findings in an Adriamycin-induced EA-TEF fetal rat model have similarly shown an abnormal distribution of nerve tissue in the esophagus [40] and inherent abnormalities in the branching pattern of the vagus nerves [41].

Postsurgical Dysmotility

On the other hand, the dysmotility may be caused by the dissection during surgery itself damaging the vagal nerve and its esophageal branches [42]. Indeed, bilateral cervical vagotomy above the origin of the pharyngoesophageal branches abolishes peristalsis in the striated muscle esophagus [43]. However, unilateral vagotomy has no effect on peristalsis, presumably because of extensive crossover of vagal innervation within the esophageal wall [44]. Surgery may also result in an extensive mobilization and denervation of the esophagus. Shono et al. demonstrated, in two patients with pure EA studied before surgery, coordinated peristalsis between the proximal and the distal esophagus as well as a normal LES reflex relaxation suggesting that surgery may alter esophageal motility [45]. However, this is not supported by experimental animal studies where transection and anastomosis of the esophagus did not cause severe esophageal dysmotility [46].

Nissen and EA

Nissen fundoplication may exacerbate the dysmotility, and careful attention must be considered for its indication. It is performed in about 9–28% of cases [4, 5, 10, 47]. The fundoplication creates a mechanical obstruction for those patients with a dyskinetic esophagus which cannot generate the pressure to open the new sphincter, and dysphagia may worsen [48]. Some authors have suggested that an anti-reflux procedure may be considered if, despite medical therapy, there is life-threatening or life-limiting symptoms (resistant esophageal strictures, recurrent respiratory symptoms, failure to grow, or severe esophagitis) [15, 21, 48].

References

1. Castilloux J, Noble AJ, Faure C. Risk factors for short- and long-term morbidity in children with esophageal atresia. J Pediatr. 2010;156:755–60.
2. Kovesi T, Rubin S. Long-term complications of congenital esophageal atresia and/or tracheoesophageal fistula. Chest. 2004;126:915–25.
3. Engum SA, Grosfeld JL, West KW, Rescorla FJ, Scherer III LR. Analysis of morbidity and mortality in 227 cases of esophageal atresia and/or tracheoesophageal fistula over two decades. Arch Surg. 1995;130:502–8. discussion 508–9.
4. Konkin DE, O'Hali WA, Webber EM, Blair GK. Outcomes in esophageal atresia and tracheoesophageal fistula. J Pediatr Surg. 2003;38:1726–9.
5. Little DC, Rescorla FJ, Grosfeld JL, West KW, Scherer LR, Engum SA. Long-term analysis of children with esophageal atresia and tracheoesophageal fistula. J Pediatr Surg. 2003;38:852–6.
6. Deurloo JA, Ekkelkamp S, Taminiau JA, Kneepkens CM, ten Kate FW, Bartelsman JF, Legemate DA, Aronson DC. Esophagitis and Barrett esophagus after correction of esophageal atresia. J Pediatr Surg. 2005;40:1227–31.
7. Koivusalo A, Pakarinen MP, Rintala RJ. The cumulative incidence of significant gastrooesophageal reflux in patients with oesophageal atresia with a distal fistula—a systematic clinical, pH-metric, and endoscopic follow-up study. J Pediatr Surg. 2007;42:370–4.
8. Taylor AC, Breen KJ, Auldist A, Catto-Smith A, Clarnette T, Crameri J, Taylor R, Nagarajah S, Brady J, Stokes K. Gastroesophageal reflux and related pathology in adults who were born with esophageal atresia: a long-term follow-up study. Clin Gastroenterol Hepatol. 2007;5:702–6.
9. Lindahl H, Rintala R. Long-term complications in cases of isolated esophageal atresia treated with esophageal anastomosis. J Pediatr Surg. 1995;30:1222–3.
10. Somppi E, Tammela O, Ruuska T, Rahnasto J, Laitinen J, Turjanmaa V, Jarnberg J. Outcome of patients operated on for esophageal atresia: 30 years' experience. J Pediatr Surg. 1998;33:1341–6.
11. Okada A, Usui N, Inoue M, Kawahara H, Kubota A, Imura K, Kamata S. Esophageal atresia in Osaka: a review of 39 years' experience. J Pediatr Surg. 1997;32:1570–4.
12. Sistonen SJ, Koivusalo A, Nieminen U, Lindahl H, Lohi J, Kero M, Karkkainen PA, Farkkila MA, Sarna S, Rintala RJ, Pakarinen MP. Esophageal morbidity and function in adults with repaired esophageal atresia with tracheoesophageal fistula: a population-based long-term follow-up. Ann Surg. 2010;251:1167–73.
13. Frohlich T, Otto S, Weber P, Pilic D, Schmidt-Choudhury A, Wenzl TG, Kohler H. Combined esophageal multichannel intraluminal impedance and pH monitoring after repair of esophageal atresia. J Pediatr Gastroenterol Nutr. 2008;47:443–9.
14. Mousa H. Clinical review: esophageal impedance monitoring for gastroesophageal reflux. J Pediatr Gastroenterol Nutr. 2011;52(2):129–39.
15. Orringer MB, Kirsh MM, Sloan H. Long-term esophageal function following repair of esophageal atresia. Ann Surg. 1977;186:436–43.
16. Duranceau A, Fisher SR, Flye M, Jones RS, Postlethwait RW, Sealy WC. Motor function of the esophagus after repair of esophageal atresia and tracheoesophageal fistula. Surgery. 1977;82:116–23.
17. Montgomery M, Escobar-Billing R, Hellstrom PM, Karlsson KA, Frenckner B. Impaired gastric emptying in children with repaired esophageal atresia: a controlled study. J Pediatr Surg. 1998;33:476–80.
18. Romeo C, Bonanno N, Baldari S, Centorrino A, Scalfari G, Antonuccio P, Centonze A, Gentile C. Gastric motility disorders in patients operated on for esophageal atresia and tracheoesophageal fistula: long-term evaluation. J Pediatr Surg. 2000;35:740–4.
19. Faure C. Endoscopic features in esophageal atresia: from birth to adulthood. J Pediatr Gastroenterol Nutr. 2011;52 Suppl 1:S20–2.
20. Tomaselli V, Volpi ML, Dell'Agnola CA, Bini M, Rossi A, Indriolo A. Long-term evaluation of esophageal function in patients treated at birth for esophageal atresia. Pediatr Surg Int. 2003;19:40–3.
21. Tovar JA, Diez Pardo JA, Murcia J, Prieto G, Molina M, Polanco I. Ambulatory 24-hour manometric and pH metric evidence of permanent impairment of clearance capacity in patients with esophageal atresia. J Pediatr Surg. 1995;30:1224–31.

22. Koivusalo A, Pakarinen MP, Turunen P, Saarikoski H, Lindahl H, Rintala RJ. Health-related quality of life in adult patients with esophageal atresia—a questionnaire study. J Pediatr Surg. 2005;40:307–12.
23. Batres LA, Liacouras C, Schnaufer L, Mascarenhas MR. Eosinophilic esophagitis associated with anastomotic strictures after esophageal atresia repair. J Pediatr Gastroenterol Nutr. 2002;35:224–6.
24. Holschneider P, Dubbers M, Engelskirchen R, Trompelt J, Holschneider AM. Results of the operative treatment of gastroesophageal reflux in childhood with particular focus on patients with esophageal atresia. Eur J Pediatr Surg. 2007;17:163–75.
25. Michaud L, Sfeir R, Couttenier F, Turck D, Gottrand F. Dumping syndrome after esophageal atresia repair without antireflux surgery. J Pediatr Surg. 2010;45:E13–5.
26. Dutta HK, Grover VP, Dwivedi SN, Bhatnagar V. Manometric evaluation of postoperative patients of esophageal atresia and tracheo-esophageal fistula. Eur J Pediatr Surg. 2001;11:371–6.
27. Romeo G, Zuccarello B, Proietto F, Romeo C. Disorders of the esophageal motor activity in atresia of the esophagus. J Pediatr Surg. 1987;22:120–4.
28. Montgomery M, Witt H, Kuylenstierna R, Frenckner B. Swallowing disorders after esophageal atresia evaluated with videomanometry. J Pediatr Surg. 1998;33:1219–23.
29. Hoffman I, De Greef T, Haesendonck N, Tack J. Esophageal motility in children with suspected gastroesophageal reflux disease. J Pediatr Gastroenterol Nutr. 2010;50(6):601–8.
30. Dutta HK, Rajani M, Bhatnagar V. Cineradiographic evaluation of postoperative patients with esophageal atresia and tracheoesophageal fistula. Pediatr Surg Int. 2000;16:322–5.
31. Bozinovski J, Poenaru D, Paterson W, Kamal I. Esophageal aperistalsis following fundoplication in a patient with trisomy 21. Pediatr Surg Int. 1999;15:510–1.
32. Biller JA, Allen JL, Schuster SR, Treves ST, Winter HS. Long-term evaluation of esophageal and pulmonary function in patients with repaired esophageal atresia and tracheoesophageal fistula. Dig Dis Sci. 1987;32:985–90.
33. Lemoine C, Aspirot A, Le Henaff G, Piloquet H, Lévesque D, Miguère L, Morris M, Faure C. Characterization of esophageal motility following esophageal atresia repair using high-resolution esophageal manometry. Neurogastroenterol Motil. 2011;23(S1):41A.
34. Gundry SR, Orringer MB. Esophageal motor dysfunction in an adult with a congenital tracheoesophageal fistula. Arch Surg. 1985;120:1082–3.
35. Heitmiller RF, Nikoomanesh P, Ravich WJ. Esophageal motility in an adult with a congenital H-type tracheoesophageal fistula. Dysphagia. 1990;5:138–41.
36. Nakazato Y, Wells TR, Landing BH. Abnormal tracheal innervation in patients with esophageal atresia and tracheoesophageal fistula: study of the intrinsic tracheal nerve plexuses by a microdissection technique. J Pediatr Surg. 1986;21:838–44.
37. Dutta HK, Mathur M, Bhatnagar V. A histopathological study of esophageal atresia and tracheoesophageal fistula. J Pediatr Surg. 2000;35:438–41.
38. Boleken M, Demirbilek S, Kirimiloglu H, Kanmaz T, Yucesan S, Celbis O, Uzun I. Reduced neuronal innervation in the distal end of the proximal esophageal atretic segment in cases of esophageal atresia with distal tracheoesophageal fistula. World J Surg. 2007;31:1512–7.
39. Li K, Zheng S, Xiao X, Wang Q, Zhou Y, Chen L. The structural characteristics and expression of neuropeptides in the esophagus of patients with congenital esophageal atresia and tracheoesophageal fistula. J Pediatr Surg. 2007;42:1433–8.
40. Qi BQ, Uemura S, Farmer P, Myers NA, Hutson JM. Intrinsic innervation of the oesophagus in fetal rats with oesophageal atresia. Pediatr Surg Int. 1999;15:2–7.
41. Qi BQ, Merei J, Farmer P, Hasthorpe S, Myers NA, Beasley SW, Hutson JM. The vagus and recurrent laryngeal nerves in the rodent experimental model of esophageal atresia. J Pediatr Surg. 1997;32:1580–6.
42. Davies MR. Anatomy of the extrinsic motor nerve supply to mobilized segments of the oesophagus disrupted by dissection during repair of oesophageal atresia with distal fistula. Br J Surg. 1996;83:1268–70.
43. Ueda M, Schlegel JF, Code CF. Electrical and motor activity of innervated and vagally denervated feline esophagus. Am J Dig Dis. 1972;17:1075–88.
44. Roman C. Nervous control of peristalsis in the esophagus. J Physiol Paris. 1966;58:79–108.
45. Shono T, Suita S, Arima T, Handa N, Ishii K, Hirose R, Sakaguchi T. Motility function of the esophagus before primary anastomosis in esophageal atresia. J Pediatr Surg. 1993;28:673–6.
46. Haller Jr JA, Brooker AF, Talbert JL, Baghdassarian O, Vanhoutte J. Esophageal function following resection. Studies in newborn puppies. Ann Thorac Surg. 1966;2:180–7.
47. Chetcuti P, Phelan PD. Gastrointestinal morbidity and growth after repair of oesophageal atresia and tracheo-oesophageal fistula. Arch Dis Child. 1993;68:163–6.
48. Curci MR, Dibbins AW. Problems associated with a Nissen fundoplication following tracheoesophageal fistula and esophageal atresia repair. Arch Surg. 1988;123:618–20.

Anorectal Malformations

26

Jose M. Garza and Ajay Kaul

Anorectal malformations (ARM) are a spectrum of congenital abnormalities of distal hindgut development in which the gastrointestinal tract ends blindly or opens ectopically with a fistula to the skin or into the genitourinary tract. ARM affect about 2–5 per 10,000 live births, an incidence similar to that of Hirschsprung's disease [1]. Males are affected more frequently than females [2]. The most frequent malformation in males involves a rectourethral fistula and in girls a vestibular fistula. The term ARM is often erroneously used synonymously with "imperforate anus."

Embryology and Genetics of ARM

The distal colon, the rectum, and the anal canal above the dentate line are all derived from the hindgut. Before the fifth week of gestation, the intestinal and urogenital tracts terminate in a common cavity called cloaca (Fig. 26.1a). At the sixth week, the urorectal septum migrates caudally in the cloaca and the two tracts are separated (Fig. 26.1b), and during the tenth week, the perineal body is formed and the cloacal sphincter is separated by the perineal body into urogenital and anal portions (Fig. 26.1c) [3]. It has been postulated that failures in this process of normal development lead to the various forms of anorectal malformations, from simple to complex. Prenatal demonstration of the fetal anal sphincter on ultrasound is consistently possible at 23–24 weeks and has been shown to develop in a predictable pattern [4]. Although prenatal diagnosis is possible, most of these malformations are diagnosed at or soon after birth.

ARM have been associated with many different genetic or inherited conditions such as Townes-Brocks syndrome, Currarino triad, Pallister-Hall syndrome, Johanson-Blizzard syndrome, Down syndrome, trisomies 18 and 12, as well in individuals with VACTERL association [1]. There are several reports of increased incidence of nonsyndromic or isolated ARMs in family members, especially in siblings. Recurrence rates of up to 3–4% in full siblings and approximately 2% in first-degree relatives have been reported [1].

Classification of ARM

There is currently no consensus on the classification of ARMs. The Wingspread classification of anorectal malformations has been the most common classification described internationally. ARMs are usually categorized according to the level of the

J.M. Garza, M.D., M.S.
Gastroenterology, Heptology and Nutrition Division, Pediatrics Department, Cincinnati Children's Hospital Medical Center, Cincinnati, OH, USA

A. Kaul, M.D. (✉)
Professor of Clinical Pediatrics,
Director of Neuro-Gastroenterology Program,
Director of GI Operations at Liberty Campus,
Cincinnati Children's Hospital Medical Center,
3333 Burnet Ave (ML 2010), Cincinnati, OH 45229, USA
e-mail: ajay.kaul@cchmc.org

C. Faure et al. (eds.), *Pediatric Neurogastroenterology: Gastrointestinal Motility and Functional Disorders in Children*, Clinical Gastroenterology,
DOI 10.1007/978-1-60761-709-9_26, © Springer Science+Business Media New York 2013

a

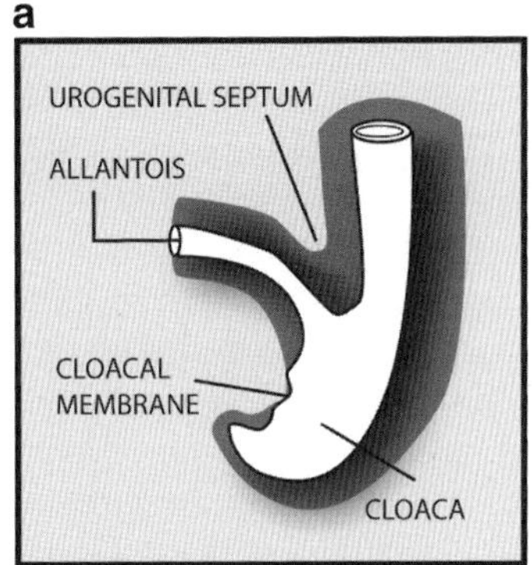

b

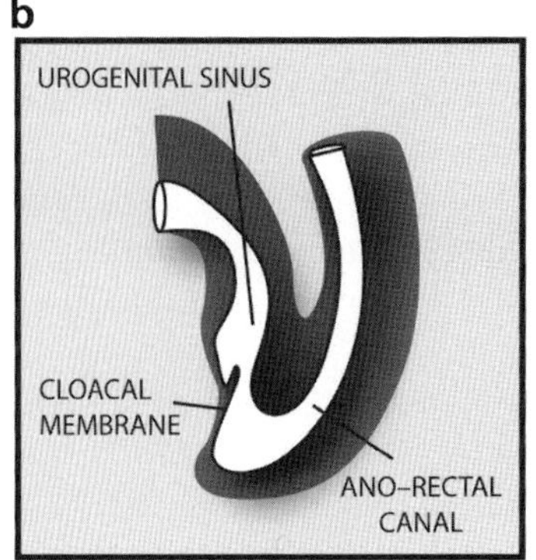

c

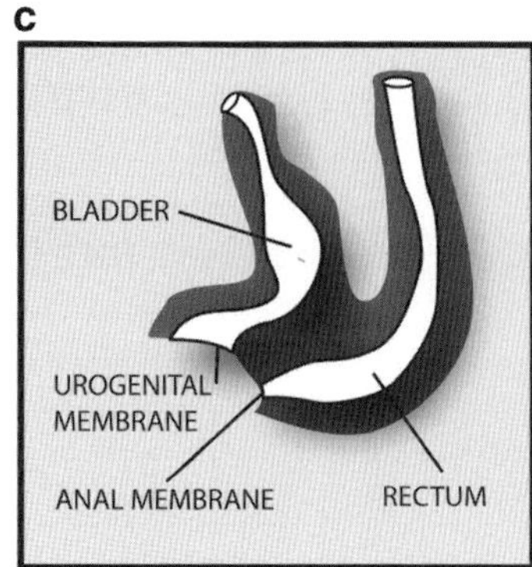

Fig. 26.1 Embryology

rectal pouch relative to the levator ani muscles into high, intermediate, and low anomalies, with special groups established for cloacal and rare malformations [5]. An international conference for the development of standards in the treatment of anorectal malformation was organized at Krickenbeck Castle, Germany, and a modification of the classification was proposed [5]. The major clinical groups were classified as perineal (cutaneous) fistulas, rectourethral fistulas (prostatic and bulbar), rectovesical fistulas, vestibular fistulas, cloacal malformations, patients with no fistula, and anal stenosis. Rare and regional variants were subclassified as pouch colon, rectal atresia/stenosis, rectovaginal fistulas, H-type fistulas, and others [5].

Perineal (Cutaneous) Fistula (Fig. 26.2a, b)

This is a very low malformation in which the rectum passes normally through much of the sphincter complex. The lowest part of the rectum is anteriorly deviated and ends as a perineal fistula anterior to the center of the external sphincter. In males, this fistula can open anywhere between the anus to the ventral portion of the penis. In females, the anterior rectal wall and the posterior vaginal wall are completely separated [2].

Rectourethral Fistula (Fig. 26.2c)

The rectum descends partially through the sphincter muscle, but at some point, it deviates anteriorly and connects with the urethra, most frequently the bulbar urethra. Quality of muscle is usually good in bulbar urethra with a better potential because it has already passed through much of the levator ani and muscle complex mechanism [2].

Rectum-Bladder Neck Fistula (Fig. 26.2d)

In this defect, the levator ani muscle complex and external sphincter are usually underdeveloped with a high association with abnormal sacrum and flat bottom. About 90% of infants with this anomaly have other congenital defects. Continence is usually poor [2].

Vestibular Fistula (Fig. 26.2e)

This is the most common ARM in females. The rectum is anteriorly deviated at a higher level and opens immediately behind the hymen into the vestibule. Most patients have a normal appearing sacrum, adequate innervations, and normal-looking perineum. This malformation is frequently misdiagnosed as a rectovaginal fistula. This defect has excellent potential for bowel control [2].

Persistent Cloaca (Fig. 26.2f)

Cloacae represent a wide array of defects with presence of a single perineal orifice as the

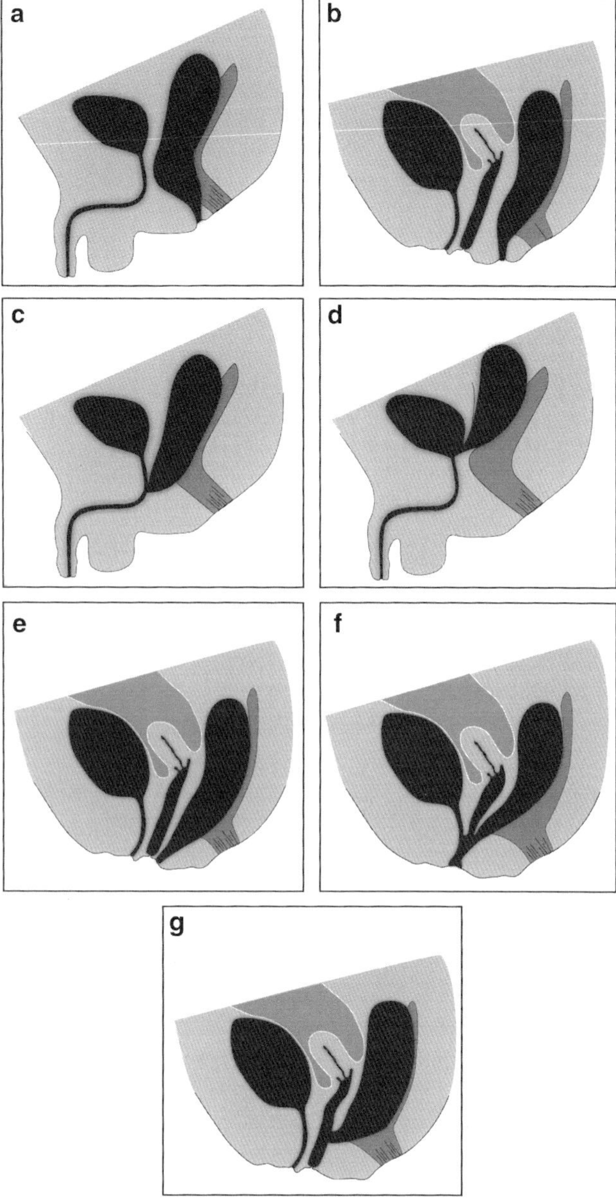

Fig. 26.2 Anorectal malformations (**a**) perineal fistula in a male, (**b**) perineal fistula in a female, (**c**) rectourethral fistula, (**d**) rectum-bladder neck fistula, (**e**) vestibular fistula, (**f**) persistent cloaca, (**g**) rectovaginal fistula

common denominator. The length of the common channel varies from 1 to 10 cm with an average of approximately 3 cm. It is unclear why 30% have a dilated vagina filled with fluid, urine, or mucus (hydrocolpos) since the common channel is almost never atretic. Hydrocolpos can compress the trigone of the bladder anteriorly producing ureterovesical obstruction, megaureter, and hydronephrosis. Alternatively, it may become infected leading to pyocolpos and potentially perforate [6]. The diagnosis of cloaca is a clinical one made by identifying a single perianal orifice with no evidence of vagina or rectum. Sometimes, one finds hypertrophic folds of skin in the area of the single perineal orifice, which gives a false impression of a phallus which is likely why some patients are misdiagnosed with disorders of sexual development. Associated congenital defects are common, and it is vital to recognize urological abnormalities [6].

Rectovaginal Fistula (Fig. 26.2g)

Very unusual malformation in females, the higher the malformation is, the shorter the common wall between the rectum and vagina; one cannot see the fistula orifice by inspection, and the meconium seems to come from within the vagina [2].

Anorectal Agenesis Without Fistula

This defect is relatively less common and constitutes about 5% of anorectal malformations. About half of these children have Down syndrome. Over 90% of children with Down syndrome who have an anorectal malformation have this particular defect. Of these, 80% tend to have voluntary bowel control later in life and usually have good muscle quality and a well-developed sacrum [2].

Anal Stenosis

In this type of defect, there is a ring of fibrous tissue located at the anal verge that causes a stricture resulting in varying degrees of functional abnormality. The presenting symptom is constipation with "thin" feces. Most of these only need to be serially dilated and generally have a good outcome [2].

Long-Term Outcomes in ARM

Anorectal malformations include a spectrum of rare congenital defects involving the developing hindgut. It is estimated that about 64% of children with ARM have other defects, and 15% have a chromosomal abnormality [7]. The most common associated abnormalities involve the urinary tract (40%). The underlying etiology for these varied defects is not known. Improved surgical techniques and care after reconstruction have improved survival to nearly 100%. The primary goal for the surgeon during reconstruction of these anomalies is to preserve fecal and urinary continence. Despite this, there is variable long-term morbidity associated with these disorders. Traditionally, long-term prognosis was based on the type of defect: best prognosis with low defects and worst with high defects and cloacal malformations. While this may be a good rule of thumb, predicting prognosis in children with ARM is often complicated. In addition to the type of defect, there are other factors that potentially impact outcomes. These include surgical technique and experience, immediate postsurgical care, presence of other comorbidities, child's level of cognitive functioning and coping skills, ongoing medical care, and social support.

Constipation and fecal soiling are common long-term defecatory problems reported in children after ARM repair. The etiologies include anal sphincter dysfunction (congenital or acquired), megarectum (associated with sacral anomalies or acquired), and colonic dysmotility (hyperactivity or ineffective colonic contractions) [8–11]. Untreated constipation can lead to megarectum and overflow incontinence ("pseudo-incontinence"). It is important to distinguish constipation with overflow incontinence from true fecal incontinence as the underlying etiology, and therefore their management, is different [12, 13]. The evaluation of such a patient should include radiographic studies to define anatomy, anorectal, and colonic manometry to study anal sphincter and colonic function [14–17]. On occasion, imaging studies of the lower spine and pelvis may be indicated.

The long-term outcomes data on children with ARM are inconsistent at best. Additionally, definitions and methodologies used to study this complex issue vary widely between studies, so correlations between defecatory functioning and quality of life are conflicting. From a review of published studies, Hartman et al. tried to examine disease-specific functioning and quality of life in patients with ARM across different developmental stages. They concluded that even though adolescents reported better fecal functioning, they had more psychosocial quality of life problems than their younger counterparts [18]. In an earlier study, the same group reported that even though patients with ARM and Hirschsprung's disease had comparable quality of life, those with an

Table 26.1 Initial work-up

Place an NG tube to r/o esophageal atresia
Echocardiogram to rule out cardiac conditions
Kidney or bladder US to r/o presence of hydronephrosis and megaureters
Pelvic US, rule out hydrocolpos
Spinal US to evaluate for tethered cord
Plain abdominal X-ray sacrum and sacral ratio

ARM reported additional pain and limitations in role functioning due to physical problems [19]. Another study on 10-year outcomes of children that had posterior sagittal anorectoplasty for ARM reported fecal continence in 58–90% of patients depending upon the severity of the anomaly [20]. A long-term outcome study from Japan reported that only 21% adolescents who had corrective surgery for Hirschsprung's disease had completely normal bowel function [21]. In a review of one of the largest series of 1,192 patients with ARM, Pena and Hong reported that only 37% had complete continence [22].

With regard to urinary and renal function, common anomalies include renal dysgenesis, ectopic and duplex kidneys, vesicoureteric reflux, fistulae, and neurogenic bladder. Inadvertent injury to the urinary tract during surgery, especially in males with a high ARM that undergo a pull through procedure, can be as high as 11% [23]. Urinary incontinence is the most frequent long-term complication noted in this subset, and the rates may vary from less than 10% to 69% (in those with a long common channel cloaca) [24]. Neuropathic bladder is usually encountered in those with a cloacal defect and associated sacral abnormalities. The rate of renal failure in this setting is quite high (50%), with some patients requiring a renal transplant (6%) [25]. There is a small but definite risk for sexual dysfunction and infertility due to genital and sacral anomalies or iatrogenic injury during reconstruction.

Behavioral and psychological problems are known to exist in children with chronic disorders, and it is no surprise that 35–58% adolescents with ARM carry a psychiatric diagnosis [26, 27]. Fecal soiling and intrusive procedures such as repeated anal dilations or enemas have been implicated with changes in self-esteem, body image, and future relationships.

Due to the potential involvement of multiple organ systems in a child born with an ARM, a multidisciplinary approach to evaluation and management is imperative for best outcomes (Table 26.1). Since surgical reconstruction may need to be done in a step-wise manner and involve several surgical disciplines, including colorectal surgeons, urologists, and gynecologists, a coordinated effort to plan surgeries is critical. Additional medical specialists may need to be engaged after the initial reconstruction to address any potential complications with long-term effects. These personnel include primary care providers, gastroenterologists, and psychologists. Even though outcomes of children born with ARM have significantly improved over the recent decades, even better long-term outcomes are possible and may be accomplished by standardizing their care at specialized centers.

References

1. Mundt E, Bates MD. Genetics of Hirschsprung disease and anorectal malformations. Semin Pediatr Surg. 2010;19:107–17.
2. Pena A, Levitt M. Pediatric surgical problems. In: Corman ML, editor. Colon and rectal surgery. Philadelphia, PA: Lippincott Williams & Wilkins; 2005. p. 555–605.
3. Wexner SD, Jorge JM. Anatomy and embryology of the anus, rectum and colon. In: Corman ML, editor. Colon and rectal surgery. Philadelphia, PA: Lippincott Williams & Wilkins; 2005. p. 1–28.
4. Moon MH, Cho JY, Kim JH, et al. In-utero development of the fetal anal sphincter. Ultrasound Obstet Gynecol. 2010;35:556–9.
5. Holschneider A, Hutson J, Pena A, et al. Preliminary report on the International Conference for the Development of Standards for the Treatment of Anorectal Malformations. J Pediatr Surg. 2005;40:1521–6.
6. Levitt MA, Pena A. Cloacal malformations: lessons learned from 490 cases. Semin Pediatr Surg. 2010;19:128–38.
7. Cuschieri A. Anorectal anomalies associated with or as part of other anomalies. Am J Med Genet. 2002;110:122–30.
8. Rintala RJ, Pakarinen MP. Imperforate anus: long- and short-term outcome. Semin Pediatr Surg. 2008;17:79–89.
9. Burjonrappa S, Youssef S, Lapierre S, et al. Megarectum after surgery for anorectal malformations. J Pediatr Surg. 2010;45:762–8.

10. Athanasakos EP, Ward HC, Williams NS, et al. Importance of extrasphincteric mechanisms in the pathophysiology of faecal incontinence in adults with a history of anorectal anomaly. Br J Surg. 2008;95:1394–400.
11. Kaul A, Garza JM, Connor FL, et al. Colonic hyperactivity results in frequent fecal soiling in a subset of children after surgery for Hirschsprung disease. J Pediatr Gastroenterol Nutr. 2011;52:433–6.
12. Gariepy CE, Mousa H. Clinical management of motility disorders in children. Semin Pediatr Surg. 2009;18:224–38.
13. Zundel S, Obermayr F, Schaefer JF, et al. Hirschsprung disease associated with total colonic agenesis and imperforate anus—case report and review of the literature. J Pediatr Surg. 2010;45:252–4.
14. Senel E, Demirbag S, Tiryaki T, et al. Postoperative anorectal manometric evaluation of patients with anorectal malformation. Pediatr Int. 2007;49:210–4.
15. Rintala RJ. Fecal incontinence in anorectal malformations, neuropathy, and miscellaneous conditions. Semin Pediatr Surg. 2002;11:75–82.
16. Keshtgar AS, Athanasakos E, Clayden GS, et al. Evaluation of outcome of anorectal anomaly in childhood: the role of anorectal manometry and endosonography. Pediatr Surg Int. 2008;24:885–92.
17. Heikenen JB, Werlin SL, Di Lorenzo C, et al. Colonic motility in children with repaired imperforate anus. Dig Dis Sci. 1999;44:1288–92.
18. Hartman EE, Oort FJ, Aronson DC, et al. Quality of life and disease-specific functioning of patients with anorectal malformations or Hirschsprung's disease: a review. Arch Dis Child. 2011;96:398–406.
19. Hartman EE, Oort FJ, Aronson DC, et al. Critical factors affecting quality of life of adult patients with anorectal malformations or Hirschsprung's disease. Am J Gastroenterol. 2004;99:907–13.
20. Hassett S, Snell S, Hughes-Thomas A, et al. 10-year outcome of children born with anorectal malformation, treated by posterior sagittal anorectoplasty, assessed according to the Krickenbeck classification. J Pediatr Surg. 2009;44:399–403.
21. Ieiri S, Nakatsuji T, Akiyoshi J, et al. Long-term outcomes and the quality of life of Hirschsprung disease in adolescents who have reached 18 years or older—a 47-year single-institute experience. J Pediatr Surg. 2010;45:2398–402.
22. Pena A, Hong A. Advances in the management of anorectal malformations. Am J Surg. 2000;180:370–6.
23. Misra D, Chana J, Drake DP, et al. Operative trauma to the genitourinary tract in the treatment of anorectal malformations: 15 years' experience. Urology. 1996;47:559–62.
24. Pena A. Anorectal malformations. Semin Pediatr Surg. 1995;4:35–47.
25. Warne SA, Wilcox DT, Ledermann SE, et al. Renal outcome in patients with cloaca. J Urol. 2002;167:2548–51. discussion 51.
26. Ludman L, Spitz L, Kiely EM. Social and emotional impact of faecal incontinence after surgery for anorectal abnormalities. Arch Dis Child. 1994;71:194–200.
27. Diseth TH, Emblem R. Somatic function, mental health, and psychosocial adjustment of adolescents with anorectal anomalies. J Pediatr Surg. 1996;31:638–43.

Small Bowel and Colonic Dysfunction After Surgery

27

Roberto Gomez, H. Nicole Lopez, and John E. Fortunato

Introduction

Surgery of the small intestine and colon is commonly performed in children for a variety of indications ranging from congenital anatomic abnormalities to need for enteral feeding access to underlying motility disorders. Under most circumstances, nonemergent operations allow time for a multidisciplinary team approach between surgeons and gastroenterologists to devise a thorough preoperative diagnostic strategy. Unfortunately, abdominal catastrophes such as malrotation with volvulus often preclude the luxury of time before surgery necessitating a strong relationship between surgeon and gastroenterologist to address the potential consequences of such an event. Under both circumstances, the motility of the small bowel and colon remains a critical feature that often predicts the success of an operation and, most importantly, the prognosis of the patient. This chapter aims to address several of the more prevalent motility disorders observed in children after small bowel and colonic surgery.

R. Gomez, M.D.
Pediatric Gastroenterology Department, Wake Forest University, Winston-Salem, NC, USA

H.N. Lopez, M.D.
Pediatrics Department, Wake Forest University School of Medicine, Winston-Salem, NC, USA

J.E. Fortunato, M.D. (✉)
Department of Pediatrics, Wake Forest University, Medical Center Blvd, Winston-Salem, NC 27157, USA
e-mail: jfortuna@wfubmc.edu

Small Bowel Motility After Resection

Resection of all or part of the small bowel may be necessary for conditions including *surgical emergencies* such as bowel ischemia or necrosis from volvulus and perforation; *congenital anomalies* such as intestinal atresia, malrotation, and gastroschisis; or *acquired etiologies* encompassing stricturing Crohn's disease, ulcerative colitis, severe necrotizing enterocolitis, intestinal pseudoobstruction, or abdominal trauma. Preservation of bowel length, particularly the small intestine, is critical to insure adequate absorption of nutrients, fluids, and electrolytes but is contingent on circumstances such as extent of the necrosis or ischemia. The consequences of a more extensive resection of small bowel include symptoms such as frequent diarrhea, malnutrition, and bloating due to bacterial overgrowth and may result in the need for parental nutrition with its associated complications.

Small intestinal resections are classified into three categories based on length of residual small bowel: short resection with 100–150-cm length remaining, large resection with 40–100 cm remaining, and massive resection with 40 cm or less remaining. In general, massive resections particularly in the context of an absent ileocecal valve are associated with inability to wean completely from

C. Faure et al. (eds.), *Pediatric Neurogastroenterology: Gastrointestinal Motility and Functional Disorders in Children*, Clinical Gastroenterology,
DOI 10.1007/978-1-60761-709-9_27, © Springer Science+Business Media New York 2013

parenteral nutrition [1]. The absence of ileocecal valve has been associated with increased diarrhea and small bowel bacterial overgrowth (SBBO).

While mucosal adaptation has been extensively studied, there is a paucity of data regarding changes in motility after small intestinal resection. A better functional outcome is associated with proximal compared to distal resection, which may be related to both the adaptive capacity and intrinsic properties of the jejunum and ileum. Adaptation involves all layers of the bowel wall, including intestinal smooth muscle. The intestinal smooth muscle is coordinated by both hormonal and neuronal components which regulate the transit of intestinal contents through the gastrointestinal tract [2]. Activation of this complex circuitry allows changes in the peristaltic reflex to modulate the intestinal motility pattern from propagative to segmenting. This is accomplished through a complex integration of signals that trigger a jejunal and ileal break mechanism in response to nutrients, most notably fats. Mediators involved in this response include peptide YY, chemosensitive afferent neurons, noradrenergic nerves, myenteric serotonergic neurons, and opioid neurons [3]. Following proximal resection of small bowel, for example, it has been demonstrated that the postprandial motilin response is decreased, whereas transient increases in neurotensin and peptide YY have been noted after distal resection [4].

After intestinal loss, a combination of shorter bowel length and disruption of normal physiological mechanisms may lead to poor absorption and malnutrition. Increased contractile response and proliferative changes in intestinal smooth muscle cells may contribute to the compensatory adaptive mechanism to slow intestinal transit and improve nutrient absorption. While the cellular mechanism for this process is not well defined, mechanisms such as epidermal growth factor receptor signaling have been shown to play a role in adaptation of the smooth muscle cellular compartment [2].

Little is known about changes in the migrating motor complex (MMC) after resection. Animal studies often reveal conflicting results with a broad spectrum of motility changes depending on the extent and location of resection. For example, after extensive distal small bowel resection, postoperative changes such as decreased MMC velocity and longer intervals between MMCs during fasting with slight recovery of propagation frequency in the chronic phase have been observed [5, 6]. Findings such as shorter phase I duration and discoordinate clustered MMC activity have also been seen using the same model [7]. There are very limited motility studies in humans after small bowel resection [8–10]. With extensive distal resection, motility changes include shorter duration and more frequent MMCs as well as a reduction in phase 2 activity; however, limited ileal resection does not result in detectable manometric changes of jejunal motility [9]. The postprandial motor response is not well defined, but appears to be shorter in patients after resection [10].

Intestinal Lengthening

Various surgical procedures, including Bianchi intestinal lengthening and serial transverse enteroplasty (STEP), have been developed to address the anatomic and physiological consequence of short bowel syndrome [11, 12]. These consequences include reduced intestinal length, decreased mucosal surface area, rapid intestinal transit, and ineffective peristalsis. Bianchi isoperistaltic bowel lengthening entails longitudinal division of the bowel with isoperistaltic end-to-end anastomosis effectively doubling the length of that portion of the bowel. The STEP procedure involves the sequential linear stapling of the dilated small bowel from alternating directions perpendicular to the long axis of the intestine [12].

Both the Bianchi and STEP have been shown to successfully result in increased caloric absorption and improved intestinal motility [13, 14]. After Bianchi, increased tolerance of enteral feeds, improved growth, and decreased frequency of catheter infections have been reported [15]. Significant improvement in stool counts, intestinal transit time, D-xylose absorption, and fat absorption resulting in discontinuation of parenteral nutrition has also been observed [15, 16]. Longitudinal intestinal lengthening and tailoring has also been associated with normalization in liver enzymes in patients weaned from parental nutrition [17]. Limitations of the Bianchi procedure include its technical difficulty, involvement of at least one intestinal anastomosis, and risk to the mesenteric blood supply. It is also best performed if the bowel is symmetrically dilated. Some complications such as ileal valve prolapse and recurrent small bowel dilatation have been reported after the operation [14].

STEP has become widely accepted among pediatric surgeons as it is technically easier to perform than longitudinal bowel lengthening and preserves the natural mesenteric vasculature to the intestine [18]. STEP has been shown to improve weight retention, nutritional status, and intestinal absorptive capacity in an animal model [19]. Phase III of the MMC appeared to be preserved in animals with STEP after resection and anastomosis with the same mean amplitude and frequency after octreotide as well as motility index compared to controls [12]. Nonspecific abnormalities observed in both groups included simultaneous or tonic contractions as well as contractions present in only proximal or distal segments. The duration of phase III after octreotide was also increased in STEP animals [12]. In patients with severe ischemia even after the STEP procedure, the intestinal motility continues to be affected, and it correlates with feeding intolerance and TPN dependency (Fig. 27.1).

Intestinal Transplantation

Intestinal transplantation has become an increasingly accepted treatment for children with intestinal failure with 3- and 5-year survival rates of 84% and 77%, respectively, with most patients becoming independent of TPN [20]. The most frequent cause of intestinal failure is short-gut syndrome (SGS) defined by malabsorption, malnutrition, and growth retardation secondary to extensive loss of intestinal length or functional gut mass [21, 22]. Gastroschisis, volvulus, necrotizing enterocolitis, intestinal atresia, chronic intestinal pseudoobstruction, and congenital enteropathy are frequent conditions associated with SGS [20].

Small bowel or multivisceral organ transplantation is often necessary for children after massive intestinal resection including those with less than 25 cm of small bowel without ileocecal valve, congenital intractable mucosal disorders, persistent hyperbilirubinemia, and diminishing venous access, often associated with recurrent episodes of sepsis [23, 24]. The role of performing small bowel motility studies as a gauge to determine whether intestinal transplantation should be undertaken is unclear, but has been proposed as a potential prognostic tool [25]. Most studies have focused on the impact on intestinal motility after transplantation [26].

After intestinal transplantation, maintenance of intestinal motility with coordinated smooth muscle function and adequate absorptive capability is paramount. Animal models have confirmed that intrinsic nerves are generally preserved after transplantation [27, 28]. The consequence of extrinsic denervation from the small bowel may lead to poor functioning of the grafted intestine. In a canine model, for instance, body weight and serum albumin levels remain stable after autotransplantation. However, transplanted animals demonstrated significant defects in fat and D-xylose absorption compared to controls, possibly attributed to overgrowth in fecal flora [27]. In a similar model, dogs undergoing autotransplantation experienced rapid intestinal transit compared to short-gut animals which may suggest that adaptive responses of the transplanted intestine may be impaired by neuromuscular injury associated with denervation or ischemia [29].

Intestinal motility after small bowel transplantation has been studied in children using antroduodenal manometry [26]. Interdigestive phase III motor activity with normal manometric characteristics was seen as early as 3 months post transplantation in the majority of patients. However, disruption of an orderly MMC was noted across the anastomosis as well as abnormal postprandial motility, which may in part be responsible for abnormal intestinal transit and poor absorption [26]. These studies emphasize how little is known about the effect of small bowel transplantation on motility and underscore the need for future prospective research.

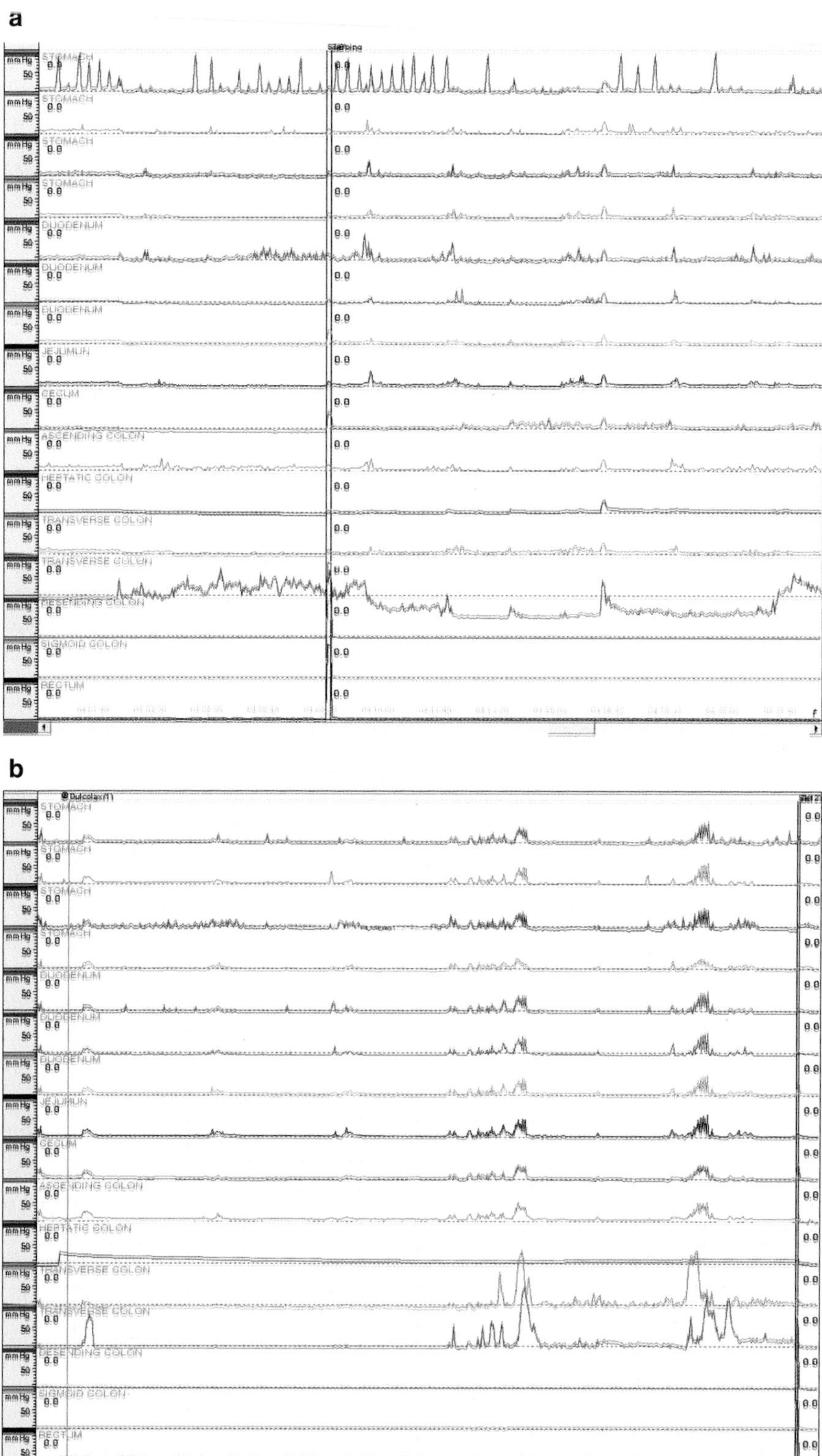

Fig. 27.1 Small bowel and colonic motility in a 4-year-old boy with a medical history of NEC, small bowel syndrome, and post-STEP procedure. (**a**) Presence of simultaneous contractions in the antrum and small bowel in the first eight channels. (**b**) HAPCs in the sigmoid after bisacodyl stimulation (*arrow*). Courtesy of Dr. Carlo Di Lorenzo and Dr. Hayat Mousa Nationwide Children's Hospital

Roux-en-Y Jejunostomy and Bariatric Surgery

Roux-en-Y gastrojejunostomy has been employed in both children and adults for a variety of indications including postgastrectomy for peptic ulcer disease, as a component of bariatric surgery, and for jejunal feeding access [29]. The technique limits reflux of bile into the gastric remnant and esophagus. Common postoperative symptoms attributed to secondary dysmotility include abdominal fullness, distension, pain, nausea, and vomiting [30]. These symptoms are likely the result of interrupted slow-wave electrical conduction which occurs after transecting the jejunum resulting in shortened phase III MMC duration and abnormal motor response to meals [31]. The consequence of disruption of the enteric nervous system may include serious conditions such as ascending cholangitis due to stasis of bowel contents in the proximal limb of the roux segment, known as blind-loop syndrome [32].

It has been shown in both adults and animals that using an "uncut" Roux-en-Y technique may avoid the problems observed with jejunal transection by prolonging the phase III MMC, thereby enhancing digestive clearance [32]. While gastrectomy is uncommon in children, there has been an increase in pediatric gastric surgery to treat obesity particularly in adolescents [33]. Both laparoscopic adjustable gastric banding and laparoscopic Roux-en-Y gastric bypass have been performed in children, but there is a paucity of data examining the effects of these operations on gut motility. Overall, there seems to be an improvement in health-related quality of life based on early studies, which may suggest limited disturbances in motility in these patients [34].

Congenital Diaphragmatic Hernia

Congenital diaphragmatic hernia (CDH) is a developmental defect present in less than 1 of 1,000 live births resulting in herniation of abdominal viscera into the chest [35, 36]. It is associated with other anatomic malformations in 30% of the patients resulting in increased mortality [37, 38]. Long-term gastrointestinal problems, most notably refractory gastroesophageal reflux disease (GERD), have been described in patients with prior CDH repair [39]. In a recent multivariate analysis, the incidence of GERD was shown to be 39% immediately after repair and 16% 12–18 years after repair. Patients with an intrathoracic stomach and patch closure of the diaphragm seemed to demonstrate the most significant reflux symptoms in the early postoperative period [40].

Reports of intestinal motility disorders in patients with CDH are limited. However, foregut dysmotility has been postulated after CDH repair as evidenced by persistent upper GI symptoms noted in association with abnormal gut fixation seen in nearly 10% of patients [41]. For example, antral hypomotility with low-amplitude and prolonged phase III contractions has been observed after CDH repair manifesting as symptoms of severe gastroesophageal reflux and delayed gastric emptying scintigraphy testing [42].

Gastroschisis

Gastroschisis is a full-thickness defect in the abdominal wall usually adjacent to the insertion of the umbilical cord with an incidence between 0.4 and 3 per 10,000 births [43]. A variable amount of intestine and abdominal organs may herniate through this defect without the protective covering of the peritoneal sac [44]. Ten percent of infants with gastroschisis develop ischemic injury to the bowel due to vascular insufficiency which may result in intestinal stenosis or atresia [43, 45]. Gastroschisis represents one of the major causes of intestinal failure often necessitating consideration of intestinal transplantation. Approximately 40% of patients with gastroschisis require parenteral nutrition by the age of 4 months and 10% by the age of 2 years [46].

Patients with gastroschisis tend to have persistent gut dysmotility with symptoms suggestive of intestinal pseudoobstruction [47]. Even after repair with adequate bowel length, these patients have evidence of profound feeding problems, increased hospitalizations, and mortality [48, 49]. Many of these patients with feeding problems may have neuropathic predominant changes based on antroduodenal manometry (Gomez et al. unpublished case series). Interestingly, in postnatal autopsy studies, there is no evidence of ganglion cell or generalized myenteric nervous system abnormalities to explain the motility disorders that often accompany cases of gastroschisis [50].

Motility Disorders After Repair of Malrotation and Intestinal Atresia

Malrotation is defined by the absence of midgut rotation before reentering the abdominal cavity during the 12th week of gestation [51]. By this time in embryonic development, the neurons forming the ENS have already migrated from the neural crest to the intestine. Surgical correction (Ladd's procedure) involves division of a fibrous stalk of peritoneal tissue attaching the cecum to the abdominal wall, known as Ladd's bands; widening the small bowel mesentery; appendectomy; and appropriate placement of the colon. Small bowel motility abnormalities including complete absence of motor activity, low-amplitude or slow-frequency contractions, and slow propagation of phase III of the MMCs have been described after performing a Ladd's procedure for these patients [52]. These manometric abnormalities have been associated in some patients with histological changes such as distended neuronal axon hypoganglionosis or vacuolated nerve tracts in the small bowel [53].

Intestinal atresia is a frequent cause of bowel obstruction in neonates. Operative management includes resection of the atresia with primary bowel anastomosis, resection with tapering enteroplasty, temporary ostomy with intestinal resection, enterostomy with web excision, and longitudinal intestinal lengthening procedures. After surgical correction, symptoms of adhesive bowel obstruction occur in close to 25% of the patients with prolonged adynamic ileus in 9% and enterostomy prolapse in 2% [54]. Prolonged small bowel obstruction due to atresia or malrotation can lead to severe refeeding problems in the neonatal period. Cezard et al. described a form of postobstructive enteropathy (POE) of the apparently normal small intestine segment proximal to the obstruction. POE patients showed significant abnormal peristalsis as characterized by barium and carmine transit times. Small bowel manometric recordings are characterized by an absence or abnormal phase III of the migrating motor complex and decreased motility index of the small intestine above the obstruction [55, 56].

Colectomy and Partial Colonic Resection

Colonic resection in children is reserved for chronic conditions such as refractory ulcerative colitis, Crohn's colitis, familial adenomatous polyposis, severe constipation, Hirschsprung's disease, and debilitating motility disorders such as intestinal pseudoobstruction. Small bowel and residual colonic function is contingent on the region and extent of colonic resection as well as the underlying pathology necessitating surgery. As an example, subtotal colectomy is a surgical option to treat severe cases of constipation associated with colonic dilatation. While extensive resection of colon may accomplish reduction in intestinal transit time, it may not eliminate symptoms of pain and bloating suggesting the possibility of a more generalized motor disorder of the gut [57]. Colectomy in these patients may also be associated with uncontrolled diarrhea and fecal incontinence as well as relapsing constipation [58].

The difficulties associated with subtotal colectomy may be due to the adaptive changes in the MMC resulting in increased anaerobic bacterial colonization of the small intestine [59]. Partial colonic resection may alleviate some of symptoms observed after subtotal colectomy particularly if performed in conjunction with preoperative motor assessment including Sitz markers, scintigraphy, and antroduodenal and colonic manometry [60–62].

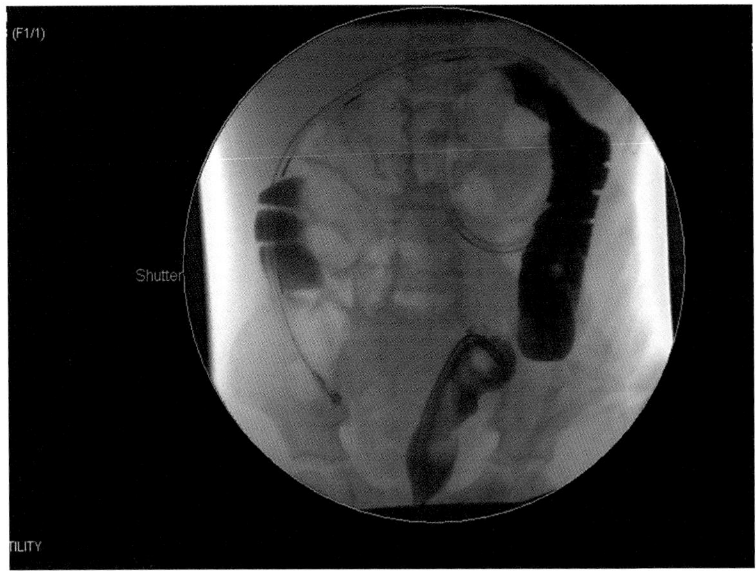

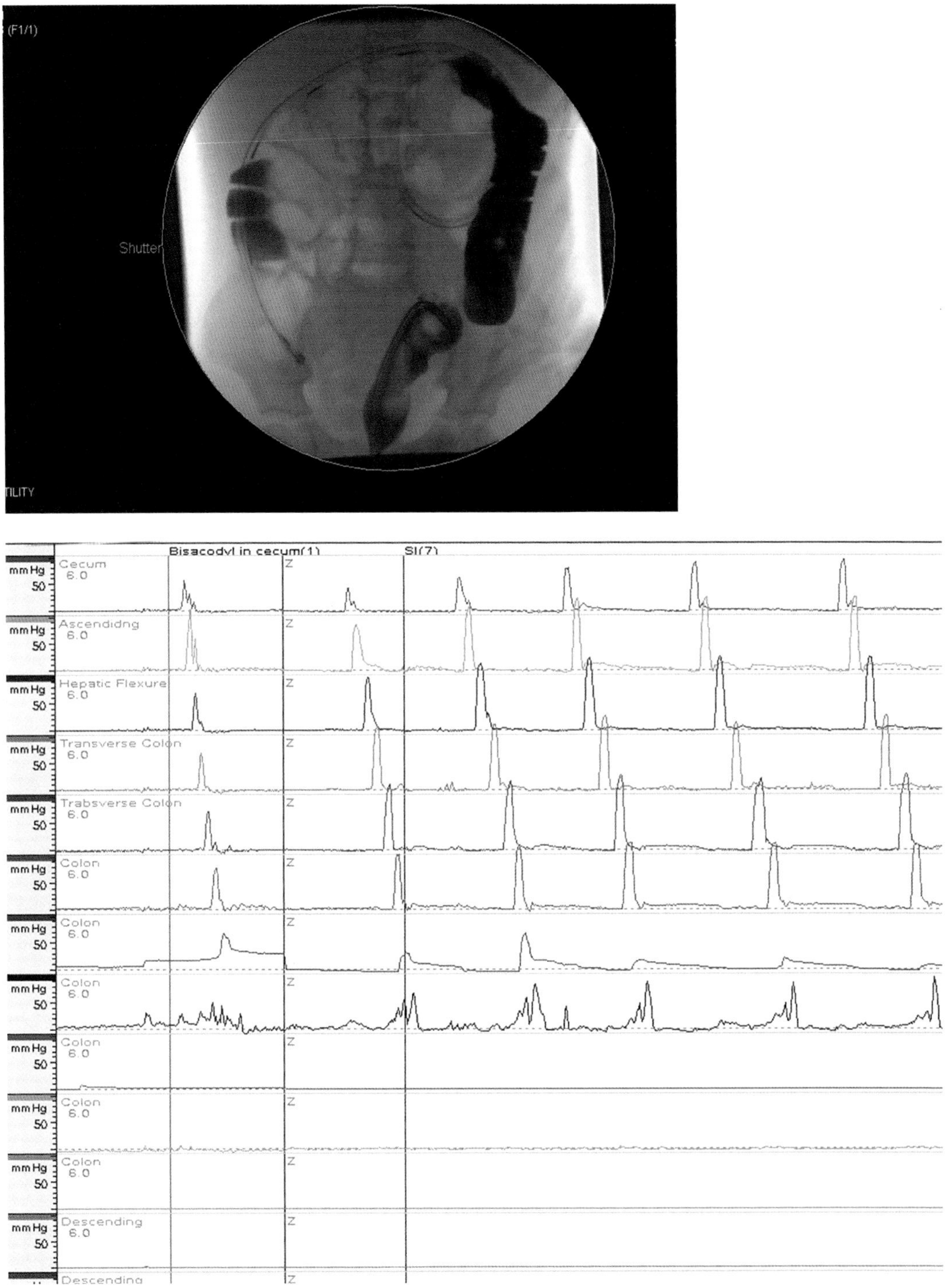

Fig. 27.2 Example of two manometry catheters placed in a retrograde fashion from a colostomy and from the anus. The top panel shows the radiology image of the two manometry catheters. The bottom panel shows the manometry study. There is evidence of propulsive contractions proximal to a diverting colostomy (top 8 channels in the manometry tracing) and absent motility in the distal 4 channels in the distal colonic segment

In patients with refractory constipation and colonic dilatation, colonic and antroduodenal manometry may be key diagnostic tests to determine the optimal surgical approach [62–64]. In the absence of demonstrable colonic motility, a decompressive ileostomy or proximal colostomy for several months may allow improvement in the degree of colonic dilatation with return of some degree of motor function in the distal, diverted colon [62, 64]. Performing a subsequent colonic manometry study after a diverting ileostomy or colostomy may allow a more objective surgical decision between ostomy takedown and reanastomosis alone versus reanastomosis combined with partial resection of colon particularly in the context of adequate small bowel motility (Fig. 27.2). A permanent ileostomy may be indicated in the context of persistently absent colonic high-amplitude propagating contractions (HAPCs) particularly in association with abnormal small bowel motility [62].

Summary

The need for small bowel and colonic surgery for a variety of indications is a common occurrence in children. The impact of operative manipulation and interventions on subsequent gut motility may have serious implications in terms of the functional capacity of the remaining intestine to effectively absorb nutrients without gastrointestinal symptoms. Thus, motility testing in children whether performed in the preoperative or postoperative phase of management may play a significant role in the surgical decision-making process. Future studies are needed to better discern the underlying mechanisms responsible for motility problems observed after small intestine and colonic surgery.

References

1. Goulet O, Ruemmele F, Lacaille F, et al. Irreversible intestinal failure. J Pediatr Gastroenterol Nutr. 2004; 38(3):250–69.
2. Martin CA, Bernabe KQ, Taylor JA, et al. Resection-induced intestinal adaptation and the role of enteric smooth muscle. J Pediatr Surg. 2008;43(6):1011–7.
3. Van Citters GW, Lin HC. Ileal brake: neuropeptidergic control of intestinal transit. Curr Gastroenterol Rep. 2006;8(5):367–73.
4. Thompson JS, Quigley EM, Adrian TE. Factors affecting outcome following proximal and distal intestinal resection in the dog: an examination of the relative roles of mucosal adaptation, motility, luminal factors, and enteric peptides. Dig Dis Sci. 1999;44(1):63–74.
5. Uchiyama M, Iwafuchi M, Matsuda Y, et al. Intestinal motility after massive small bowel resection in conscious canines: comparison of acute and chronic phases. J Pediatr Gastroenterol Nutr. 1996;23(3):217–23.
6. Uchiyama M, Iwafuchi M, Ohsawa Y, et al. Intestinal myoelectric activity and contractile motility in dogs with a reversed jejunal segment after extensive small bowel resection. J Pediatr Surg. 1992;27(6):686–90.
7. Quigley EM, Thompson JS. The motor response to intestinal resection: motor activity in the canine small intestine following distal resection. Gastroenterology. 1993;105(3):791–8.
8. Scolapio JS, Camilleri M, Fleming CR. Gastrointestinal motility considerations in patients with short-bowel syndrome. Dig Dis. 1997;15(4–5):253–62.
9. Remington M, Malagelada JR, Zinsmeister A, et al. Abnormalities in gastrointestinal motor activity in patients with short bowels: effect of a synthetic opiate. Gastroenterology. 1983;85(3):629–36.
10. Schmidt T, Pfeiffer A, Hackelsberger N, et al. Effect of intestinal resection on human small bowel motility. Gut. 1996;38(6):859–63.
11. Bianchi A. Intestinal loop lengthening–a technique for increasing small intestinal length. J Pediatr Surg. 1980;15(2):145–51.
12. Kim HB, Fauza D, Garza J, et al. Serial transverse enteroplasty (STEP): a novel bowel lengthening procedure. J Pediatr Surg. 2003;38(3):425–9.
13. Figueroa-Colon R, Harris PR, Birdsong E, et al. Impact of intestinal lengthening on the nutritional outcome for children with short bowel syndrome. J Pediatr Surg. 1996;31(7):912–6.
14. Javid PJ, Kim HB, Duggan CP, et al. Serial transverse enteroplasty is associated with successful short-term outcomes in infants with short bowel syndrome. J Pediatr Surg. 2005;40(6):1019–23.
15. Weber TR, Powell MA. Early improvement in intestinal function after isoperistaltic bowel lengthening. J Pediatr Surg. 1996;31(1):61–3.
16. Weber TR. Isoperistaltic bowel lengthening for short bowel syndrome in children. Am J Surg. 1999;178(6): 600–4.
17. Reinshagen K, Zahn K, Buch C, et al. The impact of longitudinal intestinal lengthening and tailoring on liver function in short bowel syndrome. Eur J Pediatr Surg. 2008;18(4):249–53.
18. Modi BP, Javid PJ, Jaksic T, et al. First report of the international serial transverse enteroplasty data registry: indications, efficacy, and complications. J Am Coll Surg. 2007;204(3):365–71.

19. Chang RW, Javid PJ, Oh JT, et al. Serial transverse enteroplasty enhances intestinal function in a model of short bowel syndrome. Ann Surg. 2006;243(2): 223–8.
20. Avitzur Y, Grant D. Intestine transplantation in children: update 2010. Pediatr Clin North Am. 2010;57(2): 415–31. table.
21. Galea MH, Holliday H, Carachi R, et al. Short-bowel syndrome: a collective review. J Pediatr Surg. 1992;27(5):592–6.
22. Georgeson KE, Breaux Jr CW. Outcome and intestinal adaptation in neonatal short-bowel syndrome. J Pediatr Surg. 1992;27(3):344–8.
23. Beath S, Pironi L, Gabe S, et al. Collaborative strategies to reduce mortality and morbidity in patients with chronic intestinal failure including those who are referred for small bowel transplantation. Transplantation. 2008;85(10):1378–84.
24. Kaufman SS, Atkinson JB, Bianchi A, et al. Indications for pediatric intestinal transplantation: a position paper of the American Society of Transplantation. Pediatr Transplant. 2001;5(2):80–7.
25. Mousa H, Bueno J, Griffiths J, et al. Intestinal motility after small bowel transplantation. Transplant Proc. 1998;30(6):2535–6.
26. Johnson CP, Sarna SK, Zhu YR, et al. Effects of intestinal transplantation on postprandial motility and regulation of intestinal transit. Surgery. 2001;129(1):6–14.
27. Kiyochi H, Ono A, Miyagi K, et al. Extrinsic reinnervation one year after intestinal transplantation in rats. Transplant Proc. 1996;28(5):2542.
28. Kiyochi H, Ono A, Yamamoto N, et al. Extrinsic nerve preservation technique for intestinal transplantation in rats. Transplant Proc. 1995;27(1):587–9.
29. Le Blanc-Louvry I, Ducrotte P, Peillon C, et al. Roux-en-Y limb motility after total or distal gastrectomy in symptomatic and asymptomatic patients. J Am Coll Surg. 2000;190(4):408–17.
30. Zhang YM, Liu XL, Xue DB, et al. Myoelectric activity and motility of the Roux limb after cut or uncut Roux-en-Y gastrojejunostomy. World J Gastroenterol. 2006;12(47):7699–704.
31. Le Blanc-Louvry I, Ducrotte P, Lemeland JF, et al. Motility in the Roux-Y limb after distal gastrectomy: relation to the length of the limb and the afferent duodenojejunal segment—an experimental study. Neurogastroenterol Motil. 1999;11(5):365–74.
32. Klaus A, Weiss H, Kreczy A, et al. A new biliodigestive anastomosis technique to prevent reflux and stasis. Am J Surg. 2001;182(1):52–7.
33. Jen HC, Rickard DG, Shew SB, et al. Trends and outcomes of adolescent bariatric surgery in California, 2005–2007. Pediatrics. 2010;126(4):e746–53.
34. Loux TJ, Haricharan RN, Clements RH, et al. Health-related quality of life before and after bariatric surgery in adolescents. J Pediatr Surg. 2008;43(7):1275–9.
35. Harrison MR, Bjordal RI, Langmark F, et al. Congenital diaphragmatic hernia: the hidden mortality. J Pediatr Surg. 1978;13(3):227–30.
36. Skari H, Bjornland K, Haugen G, et al. Congenital diaphragmatic hernia: a meta-analysis of mortality factors. J Pediatr Surg. 2000;35(8):1187–97.
37. Cannon C, Dildy GA, Ward R, et al. A population-based study of congenital diaphragmatic hernia in Utah: 1988–1994. Obstet Gynecol. 1996;87(6): 959–63.
38. Moore A, Umstad MP, Stewart M, et al. Prognosis of congenital diaphragmatic hernia. Aust N Z J Obstet Gynaecol. 1998;38(1):16–21.
39. Vanamo K, Rintala RJ, Lindahl H, et al. Long-term gastrointestinal morbidity in patients with congenital diaphragmatic defects. J Pediatr Surg. 1996;31(4): 551–4.
40. Peetsold MG, Kneepkens CM, Heij HA, et al. Congenital diaphragmatic hernia: long-term risk of gastroesophageal reflux disease. J Pediatr Gastroenterol Nutr. 2010;51(4):448–53.
41. Kieffer J, Sapin E, Berg A, et al. Gastroesophageal reflux after repair of congenital diaphragmatic hernia. J Pediatr Surg. 1995;30(9):1330–3.
42. Arena F, Romeo C, Baldari S, et al. Gastrointestinal sequelae in survivors of congenital diaphragmatic hernia. Pediatr Int. 2008;50(1):76–80.
43. Kilby MD. The incidence of gastroschisis. BMJ. 2006;332(7536):250–1.
44. Ledbetter DJ. Gastroschisis and omphalocele. Surg Clin North Am. 2006;86(2):249–60. vii.
45. Vermeij-Keers C, Hartwig NG, van der Werff JF. Embryonic development of the ventral body wall and its congenital malformations. Semin Pediatr Surg. 1996;5(2):82–9.
46. Hoyme HE, Higginbottom MC, Jones KL. The vascular pathogenesis of gastroschisis: intrauterine interruption of the omphalomesenteric artery. J Pediatr. 1981;98(2):228–31.
47. Phillips JD, Raval MV, Redden C, et al. Gastroschisis, atresia, dysmotility: surgical treatment strategies for a distinct clinical entity. J Pediatr Surg. 2008;43(12): 2208–12.
48. Snyder CL, Miller KA, Sharp RJ, et al. Management of intestinal atresia in patients with gastroschisis. J Pediatr Surg. 2001;36(10):1542–5.
49. Hoehner JC, Ein SH, Kim PC. Management of gastroschisis with concomitant jejuno-ileal atresia. J Pediatr Surg. 1998;33(6):885–8.
50. Kato T, Tzakis AG, Selvaggi G, et al. Intestinal and multivisceral transplantation in children. Ann Surg. 2006;243(6):756–64.
51. Durkin ET, Lund DP, Shaaban AF, et al. Age-related differences in diagnosis and morbidity of intestinal malrotation. J Am Coll Surg. 2008;206(4):658–63.
52. Penco JM, Murillo JC, Hernandez A, et al. Anomalies of intestinal rotation and fixation: consequences of late diagnosis beyond two years of age. Pediatr Surg Int. 2007;23(8):723–30.
53. Devane SP, Coombes R, Smith VV, et al. Persistent gastrointestinal symptoms after correction of malrotation. Arch Dis Child. 1992;67(2):218–21.

54. la Vecchia LK, Grosfeld JL, West KW, et al. Intestinal atresia and stenosis: a 25-year experience with 277 cases. Arch Surg. 1998;133(5):490–6.
55. Cezard JP, Aigrain Y, Sonsino E, et al. Postobstructive enteropathy in infants with transient enterostomy: its consequences on the upper small intestinal functions. J Pediatr Surg. 1992;27(11):1427–32.
56. Cezard JP, Cargill G, Faure C, et al. Duodenal manometry in postobstructive enteropathy in infants with a transient enterostomy. J Pediatr Surg. 1993;28(11):1481–5.
57. Preston DM, Hawley PR, Lennard-Jones JE, et al. Results of colectomy for severe idiopathic constipation in women (Arbuthnot Lane's disease). Br J Surg. 1984;71(7):547–52.
58. Pikarsky AJ, Singh JJ, Weiss EG, et al. Long-term follow-up of patients undergoing colectomy for colonic inertia. Dis Colon Rectum. 2001;44(2): 179–83.
59. Kayama H, Koh K. Clinical and experimental studies on gastrointestinal motility following total colectomy: direct measurement (strain gauge force transducer method, barium method) and indirect measurement (hydrogen breath test, acetaminophen method). J Smooth Muscle Res. 1991;27(2):97–114.
60. You YT, Wang JY, Changchien CR, et al. Segmental colectomy in the management of colonic inertia. Am Surg. 1998;64(8):775–7.
61. Lundin E, Karlbom U, Pahlman L, et al. Outcome of segmental colonic resection for slow-transit constipation. Br J Surg. 2002;89(10):1270–4.
62. Villarreal J, Sood M, Zangen T, et al. Colonic diversion for intractable constipation in children: colonic manometry helps guide clinical decisions. J Pediatr Gastroenterol Nutr. 2001;33(5):588–91.
63. Martin MJ, Steele SR, Mullenix PS, et al. A pilot study using total colonic manometry in the surgical evaluation of pediatric functional colonic obstruction. J Pediatr Surg. 2004;39(3):352–9.
64. Martin MJ, Steele SR, Noel JM, et al. Total colonic manometry as a guide for surgical management of functional colonic obstruction: preliminary results. J Pediatr Surg. 2001;36(12):1757–63.

28 Gastric Function After Fundoplication

Samuel Nurko

Fundoplication is one of the most common operations performed in children [1–3]. It is a very successful operation to control gastroesophageal reflux, but it can be associated with significant postoperative symptoms that may limit its effectiveness [1, 2, 4].

Effect on Gastric Sensorimotor Function

Fundoplication reduces the volume of the stomach and uses most of the proximal stomach to create a wrap around the lower part of the esophagus [2, 3]. This can have a major impact on gastric function and may explain some of the postoperative symptoms that may develop [5]. There have been a few studies that have evaluated gastric accommodation, sensation, and emptying in children and adults after fundoplication. Mousa et al. [3] studied gastric compliance and gastric sensory function before and after Nissen fundoplication in children. They performed barostat studies in 13 children before surgery and repeated the test after surgery in 8. After fundoplication the patients had significantly higher minimal distending pressure values, reduced gastric compliance, and significantly higher pain scores. It can be hypothesized that the lower gastric compliance leads to stimulation of visceral efferents and heightened perception. Zangen et al. [6] showed that in 12/14 children there was a decrease in gastric volume capacity that produced retching.

Similar findings of abnormal gastric accommodation have been reported in adults. In a case controlled study, proximal gastric function was studied with the use of barostat in 12 adult patients that underwent fundoplication and compared with 12 controls [7]. It was found that there was no difference between groups in compliance during fasting. However, the adaptive relaxation in the fundoplication group was significantly less than that in controls after ingestion of a liquid meal [7]. The authors also showed that the fundal wrap is still functional and able to accommodate to pressure increments, that the stomach relaxation after a meal occurs normally, but that there was a decrease in receptive relaxation in the patients with fundoplication. Similar findings related to accommodation were reported by Vu et al. [8] who studied with a barostat 12 adult patients before and after Nissen fundoplication and compared the results with the findings on 12 healthy adults and 12 adults with GERD without surgery. The sensation of fullness was increased in the postoperative patients. Again, post-Nissen patients had normal compliance, but reduced postprandial gastric accommodation and accelerated gastric emptying.

S. Nurko, M.D., M.P.H. (✉)
Center for Motility and Functional Gastrointestinal Disorders, Children's Hospital Boston,
300 Longwood Ave, Boston, MA 02155, USA
e-mail: samuel.nurko@childrens.harvard.edu

C. Faure et al. (eds.), *Pediatric Neurogastroenterology: Gastrointestinal Motility and Functional Disorders in Children*, Clinical Gastroenterology,
DOI 10.1007/978-1-60761-709-9_28, © Springer Science+Business Media New York 2013

Other less invasive methods that indirectly assess gastric function have also been used to study gastric function after surgery. By using single-photon emission computed tomography with three-dimensional analysis, Bouras et al. [9] showed that patients post fundoplication had a postprandial/fasting gastric volume ratio that was lower than in healthy controls, again suggesting impaired gastric accommodation. By using the water load test, Remes-Troche et al. [10] found that patients with dyspeptic symptoms after fundoplication had a significantly lower drinking capacity and higher symptom scores than controls with values similar to those of patients with functional dyspepsia. They suggested that, as in functional dyspepsia, severe dyspeptic symptoms after fundoplication are associated with an impaired drinking capacity, reflecting visceral hypersensitivity or impaired gastric accommodation or both. Visceral hypersensitivity has been associated with abnormal gastric accommodation and hyperalgesia, and contributing factors to this hypersensitivity are likely to be wall tension and the function of visceral afferents [11].

The exact mechanism by which these changes in accommodation occur is not clear. There may be alterations in the proximal gastric wall function or the abnormalities may be secondary to vagal dysfunction or to the mechanical effects of the fundoplication per se [3, 5, 12]. The proximal gastric wall seems to function normally as gastric compliance and tone have been found to be normal [7, 8]. It is then possible that the surgical manipulation itself could impair autonomic pathways affecting the gastric sensorimotor function and that changes in postprandial relaxation after reflux surgery could result from alterations in neurohormonal control [5, 12]. Vagal nerve function after fundoplication has been evaluated by using different methods. By using sham-feeding-stimulated pancreatic polypeptide (PP) test before and after surgery, Devault et al. [12] showed that 5/12 with normal testing before the surgery had developed evidence of vagal dysfunction after surgery. Interestingly, there was no correlation between PP tests and the development or worsening of symptoms after surgery. In another study that evaluated vagal function by measuring PP serum changes to insulin-induced hypoglycemia, Vu et al. found that 11 of their 12 patients had a normal response [8]. Thus, it appears that the reduced gastric accommodation is probably mechanical in origin [7, 8].

Effects on Gastric Emptying

Patients with GERD frequently have delayed gastric emptying [8]. It has been reported that fundoplication may accelerate gastric emptying for both solids and liquids [7, 8, 13, 14]. Faster gastric emptying after a fundoplication is attributed to the loss of accommodation in the stomach, thereby preventing the fundus from expanding to hold the liquid portion of the meal [15]. An acceleration of gastric emptying after surgery in children has not been consistently found. Mousa et al. [3] found no significant change in emptying for both solids and liquids after surgery, although most patients had normal emptying before the surgery.

A fast gastric emptying after surgery can produce postoperative symptoms [2, 4, 12]. Diarrhea which can occur in up to 18 % of patients [12] has been correlated with rapid gastric emptying. An exaggerated fast gastric emptying for liquids may produce dumping syndrome [2, 4, 12]. Even though this occurrence is more frequent when a pyloroplasty has been performed, it has been shown to occur also in children and adults in whom no pyloroplasty was done. The pathophysiology of dumping syndrome in children is multifactorial, although its incidence and its severity appear to be proportional to the rate of emptying [16]. Fonkalsrud et al. [1] described a postoperative transient dumping syndrome in 0.9 % out of 7,467 fundoplications (0–5 %), and in a prospective study of 50 pediatric patients, Samuk et al. [17] diagnosed dumping syndrome in 30 %.

Effects on Antroduodenal Motility and Gastric Myoelectrical Activity

The effect of fundoplication on antroduodenal motility has not been clearly established. No prospective studies measuring antroduodenal motility before and after fundoplication have been reported, but studies of children and adults with postoperative problems have shown abnormal antroduodenal motility [5, 6, 18]. In one study it was shown that 25 of 28 symptomatic children after fundoplication had abnormalities. The most common abnormality found was an absence of the migrating motor complex in 12, while six had postprandial hypomotility; other nonspecific abnormalities included clustered, retrograde, and tonic contractions [18]. Similar motility abnormalities have been described in adults [5].

In another study of 14 patients with food refusal after fundoplication, an abnormal antroduodenal manometry was described in nine patients, suggesting that abnormal motility after surgery does not occur in all patients with symptoms. It is unclear if the abnormalities were present before the operation or are a result of it. Given that the abnormalities found were similar to those seen in chronic intestinal pseudo-obstruction and that not all children with postoperative symptoms have motility dysfunction, it is likely that the abnormalities predated the operation, suggesting that those children had a more generalized gastrointestinal dysfunction, and not only gastroesophageal reflux. The presence of preoperative gastric myoelectrical dysfunction has also been reported. Richards et al. measured gastric myoelectrical activity before and after fundoplication with the use of surface electrogastrography in 27 children (17 neurologically impaired and 10 neurologically normal) [19]. They found abnormal gastric electrical activity before surgery in 65 % of the neurologically impaired as compared with 20 % of the neurologically normal group. After surgery an abnormal myoelectrical activity developed in six (three in each group).

Relation of Postoperative Symptoms to Gastric Dysfunction

It has been reported that up to a third of patients develop symptoms after fundoplication [3]. Symptoms commonly seen after antireflux surgery include dysphagia, inability to belch, early satiety, bloating, dyspepsia, gas-bloat syndrome, retching, pain, feeding refusal, and diarrhea [2, 4, 6, 12]. Dysphagia can often be corrected with esophageal dilation and occasionally repeated surgery [4]. Inability to belch is an expected outcome after fundoplication and most patients learn to compensate for this symptom [4]. The development of retching, gas-bloat syndrome, early satiety, diarrhea, pain, and feeding refusal is more difficult to explain [4, 10, 20] and is probably related to the effects that the fundoplication has on the sensorimotor gastric function.

There are other factors that may predispose patients to have symptoms. The presence of a fundoplication, which both strengthens the lower esophageal sphincter and decreases transient lower esophageal sphincter relaxations [21], may prevent venting of gas from the proximal stomach and cause increased abdominal distention, particularly in patients with gastroesophageal reflux who are known to swallow large volumes of air routinely [12]. Richards et al. found that children, in whom gastric myoelectrical activity had deteriorated after surgery, developed retching postoperatively [19], and concluded that Nissen fundoplication may be followed by a progression of gastric dysrhythmias that may be associated with retching [19]. In children, another prominent symptom after fundoplication can be food refusal which can be secondary not only to gastric dysfunction but also be related to pain and behavioral issues [6].

Given that the symptoms can originate from a variety of underlying problems, it is important to clarify the pathophysiology of the symptoms in each patient [6]. Ideally, treatment has to be tailored accordingly, and a multidisciplinary team may be necessary [6]. Drugs that increase gastric accommodation may be beneficial. Given that $5HT_1$ receptors are involved in gastric accommodation, agonists such as cyproheptadine, sumatriptan, and buspirone may be used [2, 6, 10]. Prokinetics may be beneficial in those children with evidence of delayed gastric emptying. Erythromycin has been used for this purpose but it can cause increased pain and nausea [2]. Other prokinetics, like metoclopramide, cisapride, and domperidone, have limited use given their side effect profile and lack of availability in most parts of the world [2, 4, 6]. Injection of botulinum toxin into the pylorus may relieve some of the gas-bloat symptoms. Smaller meals, anticholinergics and pain modulators (like low-dose antidepressants or gabapentin), and behavioral techniques are often used [2, 6]. When symptoms related to food ingestion are particularly severe, it may be necessary to use jejunal feedings [6].

Summary and Conclusions

Fundoplication has an impact on gastric sensorimotor function. It reduces the volume of the stomach and uses most of the proximal stomach to create a wrap around the lower part of the esophagus. Studies consistently show that fundoplication accelerates the rate of gastric emptying, decreases gastric accommodation, changes distribution of intragastric food with the ingested material reaching and distending the distal stomach earlier than physiologically expected, and may produce visceral hypersensitivity. Postoperative symptoms that may be attributed to gastric sensorimotor dysfunction after surgery include inability to belch, early satiety, bloating, dyspepsia, gas-bloat syndrome, retching, pain, feeding refusal, diarrhea, and dumping. Given that the symptoms can originate from a variety of underlying problems, it is important to clarify the pathophysiology of the symptoms in each patient in order to be able to tailor therapy accordingly.

Acknowledgement Supported by grant NIH K24DK082792A.

References

1. Fonkalsrud EW, Ashcraft KW, Coran AG, Ellis DG, Grosfeld JL, Tunell WP, et al. Surgical treatment of gastroesophageal reflux in children: a combined hospital study of 7467 patients. [comment]. Pediatrics. 1998;101(3 (Pt 1)):419–22.
2. Di Lorenzo C, Orenstein S. Fundoplication: friend or foe? J Pediatr Gastroenterol Nutr. 2002;34:117–24.
3. Mousa H, Caniano DA, Alhajj M, Gibson L, Di Lorenzo C, Binkowitz L. Effect of Nissen fundoplication on gastric motor and sensory functions. J Pediatr Gastroenterol Nutr. 2006;43(2):185–9.
4. Nurko SS. Complications after gastrointestinal surgery. A medical perspective. In: Walker WA et al., editors. Pediatric gastrointestinal disease. 3rd ed. Philadelphia: B.C. Decker Inc.; 2004. p. 2111–38.
5. Stanghellini V, Malagelada JR. Gastric manometric abnormalities in patients with dyspeptic symptoms after fundoplication. Gut. 1983;24(9):790–7.
6. Zangen T, Ciarla C, Zangen S, Di Lorenzo C, Flores AF, Cocjin J, et al. Gastrointestinal motility and sensory abnormalities may contribute to food refusal in medically fragile toddlers. J Pediatr Gastroenterol Nutr. 2003;37(3):287–93.
7. Wijnhoven BP, Salet GA, Roelofs JM, Smout AJ, Akkermans LM, Gooszen HG. Function of the proximal stomach after Nissen fundoplication. Br J Surg. 1998;85(2):267–71.
8. Vu MK, Ringers J, Arndt JW, et al. Prospective study of the effect of laparoscopic hemifundoplication on motor and sensory function of the proximal stomach. Br J Surg. 2000;87:338–43.
9. Bouras EP, Delgado-Aros S, Camilleri M, Castillo EJ, Burton DD, Thomforde GM, et al. SPECT imaging of the stomach: comparison with barostat, and effects of sex, age, body mass index, and fundoplication. Single photon emission computed tomography. Gut. 2002; 51(6):781–6.
10. Remes-Troche JM, Montano-Loza A, Martinez JC, Herrera M, Valdovinos-Diaz MA. Drinking capacity and severity of dyspeptic symptoms during a water load test after Nissen fundoplication. Dig Dis Sci. 2007;52(10):2850–7.
11. Mertz H, Fullerton S, Naliboff B, Mayer EA. Symptoms and visceral perception in severe functional and organic dyspepsia. Gut. 1998;42(6):814–22.
12. DeVault KR, Swain JM, Wentling GK, Floch NR, Achem SR, Hinder RA. Evaluation of vagus nerve function before and after antireflux surgery. J Gastrointest Surg. 2004;8(7):883–8. discussion 8–9.
13. Lindeboom MY, Ringers J, van Rijn PJ, Neijenhuis P, Stokkel MP, Masclee AA. Gastric emptying and vagus nerve function after laparoscopic partial fundoplication. Ann Surg. 2004;240(5):785–90.
14. Farrell TM, Richardson WS, Halkar R, Lyon CP, Galloway KD, Waring JP, et al. Nissen fundoplication improves gastric motility in patients with delayed gastric emptying. Surg Endosc. 2001; 15(3):271–4.
15. Hinder RA, Stein HJ, Bremner CG, DeMeester TR. Relationship of a satisfactory outcome to normalization of delayed gastric emptying after Nissen fundoplication. Ann Surg. 1989;210(4):458–64. discussion 64–5.
16. Borovoy J, Furuta L, Nurko S. Benefit of uncooked corn starch in the management of children with dumping syndrome fed exclusively by gastrostomy. Am J Gastroenterol. 1998;93:814–8.
17. Samuk I, Afriat R, Horne T, Bistritzer T, Barr J, Vinograd I. Dumping syndrome following Nissen

fundoplication, diagnosis, and treatment. J Pediatr Gastroenterol Nutr. 1996;23(3):235–40.
18. DiLorenzo C, Flores A, Hyman PE. Intestinal motility in symptomatic children with fundoplication. J Pediatr Gastroenterol Nutr. 1991;12:169–73.
19. Richards CA, Andrews PL, Spitz L, Milla PJ. Nissen fundoplication may induce gastric myoelectrical disturbance in children. J Pediatr Surg. 1998; 33(12):1801–5.
20. Klaus A, Hinder RA, DeVault KR, Achem SR. Bowel dysfunction after laparoscopic antireflux surgery: incidence, severity, and clinical course. Am J Med. 2003;114(1):6–9.
21. Scheffer RC, Tatum RP, Shi G, Akkermans LM, Joehl RJ, Kahrilas PJ. Reduced tLESR elicitation in response to gastric distension in fundoplication patients. Am J Physiol Gastrointest Liver Physiol. 2003;284(5):G815–20.

Part V

Functional Gastrointestinal Disorders

29 History and Definition of the Rome Criteria

Andrée Rasquin

The history of the Rome criteria began in 1987, when Professor Aldo Torsoli proposed the use of a consensus process to define various gastrointestinal disturbances that appeared to cluster together with significant prevalence, constituting disorders. Because of the lack of reproducible anatomical or biochemical abnormalities, these complaints were considered to be of functional origin. Among them, irritable bowel syndrome (IBS) was a good example. A working team of international experts in gastroenterology was formed and its members decided to use the so-called Delphic approach, which promotes the reaching of a consensus for questions not easily addressed [1]. They applied this method to clarify gastrointestinal conditions that were not easily resolved by scientific research or literature review. It took 2–3 years for the entire consensus process to be completed. Five committees were each given a topic based on anatomical region: esophageal, gastroduodenal, intestinal, biliary, and anorectal. Within each committee, members were invited to apply their own experience and knowledge of the literature to define criteria, and their reports were subsequently merged to form a final document. Thus the Rome I symptom-based diagnostic criteria for functional gastrointestinal disorders (FGIDs) in adult patients were born and published in 1991 [2, 3]. This arduous process improved the understanding of FGIDs tremendously. It introduced clarity and consistency in deriving clinical diagnoses, which could now be made positively according to the criteria. By selecting homogenous groups of patients, it became possible to make comparisons between different treatment approaches to the often complex factors compounding the disorders. Moreover, it definitively encouraged research on pathophysiology.

In 1993, I was faced with the decision of where to spend a sabbatical year. Having spent the previous 8 years working with a multidisciplinary team to build the pediatric liver transplant program for the province of Quebec, I was convinced of the deep and effective human value that a biopsychosocial approach could bring to children with chronic disease and to their families. Despite the physical and emotional suffering that accompanied the journey through a liver transplant, children and their families were coming out of the experience with a deeper understanding and appreciation of themselves and their lives. I decided to apply the same biopsychosocial model to a group of children that we, as pediatric gastroenterologists, had been poorly prepared to treat, i.e., children with FGIDs. We were still conducting endoscopies that indeed revealed negative results and were sending these families home saying that nothing was found. After investigating different centers where I could be trained, I chose the gastroenterology unit at the University

A. Rasquin, M.D. (✉)
Division of Gastroenterology, Pediatrics Department, Chu Ste Justine, University of Montreal, 3175 Cote Ste Catherine, Montreal, QC, Canada H3T-1C5
e-mail: augustineras@videotron.ca

C. Faure et al. (eds.), *Pediatric Neurogastroenterology: Gastrointestinal Motility and Functional Disorders in Children*, Clinical Gastroenterology,
DOI 10.1007/978-1-60761-709-9_29, © Springer Science+Business Media New York 2013

of North Carolina, where Douglas Drossman had been using the biopsychosocial approach with adult patients with FGIDs. I felt that this setting would be the most appropriate place, despite the fact that I had not approached an adult patient for the last 25 years!

My experience at UNC in 1994–1995 provided me with new insight into the medical approach to FGIDs. Observing Douglas Drossman interviewing and listening to his patients was a deeply human experience, and I learned from him how to never let them feel that they had "nothing." The trust and confidence that he established was remarkable in that his patients finally felt that a doctor cared and would accompany them. This was the beginning of a healing journey for them, despite the fact that a cure was never promised [4].

Synchronicities do occur! In 1995, the revision of the Rome I symptom-based diagnostic criteria for adult FGIDs was in progress. During my stay in North Carolina, it soon became obvious that the rationale for symptom-based criteria applied equally to pediatric patients and that the participation of pediatric gastroenterologists to the Rome process could make an important contribution to the approach for children with FGIDs.

Thanks to Douglas Drossman and Enrico Corazziari, we were allowed to form an international pediatric working team. It was composed of Paul E. Hyman, Jeffrey S. Hyams, David R. Fleisher, Peter J. Milla, Annamaria Staiano, Salvatore Cucchiara, and myself. Each member produced a document that was incorporated into a manuscript. In 1996, the team met in Rome for 3 days to reach a consensus. The final version of the document was sent to six independent international experts before the final consensus report on the criteria for pediatric functional gastrointestinal disorders was presented to the adult group. They were published in 1999 and 2000 as part of the Rome II criteria [5, 6]. In this publication on the revised Rome criteria for adult patients, other chapters addressed newly developing topics, such as gut motility and sensitivity, brain/gut interaction, psychosocial aspects of FGIDs, recommendations for clinical trials and designs, and questionnaires.

The work of the pediatric working team was original in that for the first time, it proposed a classification system and symptom-based diagnostic criteria for all the gastrointestinal syndromes considered to be functional in children. It also reviewed diagnostic guidelines and treatment approaches. The effort was well received by the scientific community; to date, the publication has been cited nearly 500 times in the medical literature. The contact and sharing of experience among different working groups within the Rome structure was inspiring and proved to be a great asset to the pediatric team. It helped place the pediatric disorders within a larger perspective and reaffirmed the belief that early life experiences can have important consequences in adulthood [7]. The team decided to classify the pediatric disorders according to symptoms rather than anatomical regions. The disorders were grouped according to the following presenting symptoms: vomiting, abdominal pain, diarrhea, and defecation complaints. The team tried to take different development stages of childhood into account. Indeed, some digestive symptoms, such as regurgitation, may accompany normal development in an infant, but not at later stages of development. Some symptoms could be indicative of maladaptive behavior, as in the case of a child with retentive fecal soiling. Age limits were defined for certain syndromes, such as IBS and dyspepsia, recognizing that after a certain age, the child can be a reliable self-reporter of symptoms. Particular emphasis was put on the child's psychosocial context; it was recognized that the decision to report symptoms generally lies with parents and that their own private issues and fears can influence their children's symptom presentation.

This effort at classification was a first attempt and, obviously, far from perfect. There were little evidence-based data available, obliging team members to rely mainly on their experience. Furthermore, at that time, the team was limited to six members, whose task was to define all functional disorders, and it excluded the participation of several excellent experts in each domain. The team was neither multinational nor multidisciplinary and did not include infantile neurophysiologists and pediatric psychologists. However,

Table 29.1 Pediatric functional gastrointestinal disorders

(A) Neonates and toddlers	
Infant regurgitation	Functional diarrhea
Infant rumination syndrome	Infant dyschezia
Cyclic vomiting syndrome	Functional constipation
Infant colic	
(B) Children and adolescents	
Vomiting and aerophagia	Abdominal pain-related FGIDs
Adolescent rumination syndrome	Functional dyspepsia
Cyclic vomiting syndrome	Irritable bowel syndrome
Aerophagia	Abdominal migraine
Constipation and incontinence	Childhood functional abdominal pain
Functional constipation	Childhood functional abdominal pain syndrome
Nonretentive fecal incontinence	

the team felt that it was a good starting point and that the advantages of being part of the Rome process far exceeded its drawbacks.

Studies supporting the validity of the pediatric criteria were published as early as 2001 [8, 9]. However, since the criteria were defined by consensus, validation studies were needed to confirm that the disorders did indeed exist in the patient population. The preliminary steps consisted of establishing a questionnaire based on the disorders and validating its use among adolescents with digestive complaints and their parents. This validation was performed and published in 2005 [10, 11]. The development and validation of the questionnaire promoted further research, facilitated clinical trials, and helped in the subsequent revision of the pediatric criteria.

The Rome III pediatric criteria were published in 2006 (Table 29.1) [12, 13]. For this task, two pediatric working teams, consisting of six members each, were created. It was decided to divide pediatric FGIDs into two groups, according to the developmental stage of their occurrence: (1) neonates and toddlers and (2) children and adolescents. This time, experts from yet other countries participated and a pediatric psychologist was included. This work led to another 540 citations in the medical literature during the following years. The use of the Rome III criteria has been encouraged and the biopsychosocial approach has been highly recommended [14]. The Rome III criteria were shown to be more inclusive for children with abdominal pain-related FGIDs, but further refinement is still required, since inter-rater reliability among pediatric gastroenterologists remains only fair to moderate [15, 16]. The criteria have helped in the design of multicenter clinical trials and research on pathophysiology [17–21]. However, pediatric studies remain very modest in comparison to the recent dramatic research advances in neuroscience [22].

The number of publications using the pediatric Rome III criteria has been growing more recently in various countries and continents. This should permit comparisons between children from different cultural origins in the future, an exploration that has already been promoted in the document of the Rome III criteria [12]. Along with sections on pharmacology and pharmacokinetics of medications for FGIDs, a new chapter appeared concerning the respective influences of gender, age, society, and culture on symptom presentation and clinical approaches. This topic in particular was recently examined at our university in collaboration between the Departments of Pediatrics and Anthropology and is reported upon in another chapter of this book. Suffice to say that the study of cultural aspects of abdominal pain-related FGIDs was very interesting. It certainly helped me realize the extent to which my own interviews were devoid of cultural inquiry.

Using the Rome criteria and a biopsychosocial approach will undoubtedly help physicians caring for children. Recently, I have become deeply concerned by the increasing level of diffuse anxiety in children in general and in those with FGIDs in particular. Children are increasingly aware of global violence, threats, and catastrophes, and many experience these events through different forms of media. Children's involvement in saving the planet is regularly addressed at school, and their concerns and anxieties are growing. I am convinced that physicians must address this issue as well as better understand how cultural origins influence children's and families' ways of coping.

Advances in neurogastroenterology, which explore the brain/gut axis and the transfer of information through the autonomic, neuroendocrine, and immune systems, have brought new knowledge about the influence of psychosocial factors on physical symptoms [23, 24]. More recently, features of IBS occurring after an infectious episode have been shown in some patients to overlap with those of inflammatory bowel diseases. With these advances, the frontiers between organic and functional are becoming thinner, challenging our present dualistic view [25]. How long the Rome criteria will remain a useful clinical tool before FGIDs become "organic" is indeed a challenging question. Meanwhile, I remain convinced that these criteria constitute a valuable tool for both research and clinical approaches to FGIDs in children and that their use should be promoted among physicians [26].

References

1. Milholland AV, Wheeler SG, Heieck JJ. Medical assessment by a Delphi group opinion technic. N Engl J Med. 1973;288:1272–5.
2. Thompson WG. The road to rome. Gastroenterology. 2006;130:1552-6.
3. Drossman DA, Richter JE, Talley NJ, et al. The functional gastrointestinal disorders: diagnosis, pathophysiology and treatment: a multinational consensus. Boston; 1994. 370 p.
4. Wong RK, Tan JS, Drossman DA. Here's my phone number, don't call me: physician accessibility in the cell phone and e-mail era. Dig Dis Sci. 2010;55:662–7.
5. Rasquin-Weber A, Hyman PE, Cucchiara S, et al. Childhood functional gastrointestinal disorders. Gut. 1999;45 Suppl 2:II60–8.
6. Hyman PE, Rasquin-Weber A, Fleisher D, et al. Childhood functional gastrointestinal disorders. In: Drossman D, editor. The functional gastrointestinal disorders. McLean, VA: Degnon Associates; 2000. p. 533–75.
7. Milla PJ. Irritable bowel syndrome in childhood. Gastroenterology. 2001;120:287–90.
8. Van Ginkel R, Voskuijl WP, Benninga MA, et al. Alterations in rectal sensitivity and motility in childhood irritable bowel syndrome. Gastroenterology. 2001;120:31–8.
9. Di Lorenzo C, Youssef NN, Sigurdsson L, et al. Visceral hyperalgesia in children with functional abdominal pain. J Pediatr. 2001;139:838–43.
10. Caplan A, Walker L, Rasquin A. Development and preliminary validation of the questionnaire on pediatric gastrointestinal symptoms to assess functional gastrointestinal disorders in children and adolescents. J Pediatr Gastroenterol Nutr. 2005;41:296–304.
11. Caplan A, Walker L, Rasquin A. Validation of the pediatric Rome II criteria for functional gastrointestinal disorders using the questionnaire on pediatric gastrointestinal symptoms. J Pediatr Gastroenterol Nutr. 2005;41:305–16.
12. Di Lorenzo C, Rasquin A, Forbes D, et al. Childhood functional gastrointestinal disorders: child/adolescent. In: Drossman A, editor. The functional gastrointestinal disorders. Durham, NC: BW&A Books Inc.; 2006. p. 723–7.
13. Rasquin A, Di Lorenzo C, Forbes D, et al. Childhood functional gastrointestinal disorders: child/adolescent. Gastroenterology. 2006;130:1527–37.
14. Hyman PE. Will the Rome criteria help pediatrics? J Pediatr Gastroenterol Nutr. 2008;47:700–3.
15. Baber KF, Anderson J, Puzanovova M, et al. Rome II versus Rome III classification of functional gastrointestinal disorders in pediatric chronic abdominal pain. J Pediatr Gastroenterol Nutr. 2008;47:299–302.
16. Chogle A, Dhroove G, Sztainberg M, et al. How reliable are the Rome III criteria for the assessment of functional gastrointestinal disorders in children? Am J Gastroenterol. 2010;105:2697–701.
17. Saps M, Youssef N, Miranda A, et al. Multicenter, randomized, placebo-controlled trial of amitriptyline in children with functional gastrointestinal disorders. Gastroenterology. 2009;137:1261–9.
18. Saps M, Pensabene L, Turco R, et al. Rotavirus gastroenteritis: precursor of functional gastrointestinal disorders? J Pediatr Gastroenterol Nutr. 2009;49:580–3.
19. Saps M, Pensabene L, Di Martino L, et al. Post-infectious functional gastrointestinal disorders in children. J Pediatr. 2008;152:812–6.
20. Halac U, Noble A, Faure C. Rectal sensory threshold for pain is a diagnostic marker of irritable bowel syndrome and functional abdominal pain in children. J Pediatr. 2010;156:60–5.
21. Shulman RJ, Eakin MN, Czyzewski DI, et al. Increased gastrointestinal permeability and gut inflammation in children with functional abdominal pain and irritable bowel syndrome. J Pediatr. 2008;153:646–50.

22. Youssef NN, Di Lorenzo C. Pediatric gastrointestinal motility—future directions and challenges. Dig Dis. 2006;24:308–12.
23. Lane RD, Waldstein SR, Chesney MA, et al. The rebirth of neuroscience in psychosomatic medicine. Part I: Historical context, methods, and relevant basic science. Psychosom Med. 2009;71:117–34.
24. Lane RD, Waldstein SR, Critchley HD, et al. The rebirth of neuroscience in psychosomatic medicine. Part II: Clinical applications and implications for research. Psychosom Med. 2009;71:135–51.
25. Grover M, Herfarth H, Drossman DA. The functional-organic dichotomy: postinfectious irritable bowel syndrome and inflammatory bowel disease-irritable bowel syndrome. Clin Gastroenterol Hepatol. 2009;7:48–53.
26. Hyman PE, Monagas J. Rectal perceptual hypersensitivity: a biomarker for pediatric irritable bowel syndrome. J Pediatr. 2010;156:5–7.

Infant Regurgitation and Pediatric Gastroesophageal Reflux Disease

30

Yvan Vandenplas, Bruno Hauser, Thierry Devreker, and Silvia Salvatore

Definitions

Determination of the exact prevalence of gastroesophageal reflux (GER) and GER disease (GERD) at any age is virtually impossible for many reasons: most reflux episodes are asymptomatic, symptoms and signs are nonspecific, and self-treatment is common. "Physiologic GER" is GER associated with absence of symptoms, or during the first months of life accompanied with regurgitation, and occasionally with vomiting. Regurgitation, spitting up, possetting, and spilling are synonyms and are defined as the passage of refluxed gastric contents into the pharynx and sometimes expelled out of the mouth [1]. Regurgitation is distinguished from vomiting by the absence of a central nervous system emetic reflex, retrograde upper intestinal contractions, nausea, and retching. Vomiting is defined as expulsion with force of the refluxed gastric contents from the mouth [2, 3]. Vomiting associated with reflux is likely the result of the stimulation of pharyngeal sensory afferents by refluxed gastric contents. Rumination is the consequence of a contraction of the abdominal muscles resulting in the habitual regurgitation of recently ingested food that is subsequently spitted up or reswallowed.

GERD is a spectrum of a disease that can best be defined as manifestations causing esophageal or extraesophageal troublesome symptoms or esophageal or adjacent organ injury secondary to the reflux of gastric contents into the esophagus or, beyond, into the oral cavity or airways. To be defined as GERD, reflux symptoms must be troublesome to the infant, child, or adolescent and not simply troublesome for the caregiver [4]. Environmental and genetic factors are indentified as predisposing factors [2].

Transient lower esophageal sphincter relaxations (TLESRs) are the most frequent and important pathophysiologic mechanism causing GER at any age, from prematurity into adulthood [5, 6]. More information on pathophysiology can be found elsewhere [5].

Symptoms of GERD

While reflux occurs physiologically at all ages, there is also at all ages a continuum between physiologic GER and GERD [2]. Less than 10%

Y. Vandenplas, M.D., Ph.D. (✉)
Pediatrics, Universitair Ziekenhuis Brussel, Laarbeeklaan 101, 1090, Brussels, Belgium
e-mail: yvan.vandenplas@uzbrussel.be

B. Hauser, M.D.
Paediatrics Department, Paediatric Gastroenterology Hepatology and Nutrition Division, Universitair Kinderziekenhuis Brussel, Brussels, Belgium

T. Devreker, M.D.
Pediatric Gastroenterology Department, Universitair Kinderziekenhuis Brussel, Brussels, Belgium

S. Salvatore, M.D.
Pediatric Department, University of Insubria, Ospedale "F. Del Ponte", Varese, Italy

C. Faure et al. (eds.), *Pediatric Neurogastroenterology: Gastrointestinal Motility and Functional Disorders in Children*, Clinical Gastroenterology,
DOI 10.1007/978-1-60761-709-9_30, © Springer Science+Business Media New York 2013

Table 30.1 Symptoms and signs that may be associated with gastroesophageal reflux

Symptoms
Recurrent regurgitation with/without vomiting
Weight loss or poor weight gain
Irritability in infants
Ruminative behavior
Heartburn or chest pain
Hematemesis
Dysphagia, odynophagia
Wheezing
Stridor
Cough
Hoarseness
Signs
Esophagitis
Esophageal stricture
Barrett's esophagus
Laryngeal/pharyngeal inflammation
Recurrent pneumonia
Anemia
Dental erosion
Feeding refusal
Dystonic neck posturing (Sandifer syndrome)
Apnea spells

Apparent life-threatening events (ALTE). Adapted from Vandenplas, Rudolph CD, Di Lorenzo C, Hassall E., et al. Pediatric gastroesophageal reflux clinical practice guidelines; joint recommendations of the North American Society for Pediatric Gastroenterology, Hepatology, and Nutrition (NASPGHAN) and the European Society Pediatric Gastroenterology, Hepatology, and Nutrition (ESPGHAN). J Pediatr Gastroneterol Nutr 2009;49(4):498–547

of infants and children have (acid and troublesome) GERD [7]. The presenting symptoms of GERD differ according to age. Possible associations exist between GERD and hiccups, chronic cough, chest pain, hoarseness, recurrent otitis media, asthma, pneumonia, bronchiectasis, apparent life-threatening events (ALTE), laryngotracheitis, sinusitis, and dental erosions (Table 30.1), but causality or temporal association has not been established for many of these signs and symptoms [8].

Uncomplicated Regurgitation

Regurgitation is the most common presentation of infantile GER and is usually but not always effortless. Regurgitation is neither necessary nor sufficient to diagnose GERD, because it is not sensitive or specific [4]. Excessive regurgitation is one of the symptoms of GERD, but the terms regurgitation and GERD should not be used as synonyms. Up to 70% of healthy infants have daily physiologic regurgitation, resolving without intervention from the age of 6 months onward. Frequent regurgitation, defined as >4 times per day, occurs in about 20% of infants during the first months of life. By 12–14 months of age, regurgitation has disappeared in over 95% [9, 10]. A prospective study confirmed disappearance of regurgitation before 12 months, although the prevalence of feeding refusal, duration of meals, parental feeding-related distress, and impaired quality of life was related to the earlier frequency of regurgitation and persisted even after the disappearance of the regurgitation [11]. Regurgitation is frequent in infants because of the large liquid volume intake, the limited capacity of the esophagus (10 ml in newborn infants), and the horizontal position of infants. Infants ingest per kg bodyweight more than twice the volume that adults do (100–150 ml/kg/day compared to 30–50 ml/kg/day), causing more gastric distention, and as a consequence more TLESRs. Feeding frequency is also higher in infants than in adults, resulting in more postprandial periods during which TLESRs are more common. Irritability may accompany regurgitation and vomiting; however, in the absence of other warning symptoms (Table 30.2), it is not an indication for extensive testing [1]. Parental coping capacity or anxiousness usually determines if a physician is consulted or not. Infant regurgitation is a benign condition with a good prognosis, needing no other intervention than parental education and anticipatory guidance, and if necessary, intervention on feeding volume, frequency, and composition will contribute to parental reassurance. Overfeeding exacerbates recurrent regurgitation. Thickened or anti-regurgitation formula decreases overt regurgitation [1].

Table 30.2 Warning signals requiring investigation in infants with regurgitation or vomiting

Bilious vomiting
GI bleeding
– Hematemesis
– Hematochezia
Consistently forceful vomiting
Onset of vomiting after 6 months of life
Failure to thrive
Diarrhea
Constipation
Fever
Lethargy
Hepatosplenomegaly
Bulging fontanelle
Macro-/microcephaly
Seizures
Abdominal tenderness or distension
Documented or suspected genetic/metabolic syndrome

Adapted from Vandenplas, Rudolph CD, Di Lorenzo C, Hassall E., et al. Pediatric gastroesophageal reflux clinical practice guidelines; joint recommendations of the North American Society for Pediatric Gastroenterology, Hepatology, and Nutrition (NASPGHAN) and the European Society Pediatric Gastroenterology, Hepatology, and Nutrition (ESPGHAN). J Pediatr Gastroneterol Nutr 2009;49(4):498–547

Recurrent Regurgitation/Vomiting and Poor Weight Gain

Although usually regurgitation causes little more than a nuisance, regurgitation of large amount of ingested food may result in caloric insufficiency and malnutrition. Poor weight gain is a crucial warning sign that necessitates clinical evaluation and testing. Hospitalization may be needed. Some infants have no apparent abnormalities and end up being diagnosed as suffering from "nonorganic failure to thrive" ("NOFTT"), a "disorder" that sometimes is attributed to social/sensory deprivation and socioeconomic or primary maternal-child problems. GERD is only one of the many etiologies of "feeding problems" during infancy. Poor weight gain, feeding refusal, back arching, irritability, and sleep disturbances have been reported to be related as well as unrelated to GERD [12].

GER(D) and Distressed Behavior

The concept that infant irritability and sleep disturbances are manifestations of GER is largely derived from adult data [1]. The same amount of distress and crying may be deemed by some parents as easily acceptable while it may be unbearable for others. Many factors, such as dietary protein milk allergy and exposure to tobacco smoke, may cause infant irritability. There is substantial interindividual variability and some healthy infants may cry up to 6 h a day.

In adults, "nonerosive reflux disease" ("NERD") is a widely accepted entity. Again in adults, impaired quality of life, notably regarding pain, mental health, and social function, has been demonstrated in patients with GERD, regardless of the presence of esophagitis [13]. The developing nervous system of infants seems susceptible to pain (hyper)sensitivity when in contact with acid despite the absence of tissue damage. Some adults "learn to live with their symptoms" (only half of the heartburn complainers seek medical help, although 60% take medications) and develop tolerance to long-lasting symptoms.

A relation between GER, GERD, and feeding refusal has not been established. Persistent crying, irritability, back arching, and feeding and sleeping difficulties have been proposed as equivalents of adult heartburn. However, two placebo-controlled studies with proton pump inhibitors (PPIs) in distressed infants presenting with frequent regurgitation failed to show an effect on crying superior to placebo [14, 15].

The Food and Drug Administration (FDA) has completed its review of four clinical trials evaluating the use of PPIs in infants (ages 1 month to <12 months) for the treatment of GERD and concluded that PPIs should not be administered to treat the symptoms of GERD in the otherwise healthy infant without evidence of acid-induced disease [16].

Up to date, there is no evidence that routine acid suppressive therapy is effective in infants who present only with inconsolable crying.

Symptoms of GERD and cow's milk protein allergy (CMPA) overlap [17]. CMPA and GERD may coexist or CMPA may complicate GERD [17]. Treatment of CMPA implies the use of hydrolysates (or amino acid formula). Improvement of GER(-like) symptoms with hydrolysates is not a proof that an underlying immunological disease exists, such as CMPA, since hydrolysates have a more rapid gastric emptying. A thickened hydrolysate may be helpful in regurgitating babies with CMPA (unpublished data).

GER(D) and Heartburn

Heartburn is the predominant GER symptom in adults, occurring weekly in 15–20% and daily in 5–10% of subjects. While the verbal child can communicate pain, descriptions of the intensity, location, and severity may be unreliable until the age of at least 8 years and sometimes later [4]. Diagnosis and management of GERD in older children (>12 years) and adolescents follow the recommendations for adults [1].

GERD and Esophagitis

Esophagitis is defined as visible breaks of the esophageal mucosa [1]. Children with GER symptoms present esophagitis in 15% up to 62%, Barrett's esophagus in 0.1–3%, and refractory GERD requiring surgery in 6–13% [1, 18]. Erosive esophagitis in 0–17-year-old children with GERD symptoms was reported to occur in 12.4% and to increase with age [19]. The median age of the group with erosive esophagitis was 12.7±4.9 years versus 10.0±5.1 years in patients without [19]. The incidence of erosive esophagitis was only 5.5% in those younger than 1 year [19]. Obviously, patient selection and recruitment, differences in definition of esophagitis, and availability of self-treatment may affect these data. In nonverbal infants, behaviors suggesting esophagitis include crying, irritability, sleep disturbance, and "colic." Infants may also appear very hungry for the bottle until their first swallows and then become irritable and refuse to drink.

Dysphagia is a typical symptom of children with eosinophilic esophagitis (EoE) or esophageal strictures but has also been linked to esophagitis. The impressive rise in prevalence of EoE is still poorly understood [20], and difficulties in distinguishing EoE from reflux esophagitis are common. In reflux esophagitis, the eosinophilic infiltrate is in theory limited to less than 5/per high power field (HPF) with 85% positive response to GER treatment, compared to primary EoE with >20 eosinophils per HPF. Demonstration of failure of PPI treatment as a condition needed to diagnose EoE brought reflux esophagitis back in the picture [21]. Patients with allergic esophagitis are typically younger and have atopic features (allergic symptoms or positive allergic tests), but no specific symptoms. Atopic features are reported in more than 90% and peripheral eosinophilia in 50% of patients.

GER(D) and Extraesophageal Manifestations

GER(D) and Reactive Airway Disease

Although an etiologic role for GER in reactive airway disease has not been demonstrated, different pathophysiologic mechanisms have been proposed: direct aspiration, vagal-mediated bronchial and laryngeal spasm, and neurally mediated inflammation. Chronic pulmonary hyperinflation predisposes to GER. An association between asthma and reflux measured by pH or impedance probe has been reported in many studies [8]. Wheezing appears more related to GERD if it is nocturnal. There are no diagnostic studies that help in selecting patients in whom reflux treatment may result in a reduction of asthma medication, if there are such patients at all [1, 8]. In a series of 46 children with persistent moderate asthma despite use of bronchodilators, inhaled corticosteroids, and leukotriene antagonists, 59% (27/46) had an abnormal pH-metry [22]. Reflux treatment resulted in a significant reduction in asthma medication. Patients with a normal pH-metry were randomized to placebo or reflux treatment: 25% (2 of only 8 children) of the treated patients could reduce their asthma medication, while this was not possible in any patient on placebo [22]. Another study found omeprazole ineffective in improving asthma symptoms and parameters in children with asthma [23]. In patients with reactive airway disease, a "negative symptom association probability" does not exclude a causal role for GER since a threshold "amount" of reflux may be necessary to start airway inflammation.

GER(D) and Recurrent Pneumonia

GER causing recurrent pneumonia has been reported with an incidence as low as 6% [24]. No test can determine whether reflux is causing recurrent pneumonia. A new technique to record pharyngeal reflux has been developed (Restech®), with promising results needing confirmation [25]. However, according to recent data from our unit (yet unpublished), there is no correlation between results of Restech® and multichannel intraluminal impedance monitoring (MII).

The sensitivity and specificity of lipid-laden macrophages for GER(D) is poor. The measurement of pepsin in bronchial aspirate seems to be more promising, although with substantial overlap between patients and controls [26]. One study evaluating nuclear scintigraphy with late imaging reported that 50% of patients with a variety of respiratory symptoms had pulmonary aspiration after 24 h [27]. But aspiration also occurs in healthy subjects, especially during sleep [1]. Moreover, later studies failed to reproduce these findings [28]. Pathologic acid reflux occurs in the majority of CF patients, even before respiratory symptoms develop [1].

GER(D) and ENT Manifestations

Several studies have detected pepsin in the middle-ear fluid, albeit with a huge variation in incidence (14–73%) [1]. Bile acids have also been detected in middle-ear liquid, in higher concentrations than in serum [29]. However, several epidemiologic studies suggest a low incidence of reflux symptoms in patients with recurrent middle-ear infections. Data from several placebo-controlled studies and meta-analyses uniformly have shown no effect of antireflux therapy on upper airway symptoms or signs [1]. The presence of pepsin and bile in middle-ear fluid might as well be the consequence of reflux (and vomiting) at the moment of the acute middle-ear infection rather than proof that chronic GER may be responsible for the chronic middle-ear problem.

GER(D) and Dental Erosions

Young children and children with neurologic impairment appear to be at greatest risk to have dental erosions caused by GER. Juice drinking, bulimia, and racial and genetic factors that affect dental enamel and saliva might be confounding variables that have been insufficiently considered [1]. There have been no long-term (intervention) follow-up studies in high-risk populations.

GER(D) and Sandifer Syndrome

Sandifer syndrome (spasmodic torsional dystonia with arching of the back and opisthotonic posturing, mainly involving the neck and back) is an uncommon but specific manifestation of GERD.

GER(D) and Apnea, ALTE, and SIDS

The literature can best be summarized as follows: most series fail to show a temporal association between GER and pathologic apnea, apparent life-threatening events (ALTE), and bradycardia [1]. However, a relation between GER and short, physiologic apnea has been shown [30, 31]. There are well-described cases or small series that demonstrate that pathologic apnea can occur as a consequence of GER.

GER(D) and Neurologic Impairment

The neurologic impaired child is known to be at risk for increased GER and GERD. Diagnosis of GERD in these children is often challenging due to their underlying conditions. Whether this group of patients has more severe reflux disease, has less effective defense mechanisms, or presents with more severe symptoms because of the inability to express and/or recognize symptoms remains open for debate. Response to treatment, both medical and surgical, is poor in the neurological impaired child compared to the neurologic normal child.

GER(D) and Other Risk Groups

Symptomatic GER is estimated to occur in 30–80% of children who have undergone repair of esophageal atresia [32]. Children with congenital abnormalities, such as hiatal hernia and malrotation, or who have had major thoracic or abdominal surgery are at risk for developing severe GERD. Although there is abundant literature on increased prevalence of GER in overweight and obese adults, data in children are scarce. There are no data in literature suggesting that preterm babies have more (severe) reflux than term-born babies, although many premature babies are treated for reflux. The role of reflux in patients with bronchopulmonary dysplasia and other chronic respiratory disorders is not clear.

GERD and Complications

Barrett's esophagus, strictures, and esophageal adenocarcinoma are complications of chronic severe GERD. Barrett's esophagus is a premalignant condition in which metaplastic specialized columnar epithelium with goblet cells is present in the tubular esophagus. In a series including 402 children with GERD without neurological or congenital anomalies, no case of Barrett's esophagus was detected [18]. In another series including 103 children with long-lasting GERD and not previously treated with H_2-receptor antagonists (H_2RAs) or PPIs, Barrett's esophagus was detected in 13%. An esophageal stricture was present in 5 of the 13 patients with Barrett's (38%) [33]. Reflux symptoms during childhood were not found to be different in adults without than in adults with Barrett's [34]. Barrett's has a male predominance and increases with age. Patients with short segments of columnar-lined esophagus and intestinal metaplasia have been found to have similar esophageal acid exposure but significantly higher frequency of abnormal bilirubin exposure and longer median duration of reflux symptoms than patients without intestinal metaplasia [35]. There is a genetic predisposition in families in patients with Barrett's esophagus and esophageal carcinoma [1].

Peptic ulcer and esophageal and gastric neoplastic changes in children are extremely rare. In adults, a decreased prevalence of gastric cancer and peptic ulcer with an opposite increase of esophageal adenocarcinoma and GERD has been noted over the last 30 years [36]. This has been attributed to several independent factors, such as changes in dietary habits such as a higher fat intake, an increased incidence of obesity, and a decreased incidence of Helicobacter pylori infection [36]. Frequency, severity, and duration of reflux symptoms are related to the risk of developing esophageal cancer. Among adults with longstanding and severe reflux, the odds ratios are 43.5 for esophageal adenocarcinoma and 4.4 for adenocarcinoma at the cardia [37]. It is unknown whether mild esophagitis or GER symptoms persisting from childhood are related to an increased risk for severe complications in adults.

Diagnosis

Diagnostic procedures will not be discussed in detail. History in children is difficult to obtain and considered poorly reliable up to the age of minimally 8 or even 12 years old [1]. Orenstein developed the "infant GER questionnaire" (I-GERQ) [38]. But, the I-GERQ cutoff score failed to identify 26% of infants with GERD and was positive in 81% of infants with normal esophageal histology and normal pH-metry [39]. Barium contrast radiography, nuclear scintiscanning, and ultrasound are techniques evaluating postprandial reflux and provide limited information on gastric emptying. Barium studies are not recommended as first-line investigation to diagnose GERD, but are of importance to diagnose anatomic abnormalities such as hiatal hernia, malrotation, duodenal web, and stenosis and may suggest functional abnormalities such as esophageal achalasia. The results of ultrasound are investigator dependent, and a relation between reflux detected on ultrasound and symptoms has not been established [1]. Manometry does not demonstrate reflux, but has been instrumental to uncover pathophysiologic mechanisms causing reflux and is indicated in the diagnosis of specific conditions such as achalasia [1]. Experience in children with spectrophotometric esophageal probes to detect bilirubin is still very limited. Orel and coworkers found that some children with esophagitis suffer bile reflux [40].

Modern endoscopes are so miniaturized that endoscoping preterm infants of less than 1,000 g has become technically easy. Macroscopic lesions associated with GERD include erosions, exudate, ulcers, structures, and hiatal hernia. "Erythema" of the distal esophagus in young infants is a normal finding because of the increased number of small blood vessels at the cardiac region. Endoscopy may also show a "sliding hernia," stomach that is protruding in the esophagus during belching, influenced by the amount of insufflated air during endoscopy. Recent consensus guidelines define reflux esophagitis as the presence of endoscopically visible breaks in the esophageal mucosa at or immediately above the GE junction [1, 4]. Endoscopy-negative reflux disease is common. There is a poor correlation between the severity of symptoms and presence and absence of esophagitis. There is insufficient evidence to support the use of histology to diagnose or exclude GERD. Biopsies of duodenal, gastric, and esophageal mucosa are mandatory to exclude other diseases [1]. More detailed information on pros and cons of histology can be found in recent consensus papers [1, 4].

Ambulatory 24-h esophageal pH monitoring measures the incidence and duration of acid reflux, while impedance measures all reflux episodes, if they are accompanied by a bolus. Esophageal pH-metry is the best method to measure acid in the esophagus, but not all reflux causing symptoms is acid and not all acid reflux is causing symptoms. Both hardware (electrodes, devices) and software influence the results [41, 42]. Although normal ranges have been established for pH-metry, it should be remembered that they are hard- and software dependent and have been established with glass electrodes. Intraluminal impedance measures electrical potential differences and is becoming of increasing interest (see below).

All GER investigation techniques test different aspects of reflux. Therefore, it is not unexpected that the correlation among the results of the different techniques is poor. There is no "always-best" investigation technique to diagnose GER(D). "Logic" (but not evidence-based medicine) suggests that if the question asked is "does this patient have esophagitis?" then endoscopy with biopsy is the best technique. If it is in the interest of the patient to measure acid GER episodes, 24-h pH-metry is the preferred technique. If it is important to measure "all episodes of reflux," multichannel intraluminal impedance (MII) seems to be the investigation of choice. However, postprandial reflux is mainly weakly acid or alkaline, and postprandial reflux was in general considered to be not clinically relevant, and most techniques measuring postprandial reflux (barium swallow, ultrasound, scintiscanning) are often not recommended for this reason. As long as therapeutic options are mainly limited to acid-reducing medication, one may question if it is really relevant to measure weakly acid and alkaline reflux.

Esophageal Impedance Recording

The measurement of reflux by MII is not pH dependent, but in combination with pH-metry, it allows detection of acid (pH<4.0), weakly acid (pH 4.0–7.0), and alkaline reflux (pH>7).

Experience has shown that impedance needs to be performed in combination with pH-metry, since pH-only events occur (mainly during the night and mainly in young infants). Also gas reflux can be measured, since liquid reflux causes a drop in impedance and gas reflux an increase. Obviously, "more" reflux episodes are detected with impedance pH-metry than with pH-metry alone, but the question remains at this moment unanswered if "more is always necessary or better." Recent (yet unpublished) research showed a very high intra- and interobserver variability between "experts." The major clinical interest of impedance seems to be demonstration of symptom association, but normal data and validation of symptom association parameters in children are missing. Interestingly, pH-only episodes, reflux episodes detected with pH-metry but not with impedance (drop in pH without bolus movement), occur in young children [43]. A major difference between pH-metry and impedance regards the "nature" of the reflux: pH-metry measures the chemical clearance of the esophagus, while impedance measure the bolus (volume) clearance. In general, chemical clearance is much slower than bolus clearance.

Impedance Studies in Newborns

A number of studies have studied the number of reflux episodes as primary outcome. In 52 symptomatic preterm infants, 24-h MII-pH detected 2,834 GER episodes: 2162 (76%) nonacid and 672 (24%) acid. The acid bolus exposure index was 0.28% (0.02–2.73%), and the nonacid bolus exposure index was 1.03% (0.06–38.15%). By considering only pH sensor (pH-monitoring analysis), an average of 53.2 AR episodes were detected and esophageal exposure to acid was 11% (or thus more than 30 times higher than with impedance) [44]. The influence of feeding on the number of reflux episodes was analyzed in a number of reports. In 21 healthy preterm newborns, in which the nasogastric feeding tube was replaced by a feeding-impedance catheter, the number of acid reflux episodes per hour was higher during fasting than during feeding periods. Conversely, the number of weakly acid reflux episodes per hour was significantly higher in feeding than in fasting periods [45]. In 17 symptomatic preterm newborns fed naïve and fortified human milk, pH-MII revealed an inverse correlation between naïve human milk protein content and acid reflux index (RIpH: $P=0.041$, $\rho=-0.501$). After fortification, osmolality often exceeded the values recommended for infant feeds, and a statistically significant ($P<0.05$) increase in nonacid reflux indexes was observed [46].

MII-pH was combined with epigastric impedance for 3 h in 30 newborns referred for apparent life-threatening events (ALTE) and signs of GERD [47]. An inverse correlation was evident for reflux frequency and gastric emptying velocity ($r^2=0.94$; $P<0.001$) and between acid refluxes and the gastric filling state ($r^2=0.95$; $P<0.001$), whereas a positive correlation was found between the reflux level and the gastric filling state ($r^2=0.52$; $P<0.05$) [47].

Other studies analyzed the relation in time between reflux episodes and extraesophageal manifestations, such as apnea. Corvaglia et al. investigated 52 preterm infants and showed that 154 (14%) apneas out of 1,136 were related in time to GER. The frequency of apnea during the 1-min time around the onset of GER (within 30 s before and after) was significantly higher than the apnea frequency detected in GER-free periods ($P=0.03$). Furthermore, the frequency of apnea in the 30 s after GER (GER-triggered apneas) was greater than that detected in the 30 s before ($P=0.01$). This suggests that a number of apneas are induced by GER [48]. In a small group of 6 premature infants with apnea or hypoxemia not responsive to caffeine treatment, a total of 405 reflux events [306 (76%) weakly acid and 99 acid refluxes] and 142 apneas were detected. The sub-analysis based on chemical composition and duration of refluxate showed that the frequency of apneas associated with weakly acid reflux events was significantly greater than the one calculated for reflux-free period [0.416/min (0.00–1.30) vs. 0.016/min (0.003–0.028), respectively; $P<0.05$] and that the frequency of apneas occurring during reflux events longer than 30s was significantly higher than those occurring during shorter reflux events (22 vs. 11%; $P<0.004$) [49].

The relation between body position and reflux episodes was evaluated in a number of studies. In 10 healthy preterm infants, a "crossover position study" and postprandial evaluation showed more liquid GER in the right than in the left lateral position. Gastric emptying was faster in the right than in the left lateral position [50]. Similar findings were reported by another group in 22 preterm babies presenting with regurgitation and postprandial desaturations: the number of acid and nonacid reflux episodes was significantly lower when the subjects were in the prone and left-side sleeping position in comparison to the supine and right-side positions [51]. The left-side position showed the lowest esophageal acid exposure in the early postprandial period, whereas in the prone position acid reflux was smallest in the late postprandial period [51].

Using an esophageal impedance-manometry catheter incorporating an intragastric infusion port, it was shown in 8 preterm infants that more transient lower esophageal sphincter relaxations (TLESRs) were triggered in the right lateral position compared to the left lateral position. First TLESR occurred at a significantly lower infused volume and percentage of feed in right compared with left lateral position. TLESRs and GER were triggered at small volumes, unlikely to induce gastric distension [52].

MII-pH was carried out in 13 newborns receiving 0.3 mg per kg domperidone and in 13 controls. Each newborn was compared to the control nearest in postconceptional age. GER episodes per hour increased significantly compared to the baseline in the domperidone group, whereas there were no differences in the maximum proximal extent reached by the refluxes. The authors speculated that the paradoxical increase in the number of GER episodes could be the expression of a domperidone-induced amplification of the motor incoordination of the neonatal gastroesophageal tract [53].

In 26 preterm infants and term neonates, esomeprazole (0.5 mg/kg once daily for 7 days) produced no change in bolus reflux characteristics (frequency, content, extent, and clearance time) despite significant acid suppression (reduced number of episodes and reflux index) and clinical improvement (reduced number of symptoms recorded) [54].

Studies in Infants

Several studies report that in infants significantly more acid reflux is detected with "classic pH-monitoring analysis" (pH<4.0) than with "impedance" (bolus detection with a pH<4.0). In other words, there is a substantial difference between chemical and bolus reflux. Woodley et al. analyzed the tracings of 14 infants. Significantly fewer (~ 25%) acid reflux episodes were detected using MII-pH when compared to pH monitoring alone. Estimates of esophageal acid exposure using pH monitoring alone were twofold higher than with impedance criteria: 71.8% of the acid reflux episodes detected by pH monitoring could not be confirmed by combined MII-pH [55]. Di Fiore and coworkers analyzed impedance tracings obtained in 80 preterm and 39 term infants: 59% out of 2,572 events detected by pH were not identified by MII. A significant higher incidence of these pH-only events occurred in preterm versus term infants. The two major identified reasons for this discrepancy were absence of change in impedance and failure to meet MII scoring criteria [56]. In 12 symptomatic infants, MII-pH revealed that total acid GER episodes, total acid reflux exposure time, and acid episodes lasting 5 min or longer were largely a function of classic 2 phase (acid reflux episode with bolus component and bolus clearance time shorter than acid clearance time) and of pH-only acid GER types [57].

MII-pH tracings from 12 symptomatic infants showed that mean duration of volume clearance was much shorter than chemical clearance [58]. Volume clearance did not change throughout the feeding cycle, but chemical clearance was significantly prolonged during fasting compared with feeding and first postprandial hour. The authors speculated that inefficient chemical clearance during fasting is likely due to reduced efficiency of acid clearance mechanisms that could include salivation, swallowing, peristalsis, and/or intraluminal secretion [58].

In 9 infants with chronic lung disease, a total of 511 AR events were temporally (2-min window) associated with symptoms in only 1 patient in 3, and an SSI of 77% was noted when AR reached the pharynx (11% respiratory, 17% sensory, and 12% movements associated). A 3.5-fold higher correlation between reflux episodes and symptoms was found if acid clearance time was prolonged [59].

In 16 infants with a diagnosis of ALTE (mean of age 3 months), 23.4 reflux episodes were recorded with pH monitoring, whereas the number of reflux episodes obtained with impedance was 70.9, with 36.2% acid and 63.8% weakly acid reflux episodes. In only one patient, 4 apneas were associated with GER (3 nonacid and one acid) resulting in a statistically positive relation (SI>or=50%; SSI>or=10%) [60].

Studies in Children

In 75 infants and children, aged from 9 days to 12 years, 2,247 reflux events were detected by MII, while only 967 reflux events were detected by pH-metry. Nonacid reflux was more predominant during postprandial periods ($P<0.001$). The symptom index was higher if reflux was measured with MII-pH (31.1%) than with pH probe (8.2%) [61]. In a 12-h MII-pH study, Del Buono confirmed an increased number of reflux episodes (both acid and nonacid) and median height of reflux events in 9/16 neurological impaired children fed through a nasogastric tube, in comparison to the orally fed subgroup [62]. In 50 patients (29 infants and 21 children) MII detection of all bolus GER yielded a significantly greater number of patients that were symptom positive: 36 (72%) compared with 25 (50%) with standard pH monitoring. Symptoms of cough, pain irritability/crying, sneeze, nausea, choking, back arching, heartburn, hiccups, stridor, and bad breath were included for analysis [63].

The presence or absence of esophagitis does not seem to be related to the results of MII-pH [64]. Recently, data were published obtained in a large population of 291 children referred for suspected GERD, and sensitivity and diagnostic accuracy of MII-pH versus pH monitoring and symptom association were determined [65]. MII-pH detected 13,631 reflux episodes, 6,260 (46%) of which were nonacid. The prevalence of weakly acid reflux during 24 h and during postprandial periods as well as the proximal extension of the refluxates was significantly greater in infants than in children. The diagnostic accuracy of combined MII-pH in revealing reflux episodes, and specifically AR, was significantly higher in infants than in children. The authors concluded that the addition of MII to conventional pH monitoring significantly increased the diagnostic yield of symptom association analysis in revealing an association between extraesophageal symptoms and reflux, irrespective of age, whereas in studying typical symptoms this was true only for infants [65].

However, recent information showed that baseline impedance is lower in the presence of esophagitis than in patients with normal esophageal mucosa. As a consequence, baseline impedance (BImp) reflects esophageal mucosal integrity [66–68]. In rabbits, esophagitis was shown to decrease BImp with about 1/3rd compared to the BImp in healthy controls [66]. The measurement of BImp may increase the information obtained from a MII-pH recording and thus bring possible clinical advantage [68].

In 50 children undergoing both MII-pH and bronchoscopy, there was no significant correlation between the lipid-laden macrophage index and the number of reflux episodes. In the subgroup of patients who underwent fundoplication for intractable respiratory disease, there was no significant difference in any of the reflux parameters between patients who did and did not experience clinical improvement after fundoplication [69].

In a more recent study, 21 children with a diagnosis of bronchial asthma, recurrent lung consolidations, and recurrent laryngotracheitis underwent MII-pH, fiber-optic bronchoscopy, and bronchoalveolar lavage. The number of nonacid reflux episodes and the number of those reaching the proximal esophagus were significantly higher in patients with recurrent lung consolidations than in those with bronchial asthma and laryngotracheitis. Bronchoalveolar lavage studies showed a significantly higher lipid-laden macrophage content in children with recurrent lung consolidations than in those with bronchial asthma and laryngotracheitis. The lipid-laden macrophage content correlated significantly with the total number of reflux episodes ($r=0.73$) and with those reaching the proximal esophagus ($r=0.67$). Finally, the lipid-laden macrophage content correlated with the number of nonacid reflux episodes ($r=0.61$), with those reaching the proximal esophagus ($r=0.64$) and with the percentage of bronchoalveolar neutrophils ($r=0.7$) [70].

Treatment Options

Because symptoms of GER and GERD are frequent and nonspecific, especially during infancy, and because there is no "golden-standard" diagnostic technique, many infants and children are exposed to empiric antireflux treatment. Therapeutic options vary from reassurance, nutritional and positional treatment, and administration of prokinetic and acid-reducing medications to surgery (Table 30.3). Physiologic GER does not need medical treatment. Therapeutic intervention should always be a balance between intended improvement of symptoms and risk for side effects.

Complications of Nonintervention

Although data on the natural evolution of regurgitation are now available, there are only limited data on the natural history of GERD in infants and children because most patients receive treatment. Recent data suggest a decreased quality of life in a number of parents of infants presenting with frequent regurgitation, even if the regurgitation has disappeared [11]. Although symptoms improved in more than half of the infants with reflux esophagitis followed longitudinally for 1 year without pharmacotherapy, histology remained abnormal in all [71]. It is not known if treatment of GER during infancy changes the long-term outcome and GERD in adults.

Non-pharmacologic and Nonsurgical Therapies for GER

The most common reason to seek medical help for parents of young infants with suspected GERD is frequent regurgitation and infant distress. Because infants with physiologic regurgitation are difficult to distinguish from infants with mild to moderate GERD symptoms, non-pharmacologic treatment (reassurance, dietary and positional treatment) is considered the appropriate first approach. Observation of feeding and handling of the child during and after feedings is essential. Many infants are overfed or fed with an inappropriate technique [1]. Reassurance while showing compassion for the impaired quality of life is of importance [1].

Many infants presenting with frequent regurgitation have a distressed behavior and are irritable. A thickened or commercialized anti-regurgitation formula (not antireflux formula!) decreases visual regurgitation, but does not systematically decrease (acid) reflux [72]. However, data from three independent studies suggest acid reflux is actually reduced with cornstarch thickened formula [73]. Commercialized thickened formula is preferred to thickening agents added to formula at home; the nutritional content of the thickening agent and its effect on osmolality have been taken in account in the commercialized formula [1]. Dietary protein allergy may be a cause of reflux, regurgitation, and vomiting, often accompanied by distressed behavior [1, 2]. Ongoing studies suggest promising results with thickened extensive hydrolysates (unpublished data).

Sleeping positions that have been suggested to reduce GER include prone, left side after feeding, and supine 40° anti-Trendelenburg. Prone position is considered obsolete in infants because of the increased risk of sudden infant death (SID). Van Wijk et al. concluded that biggest benefit

Table 30.3 Schematic therapeutic approach in 2011

Phase 1	Parental reassurance. Observation. Lifestyle changes. Exclude overfeeding
Phase 2	Dietary treatment (decrease regurgitation). Thickened formula, thickening agents, extensive hydrolysates, or amino acid-based formula in cow's milk allergy. Positional treatment (°)
Phase 3	For immediate symptom relief: alginates (some efficacy in moderate GERD), antacids only in older children
Phase 4	Proton pump inhibitors (drug of choice in severe GERD; more safety data needed). H_2-receptor antagonists less effective than PPIs
Phase 5	Prokinetics (but not one product available on the market in 2010 has been shown to be effective) would treat pathophysiologic mechanism of GERD
Phase 6	Laparoscopic surgery

Efficacy and safety data in infants and children for most anti-GER medication is limited (°): data on 40 ° supine sleeping position in infants are limited Adapted from Vandenplas, Rudolph CD, Di Lorenzo C, Hassall E., et al. Pediatric gastroesophageal reflux clinical practice guidelines; joint recommendations of the North American Society for Pediatric Gastroenterology, Hepatology, and Nutrition (NASPGHAN) and the European Society Pediatric Gastroenterology, Hepatology, and Nutrition (ESPGHAN). J Pediatr Gastroneterol Nutr 2009;49(4):498–547

was achieved with a strategy of right lateral positioning for the first postprandial hour with a position change to the left thereafter to promote gastric emptying and reduce liquid GER in the late postprandial period [50]. However, at least two independent studies reported a significantly increased risk of SID in the side compared to the supine sleeping position. The results of a pilot study with the "Multicare-AR Bed®" suggest that a specially made bed that nurses the infant at 40° supine body position reduces regurgitation, acid reflux (measured with pH monitoring), and reflux-associated symptoms (evaluated with the I-GERQ) [74].

Prokinetics and Other Nonacid-Reducing/Blocking Medication

From the pathophysiologic point of view, prokinetics seem the most logic therapeutic approach to treating GERD. Unfortunately, according to the NASPGHAN-ESPGHAN guidelines, the adverse events of currently available prokinetics, including metoclopramide, domperidone, and cisapride, outweigh their potential benefit, since the latter was never clearly demonstrated [1]. Bethanechol, a direct cholinergic agonist, studied in a few controlled trials has uncertain efficacy and a high incidence of side effects in children with GERD. Baclofen is a gamma-aminobutyric acid (GABA)-B receptor agonist used to reduce spasticity in neurologically impaired patients. Baclofen was shown to reduce the number of TLSERs and acid GER during a 2-h test period and to accelerate gastric emptying [75]. The data on baclofen are still very limited and the number of adverse events does not justify yet its widespread use. A baclofen was originally considered as possibly more promising, but results are disappointing as well. M0003 (Movetis) is a "next generation gastrokinetic." M0003 is a specific and high-affinity 5-HT4 agonist for the treatment of upper GI disorders, focusing initially on severe gastroparesis and pediatric reflux in children. Today, the drug is still in the phase of development, and clinical trials in children have not yet started.

(Alginate-)Antacids and Mucosaprotectors

The key therapeutic advantage of antacids is their rapid onset of action, within minutes from ingestion. These products have mainly been validated in adults. Results showed a marginal but significant difference between Gaviscon infant and placebo in average reflux height (being better for placebo!) and raise questions regarding any perceived clinical benefit of its use [76]. Data on compliance in infants and children (these products have a poor taste) and side effects (many antacids have a high aluminum content) are missing. Extrapolating from adult data, one may conclude that it is unlikely that mucosaprotectors would be effective in children.

H²-Receptor Antagonists (H2RAs) and Proton Pump Inhibitors (PPI)

Since PPIs are more effective acid suppressing agents than H_2RAs, PPIs are often considered the preferred option for treatment of GERD in children and adults. PPIs are prodrugs since protonation of the molecule in highly acidic environments is necessary for their action. PPIs must be taken once a day, before breakfast, and must be protected from gastric acid by enteric coating. The achievement of "maximal acid suppressant effect" can take up to 4 days. The granules and tablets should not be crushed, chewed, or dissolved as gastric acid secretion may alter the drugs. If the microgranules are enteric coated, the capsules can be opened and administered orally or via a feeding tube, in suspension in an acidic medium such as fruit juice, yogurt, or apple sauce. A "homemade" liquid formulation, produced by dissolving the granula, not the microgranula, in 8.4% bicarbonate solution has been used in some reports [1]. Omeprazole and esomeprazole are approved in the USA and Europe for use in children older than 1 year of age; in the USA, lansoprazole is approved as well. In uncontrolled trials and case reports, omeprazole was used in dosage between 0.2 and 3.5 mg/kg/day for periods ranging from 14 days to 36 months. Lansoprazole, omeprazole, and pantoprazole are metabolized by a genetically polymorphic enzyme, CYP2C19, absent in approximately 3% of Caucasians and 20% of Asians. Salivary secretion is decreased with omeprazole (and increased with cisapride).

There are four main categories of adverse effects related to PPI: idiosyncratic reactions, drug-drug interactions, drug-induced hypergastrinemia, and drug-induced hypochlorhydria [1]. Idiosyncratic reactions occur in up to 12–14% of children taking PPIs: headache, diarrhea, constipation, and nausea [1]. Acid suppression, or hypochlorhydria, causes abnormal gastrointestinal flora and bacterial overgrowth [1]. As a consequence, the prevalence of infectious respiratory and gastrointestinal tract infections is increased [1].

Surgery and Therapeutic Endoscopic Procedures

Therapeutic endoscopic procedures are rarely indicated and should only be performed where there is evidence of experience. Most of the literature on surgical therapy in children with GERD consists of retrospective case series in which documentation of the diagnosis of GERD and details of previous medical therapy are deficient, making it difficult to assess the indications for and responses to surgery [1]. Adult series report that between 37% and 62% of patients are taking PPI a few years after the surgery [77, 78]. Different antireflux surgical approaches do exist. In general, experience seems to be the best guidance for choosing the preferred technique. While antireflux surgery in certain groups of children may be of considerable benefit, a failure rate of up to 22% has been reported [1]. Children with underlying conditions predisposing to the most severe GERD comprise a large percentage of many surgical series. Total esophagogastric dissociation is an operative procedure that is useful in selected children with neurologic impairment or other conditions causing life-threatening aspiration during oral feedings.

References

1. Vandenplas Y, Rudolph CD, Di Lorenzo C, Hassall E, Liptak G, Mazur L, Sondheimer J, Staiano A, Thomson M, Veereman-Wauters G, Wenzl TG. Pediatric Gastroesophageal Reflux Clinical Practice Guidelines: Joint Recommendations of the North American Society of Pediatric Gastroenterology, Hepatology, and Nutrition and the European Society of Pediatric Gastroenterology, Hepatology, and Nutrition. J Pediatr Gastroenterol Nutr. 2009;49:498–5472.
2. Stanford EA, Chambers CT, Craig KD. The role of developmental factors in predicting young children's use of a self-report scale for pain. Pain. 2006;120:16–23.

3. von Baeyer CL, Spagrud LJ. Systematic review of observational (behavioral) measures of pain for children and adolescents aged 3 to 18 years. Pain. 2007;127:140–50.
4. Sherman PM, Hassall E, Fagundes-Neto U, Gold BD, Kato S, Koletzko S, Orenstein S, Rudolph C, Vakil N, Vandenplas Y. A global, evidence-based consensus on the definition of gastroesophageal reflux disease in the pediatric population. Am J Gastroenterol. 2009;104:1278–95.
5. Vandenplas Y, Hassall E. Mechanisms of gastroesophageal reflux and gastroesophageal reflux disease. J Pediatr Gastroenterol Nutr. 2002;35:119–36.
6. Omari TI, Benninga MA, Barnett CP, Haslam RR, Davidson GP, Dent J. Characterization of esophageal body and lower esophageal sphincter motor function in the very premature neonate. J Pediatr. 1999;135:517–21.
7. Vandenplas Y, Goyvaerts H, Helven R. Gastroesophageal reflux, as measured by 24-hours pH-monitoring, in 509 healthy infants screened for risk of sudden infants death syndrome. Pediatrics. 1991;88:834–40.
8. Tolia V, Vandenplas Y. Systematic review: the extra-oesophageal symptoms of gastro-oesophageal reflux disease in children. Aliment Pharmacol Ther. 2009;29:258–72.
9. Hegar B, Dewanti NR, Kadim M, Alatas S, Firmansyah A, Vandenplas Y. Natural evolution of regurgitation in healthy infants. Acta Paediatr. 2009;98:1189–93.
10. Nelson SP, Chen EH, Syniar GM. Prevalence of symptoms of gastroesophageal reflux in infancy. Arch Pediatr Adolesc Med. 1997;151:569–72.
11. Nelson SP, Chen EH, Syniar GM. One year follow-up of symptoms of gastroesophageal reflux during infancy. Pediatrics. 1998;102:e67.
12. Heine RG, Jaquiery A, Lubitz L, et al. Role of gastro-oesophageal reflux in infant irritability. Arch Dis Child. 1995;73:121–5.
13. Nandurkar S, Talley NJ. Epidemiology and natural history of reflux disease. Bailliere's Clin Gastroenterol. 2000;14:743–57.
14. Moore DJ, Tao BS, Lines DR, Hirte C, Heddle ML, Davidson GP. Double-blind placebo-controlled trial of omeprazole in irritable infants with gastroesophageal reflux. J Pediatr. 2003;143:219–23.
15. Orenstein SR, Hassall E, Furmaga-Jablonska W, Atkinson S, Raanan M. Multicenter, double-blind, randomized, placebo-controlled trial assessing the efficacy and safety of proton pump inhibitor lansoprazole in infants with symptoms of gastroesophageal reflux disease. J Pediatr. 2009;154:514–20.
16. Chen IL, Gao WY, Johnson AP, Niak A, Troiani J, Korvick J, Snow N, Estes K, Taylor A, Griebel D. Proton pump inhibitor use in infants: FDA reviewer experience. J Pediatr Gastroenterol Nutr. 2011;54(1):8–14.
17. Salvatore S, Vandenplas Y. Gastroesophageal reflux and cow's milk allergy: is there a link? Pediatrics. 2002;110:972–84.
18. El-Serag HB, Bailey NR, Gilger M, Rabeneck L. Endoscopic manifestations of gastroesophageal reflux disease in patients between 18 months and 25 years without neurological deficits. Am J Gastroenterol. 2002;97:1635–9.
19. Gilger MA, El-Serag HB, Gold BD, Dietrich CL, Tsou V, McDuffie A, Shub MD. Prevalence of endoscopic findings of erosive esophagitis in children: a population-based study. J Pediatr Gastroenterol Nutr. 2008;47:141–6.
20. Spergel JM, Brown-Whitehorn TF, Beausoleil JL, Franciosi J, Suker M, Verma R, Liacouras CA. 14 years of eosinophilic esophagitis: clinical features and prognosis. J Pediatr Gastroenterol Nutr. 2009;48:30–6.
21. Furuta GT, Liacouras CA, Collins MH, Gupta SK, Justinich C, Putnam PE, Bonis P, Hassall E, Straumann A, Rothenberg ME. First International Gastrointestinal Eosinophil Research Symposium (FIGERS) Subcommittees. Eosinophilic esophagitis in children and adults: a systematic review and consensus recommendations for diagnosis and treatment. Gastroenterology. 2007;133:1342–63.
22. Khoshoo V, Le T, Haydel Jr RM, Landry L, Nelson C. Role of GER in older children with persistent asthma. Chest. 2003;123:1008–13.
23. Stordal K, Johannesdottir GB, Bentsen BS, Knudsen PK, Carlsen KC, Closs O, Handeland M, Holm HK, Sandvik L. Acid suppression does not change respiratory symptoms in children with asthma and gastro-oesophageal reflux disease. Arch Dis Child. 2005;90:956–60.
24. Button BM, Roberts S, Kotsimbos TC, Levvey BJ, Williams TJ, Bailey M, Snell GI, Wilson JW. Gastroesophageal reflux (symptomatic and silent): a potentially significant problem in patients with cystic fibrosis before and after lung transplantation. J Heart Lung Transplant. 2005;24:1522–9.
25. Ayazi S, Lipham JC, Hagen JA, Tang AL, Zehetner J, Leers JM, Oezcelik A, Abate E, Banki F, DeMeester SR, DeMeester TR. A new technique for measurement of pharyngeal pH: normal values and discriminating pH threshold. J Gastrointest Surg. 2009;13:1422–9.
26. Starosta V, Kitz R, Hartl D, Marcos V, Reinhardt D, Griese M. Bronchoalveolar pepsin, bile acids, oxidation, and inflammation in children with gastroesophageal reflux disease. Chest. 2007;132:1557–64.
27. Ravelli AM, Panarotto MB, Verdoni L, Consolati V, Bolognini S. Pulmonary aspiration shown by scintigraphy in gastroesophageal reflux-related respiratory disease. Chest. 2006;130:1520–6.
28. Morigeri C, Bhattacharya A, Mukhopadhyay K, Narang A, Mittal BR. Radionuclide scintigraphy in the evaluation of gastroesophageal reflux in symptomatic and asymptomatic pre-term infants. Eur J Nucl Med Mol Imaging. 2008;35:1659–65.
29. Klokkenburg JJ, Hoeve HL, Francke J, Wieringa MH, Borgstein J, Feenstra L. Bile acids identified in middle ear effusions of children with otitis media with effusion. Laryngoscope. 2009;119:396–400.

30. Wenzl TG, Schenke S, Peschgens T, Silny J, Heimann G, Skopnik H. Association of apnea and nonacid gastroesophageal reflux in infants: Investigations with the intraluminal impedance technique. Pediatr Pulmonol. 2001;31:144–9.
31. Sacre L, Vandenplas Y. Gastroesophageal reflux associated with respiratory abnormalities during sleep. J Pediatr Gastroenterol Nutr. 1989;9:28–33.
32. Fonkalsrud EW, Ament ME. Gastroesophageal reflux in childhood. Curr Probl Surg. 1996;33:1–70.
33. Krug E, Bergmeijer JH, Dees J. Gastroesophageal reflux and Barrett's esophagus in adults born with esophageal atresia. Am J Gastroenterol. 1999;94:2825–8.
34. Hassall E. Barrett's esophagus: new definitions and approaches in children. J Pediatr Gastroenterol Nutr. 1993;16:345–64.
35. Oberg S, Peters JH, DeMeester TR, Lord RV, Johansson J, DeMeester SR, Hagen JA. Determinants of intestinal metaplasia within the columnar-lined esophagus. Arch Surg. 2000;135:651–6.
36. Sonnenberg A, El-Serag HB. Clinical epidemiology and natural history of gastroesophageal reflux disease. Yale J Biol Med. 1999;72:81–92.
37. Lagergren J, Bergstrom R, Lindgren A, Nyrén O. Symptomatic gastroesophageal reflux as a risk factor for esophageal adenocarcinoma. N Engl J Med. 1999;340:825–31.
38. Orenstein SR, Cohn JF, Shalaby T. Reliability and validity of an infant gastroesophageal questionnaire. Clin Pediatrics. 1993;32:472–84.
39. Salvatore S, Hauser B, Vandemaele K, Novario R, Vandenplas Y. Gastroesophageal reflux disease in infants: how much is predictable with questionnaires, pH-metry, endoscopy and histology? J Pediatr Gastroenterol Nutr. 2005;40:210–5.
40. Orel R, Brecelj J, Homan M, Heuschkel R. Treatment of oesophageal bile reflux in children: the results of a prospective study with omeprazole. J Pediatr Gastroenterol Nutr. 2006;42:376–83.
41. Vandenplas Y, Badriul H, Verghote M, Hauser B, Kaufman L. Glass and antimony electrodes for oesophageal pH monitoring in distressed infants: how different are they? Eur J Gastroenterol Hepatol. 2004;16:1325–30.
42. Hemmink GJ, Weusten BL, Oors J, Bredenoord AJ, Timmer R, Smout AJ. Ambulatory oesophageal pH monitoring: a comparison between antimony, ISFET, and glass pH electrodes. Eur J Gastroenterol Hepatol. 2010;22:572–7.
43. Rosen R, Lord C, Nurko S. The sensitivity of multichannel intraluminal impedance and the pH probe in the evaluation of gastroesophageal reflux in children. Clin Gastroenterol Hepatol. 2006;4:167–72.
44. Corvaglia L, Mariani E, Aceti A, Capretti MG, Ancora G, Faldella G. Combined oesophageal impedance-pH monitoring in preterm newborn: comparison of two options for layout analysis. Neurogastroenterol Motil. 2009;21:1027–e81.
45. Moya MJ, Cabo JA, Macías MC. Fernández Pineda I, Granero R, López-Alonso M. Pandrial gastroesophageal reflux in healthy preterm infants. Cir Pediatr. 2006;19:236–40.
46. Aceti A, Corvaglia L, Paoletti V, Mariani E, Ancora G, Galletti S, Faldella G. Protein content and fortification of human milk influence gastroesophageal reflux in preterm infants. J Pediatr Gastroenterol Nutr. 2009;49:613–8.
47. Cresi F, de Sanctis L, Savino F, Bretto R, Testa A, Silvestro L. Relationship between gastro-oesophageal reflux and gastric activity in newborns assessed by combined intraluminal impedance, pH metry and epigastric impedance. Neurogastroenterol Motil. 2006;18:361–8.
48. Corvaglia L, Zama D, Gualdi S, Ferlini M, Aceti A, Faldella G. Gastro-oesophageal reflux increases the number of apnoeas in very preterm infants. Arch Dies Child Fatal Neonatal Ed. 2009;94:F188–92.
49. Magistà AM, Indrio F, Baldassarre M, Bucci N, Menolascina A, Mautone A, Francavilla R. Multichannel intraluminal impedance to detect relationship between gastroesophageal reflux and apnoea of prematurity. Dig Liver Dies. 2007;39:216–21.
50. Van Wijk MP, Benninga MA, Dent J, Lontis R, Goodchild L, McCall LM, Haslam R, Davidson GP, Omari T. Effect of body position changes on postprandial gastroesophageal reflux and gastric emptying in the healthy premature neonate. J Podiatry. 2007;151:585–90.
51. Corvaglia L, Rotatori R, Ferlini M, Aceti A, Ancora G, Faldella G. The effect of body positioning on gastroesophageal reflux in premature infants: evaluation by combined impedance and pH monitoring. J Pediatr. 2007;151:591–6.
52. van Wijk MP, Benninga MA, Davidson GP, Haslam R, Omari TI. Small volumes of feed can trigger transient lower esophageal sphincter relaxation and gastroesophageal reflux in the right lateral position in infants. J Pediatr. 2010;156:744–8.
53. Cresi F, Marinaccio C, Russo MC, Miniero R, Silvestro L. Short-term effect of domperidone on gastroesophageal reflux in newborns assessed by combined intraluminal impedance and pH monitoring. J Perinatol. 2008;28:766–70.
54. Omari T, Lundborg P, Sandström M, Bondarov P, Fjellman M, Haslam R, Davidson G. Pharmacodynamics and systemic exposure of esomeprazole in preterm infants and term neonates with gastroesophageal reflux disease. J Pediatr. 2009;155:222–8.
55. Woodley FW, Mousa H. Acid gastroesophageal reflux reports in infants: a comparison of esophageal pH monitoring and multichannel intraluminal impedance measurements. Dig Dis Sci. 2006;51:1910–6.
56. Di Fiore JM, Arko M, Churbock K, Hibbs AM, Martin RJ. Technical limitations in detection of gastroesophageal reflux in neonates. J Pediatr Gastroenterol Nutr. 2009;49:177–82.

57. Woodley FW, Hayes J, Mousa H. Acid gastroesophageal reflux in symptomatic infants is primarily a function of classic 2-phase and pH-only acid reflux event types. J Pediatr Gastroenterol Nutr. 2009;48:550–8.
58. Woodley FW, Fernandez S, Mousa H. Diurnal variation in the chemical clearance of acid gastroesophageal reflux in infants. Clin Gastroenterol Hepatol. 2007;5:37–43.
59. Jadcherla SR, Gupta A, Fernandez S, Nelin LD, Castile R, Gest AL, Welty S. Spatiotemporal characteristics of acid refluxate and relationship to symptoms in premature and term infants with chronic lung disease. Am J Gastroenterol. 2008;103:720–8.
60. Cendón RG, Jiménez MJ, Valdés JA. Fernández Pineda I, Limousin IT, López-Alonso M. Intraluminal impedance technique in the diagnosis of apparent life-threatening events (ALTE). Cir Pediatr. 2008;21:11–4.
61. Lee SH, Jang JY, Yoon IJ, Kim KM. Usefulness of multichannel intraluminal impedance-pH metry in children with suspected gastroesophageal reflux disease. Korean J Gastroenterol. 2008;52:9–15.
62. Del Buono R, Wenzl TG, Rawat D, Thomson M. Acid and non-acid gastro-esophageal reflux reflux in neurologically impaired children: investigation with the multiple intraluminal impedance procedure. J Pediatr Gastroenterol Nutr. 2006;43:331–5.
63. Loots CM, Benninga MA, Davidson GP, Omari TI. Addition of pH-impedance monitoring to standard pH monitoring increases the yield of symptom association analysis in infants and children with gastroesophageal reflux. J Pediatr. 2009;154:248–52.
64. Salvatore S, Hauser B, Devreker T, Arrigo S, Marino P, Citro C, Salvatoni A, Vandenplas Y. Esophageal impedance and esophagitis in children: any correlation? J Pediatr Gastroenterol Nutr. 2009;49:566–70.
65. Francavilla R, Magistà AM, Bucci N, Villirillo A, Boscarelli G, Mappa L, Leone G, Fico S, Castellaneta S, Indrio F, Lionetti E, Moramarco F, Cavallo L. Comparison of esophageal pH and multichannel intraluminal impedance testing in pediatric patients with suspected gastroesophageal reflux. J Pediatr Gastroenterol Nutr. 2010;50:154–60.
66. Farré R, Blondeau K, Clement D, et al. Evaluation of Esophageal Mucosa Integrity "In Vivo". Validation of basal Iintraluminal impedance measurements to assess non-erosive changes induced by esophageal acid exposure in rabbit and healthy human subjects. Gastroenterology. 2010;138:s555.
67. Kessing BF, Bredenoord AJ, Weijenborg PW, Hemmink GJM, Loots CM, Smout AJPM. Esophageal acid exposure decreases intraluminal baseline impedance levels. Am J Gastroenterol. 2011;106(12):2093–7.
68. Loots MC, Van Wijk MP, Smits JM, et al. Measurement of mucosal conductivity using multichannel intraluminal impedance; a potential marker of mucosal integrity that is restored in infants receiving acid suppression therapy. J Pediatr Gastroenterol Nutr. 2011;53:120–3.
69. Rosen R, Fritz J, Nurko A, Simon D, Nurko S. Lipid-laden macrophage index is not an indicator of gastroesophageal reflux-related respiratory disease in children. Pediatrics. 2008;121:e879–84.
70. Borrelli O, Battaglia M, Galos F, Aloi M, De Angelis D, Moretti C, Mancini V, Cucchiara S, Midulla F. Non-acid gastro-oesophageal reflux in children with suspected pulmonary aspiration. Dig Liver Dis. 2010;42:115–21.
71. Orenstein SR, Shalaby TM, Kelsey SF, Frankel E. Natural history of infant reflux esophagitis: symptoms and morphometric histology during one year without pharmacotherapy. Am J Gastroenterol. 2006;101:628–40.
72. Horvath A, Dziechciarz P, Szajewska H. The effect of thickened-feed interventions on gastroesophageal reflux in infants: systematic review and meta-analysis of randomized, controlled trials. Pediatrics. 2008;122:e1268–77.
73. Vandenplas Y. Thickened infant formula does what it has to do: decrease regurgitation. Pediatrics. 2009;123:e549–50.
74. Vandenplas Y, De Schepper J, Verheyden S, Franckx J, Devreker T, Peelman M, Denayer E, Hauser B. A preliminary report on the efficacy of the "Multicare AR-Bed(R)" in 3 weeks—3 month old infants on regurgitation, associated symptoms and acid reflux. Arch Dis Child. 2010;95:26–30.
75. Omari TI, Benninga MA, Sansom L, Butler RN, Dent J, Davidson GP. Effect of baclofen on esophagogastric motility and gastroesophageal reflux in children with gastroesophageal reflux disease: a randomized controlled trial. J Pediatr. 2006;149:468–74.
76. Del Buono R, Wenzl TG, Ball G, Keady S, Thomson M. Effect of Gaviscon Infant on gastro-oesophageal reflux in infants assessed by combined intraluminal impedance/pH. Arch Dis Child. 2005;90:460–3.
77. Spechler SJ, Lee E, Ahnen D, Goyal RK, Hirano I, Ramirez F, Raufman JP, Sampliner R, Schnell T, Sontag S, Vlahcevic ZR, Young R, Williford W. Long-term outcome of medical and surgical therapies for gastroesophageal reflux disease: follow-up of a randomized controlled trial. JAMA. 2001;285:2331–8.
78. Wijnhoven BP, Lally CJ, Kelly JJ, Myers JC, Watson DI. Use of antireflux medication after antireflux surgery. J Gastrointest Surg. 2008;12:510–7.

Infant Colic

31

David R. Fleisher

Definition

There is no universally accepted definition of infant colic [1] because there is no agreement on its nature or pathogenesis. The definition used in the present discussion is crying during the first 3 months of life for 3 or more hours per day on 3 or more days per week in infants who do not suffer other conditions that may cause prolonged crying, e.g., organic diseases, hunger, or neglect [2–4]. This definition is heuristic, with elements chosen for the purpose of defining a population to be studied.

Although there is no proof that colicky crying is caused by pain in the abdomen or any other part of the infant's body [5], nevertheless, it is widely believed that the cause of colicky crying is abdominal pain of intestinal origin [6]. As a result, infants with seemingly refractory colic are referred to pediatric gastroenterologists often enough to justify including infant colic on the list of pediatric functional gastrointestinal disorders [7].

Colicky crying is best considered within the context of "normal" infant crying during the first year. All infants cry. Brazelton's data [8], confirmed 28 years later by Barr [9], demonstrated what is referred to as "the crying curve." During the first 3 months, infants generally cry more than at any other time in their lives. Crying increases during the first month, peaks during the second month, and tends to decline thereafter. It tends to be greater in late afternoons and evenings [8, 9]. This temporal pattern of crying by infants generally is similar to the usual course of crying by colicky infants. The question remains as follows: is colicky crying etiologically different from the crying of noncolicky infants, or is it the same but at the upper end of the normal crying curve? Surprisingly, the frequency of onset of crying bouts in colicky infants is similar to that of infants in general [10], but the duration of their crying bouts is longer and they are less consolable [11]. Typical colicky crying is high pitched. Bouts may begin suddenly, without warning, and have a rapid crescendo toward peak intensity, accompanied by clinched fists, drawn-up knees, and generally increased muscle tone [12].

D.R. Fleisher, M.D. (✉)
Pediatric Gastroenterology Division, Department of Child Health, University of Missouri School of Medicine, 705 Centennial Court, Columbia, MO 65203-2993, USA
e-mail: fleisherd@health.missouri.edu

Epidemiology

Colic is virtually unknown in some primitive and traditional societies in which an infant's cry is treated as an emergency signal and responded to immediately [10]. Western societies provide less cultural reinforcement of rapid, intuitive parental responses to the crying of young infants, and their crying is more likely to be viewed as a medical problem [13, 14]. Although estimates of the prevalence of colic vary between 9 and 40% [15, 16], it is generally reported to occur in about 20% of infants [12, 17]. Colic affects infants of all

C. Faure et al. (eds.), *Pediatric Neurogastroenterology: Gastrointestinal Motility and Functional Disorders in Children*, Clinical Gastroenterology,
DOI 10.1007/978-1-60761-709-9_31, © Springer Science+Business Media New York 2013

socioeconomic classes equally, boys as often as girls and breast-fed as often as bottle-fed infants [16–18]. It is unrelated to a family history of allergy [16, 17]. There is conflicting evidence regarding the effects of prolonged labor, forceps delivery, and epidural anesthesia as predisposing factors to colic [19, 20]. These events may have transient or persistent noxious effects on the central nervous system which may cause intractable crying of organic etiology, different (by definition [2]) from the colicky crying of well babies.

Some infants with intrauterine growth retardation are born with diminished muscle tone, activity, and social responsiveness; they are unusually quiet and prefer to be left alone during the first two weeks. Thereafter, they may have long bouts of inconsolable crying which have been attributed to "neurophysiologic hypersensitivity" [21]. The relevance of this syndrome to ordinary "3 months colic" is unknown.

Differential Diagnosis of Prolonged Crying in Young Infants

Persistent and recurrent crying in early infancy may be a sign of cow's milk protein intolerance [22–25], reflux esophagitis [26], fructose intolerance, infant abuse, congenital central nervous system abnormalities, infant migraine, urinary tract infection, anomalous left coronary artery, intestinal volvulus, and other illnesses [27]. The diseases that may be misdiagnosed as infant colic usually lack its typical temporal pattern and temporary responses to effective soothing maneuvers [28, 29]. Whereas the diagnosis of organic causes of persistent crying may be confirmed by technologic tests, there is no test by which infant colic can be ruled in or ruled out.

Is colicky crying essentially different from that of the 25% of "normal" babies who cry more than 2 and 3 h per day [8, 12]? Or is it simply crying of the highest intensity, acoustically indistinguishable from crying caused by acute pain, hunger, or loneliness [28, 29]? Are the activities that accompany the crying of colic specific to colic or are they nonspecific motor accompaniments of intense crying of any cause [30]?

Research on infant colic has taken two main paths: one is based on the presumption that infant colic is (a) caused by pain, (b) that the pain is intra-abdominal, and (c) that it originates in the gastrointestinal tract. The other path is based on the presumption that colicky crying has a neurodevelopmental basis, not caused by pain or organic disease of any kind—that "colic is something that infants do, rather than a condition they have" [31].

Research based on the presumption that colic is due to abdominal pain has shown statistically significant physiologic differences between populations of colicky infants and infants who do not cry excessively. Whether these physiologic characteristics of colicky infants cause their crying, result from crying, or are produced concurrently by whatever causes the crying is an unsolved question [5, 12, 22, 23, 32–38]. Suffice to say that none of these abnormalities explain the temporal pattern or the effectiveness of soothing measures that would not be expected to relieve abdominal pain. And none have thus far led to an etiologic cure for colic [23, 24, 37].

The neurodevelopmental hypothesis is ontological. The fetus is in an almost constant steady state. Once out of the womb, however, the neonate loses its unchanging environment and is accosted by new experiences, such as hunger, thirst, visual stimulation, environmental excitement, temperature changes, and tactile experiences, to name a few. Once out of the womb, when the neonate experiences a state of feeling hungry, it reacts by making the transition to the feeding state. It is hypothesized that "colic" is the behavior of infants who have difficulty making transitions from one state to another [14]. Difficulty in state transitions might cause a baby, who is crying because it is hungry, to suck a few times when put to the breast, then pull away, arch backward, and fuss. The fussing rapidly intensifies into "colicky" crying which makes feeding temporarily impossible and can persist, even though the infant is still hungry. Similarly, a sleepy baby might be unable to make a smooth transition from being awake but sleepy to falling asleep.

Colicky infants tend to be more reactive to sensory stimuli as well as more difficult to soothe [39]. Therefore, removing distracting stimuli from the environment may make state transitions easier. This is exemplified by the infant whose nighttime feedings were made easier while being gently carried about in a dark, quiet room.

Although the duration and intensity of an infant's crying can be modified by soothing techniques, the pattern of crying during the first 3 months, referred to as "the normal crying curve," cannot be modified [1, 9]. As stated by Miller and Barr, "...crying—including that which is said to be typical of colic—may be better understood as a behavioral state that is non-specific to any one of a number of causes. Rather, those infants whose crying is labeled as colic may represent individual irritability and difficulty with state regulation, in which the cry state is more readily provoked and intractable once established [1]."

How Does Colic Subside?

At about 2–3 months of age, infants become more attentive and socially responsive. This developmental shift accompanies their acquisition of an awareness of the distinction between "self" and "other" [40]. They become better able to sooth themselves, more adaptive, and able to interact and give pleasure to their caregivers [1, 41]. These developmental shifts occur at about the age that colic subsides. One hypothesis for the disappearance of colic is that the developmental advances that occur at 2–3 months enhance their ability to manage state transitions and enable the infant to more effectively self-sooth and evoke desired behaviors from caregivers. These new abilities provide the infant with options for tension resolution other than crying. Developmental advances are smoother and accompanied by less crying if the infant's temperament is easy and the mother is caring, intuitive, and self-confident and when the dyadic relationship between them proceeds with smooth reciprocity [42, 43].

Parents may bring to the colic syndrome difficulties of their own which may present the clinician with therapeutic opportunities. Emotional tension and depression during pregnancy, adverse experiences during labor and delivery, and postpartum depression are associated with a greater prevalence of colic [20, 44–46]. Excessive crying may exacerbate maternal depression or anxiety and distort the mother's perception of what might be ordinary crying behavior [3, 45, 47].

Management

Parents who view their infant's colic as a temporary, benign pattern of behavior don't seek medical attention or, if they do, need only be effectively reassured that their baby is well [48]. However, colic can present as a crisis when the crying seems uncontrollable, when all attempts at "curing" the infant have failed, and when parents feel overwhelmed, angry, and guilty [43, 49].

The goal of management should not be to abolish the crying; nothing of what is known about the physiology of colicky infants has led to a "cure." Antispasmodics, sedatives, simethicone, formula changes, fiber supplements, and other measures based on the assumption that the crying is due to gut pain have produced little or no benefit beyond their placebo affects in most infants [38, 50–53]. A more realistic goal is helping parents through the difficult early months of their infant's development [50, 54].

Less effective management strategies involve trying a succession of harmless formulas and medications of little or no efficacy [5, 55]. Colic is a time-limited condition, highly responsive to placebo [56]. Sooner or later, one of the trial measures will "work." Sequential prescriptions give parents "something to do" in the meantime. The advantage of this approach is that it requires little of the clinician's time. One of its disadvantages is that treatments carry with them the implication that something "wrong" is being treated, and this iatrogenic stigma is reinforced when whatever is "wrong" is "cured" by a medical prescription [57]. Another disadvantage is its impact on parents whose hopes may turn to anxious despair each time a treatment fails.

The following *elements of management* are derived from frequently encountered themes during my experience with about 350 infants referred for symptoms of infant colic that were refractory to previous management.

Acknowledge the Difficulty and Importance of Their Problem

Previous clinicians may have told them that their infant has colic, that it is not serious, that it will go away, and that all that they need to do is be patient. If the parents had been able to accept such statements, they would not have come for another opinion. They need to hear that, regardless of what the term "colic" implies, it can cause great suffering and disruption of family life [43, 49, 58].

Finding and Modeling Calming Methods

A crying bout is an opportunity for the clinician to model comforting procedures, e.g., rocking and patting and responding quickly before the bout gains momentum. Successful modeling of soothing procedures should be done as a diagnostic procedure to discover what is effective, being careful to avoid the false implication that the clinician is a more competent caregiver [59].

Dismantling the Pain Theory Is Essential to Management

If the parents cannot see their child's crying as anything other than pain behavior, then, regardless of how much we tell them that colic is safe and will soon subside, they won't be satisfied. Competent parents cannot put up with watching their infant suffer pain they feel powerless to relieve. They want relief and they insist that it be given immediately. Demerol has been recommended for otherwise intractable colic, and the use of a narcotic analgesic is humane and appropriate *if* one accepts that "colic is pain" [55].

The possibility that colicky crying might *not* be due to abdominal pain is counterintuitive. Parents may have difficulty relinquishing the pain paradigm [54]. Up to this point, they may have had no other explanation for the crying, and to experience it without any explanation is to suffer existential anxiety. Good communication skills enable the clinician to make the developmental paradigm believable. Parents would probably feel better if they believe that their infants' crying is part of normal development rather than an abnormal affliction [60]. Satisfying their need to feel better about their infant helps them shift to a less troubling explanation of why their infant cries.

Affirm the Baby's Excellent Health and Great Promise

The crying is due not to a sickness or defect, but to the fact that he or she may be the kind of a normal baby that is more receptive and intensely reactive to what goes on in the environment [39]. Although such temperament characteristics make the infant more challenging and less pleasurable during the first 2–4 months, these same characteristics may make his or her personality and developmental progress more exciting and pleasurable once they get through this difficult period [61].

Affirm the Excellent Prognosis

Infant colic subsides by or before 3–4 months of age in most cases. Give the parents "light at the end of their tunnel." Coping is much more difficult without it. Carey has stated that "Optimism makes a big difference. Any treatment of colic that is accompanied by indifference or pessimism will almost certainly fail. The enthusiasm of the clinician matters enormously" [62].

Teaching Techniques for Controlling Colicky Crying

None of the above concepts will do much good if the parents don't have practical methods for controlling crying bouts. Tolerance for their baby's crying wanes rapidly. Review the list of common techniques: rocking, secure swaddling, rhythmic rolling back and forth in a pram, car rides, monotonous noise, windup swings, and many more. Bouts of crying gain momentum rapidly but are easier to stop if soothing measures are applied promptly [10, 54, 63].

Making Caregiving Easier

Advice should be individualized; find out what has worked in the past. Avoid stock recommendations regarding feeding, burping, or holding techniques, especially if they increased the baby's or the mother's discomfort [59]. For example, burping after every ounce of feed is a recommendation based on the unsubstantiated notion that swallowed air causes colic. In practice, these repeated interruptions make feedings frustrating for both infant and mother [64]. When infants accumulate air in their stomachs sufficient to cause a feeling of fullness, they spontaneously stop sucking. These pauses are ideal times to burp the baby; otherwise, he or she will experience sudden deprivations of feeding satisfaction as the mother tries to get the baby to eructate small amounts of swallowed air. Colicky babies tend to show more frequent dissatisfaction during feedings than noncolicky babies [32]. The imposition of frequent, arbitrary interruptions which ignore the infant's cues invites trouble. Should parents be advised to feed on demand or according to a schedule? Should they be told to let their baby cry or never let it cry? These questions have no "correct" answers [5]. The best way is usually the easiest way. What might be easiest for one mother might be impossibly difficult for another. Find out what is easiest for each individual infant–mother couple and support them in doing it *their easy way*. Recognize the distinction between pediatric judgment and parental judgment; respect and support the parents' judgment. Infants cannot be spoiled by being held or fed liberally [54]. However, caregiving can be "spoiled" if parents ignore their own sense of what creates distress and comfort in their infant or themselves [65].

Address the Parents' Needs

Parents may minimize or deny their stress and fatigue. They invariably provide ample evidence of it during the clinical interview. Notice it, reflect upon it, and emphasize its corrosive effect on their well-being and the overriding importance of recognizing it before it becomes disabling.

Three practices can help prevent depletion of their emotional and physical strength: *free time* [14, 49, 66], *a rescue mechanism* [49], and, for parents of infants who cry during the night, *guaranteed sleep*.

Free time is defined as scheduled windows of time during which the mother can withdraw from caring for her infant, leave the caregiving milieu, and engage in recreational activities she enjoys so that, when the interval of time-off is over, she may return to her infant refreshed. Several conditions are necessary for free time to work: (a) their duration and frequency aren't as important as whether or not they are *scheduled*. Coping with demanding tasks is made easier if one knows when a break will come. (b) The surrogate caregiver must be someone the parents feel is experienced, caring, and able to cope with a severe bout of crying. Strangers or immature babysitters won't do because the mother won't be able to focus on herself if she has to worry about her baby while she is out. (c) The surrogate caregiver needs to know that the mother will return at the promised time in order for him or her to do their job well. (d) The clinician must admonish the mother to do something that may be difficult for her, namely, to put the baby out of her thoughts; forget, as much as possible, that she is a parent; and enjoy the time for herself so that she can return from her brief absence with renewed feelings of being in love with her baby. The greatest obstacle to implementation of free time is the mother's feeling that "forgetting about" her baby and focusing on her own pleasure is unconscionable. The clinician must help her overcome her potential guilt by emphasizing that, when properly done, her free time is necessary and beneficial to her baby and to the entire family as well.

A *rescue mechanism* is defined as having a prearranged contingency plan for her husband, a trusted relative, or a friend who will come to her assistance immediately should she begin to feel overwhelmed by the demands of her infant. Like panic, feelings of becoming overwhelmed are unpredictable and may develop quite rapidly. They should be viewed as a genuine emergency.

The more confidence the mother has that help will come should she need it, the less vulnerable she will feel and the less likely she would use the rescue mechanism [41].

Guaranteed sleep is useful for parents of colicky infants who cry during the night. Either one parent (usually the mother) is designated as caregiver during the night or both parents respond simultaneously, all night long, whenever the baby needs comforting. The former arrangement may be unfair and lead to feelings of resentment. The latter practice deprives both parents of sleep. They should consider dividing the night into two 4-h shifts. The parent who is "off" can go on sleeping, while the parent who is "on" knows that when his or her 4-h shift is over, it is their turn to sleep. Four hours of guaranteed sleep is probably more restful than 8 h of apprehensive dozing in anticipation of the infant's next bout of crying.

Understanding the Infant's Needs

Many babies cry for several minutes or more prior to falling asleep. Wolff described a noncolicky infant who routinely needed to cry for awhile in order to fall asleep [30]. When he experimentally interrupted this necessary period of crying by applying soothing maneuvers, the infant stopped crying only to begin the obligatory crying period again as soon as the soothing maneuver was discontinued. The sequence (resumed crying interrupted by promptly applied soothing) could be repeated in an "on–off–on–off" pattern for half an hour or more. However, when the infant was allowed to cry without interruption, the crying subsided spontaneously within a few minutes as the infant lapsed into deep sleep.

By contrast, colicky babies don't stop crying. Their crying increases in intensity and may persist for hours. Both types of babies—those with ordinary crying and those with colicky crying—are similar in that they may respond to repeated applications of comforting maneuvers with an "on–off–on–off" response pattern. They differ, however, in their ability to get themselves to sleep; the noncolicky baby is able to make this transition into sleep and thereby stop crying; the colicky baby is not yet able to make this transition and therefore continues to cry to an extent that may result in a self-perpetuated state of sleepless crying.

Recognition of such state-transition-associated crying patterns is important because colicky infants improve with time in their ability to go to sleep. As they master this skill, their requirement for comforting changes from needing prolonged soothing, in order to prevent crying from interfering with falling asleep, to being permitted a period of uninterrupted crying during which they successfully *get themselves* to sleep. If the recently colicky infant continues to receive prompt comforting with each bout of state-transition-associated crying, it may interfere with its acquisition of improved self-regulation and self-soothing [49, 67]. As the colicky baby approaches the age of 3 months, it is advisable for the parents to experiment with letting their baby "cry itself to sleep." The end of colic is near when the baby succeeds in this.

The Supportive Role of the Clinician

Every infant–parent system is unique. Therefore, any set of recommendations for management can be no more than a point of departure from which each family develops their own ways of coping [49]. Parents need 24-h accessibility to a physician or nurse who knows them and their baby [5] so that he or she can open mindedly reassess the infant when concerns about its health arise. The physician's promise to remain accessible enables the parents to continue on task without turning to unnecessary medical diagnostic procedures or false "cures." Parents' support groups may provide an invaluable resource for deepening parents' understanding of themselves and the nurturing process [68].

The etiology of infant colic remains elusive. Nevertheless, it is almost never refractory to management, no matter how severe. If approached comprehensively, it provides clinicians with opportunities for enormous therapeutic success and satisfaction.

References

1. Miller AR, Barr RG. Infantile colic. Is it a gut issue? Pediatr Clin North Am. 1991;38(6):1497–23.
2. Wessel MA, Cobb JC, Jackson EB, Harris GS, Detwiler AC. Paroxysmal fussing in infancy, sometimes called colic. Pediatrics. 1954;14(5):421–35.
3. Carey WB. "Colic"—primary excessive crying as an infant-environment interaction. Pediatr Clin North Am. 1984;31(5):993–1005.
4. Barr RG. Colic and gas. In: Walker WA, Durie PR, Hamilton JR, et al., editors. Pediatric gastrointestinal disease. Philadelphia, PA: BC Decker; 1991. p. 56–61.
5. Treem WR. Infant colic. A pediatric gastroenterologist's perspective. Pediatr Clin North Am. 1994;41(5): 1121–38.
6. Roy CC, Silverman A, Alagille D. Pediatric clinical gastroenterology. 4th ed. St Louis: Mosby; 1995. p. 32.
7. Milla P, Hyman PE, Benninga M, Davidson G, Fleisher D, Taminau J. Infant colic. Functional gastrointestinal disorders-Rome III. McLean, VA: Degnon Associates, Inc.; 2006. p. 699–7703.
8. Brazelton TB. Crying in infancy. Pediatrics. 1962;29: 579–88.
9. Barr RG. The normal crying curve: what do we really know? Dev Med Child Neurol. 1990;32:356–62.
10. Barr RG, Konner M, Bakeman R, Adamson L. Crying in Kung San infants: a test of the cultural specificity hypothesis. Dev Med Child Neurol. 1991;33(7):601.
11. St. James-Roberts I, Hurry J, Bowyer J. Objective confirmation of crying durations in infants referred for excessive crying. Arch Dis Child. 1993;68(1):82–4.
12. Lester BM. Definition and diagnosis of colic. Colic and Excessive Crying. Report of the 105th Ross Conference on Pediatric Research, Columbus, Ohio. Ross Products Div, Abbott Laboratories; 1997. p. 18–29.
13. Sferra TJ, Heitlinger LA. Gastrointestinal gas formation and infantile colic. Pediatr Clin North Am. 1996;43(2):489–510.
14. Papousek M, von Hofacker N. Excessive crying and parenting. Colic and excessive crying. Report of the 105th Ross Conference on Pediatric Research, Columbus, Ohio. Ross Products Div., Abbott Laboratories; 1997. p. 91–101.
15. Canivet C, Hagander B, Jakobsson I, Lanke J. Infantile colic—less common than previously estimated? Acta Paediatr. 1996;85(4):454–8.
16. Stahlberg MR. Infantile colic: occurrence and risk factors. Eur J Pediatr. 1984;143(2):108–11.
17. Paradise JL. Maternal and other factors in the etiology of infantile colic: report of a prospective study of 146 infants. JAMA. 1966;197(3):191–9.
18. Lucas A, St James-Roberts I. Crying, fussing and colic behavior in breast- and bottle-fed infants. Early Hum Dev. 1998;53(1):9–18.
19. Hogdall CK, Vestermark V, Birch M, Plenov G, Toftager-Larsen K. The significance of pregnancy, delivery and postpartum factors for the development of infantile colic. J Perinat Med. 1991;19(4):251–7.
20. Thomas DB. Aetiological associations in infantile colic: an hypothesis. Aust Paediatr J. 1981;17(4):292–5.
21. Als H, Tronick E, Adamson L, Brazelton TB. The behavior of the full-term but underweight newborn infant. Dev Med Child Neurol. 1976;18(5):590–602.
22. Jakobsson I. Cow's milk protein as a cause of infantile colic. Colic and excessive crying. Report of the 105th Ross Conference on Pediatric Research, Columbus, Ohio. Ross Products Div, Abbott Laboratories; 1997. p. 39–47.
23. Thomas DW, McGilligan K, Eisenberg LD, Leiberman HM, Rissman EM. Infantile colic and type of milk feeding. Am J Dis Child. 1987;141(4):451–3.
24. Liebman WM. Infantile colic: association with lactose and milk intolerance. JAMA. 1981;245:732–3.
25. Evans RW, Fergusson DM, Allardyce RA, Taylor B. Maternal diet and infantile colic in breast-fed infants. Lancet. 1981;1(8234):1340–2.
26. Heine RG, Jaquiery A, Jubitz L, Cameron DJ, Catto-Smith AG. Role of gastro-oesophageal reflux in infant irritability. Arch Dis Child. 1995;73(2):121–5.
27. Lehtonen L, Gormally S, Barr RG. In: Barr RG, Hopkins B, Green JA, editors. Crying as a sign, a symptom and a signal. London: High Holborn House; 2000. p. 67–95.
28. Taubman B. Colic and excessive crying. Report of the 105th Ross Conference on Pediatric Research, Columbus, Ohio. Ross Products Div, Abbott Laboratories; 1997. p. 34, 160.
29. Wasz-Hockert O, Lind J, Vurenoski V, et al. The infant cry: a spectrographic and auditory analysis. Philadelphia, PA: Lippincott; 1968.
30. Wolff P. The development of behavioral states and the expression of emotions in early infancy. Chicago: U. of Chicago Press; 1987. p. 24–5, 83–4, 100.
31. Barr RG. "Colic" is something that infants do, rather than a condition they have. In: Barr RG, St James-Roberts I, Keefe MR editors. New evidence on unexplained early infant crying: its origins, nature and management. Johnson & Johnson Pediatric Institute; 2001. p. 87–104.
32. Pinyerd BJ. Mother-infant interaction and temperament when the infant has colic. In: Colic and excessive crying. Report of the 105th Ross Conference on Pediatric Research, Columbus, Ohio. Ross Products Div., Abbott Laboratories; 1997. p. 101–12.
33. Lothe L, Ivarsson SA, Ekman R, Lindberg T. Motilin and infantile colic—a prospective study. Acta Paediatr Scand. 1990;79(4):410–6.
34. Lehtonen L, Svedstrom E, Korvenranta H. Gallbladder hypocontractility in infant colic. Acta Paediatr Scand. 1994;83(11):1174–7.
35. Lehtonen L, Korvenranta H, Eerola E. Intestinal microflora in colicky and non-colicky infants: bacterial cultures and gas–liquid chromatography. J Pediatr Gastroenterol Nutr. 1994;19(3):310–4.
36. Rhoads JM, Fatheree NY, Norori J, Liu Y, Lucke JF, et al. Altered fecal microflora and increased fecal calprotectin in infants with colic. J Pediatr. 2009;155(6): 823–8. e1.

37. Treem WR, Hyams JS, Blankschen E, Etienne N, Paule CL, Borschel MW. Evaluation of the effect of a fiber-enriched formula on infant colic. J Pediatr. 1991;119(5):695–701.
38. Forsythe B. Infant formulas and colic: where are we now? In: Colic and excessive crying. Report of the 105th Ross Conference on Pediatric Research, Columbus, Ohio. Ross Products Div., Abbott Laboratories; 1997. p. 49–56.
39. Blum NJ, Taubman B, Tretina L, Heyward RY. Maternal ratings of infant intensity and distractibility: relationship with crying duration in the second month of life. Arch Peiatr Adolesc Med. 2007;156(3): 286–90.
40. Stern DN. The interpersonal world of the infant. New York: Basic Books, Inc.; 1985.p. 37–68, 9–99.
41. Schmitt BD. The prevention of sleep problems and colic. Pediatr Clin North Am. 1986;33(4):763–74.
42. Brazelton TB. Joint regulation of neonate-parent behavior. In: Tronick EZ (editor) Social interchange in infancy. Baltimore, MD: University Park Press; 1982. p. 7–22.
43. Keefe MR, Froese-Fretz A. Living with an irritable infant: maternal perspectives. MCN Am J Matern Child Nurs. 1991;16(5):255–9.
44. Rautava P, Helenius H, Lehtonen L. Psychological predisposing factors for infantile colic. Brit Med J. 1993;307(6904):600–4.
45. Miller AR, Barr RG, Eaton WO. Crying and motor behavior of six-week-old infants and postpartum maternal mood. Pediatrics. 1993;92(4):551–8.
46. Zuckerman B, Bauchner H, Parker S, Cabral H. Maternal depressive symptoms during pregnancy and newborn irritability. J Dev Behav Pediatr. 1990;11(4):190–4.
47. Lehtonen L, Korhonen T, Korvenranta H. Temperament and sleeping patterns in colicky infants during the first year of life. J Dev Behav Pediatr. 1994;15(6):416–20.
48. Fleisher D. Integration of biomedical and psychosocial management. In: Hyman PE, Dilorenzo C, editors. Pediatric gastrointestinal motility disorders. New York: Academy Professional Information Services; 1994. p. 13–31.
49. Boukydis C, High P, Cucca J, Lester B. Treatment of infants and families: the infant crying and behavior clinic model. In: Colic and excessive crying. Report of the 105th Ross Conference on Pediatric Research, Columbus, Ohio. Ross Products Div, Abbott Laboratories; 1997. p. 128–38.
50. Weissbluth M. Is there a treatment for colic? In: Colic and excessive crying. Report of the 105th Ross Conference on Pediatric Research, Columbus, Ohio, Ross Products Div, Abbott Laboratories; 1997. p. 119–23.
51. Barr RG. Herbal teas for infantile colic. J Pediatr. 1993;123(4):669. author's reply, 70–1.
52. Metcalf TJ, Irons TG, Sher LD, Young PC. Simethicone in the treatment of infant colic: a randomized, placebo-controlled, multicenter trial. Pediatrics. 1994;94(1):29–34.
53. Forsythe BW. Colic and the effect of changing formulas: a double-blind, multiple-crossover study. J Pediatr. 1989;115(4):521–6.
54. Taubman B. Clinical trial of the treatment of colic by modification of parent–infant interaction. Pediatrics. 1984;74(6):998–1003.
55. Rogers WB. Colic is pain. Pediatrics. 1996;97(4): 601–2.
56. O'Donovan JC, Bradstock AS. The failure of conventional drug therapy in the management of infantile colic. Am J Dis Child. 1979;133(10):999–1001.
57. Forsythe BW, Canny PF. Perceptions of vulnerability 3-1/2 years after problems of feeding and crying behavior in early infancy. Pediatrics. 1991;88(4): 757–63.
58. Rautava P, Lehtonen L, Helenius H, Sillanpaa M. Infantile colic: child and family three years later. Pediatrics. 1995;96(1, Pt 1):43–7.
59. High P. In: Colic and excessive crying. Report of the 105th Ross Conference on Pediatric Research. Columbus, Ohio. Ross Products Div, Abbott Laboratories; 1997. p. 127, 41-2.
60. Barr RG. Normality: a clinically useless concept—the case of infant crying and colic. J Dev Behav Pediatr. 1883;14(4):264–70.
61. Boris N. In: Colic and excessive crying. Report of the 105th Ross Conference on Pediatric Research. Columbus, Ohio. Ross Products Div, Abbott Laboratories; 1997. p. 115–6.
62. Carey WB. In: Colic and excessive crying. Report of the 105th Ross Conference on Pediatric Research. Columbus, Ohio. Ross Products Div, Abbott Laboratories; 1997. p. 144.
63. Bell SM, Ainsworth MD. Infant crying and maternal responsiveness. Child Dev. 1972;43(4):1171–90.
64. Fleisher DR. Comprehensive management of infants with gastroesophageal reflux and failure to thrive. Curr Probl Pediatr. 1995;25(8):247–53.
65. Dunn J. Distress and comfort. Cambridge, MA: Harvard U. Press; 1977. p. 22–5.
66. Barr RG. In: Walker NA, Durie PR, Hamilton JR, Walker-Smith JA, Watkins JB, editors. Pediatric gastrointestinal disease. Philadelphia, PA: BC Decker; 1996. p. 241–50.
67. Lester BM. There's more to crying than meets the ear. In: Lester BM, Boukydis C, editors. Infant crying. New York; 1985. p. 1–27.
68. Mandell D. The Red Ped groups for mothers and infants and its development into a community service program. Zero Three. 1997;17(6):44–7.

Functional Diarrhea in Toddlers (Chronic Nonspecific Diarrhea)

32

Ernesto Guiraldes and José Luis Roessler

Definition and Epidemiology

Functional diarrhea in toddlers or chronic nonspecific diarrhea (CNSD) is a frequent reason for consultation to ambulatory pediatrics and pediatric gastroenterology, being the leading cause of chronic diarrhea in otherwise well children, 1–3 years of age, from an industrialized country [1–6]. It seems to predominate in middle and upper socioeconomic strata although its exact prevalence in different regions of the world is not known. By definition, CNSD occurs without underlying, preexistent nutrient malabsorption [6].

This chapter focuses on CNSD in toddlers and older infants and excludes the protracted ("intractable") and deteriorating diarrheal syndrome, evolving from an acute diarrheal episode, and whose incidence in Western countries has sharply declined in more recent decades. This latter entity, pathophysiologically related to malnutrition and to protracted or overlapping (and often multiple) gastrointestinal infections leading to prolonged dehydration, malabsorption, and wasting, is still an important cause of secondary malnutrition and diarrheal mortality in the developing world [7, 8].

E. Guiraldes, M.D. (✉)
Pontificia Universidad Católica de Chile
and Universidad Mayor, El Bosque Sur 827,
Providencia, 7510328, Santiago, Chile
e-mail: eguirald@puc.cl

J.L. Roessler, M.D.
Pediatric Gastroenterology Division, Pediatrics
Department, Hospital Félix Bulnes, Santiago, Chile

Clinical Presentation

The consensus committee Rome III has classified CNSD within the functional digestive disorders of infancy and childhood and defined it as follows: "… CNSD is defined by daily painless recurrent passage of three or more large unformed stools for four or more weeks with onset in infancy or preschool years. There is no evidence for failure-to-thrive if the diet has adequate calories. The child appears unperturbed by the loose stools, and the symptom resolves spontaneously by school age" [6]. The Rome III diagnostic criteria proper [6] are described below, in the section "Diagnosis."

The diagnosis of CNSD should come immediately to mind in all patients 12–36 months of age, who look healthy, well nourished, and active and have a pattern of intermittent or nearly constant runny stools containing recognizable undigested vegetable matter [5]. As Hoekstra perceptively adds: "Every pediatrician knows the tableau vivant of extremely worried parents around a sparkling, healthy looking child who appears to be unaware of all the commotion" [5]. Often CNSD has begun following a viral gastroenteritis. When instructed, rather vaguely, to use

C. Faure et al. (eds.), *Pediatric Neurogastroenterology: Gastrointestinal Motility and Functional Disorders in Children*, Clinical Gastroenterology,
DOI 10.1007/978-1-60761-709-9_32, © Springer Science+Business Media New York 2013

"plenty of clear fluids," in order to prevent dehydration, parents offer recreational clear liquids time and again with the misguided belief that these constitute a physiological therapy and thus start a vicious cycle of ongoing diarrhea. Periods of improvement in stool characteristics seem to occur rather randomly while relapses may also coincide with infections (mostly upper respiratory) and other causes of biopsychosocial stress.

Pathophysiology

Given the obvious difficulty in performing prospective intervention studies on CNSD and the ethical constraints to such research, most data pertaining to this entity is retrospective (and circumstantial) and basically points to the pathogenic mechanisms discussed below.

In most cases, the mechanism of diarrhea appears, convincingly, to be related to excessive intake of fluids, particularly those with a high osmolarity, such as soft drinks and fruit juices, as well as products (and supplements) that contain fructose or sorbitol [3–5, 9]. The latter is a nonabsorbable alcohol sweetener which, when taken in certain amounts, can induce osmotic diarrhea in like fashion an excess of fructose does. Several authors have reported positive (abnormal) breath hydrogen tests after intake of fruit juices rich in fructose content, by children [10–12]. It has been suggested that in patients with CNSD, the aforementioned products generate hypermotility, a concept that is in accordance with experimental studies. A pathogenic relationship exists, too, between CNSD and the ingestion of a diet low in fat [2, 4, 5, 9], which is plausible, as fat in the diet induces a physiological slowing of intestinal transit.

Hoekstra et al. [12] have suggested that, in apple juices, in addition to fructose, the increased presence of nonabsorbable sugars resulting from the enzymatic processing of apple pulp is an important etiological factor in CNSD. The same group has discouraged the use of fructose breath tests in children suspected of CNSD because of the significant overlapping distribution of results in the control group, which would preclude any meaningful classification of abnormal vs. normal groups [12]. Lebenthal-Bendor et al. [13] studied toddlers and infants given formulae containing modified food starch (acetylated distarch phosphate) and found that this regime increased breath hydrogen and produced loose stools and, if given together with sorbitol and fructose, manifest diarrhea developed.

The limited research that has been carried out on motility and CNSD suggests that intestinal motility is disturbed in children with CNSD [14] although the available evidence does not actually prove that this is the primary mechanism of "disease." Most clinicians agree that in CNSD there is a significantly shortened time in mouth-to-anus transit [5], which would be one of the explanations for the characteristic presence of noticeable undigested vegetable material in feces. Most likely this results from a reduced colonic transit time. In children with CNSD, food may fail to interrupt the migratory motor complex (MMC: the "intestinal housekeeper," a periodic series of physiologically excitatory myoelectric and related contractile activity) [14], perhaps owing to an immature gut motor development.

It is not generally well recognized that the water content of normally looking stools is 70–75 %, while in watery stools this will be 90 %. This small increase in water content can thus make all the difference in the parental perception of health and disease [5]. In CNSD, this increase in stool water content does not entail a true malabsorptive mechanism and can be rightfully considered a "cosmetic" disorder of the stools. When the anomalous dietary patterns are corrected and the child's diet is normalized, the typical result is a sustained return to normal stools [2–6, 9].

Diagnosis

The diagnostic criteria according to the Rome III consensus [6] are as follows.

For more than 4 weeks, daily painless, recurrent passage of three or more large, unformed stools, in addition to all of these characteristics:

1. Onset of symptoms begins between 6 and 36 months of age.
2. Passage of stools occurs during waking hours.
3. There is no failure to thrive if caloric intake is adequate.

Although CNSD was described several decades ago and has recently been validated by committees of experts [6, 9], the fact is that in general pediatric practice, this is a diagnosis that often is mislabeled. Yet, the typical clinical and dietary history of toddler diarrhea, when properly elicited, should allow the practitioner to make a prompt diagnosis with minimal inconveniences and costs for the patient and family and ideally with a minimum of laboratory tests. However, the relative ease of diagnosis and simplicity of treatment of this condition are suspicious and not convincing enough to some physicians seeking a more complex pathophysiological rationale or a more "organically" based explanation. Therefore, it is not uncommon that CNSD is omitted in the differential diagnosis of children with chronic or intermittent diarrhea, and the typical symptom complex is often labeled as lactose intolerance or other enzymatic malfunction, intestinal "immaturity," food allergy, enteroparasitosis, small bowel bacterial overgrowth syndrome, or other diagnosis—popular or trendy for each geographical region or historical period [15]. These tentative diagnoses are characteristically followed by the prescription of prolonged and equally unsubstantiated dietary regimes [15] that are sometimes highly costly as well as by trials of a panoply of medications, including antibiotics, antispasmodics, or whichever product is in vogue.

While it is common in certain places that every child with chronic diarrhea is referred to a pediatric gastroenterologist, CNSD can be promptly diagnosed and treated by a proactive general practitioner or general pediatrician. The evaluation of children with chronic diarrhea requires a complete clinical history and a sound physical examination [6]. Factors that may cause or exacerbate diarrhea, such as diet, antibiotics, products with laxative effects, and past enteric infections, should be investigated. Dietary factors (already commented) are the mainstay of the history and the subsequent diagnostic rationale. When laboratory tests are performed, these should reveal no abnormalities and be consistent with a normal nutritional and absorptive status [6]. It is suggested that some alternative conditions, such as giardiasis, cryptosporidiosis, Clostridium difficile infection, and celiac disease (CD), be ruled out [6]. The latter does often cause a visible deterioration of the patient's nutritional status so it is not usually a differential diagnosis that comes to the clinician's mind faced to CNSD. However, it should be kept in mind that the nutritional and anthropometric consequences of CD may not be fully evident in the short term and that in some cases, this entity does not behave "typically" in the pediatric age range and presents in a mild fashion.

Treatment

In the absence of warning signs, the sound management of chronic nonspecific diarrhea should be based on the immediate prescription of a normal dietary regime, with a drastic reduction in the excessive fluid intake and the suppression of hyperosmolar and carbonated drinks and industrial juices mentioned above [5, 6]. It has also been suggested that frequent intake of cold fluids and ingestion of food between meals be avoided, in order to prevent a disruption on the MMC and intestinal hypermotility. A normal proportion of fat should be restored in the diet. The use of antibiotics, antidiarrheal medications, and elimination diets has no rational basis or therapeutic advantages and should thus be discouraged. Parents should be given advice and support in what regards the mechanisms and prognosis of CNSD [6] since they are typically confused and concerned at the persistence of symptoms and the lack of apparent improvement on the child's stool patterns. It is particularly important to avoid iatrogenic consequences, manifested mainly in the abuse of highly restrictive diets, which may cause nutritional deficiencies in the child and domestic disruption within the family.

References

1. Davidson M, Wasserman R. The irritable colon of childhood (chronic nonspecific diarrhea syndrome). J Pediatr. 1966;69:1027–38.
2. Cohen SA, Hendricks KM, Eastham EJ, Mathis RK, Walker WA. Chronic nonspecific diarrhea. A compli-

cation of dietary fat restriction. Am J Dis Child. 1979;133:490–2.
3. Greene HL, Ghishan FK. Excessive fluid intake as a cause of chronic diarrhea in young children. J Pediatr. 1983;102:836–40.
4. Kneepkens CMF, Hoekstra JH. Chronic nonspecific diarrhea of childhood: pathophysiology and management. Pediatr Clin N Am. 1996;43:375–90.
5. Hoekstra JH. Toddler diarrhoea: more a nutritional disorder than a disease. Arch Dis Child. 1998; 79: 2–5.
6. Hyman PE, Milla PJ, Benninga MA, Davidson GP, Fleisher DF, Taminiau J. Childhood functional gastrointestinal disorders: neonate/toddler. Gastroenterology. 2006;130:1519–26.
7. Ochoa TJ, Salazar-Lindo E, Cleary TG. Management of children with infection-associated persistent diarrhea. Semin Pediatr Infect Dis. 2004;15:229–36.
8. Fang GD, Lima AA, Martins CV, Nataro JP, Guerrant RL. Etiology and epidemiology of persistent diarrhea in northeastern Brazil: a hospital-based, prospective, case–control study. J Pediatr Gastroenterol Nutr. 1995;21:137–44.
9. Hyams J, Colletti R, Faure C, et al. Functional gastrointestinal disorders: Working Group Report of the First World Congress of Pediatric Gastroenterology, Hepatology, and Nutrition. J Pediatr Gastroenterol Nutr. 2002;35 Suppl 2:S110–7.
10. Hyams JS, Etienne NL, Leichtner AM, Theuer RC. Carbohydrate malabsorption following fruit juice ingestion in young children. Pediatrics. 1988; 82: 64–8.
11. Hoekstra JH, Van den Aker JHL, Hartemink R, Kneepkens CMF. Fruit juice malabsorption: not only fructose. Acta Paediatr. 1995;84:1241–4.
12. Hoekstra JH, Van den Aker JHL, Ghoos YF, Hartemink R, Kneepkens CMF. Fluid intake and industrial processing in apple juice induced chronic non-specific diarrhoea. Arch Dis Child. 1995;73:126–30.
13. Lebenthal-Bendor Y, Theuer RC, Lebenthal A, Tabi I, Lebenthal E. Malabsorption of modified food starch (acetylated distarch phosphate) in normal infants and in 8–24-month-old toddlers with non-specific diarrhea, as influenced by sorbitol and fructose. Acta Paediatr. 2001;90:1368–72.
14. Fenton TR, Harries JT, Milla PJ. Disordered small intestinal motility: a rational basis for toddlers' diarrhoea. Gut. 1983;24:897–903.
15. Lloyd-Still JD. Chronic diarrhea of childhood and the misuse of elimination diets. J Pediatr. 1979;95:10–3.

Functional Dyspepsia

33

Alycia Leiby and Denesh K. Chitkara

Introduction

The term "dyspepsia," originating from the Greek meaning "bad to digest," is defined as chronic or recurrent pain or discomfort centered in the upper abdomen that is characterized by symptoms of nausea, vomiting, bloating, and early satiety, all of which are usually exacerbated by food intake. Dyspepsia can also overlap with heartburn; however, heartburn alone is usually characterized as gastroesophageal reflux disease (GERD). Dyspepsia has recently been subdivided into predominant symptoms of pain in the upper abdomen, known as *epigastric pain syndrome*, versus predominant symptoms of discomfort, such as nausea, vomiting, and bloating, known as *postprandial distress syndrome*. The 2006 pediatric Rome criteria for functional dyspepsia (FD) do not distinguish between these two types though, as many young children do not fit precisely into one category or the other and there have been no studies in pediatrics validating the existence of these two entities. Essential features of FD do include persistent pain or discomfort above the umbilicus, not associated or relieved by a change of stool frequency or form, as well as a lack of evidence for inflammatory, anatomic, metabolic, or neoplastic conditions [1]. In order to satisfy the Rome criteria for FD, the pain should be present at one or more times per week for at least 2 months.

A. Leiby, M.D.
Pediatric Gastroenterology and Nutrition, Goryeb Children's Hospital, Atlantic Health, Morristown, NJ, USA

D.K. Chitkara, M.D. (✉)
Pediatric Gastroenterology and Nutrition, Goryeb Children's Hospital, Atlantic Health, Morristown, NJ, USA

Assistant Professor, Department of Pediatrics Mount Sinai School of Medicine, NY, USA

Morristown Memorial Hospital, 100 Madison Avenue, Morristown, NJ 07962, USA
e-mail: dchitkara@pol.net

Epidemiology

Upper gastrointestinal (GI) symptoms are common in children and adults. In a community-based study, 5–10% of otherwise healthy adolescents reported typical dyspeptic symptoms of nausea, heartburn, and acid brash within the past year [2]. In addition, 20% of adolescents have noted upper abdominal pain at some point during the previous year [2]. In pediatric patients who ultimately undergo an esophagogastroduodenoscopy for their symptoms, two-thirds have no evidence of mucosal inflammation and are diagnosed with FD [3]. De Giacomo et al. described a prevalence of dyspepsia of as much as 45% in a school-age population of children in Italy [4]. The annual prevalence of dyspepsia in adults in Western countries is approximately 25%, and the condition accounts for 2–5% of all primary care consultation [5]. Only approximately half of adult dyspepsia

C. Faure et al. (eds.), *Pediatric Neurogastroenterology: Gastrointestinal Motility and Functional Disorders in Children*, Clinical Gastroenterology,
DOI 10.1007/978-1-60761-709-9_33, © Springer Science+Business Media New York 2013

sufferers in Europe and the USA seek medical help for their symptoms, and yet FD remains a major source of morbidity and economic burden [5]. More importantly, dyspepsia can have a significant impact on quality of life for both children and their parents and families [6].

Pathogenesis

Dyspeptic symptoms are associated with a variety of underlying disorders, such as reflux esophagitis, peptic ulcer disease, and anatomical abnormalities. A list of the differential underlying diagnoses for dyspepsia is in Table 33.1. In a prospective audit of their patient practice, Hyams et al. characterized the underlying causes of children who presented with dyspepsia in their practice. Of the subjects who underwent evaluation with upper endoscopy, 38% had the presence of mucosal inflammation either in the esophagus, stomach, or duodenum [3]. Nine percent had *Helicobacter pylori* (*H. pylori*) with gastric inflammation [3]. The remaining 62% of children had no underlying organic, metabolic, or gastrointestinal mucosal causes identified to explain their symptoms and were characterized as having FD [3]. Similarly, in adults, the majority of individuals with symptoms of dyspepsia have FD.

The etiology of FD is best understood within the biopsychosocial model of illness. The pathophysiology of symptoms of functional dyspepsia is related to abnormalities of function in the upper gastrointestinal motor function in about 50% of adults and greater than 70% of children [7, 8]. Specifically, delayed gastric and small intestinal transit, decreased gastric accommodation, and gastric dysrhythmia [8] have been found in dyspeptic patients. In a retrospective chart review, 40% of pediatric patients with FD had slow small bowel transit as measured by radioactive egg meal and increased likelihood of bloating and abdominal pain complaints [9]. Abnormal gastric emptying has also been found by both scintigraphy and ^{13}C breath testing in multiple studies [8–10]. In addition, impaired gastric accommodation, as measured by a decreased ability of the stomach to relax in response to a meal bolus, and visceral hypersensitivity may contribute to many postprandial symptoms, particularly bloating, nausea, and early satiety [11]. Compared to healthy adults, adolescents with FD had significantly higher fasting gastric volume and lower postprandial volume change when measured by ^{99m}Tc-SPECT [10].

Table 33.1 Differential diagnosis for dyspepsia

Functional disorders
Functional dyspepsia
GERD predominant symptoms
Rumination syndrome
Post-viral gastroparesis
Abdominal migraine
Inflammatory/mucosal
Gastroesophageal reflux disease
Helicobacter pylori gastritis
Peptic ulcer
NSAID ulcer
Eosinophilic gastroenteritis
Infection: Giardia, Blastocystis hominis, Dientamoeba fragilis
Bacterial overgrowth
Inflammatory bowel disease
Menetrier's disease
Varioliform gastritis
Celiac disease
Lactose/carbohydrate malabsorption or intolerance
Henoch–Schonlein purpura
Anatomic disorders
Malrotation with/without volvulus
Duodenal web
Psychiatric disorders
Psychogenic vomiting
Depression
Somatization
Anxiety
Panic disorders
Conversion reactions
Anorexia nervosa
Others
Chronic pancreatitis
Chronic hepatitis
Ureteropelvic junction obstruction
Biliary dyskinesia
Intestinal pseudo-obstruction
Lymphoma, carcinoma

Despite the lack of mucosal inflammation in the majority of children with dyspepsia, a subset of patients has a grossly normal but microscopically inflamed duodenum and stomach. A retrospective analysis of adults with postprandial distress syndrome revealed that 47% had duodenal eosinophilia and a significant association with allergy [12]. Friesen et al. found 71% of children undergoing endoscopy for dyspepsia had duodenal eosinophilia (>10 eosinophils/hpf), and 90% of these patients responded to either a combination of H1/H2 blockade or cromolyn [13]. When compared to non-atopic children, atopic children were shown to have higher mast cell and eosinophil counts within the gastric mucosa, with mast cell activation upon cows' milk challenge [14]. Gastric dysfunction was also found in the atopic group by electrogastrography after antigen challenge. Mast cell–nerve interactions are recognized in irritable bowel syndrome and may play a role in FD [15].

An altered threshold of gut-wall receptors, an abnormal modulation in the conduction of the sensory input, or a decreased threshold for pain perception at the central level may all contribute to visceral hypersensitivity, with increased sensitivity to gastric balloon distention being specific for FD [7]. Altered motor response or altered visceral sensation to gut distention caused by substances such as lactose, fructose, fatty acids, and bile acids may explain why some patients respond clinically to dietary restrictions [16]. A wide variety of physical and psychological stress factors external to the GI tract may trigger abdominal symptoms, suggesting that dysfunction of the extrinsic innervation of the gut may also contribute to the pathogenesis of the condition. Depression and anxiety are two common comorbid conditions associated with functional GI disorders. Anxiety, particularly in hypersensitive patients, is associated with a decreased pain and discomfort threshold and decreased gastric compliance [17]. Recent evidence based on PET functional brain imaging suggests that this may be related to decreased activation of the pregenual anterior cingulate during gastric distention [18].

Clinical Presentation

Dyspepsia-associated abdominal pain is often localized to the epigastrium, in the right or left upper quadrants. In younger children, however, pain is more likely to be periumbilical. Severe epigastric pain and ulcer-like dyspepsia were significantly associated with *H. pylori* infection in children, while dysmotility-like dyspepsia was not [4]. Pain usually develops immediately after eating and persists for 3–4 h. 80% of dyspeptic patients will report more than five symptoms [19]. Nausea, pyrosis, oral regurgitation, early satiety, postprandial abdominal bloating and/or distention, excess gas with or without increased belching or flatulence, queasiness, fullness, and retching are common complaints. A history of vomiting is not uncommon. However, if vomiting is persistent and associated with "red flag" symptoms such as significant abdominal pain, hematemesis, bilious emesis, recurrent fevers, persistent weight loss, or blood in the stool, a more extensive and expedited clinical work-up is indicated [1].

Diagnosis and Evaluation

The optimal diagnostic evaluation of a child who presents with dyspepsia remains controversial. Since most patients will have functional dyspepsia, approaching the diagnosis positively facilitates optimal care. Diagnostic evaluation should be driven by an index of clinical suspicion based on pertinent alarm signs in the history and physical examination. A well-structured history, physical exam, and growth curve review is essential in patients with uninvestigated dyspepsia in order to identify those with gastroesophageal reflux disease (GERD) and exclude other structural diseases such as abdominal wall and biliary pain. It is also important to explore psychosocial factors as this can have a major impact on the success of management [1]. A reasonable initial laboratory work-up includes a full blood count, measurement of the erythrocyte sedimentation rate, chemistry profile (including liver and renal function tests), stool ova and parasite analysis, and urinalysis. Presence of *H. pylori* should be investigated for the child with severe ulcer-like dyspepsia and risk factors such as a family history of *H. pylori* and crowded or institutional living conditions [20]. The test for *H. pylori* should be a monoclonal stool antigen test, as the sensitivity and specificity may approach 100% [21], or a ^{13}C urea breath test. An upper GI series with small bowel follow-through may be indicated in children with severe abdominal pain and recurrent vomiting to rule out an anatomic disorder and/or mechanical obstruction. Serum amylase, lipase, and ultrasonography are indicated for discrete acute episodes of pain, triggered by a meal or localized to the right upper quadrants. Esophageal pH/multichannel intraluminal impedance monitoring may be useful to detect extra-esophageal manifestations of GERD and unrecognized GERD. Hydrogen breath tests may be a useful diagnostic adjunctive tool for evaluation of clinically suspected bacterial overgrowth and lactose/carbohydrate malabsorption.

In most children with dyspeptic symptoms, the likelihood of finding a mucosal abnormality is low, but patients with alarm symptoms such as weight loss, recurrent vomiting, bleeding, anemia, dysphagia, and jaundice, as well as patients frequently taking nonsteroidal anti-inflammatory drugs (NSAIDs), should be considered appropriate candidates for upper endoscopy. Endoscopy is ultimately necessary to exclude peptic ulcers, erosive esophagitis, *H. pylori* infection, gastritis, and eosinophilic esophagitis, all of which may mimic symptoms of GERD. Microscopic upper GI inflammation is common in children and adults with symptoms of dyspepsia, but its clinical significance is still unclear. These findings have been described in asymptomatic adults and patients with irritable bowel syndrome, and therefore, mild histologic gastritis or duodenitis with a macroscopically normal upper endoscopy in the absence of chronic ingestion of NSAIDs may also be consistent with a diagnosis of FD. Further evaluation of gastric and small bowel motility by scintigraphy, barostat to investigate gastric accommodation and visceral sensitivity, or manometry may be helpful to better delineate the pathophysiology of the individual's symptoms. However, these tests are invasive and should be considered as secondary or tertiary investigations in the child with atypical complaints.

Course of Illness and Prognosis

Hyams et al. described the clinical constellation and natural history of dyspepsia in children and adolescents in pediatric gastroenterology practice. A standardized questionnaire was administered by a pediatric gastroenterologist to all subjects older than 5 years of age (and their parents) treated in a referral pediatric gastroenterology practice for 1 month or more for abdominal pain or discomfort, nausea, or vomiting. Duration of symptoms of less than 1 year and vomiting were risk factors for mucosal inflammation. Follow-up at 6 months to 2 years revealed 70% of subjects were either asymptomatic or much improved regardless of the cause of dyspepsia [3]. However, the remainder had mild to no improvement or worsening of symptoms despite medical management. More recently, Miele et al. supported these findings in a prospective study of children with functional gastrointestinal disorders and found most patients improved at 3 and 12 months. Patients with FD only comprised 13% of this group, however [22].

Management

A thorough history and clinical evaluation is essential to guide management decisions and to exclude GERD and irritable bowel disease in patients with untreated dyspepsia. Historically, the initial therapy for patients with uninvestigated dyspepsia has been empirical treatment with antacids, proton pump inhibitors, and prokinetic agents, depending on symptoms. A more comprehensive approach uses the biopsychosocial model in formulating a treatment plan that involves a combination of educational, pharmacological, psychological, as well as complementary therapies (Table 33.2). Using the Rome criteria to provide a positive and expeditious diagnosis of FD helps the patient and family shift their focus away

Table 33.2 Management options for dyspepsia

1. General principles
(a) Anti-reflux measures
(b) Trigger avoidance
2. Diet
(a) Timing of meals
(b) Small, frequent meals
(c) Solid versus liquid diet
(d) Minimize high fat and excessively spicy foods
3. Pharmacology
(a) H_2 blockers—cimetidine, famotidine, ranitidine
(b) Proton pump inhibitors—omeprazole, esomeprazole, lansoprazole, pantoprazole
(c) Prokinetic agents—metoclopramide, domperidone, cisapride, erythromycin
(d) Impaired gastric accommodation—sumatriptan, buspirone
(e) Duodenal eosinophilia—montelukast
(f) Visceral hypersensitivity—amitriptyline
4. Surgical
(a) Nutritional supplementation—gastrostomy/gastrojejunostomy/jejunostomy
5. Alternative therapy
(a) Hypnotherapy
(b) Cognitive behavioral therapy
(c) Psychotherapy
(d) Acupuncture
(e) Herbal therapy—Iberogast, ginger

from continued testing and investigations to improvement of symptoms and quality of life. Determining the patient's most distressing symptom may also help to target particular treatment options and individualize therapy.

Several large studies have now shown that proton pump inhibitors (PPI) (omeprazole and lansoprazole) are more effective than H_2 antagonists in relieving symptoms of uninvestigated dyspepsia [23]. The data for omeprazole in dyspepsia indicate that patients in whom ulcer-like pain is described as the most bothersome symptom are most likely to respond to PPI therapy [24]. In these patients, full-dose omeprazole 1–2 mg/kg/day up to 40 mg daily is recommended for treatment. An empirical trial of high-dose PPI is useful to confirm the acid-related nature of dyspeptic symptoms, as patients with functional dyspepsia have been shown to have duodenal hypersensitivity to acid.

Considering that abnormal gastric emptying is often present in patients with FD, prokinetic agents are an appealing option for those with dysmotility-like symptoms, such as fullness, bloating, or early satiety. In a meta-analysis, Van Zanten et al. illustrated that both cisapride (a 5HT4 agonist) and domperidone (a dopamine antagonist) were efficacious in FD [25]. However, cisapride is no longer available through general prescription in most countries, and domperidone is currently not generally available in the USA. Metoclopramide (central and peripheral dopamine-2 antagonist) is thought to be helpful for symptoms of nausea, fullness, and bloating, but its use is limited by the neurologic side effects [26]. Low-dose erythromycin (a motilin agonist) has been shown to accelerate gastric emptying, but it also decreases gastric accommodation and may increase dyspeptic symptoms. Erythromycin also has a high occurrence of tachyphalaxis after 3–4 weeks of therapy. Medications such as sumatriptan and buspirone (5HT1 agonists) that improve gastric accommodation reflex are beginning to be evaluated for FD, but their efficacy in pediatrics has not been established [27].

Low-dose tricylic antidepressants have also been used particularly to decrease hyperalgesia and improve sleep, although the evidence for their use is stronger in irritable bowel syndrome than FD. A small study of seven adults with FD showed that all improved after 4 weeks of amitriptyline versus placebo and concluded that the increased tolerance to aversive visceral sensation was the likely mechanism [28]. Bouras et al. followed gastric sensorimotor function and postprandial symptoms in a group of 41 healthy adult volunteers given with either 25 or 50-mg amitriptyline or placebo for 2 weeks. Gastric emptying was found to be delayed in both treatment groups, without effect on gastric volume or satiation but with a significant reduction in nausea 30 min after the nutrient drink test [29]. A recent pediatric study compared amitriptyline to placebo in a mixed population of irritable bowel syndrome, FD, and functional abdominal pain in 83 children. Those that were <35 kg received 10 mg/day and those >35 kg received 20 mg/day. No difference was found between groups, but almost two-third in both groups improved, underscoring the power of placebo. Of note, anxiety scores showed significant improvement in the active treatment arm of the study.

In the subset of patients with evidence of duodenal eosinophilia [12], there is preliminary evidence to suggest that the use of montelukast, a leukotriene inhibitor, may provide benefit. Forty children with duodenal eosinophilia (>10 eosinophils/hpf) were randomized to receive 10 mg of montelukast or placebo for 2 weeks, with 62% of the treatment group showing a positive response, as measured by a rating of "improved to excellent" on a global pain relief scale, versus 32% in the placebo group [30]. The mechanism of symptom response is not clear; despite a follow-up study showing similar improvement, local eosinophilic density had not changed at the end of the trial [31].

A growing body of literature supports the use of complementary and non-pharmacologic therapy for functional GI disorders. Both hypnosis [32, 33] and guided imagery [34, 35] (a form of relaxed concentration like hypnosis) are effective and would likely be beneficial also in conjunction with conventional techniques. Biofeedback-assisted relaxation training has also been used in conjunction with standard therapy for pediatric FD with duodenal eosinophilia, showing improvement in pain intensity and duration [36]. Acupuncture may be effective for dyspeptic symptoms by improving gastric emptying and accommodation and symptoms of emesis and nausea; however, more studies are needed in this area [37, 38]. Psychological interventions, including cognitive behavioral therapy and psychotherapy, may be of particular benefit when anxiety and other psychological factors coexist [39]. A number of adult studies have looked at the use of STW 5, an herbal preparation, for FD with positive results and good safety profile [40]. This nine-herb combination, including chamomile flowers, bitter candy tuft, peppermint leaves, and licorice root, was effective in reducing the gastrointestinal symptom score in a recent multicenter, placebo-controlled, double-blind study of greater than 300 adults [41]. Ginger root also has effects on gastroduodenal motility and may be a consideration for adjunctive therapy [42, 43].

Although the evidence is not overwhelming, some patients may benefit from minimizing fatty, gaseous, and spicy foods as well as NSAID use [44] and, for those with more symptoms of dysmotility, attempting smaller, more frequent meals. Depending on the clinical setting, therapies should be considered in a systematic manner, and failure of multiple therapies should result in a referral for endoscopy.

References

1. Di Lorenzo CR, R Andree, D Forbes, E Guiraldes, J Hyams, A Staiano, LS Walker. Childhood functional gastrointestinal disorders: child/adolescent. In: Drossman DA, editor. Rome III: the functional gastrointestinal disorders, 3rd ed. McLean, VA: Degnon Associates, Inc.; 2006. p. 733–8.
2. Hyams JS, Burke G, Davis PM, Rzepski B, Andrulonis PA. Abdominal pain and irritable bowel syndrome in adolescents: a community-based study. J Pediatr. 1996;129(2):220–6.
3. Hyams JS, Davis P, Sylvester FA, Zeiter DK, Justinich CJ, Lerer T. Dyspepsia in children and adolescents: a prospective study. J Pediatr Gastroenterol Nutr. 2000; 30(4):413–8.
4. De Giacomo C, Valdambrini V, Lizzoli F, et al. A population-based survey on gastrointestinal tract symptoms and Helicobacter pylori infection in children and adolescents. Helicobacter. 2002;7(6):356–63.
5. Talley NJ. Dyspepsia: management guidelines for the millennium. Gut. 2002;50 Suppl 4:iv72–8. discussion iv79.
6. Youssef NN, Murphy TG, Langseder AL, Rosh JR. Quality of life for children with functional abdominal pain: a comparison study of patients' and parents' perceptions. Pediatrics. 2006;117(1):54–9.
7. Thumshirn M. Pathophysiology of functional dyspepsia. Gut. 2002;51 Suppl 1:i63–6.
8. Friesen CA, Lin Z, Garola R, et al. Chronic gastritis is not associated with gastric dysrhythmia or delayed solid emptying in children with dyspepsia. Dig Dis Sci. 2005;50(6):1012–8.
9. Chitkara DK, Delgado-Aros S, Bredenoord AJ, et al. Functional dyspepsia, upper gastrointestinal symptoms, and transit in children. J Pediatr. 2003;143(5):609–13.
10. Chitkara DK, Camilleri M, Zinsmeister AR, et al. Gastric sensory and motor dysfunction in adolescents with functional dyspepsia. J Pediatr. 2005;146(4):500–5.
11. Bisschops R, Karamanolis G, Arts J, et al. Relationship between symptoms and ingestion of a meal in functional dyspepsia. Gut. 2008;57(11):1495–503.
12. Walker MM, Salehian SS, Murray CE, et al. Implications of eosinophilia in the normal duodenal biopsy—an association with allergy and functional dyspepsia. Aliment Pharmacol Ther. 2010;31:1229–36.

13. Friesen CA, Sandridge L, Andre L, Roberts CC, Abdel-Rahman SM. Mucosal eosinophilia and response to H1/H2 antagonist and cromolyn therapy in pediatric dyspepsia. Clin Pediatr (Phila). 2006;45(2): 143–7.
14. Schappi MG, Borrelli O, Knafelz D, et al. Mast cell-nerve interactions in children with functional dyspepsia. J Pediatr Gastroenterol Nutr. 2008;47(4): 472–80.
15. Walker MM, Talley NJ, Prabhakar M, et al. Duodenal mastocytosis, eosinophilia and intraepithelial lymphocytosis as possible disease markers in the irritable bowel syndrome and functional dyspepsia. Aliment Pharmacol Ther. 2009;29(7):765–73.
16. Fried M, Feinle C. The role of fat and cholecystokinin in functional dyspepsia. Gut. 2002;51 Suppl 1:i54–7.
17. Van Oudenhove L, Vandenberghe J, Geeraerts B, et al. Relationship between anxiety and gastric sensorimotor function in functional dyspepsia. Psychosom Med. 2007;69(5):455–63.
18. Van Oudenhove L, Vandenberghe J, Dupont P, et al. Abnormal regional brain activity during rest and (anticipated) gastric distension in functional dyspepsia and the role of anxiety: a H(2)(15)O-PET study. Am J Gastroenterol. 2010;105(4):913–24.
19. Thomson AB, Barkun AN, Armstrong D, et al. The prevalence of clinically significant endoscopic findings in primary care patients with uninvestigated dyspepsia: the Canadian Adult Dyspepsia Empiric Treatment—Prompt Endoscopy (CADET-PE) study. Aliment Pharmacol Ther. 2003;17(12):1481–91.
20. Drumm B, Rowland M. The epidemiology of Helicobacter pylori: where to from here? J Pediatr Gastroenterol Nutr. 2003;36(1):7–8.
21. Raguza D, Machado RS, Ogata SK, Granato CF, Patricio FR, Kawakami E. Validation of a monoclonal stool antigen test for diagnosing Helicobacter pylori infection in young children. J Pediatr Gastroenterol Nutr. 2010;50(4):400–3.
22. Miele E, Simeone D, Marino A, et al. Functional gastrointestinal disorders in children: an Italian prospective survey. Pediatrics. 2004;114(1):73–8.
23. Moayyedi P, Soo S, Deeks J, Delaney B, Innes M, Forman D. Pharmacological interventions for non-ulcer dyspepsia. Cochrane Database Syst Rev. 2006;4:CD001960.
24. Talley NJ, Lauritsen K. The potential role of acid suppression in functional dyspepsia: the BOND, OPERA, PILOT, and ENCORE studies. Gut. 2002;50 Suppl 4:iv36–41.
25. Veldhuyzen van Zanten SJ, Jones MJ, Verlinden M, Talley NJ. Efficacy of cisapride and domperidone in functional (nonulcer) dyspepsia: a meta-analysis. Am J Gastroenterol. 2001;96(3):689–96.
26. FDA Requires Boxed Warning and Risk Mitigation Strategy for Metoclopramide-Containing Drugs. 2009. http://www.fda.gov/NewsEvents/Newsroom/PressAnnouncements/2009/ucm149533.htm. Accessed 27 Apr 2010.
27. Tack J. Prokinetics and fundic relaxants in upper functional GI disorders. Curr Opin Pharmacol. 2008; 8(6):690–6.
28. Mertz H, Fass R, Kodner A, Yan-Go F, Fullerton S, Mayer EA. Effect of amitriptyline on symptoms, sleep, and visceral perception in patients with functional dyspepsia. Am J Gastroenterol. 1998;93(2): 160–5.
29. Bouras EP, Talley NJ, Camilleri M, et al. Effects of amitriptyline on gastric sensorimotor function and postprandial symptoms in healthy individuals: a randomized, double-blind, placebo-controlled trial. Am J Gastroenterol. 2008;103(8):2043–50.
30. Friesen CA, Kearns GL, Andre L, Neustrom M, Roberts CC, Abdel-Rahman SM. Clinical efficacy and pharmacokinetics of montelukast in dyspeptic children with duodenal eosinophilia. J Pediatr Gastroenterol Nutr. 2004;38(3):343–51.
31. Friesen CA, Neilan NA, Schurman JV, Taylor DL, Kearns GL, Abdel-Rahman SM. Montelukast in the treatment of duodenal eosinophilia in children with dyspepsia: effect on eosinophil density and activation in relation to pharmacokinetics. BMC Gastroenterol. 2009;9:32.
32. van Tilburg MA, Chitkara DK, Palsson OS, et al. Audio-recorded guided imagery treatment reduces functional abdominal pain in children: a pilot study. Pediatrics. 2009;124(5):e890–7.
33. Vlieger AM, Menko-Frankenhuis C, Wolfkamp SC, Tromp E, Benninga MA. Hypnotherapy for children with functional abdominal pain or irritable bowel syndrome: a randomized controlled trial. Gastroenterology. 2007;133(5):1430–6.
34. Weydert JA, Shapiro DE, Acra SA, Monheim CJ, Chambers AS, Ball TM. Evaluation of guided imagery as treatment for recurrent abdominal pain in children: a randomized controlled trial. BMC Pediatr. 2006;6:29.
35. Youssef NN, Rosh JR, Loughran M, et al. Treatment of functional abdominal pain in childhood with cognitive behavioral strategies. J Pediatr Gastroenterol Nutr. 2004;39(2):192–6.
36. Schurman JV, Wu YP, Grayson P, Friesen CA. A pilot study to assess the efficacy of biofeedback-assisted relaxation training as an adjunct treatment for pediatric functional dyspepsia associated with duodenal eosinophilia. J Pediatr Psychol. 2010;35: 837–47.
37. Xu S, Hou X, Zha H, Gao Z, Zhang Y, Chen JD. Electroacupuncture accelerates solid gastric emptying and improves dyspeptic symptoms in patients with functional dyspepsia. Dig Dis Sci. 2006;51(12): 2154–9.
38. Takahashi T. Acupuncture for functional gastrointestinal disorders. J Gastroenterol. 2006;41(5):408–17.
39. Soo S, Moayyedi P, Deeks J, Delaney B, Lewis M, Forman D. Psychological interventions for non-ulcer dyspepsia. Cochrane Database Syst Rev. 2004;3:CD002301.
40. Melzer J, Rosch W, Reichling J, Brignoli R, Saller R. Meta-analysis: phytotherapy of functional dyspepsia with the herbal drug preparation STW 5 (Iberogast). Aliment Pharmacol Ther. 2004;20(11–12): 1279–87.

41. von Arnim U, Peitz U, Vinson B, Gundermann KJ, Malfertheiner P. STW 5, a phytopharmacon for patients with functional dyspepsia: results of a multicenter, placebo-controlled double-blind study. Am J Gastroenterol. 2007;102(6):1268–75.
42. Micklefield GH, Redeker Y, Meister V, Jung O, Greving I, May B. Effects of ginger on gastroduodenal motility. Int J Clin Pharmacol Ther. 1999;37(7):341–6.
43. Ghayur MN, Gilani AH. Pharmacological basis for the medicinal use of ginger in gastrointestinal disorders. Dig Dis Sci. 2005;50(10):1889–97.
44. Tack JT, NJ, Camilleri M, et al. The functional gastrointestinal disorders: functional dyspepsia. In: Drossman DA, editor. Rome III: the functional gastrointestinal disorders. McLean, VA: Virginia Degnon Associates, Inc.; 2006. p. 426–450.

Irritable Bowel Syndrome

34

Bella Zeisler and Jeffrey S. Hyams

Introduction

Chronic abdominal pain is one of the most common presenting complaints both to primary care pediatric providers and pediatric gastroenterologists. The past two decades have witnessed a dramatic change in the way chronic abdominal pain is considered, evolving from a largely pejorative psychosocial diagnosis of nonorganic pain to one in which there is increasing evidence of abnormalities in motor, sensory, autonomic, immunologic, genetic, and psychological factors resulting in disordered brain-gut communication. During this time the Rome criteria for functional gastrointestinal disorders have been developed to provide a common language describing the clinical manifestations of brain-gut disorders [1]. One such disorder, irritable bowel syndrome (IBS), commonly affects children and is the subject of this chapter. In this chapter, we will provide an overview of IBS in children while describing pathophysiological mechanisms and treatments, largely derived from adult data, which likely have pediatric applicability.

Pathophysiology of IBS

Given widely varying clinical presentations (constipation predominant (IBS-C), diarrhea predominant (IBS-D), mixed defecation pattern (IBS-M)) as well as a history of post-infectious versus not post-infectious symptom development, it is likely that multiple mechanisms contribute to the development of IBS. Whether these pathogenetic pathways are similar in children and adults is not known; though with the exception of much greater female predominance in adults, the clinical picture is quite similar. It has been suggested that noxious stimulation by gastric suction at birth may lead to long-term visceral hypersensitivity and cognitive hypervigilance resulting in a greater likelihood of developing functional intestinal disorders [2]. Physical and/or sexual trauma is a well-known risk factor for IBS in adults.

Altered Motility

Systematic studies of large numbers of children with IBS are not available. Data from adults have shown delayed colonic transit in IBS-C and accelerated colonic transit in IBS-D [3]. One study showed a disturbed rectal contractile response to meals in children with IBS [4].

B. Zeisler, M.D. • J.S. Hyams, M.D. (✉)
Division of Digestive Diseases, Hepatology, and Nutrition, Connecticut Children's Medical Center, 282 Washington Street, Hartford, CT 06106, USA
e-mail: jhyams@ccmckids.org

C. Faure et al. (eds.), *Pediatric Neurogastroenterology: Gastrointestinal Motility and Functional Disorders in Children*, Clinical Gastroenterology,
DOI 10.1007/978-1-60761-709-9_34, © Springer Science+Business Media New York 2013

Genetic Determination

The concordance rate for IBS in monozygotic twins has generally been found to be higher than in dizygotic twins. However, data suggest having a parent with IBS has a greater influence than having a twin sibling and that the heredit-ability of anxiety and depression may play large roles. It has also been proposed that gene polymorphisms involving the serotonergic, adrenergic, and opioidergic systems, as well as genes encoding proteins with neuromodulatory and immunomodulatory properties, may be important [5]. Polymorphisms in the promoter region of the serotonin reuptake transporter (SERT) protein have been associated with different forms of IBS in adults [6]. In addition, decreased measured SERT mRNA in colonic biopsy specimens has been reported in pediatric patients with IBS compared to pediatric controls, thus supporting the role of 5-HT signaling in IBS [7]. Lastly, a low prevalence of the high-producer genotype for IL-10 (an anti-inflammatory cytokine) has been noted in patients with IBS [8].

Visceral Hypersensitivity

Barostat studies have convincingly demonstrated rectal hyperalgesia in children with IBS with lowered thresholds for pain as well as abnormal pain referral after rectal distention [9, 10]. Autonomic dysfunction with increased sympathetic activity has been suggested [11].

Psychiatric Disorders and Cerebral Activation

Psychiatric disorders such as anxiety, depression, and somatization have been associated with IBS. Using advanced brain imaging techniques, differences have been shown in activation within the insula, prefrontal cortex, thalamus, and cingulate cortex in adults with IBS compared to healthy controls in response to visceral stimulation [12, 13].

Gastrointestinal Microbiota and Mucosal Immune Activation

Evidence suggests that low-grade inflammation with increased CD3+ cells, T cells, macrophages, and mast cells may play a role in IBS [14, 15]. Post-infectious IBS is well described in adults and children [16, 17]. Most published data concern IBS following bacterial infection, whereas the literature does not similarly support IBS following viral infection [18] despite anecdotal evidence to the contrary. Fecal microbiota of adults with IBS differs from healthy controls with reduced numbers of lactobacilli and *Collinsella* [19]. Controversy exists as to whether small intestinal bacterial overgrowth (SIBO) may play a role in IBS [20]; these data are largely based on lactulose breath testing rather than quantitative culture of small bowel fluid. Increased intestinal methane production has been associated with IBS-C [21]. Both oral antibiotics [22] and probiotics [23] have been shown to reduce symptoms in IBS (see below on treatment).

Epidemiology of IBS

IBS has been observed worldwide; in the United States, one study found a prevalence of 8% in middle school and 14% in high-school-aged children [24]. Up to 45% of children presenting with chronic abdominal pain in whom evaluation fails to find structural, inflammatory, or neoplastic disease have symptoms consistent with IBS [1]. Obesity has been suggested as a risk factor [25].

Clinical Manifestations

IBS is a chronic, recurring disorder involving a range of symptoms including abdominal pain or discomfort and disturbances in stool form and/or frequency. Symptoms may be severe and disabling leading to significant concern for patients, families, and practitioners. Due to extensive medical testing in patients with significant gastrointestinal complaints, monetary costs, both direct and indirect, as well as quality of life costs can be high [26, 27].

Several clinical guides have been proposed to aid practitioners in making a positive, timely diagnosis of IBS, while avoiding exhaustive medical testing that may be time consuming, expensive, and anxiety provoking. The Manning criteria published in 1978 were the first widely used validated clinical diagnostic tool for IBS [28]. Over the last decades, IBS diagnostic criteria have been refined by a succession of working teams through the Rome process, culminating in the Rome III criteria for IBS published in 2006, as a subsection of diagnostic criteria for the spectrum of functional gastrointestinal disorders. To better reflect clinical experience in pediatrics and to expedite diagnosis and treatment, there are distinct Rome III criteria for pediatrics that are more inclusive than adult criteria [29] with respect to duration of symptoms (Table 34.1).

In addition to clinical criteria for the diagnosis of IBS, the Rome III working groups have furthermore delineated 4 IBS subtypes based on stool form: IBS with constipation (IBS-C), IBS with diarrhea (IBS-D), mixed IBS (IBS-M), and un-subtyped IBS (IBS-U). Subclassification may help practitioners select more targeted therapies in clinical practice, with the caveat that symptoms may change over time and classification may not be firm.

Additional supporting symptoms not required to make the diagnosis of IBS but commonly observed include abnormal stool frequency, straining, urgency, gas bloat, passage of mucus, and sensation of incomplete evacuation. IBS has also been associated with other gastrointestinal, somatic, and psychological symptoms including upper gastrointestinal complaints (e.g., dyspepsia), fibromyalgia, headache, backache, genitourinary symptoms, anxiety, depression, and poor school performance [30].

Table 34.1 Rome III diagnostic criterion for IBS in children ages 4–18 [1]

Both of the following must include:

1. Abdominal discomfort (as defined by an uncomfortable sensation not described as pain) or pain associated with 2 or more of the following at least 25% of the time:
   - Improvement with defecation
   - Onset associated with a change is frequency of stool
   - Onset associated with a change in form (appearance) of stool
2. No evidence of an inflammatory, anatomic, metabolic, or neoplastic process that explains symptoms

Criteria must be fulfilled at least once per week for at least 2 months prior to diagnosis

Table 34.2 Alarm features in children and adolescents with abdominal pain and abnormal stool pattern [1]

- Gastrointestinal bleeding
- Perirectal disease
- Fever
- Arthritis
- Persistent vomiting
- Persistent right upper or right lower quadrant pain
- Dysphagia
- Involuntary weight loss
- Nocturnal symptoms
- Family history of inflammatory bowel disease, celiac disease, and peptic ulcer disease
- Pubertal delay

Clinical Evaluation

If the practitioner highly suspects IBS based on gastrointestinal complaints that meet Rome III criteria, and the patient exhibits no alarm signs as listed in Table 34.2, specificity for IBS is high, the diagnostic yield of further testing is generally low, and no further testing is necessary. There are limited data however, suggesting that screening for celiac disease in patients presenting with IBS symptoms may be worthwhile from a cost point of view [31, 32]. A differential diagnosis for conditions that may present similarly to IBS is provided in Table 34.3. If any red flags are raised, initial laboratory tests to consider that are relatively inexpensive and readily available include a complete blood count, erythrocyte sedimentation rate, serum aminotransferases, urinalysis, and celiac serology. The need for other diagnostic testing such as abdominal imaging, breath tests, and endoscopy will depend on the clinical judgment of the practitioner. More recently, serologic-based proprietary blood tests have been marketed to aid practitioners in the diagnosis IBS. Since there are no published data on the accuracy of these tests, their diagnostic role is not clear.

Table 34.3 Differential diagnosis of chronic abdominal pain and abnormal stool pattern

Celiac disease
Carbohydrate intolerance
Inflammatory bowel disease
Small intestinal bacterial overgrowth
Infection
Gastrointestinal polyps

Therapy

There are many approaches to the treatment of IBS involving medications, dietary manipulations, and behavioral and physical therapies. An effective treatment plan is often multifaceted and should be individually tailored and symptom directed. It must be noted that data in the pediatric literature to support the evidence-based use of any particular treatment strategy for IBS are sparse. Most therapeutic strategies are empiric and/or are extrapolated from adult studies or from studies of recurrent abdominal pain rather than irritable bowel syndrome specifically as defined by Rome criteria.

The cornerstone of successful treatment of IBS is an effective physician-patient-family relationship based on validation of pain complaints, education, and ongoing support and reassurance for the patient and family members. Realistic goals of therapy are not necessarily to eliminate symptoms, but rather to optimize patient function, quality of life, school attendance, and extracurricular participation through a biopsychosocial approach. These goals may be achieved by alleviating symptoms using appropriately selected pharmacologic and non-pharmacologic approaches, while at the same time identifying and addressing psychological comorbidities and social factors that contribute to illness behavior. In order to set realistic expectations, goals of treatment should be made clear with the patient and family from the start. Pharmaceutical and non-pharmaceutical approaches for the treatment of IBS are shown in Table 34.4.

Table 34.4 Therapeutic approaches to irritable bowel syndrome

Medications
• Antispasmodics
• Antidepressants
• Probiotics
• Antibiotics
• Melatonin
• Chloride channel agonists
• 5-HT targets (largely investigational)
• Guanylate cyclase receptor agonists (investigational)
Dietary
• Limiting possible "triggers"
• Increased fiber
Behavioral approaches
• Cognitive behavioral therapy
– Psychotherapy
– Hypnotherapy
– Guided imagery
Physical therapies
• Massage
• Acupuncture
• Reflexology

Drugs

Antispasmodics

Anticholinergic medications such as dicyclomine and hyoscyamine may produce symptom relief through inhibition of smooth muscle contraction. Despite their common use in clinical practice, pediatric studies are lacking and adult studies have not found clear efficacy [33, 34]. Anticholinergic side effects may include constipation, dry mouth, and urinary retention. Evidence has also been conflicting for the use of peppermint oil whose active ingredient, menthol, is thought to produce smooth muscle relaxation in the ileum and colon via calcium channel blocker properties. While less rigorous and/or smaller studies have yielded positive results for its use in the treatment of IBS [35–38], including one pediatric-specific study [39], other larger studies do not show efficacy [40]. However, despite a dearth of convincing evidence, peppermint oil is becoming more commonplace for the treatment of IBS likely secondary to its relatively favorable side effect profile and role as a "natural" remedy. Possible side effects of peppermint oil include rectal and esophageal burning.

Antidepressants

The mechanism of action of antidepressant medications for the treatment of IBS is not fully understood; it is likely complex, involving multiple targets on the brain-gut axis. Studies have suggested that benefit in IBS may be due to a combination of their psychotropic, neuromodulatory, and analgesic properties [41–44]. In the adult literature, there is solid evidence showing the benefit of tricyclic antidepressants (TCA) on IBS symptoms, particularly for IBS-D [45, 46]. In pediatrics, the data are limited and somewhat conflicting. One recent trial of amitriptyline for the treatment of IBS in teenagers showed overall improvement [47], whereas another recent study in a pediatric population demonstrated that amitriptyline and placebo offer similar benefit [48]. In the adult literature, there is a limited body of evidence for the use of selective serotonin reuptake inhibitors (SSRIs) in the treatment of IBS particularly for IBS-C [41, 49, 50]. However, there are no large studies for the use of SSRIs in children with IBS. In neither adult nor pediatric literature are there head-to-head trials comparing SSRIs and TCAs for use in IBS. Side effects for TCAs and SSRIs include fatigue, dizziness, headaches, cardiac dysrhythmias, and worsening depression. Constipation may be a side effect of TCAs, and diarrhea may be a side effect of SSRIs. Due to the potential side effect of cardiac dysrhythmias with TCAs and SSRIs, a baseline EKG should be considered prior to initiating therapy. Patients on antidepressant medications must be monitored carefully for signs of depression.

Probiotics

Evidence suggests that enteric flora is a regulator of mucosal inflammation and immunity, and derangements of enteric flora may contribute to IBS symptoms [14, 15]. Probiotics, which are live microorganisms capable of inducing a beneficial effect in the host, are postulated to alleviate IBS symptoms via restoration of the normal enteric flora and downregulation of mucosal inflammation. Various strains of probiotics have been studied in adults with IBS yielding mixed results. Some trials have shown benefit for the use of certain Bifidobacterium and Lactobacillus strains and VSL #3 and mixed strains of probiotics in IBS-D [23, 51–54], while other studies report negative results [55–57]. High-quality pediatric-specific studies are limited and also conflicting. While some studies of children with IBS found a modest benefit for the use of Lactobacillus GG in IBS [58, 59], a different pediatric study found that Lactobacillus GG was not superior to placebo [60]. Thus, the role of probiotics for the treatment of IBS, particularly in pediatrics, remains uncertain. In addition, the lack of quality control/quality assurance with respect to the type and number of live organisms found in the myriad probiotic products sold over the counter poses an additional challenge for their therapeutic use.

Antibiotics

With some evidence suggesting that small intestinal bacterial overgrowth (SIBO) may play a role in IBS [20], the use of antibiotics for the treatment has been investigated. Several small, short-term studies have demonstrated symptomatic improvement in adult patients with IBS treated with a course of metronidazole or the nonabsorbable antibiotic rifaximin [22, 61–63]. Large, well-designed trials that include pediatric participants are necessary to establish a definitive role for antibiotics in the treatment of IBS.

Melatonin

Melatonin is a sleep-promoting hormone primarily secreted by the brain. It has more recently been shown to be produced in the gastrointestinal tract as well, and although the mechanism remains unclear, recent investigation suggests that melatonin secretion and metabolism may be involved in the pathogenesis of IBS [64–66]. Preliminary studies have shown that administration of exogenous melatonin may have a beneficial role in IBS independent of its effect on sleep [67–69].

Chloride Channel Agonists

Lubiprostone, a bicyclic fatty acid prostaglandin E2 derivative, stimulates type 2 chloride channels in the intestine to increase fluid secretion and transit thereby improving symptoms of constipation. Lubiprostone has been US FDA approved for the treatment of adults with chronic idiopathic constipation since January 2006 and for the treatment of IBS-C in adult females since April 2008. A 2009 combined analysis of 2 phase 3, randomized, placebo-controlled studies demonstrated a higher response rate for lubiprostone compared with placebo in predominantly adult females with IBS-C [70]. Reported side effects of lubiprostone are nausea, headache, and diarrhea. Overall, the data for lubiprostone are limited and mostly available in abstract form.

5-Hydroxytryptamine (5-HT) Targets

5-HT (serotonin) is a neurotransmitter found in the gut thought to mediate gastrointestinal sensorimotor function. Recent research investigating the role of 5-HT in the pathophysiology of IBS has shown altered 5-HT signaling in the digestive mucosa [7]. As such, alosetron, a 5-HT_3 receptor antagonist, and tegaserod, a 5-HT_4 partial agonist, have been shown to be effective in the treatment of adults with IBS-D and IBS-C, respectively [71–73]. Alosetron appears to decrease visceral sensation, prolong and reduce postprandial motility, increase colonic compliance, and enhance small bowel water and salt absorption slowing down transit time [74]. Tegaserod may increase gastrointestinal motility and alter visceral sensitivity. Alosetron, released in 2000, and tegaserod, released in 2002, were subsequently withdrawn from the market shortly thereafter secondary to an association with ischemic colitis and serious adverse cardiovascular events, respectively. In the United States currently, alosetron is available for the treatment of IBS-D through restricted marketing.

Guanylate Cyclase Receptor Agonists

Linaclotide is a peptide agonist of guanylate cyclase-C. It is a first-in-class investigational drug currently in clinical development for the treatment of IBS-C. In animal studies, linaclotide has been found to stimulate intestinal fluid secretion and transit and decrease visceral hypersensitivity [75]. Human studies have shown potential benefit for constipation and IBS-C [76–78] and linaclotide recently was approved by the FDA for these indications.

Miscellaneous

Other symptom-targeted agents that are often used in patients with IBS include loperamide for the treatment of associated diarrhea and various laxatives (e.g., polyethylene glycol 3350) for the treatment of constipation. Antacids, promotility agents (e.g., metoclopramide, erythromycin), and antiemetics are used to target nausea and dyspepsia.

Dietary Approaches

Fiber

Dietary supplementation with fiber is often used as a first-line approach in patients with IBS-C, particularly in the primary care setting [79]. Fiber is postulated to shorten intestinal transit time thereby alleviating constipation and decreasing intracolonic pressure. Adult studies have shown that fiber may improve constipation but not pain associated with IBS [80–83]. In fact, the evidence suggests that insoluble fiber, in particular, may actually worsen pain in IBS due to increased gas bloat [82]. There are no pediatric-specific studies published on the use of fiber in IBS, and the limited data on the use of fiber in recurrent abdominal pain in children do not suggest clear benefit [84, 85].

Elimination Diet

Many patients perceive their IBS to be triggered by food [86, 87] and often want to discuss the role of food in their condition. In a systematic review of the literature including 7 studies that examined the severity of IBS symptoms after dietary exclusion followed by food challenge, a positive response to an elimination diet ranged from 15 to 71% [88]. Milk, wheat, eggs, and coffee were the most frequently identified offenders. As the authors of this systematic review point out, each study included had major methodological flaws, and therefore, given the difficulty for patients in maintaining elimination diets and the risk of imbalanced nutrition particularly in the pediatric population, further studies are needed to validate dietary elimination as a treatment for IBS.

There have been several recent studies linking IBS with higher food-specific IgG levels [89, 90] and positive skin prick testing [91], implicating a role for directed food elimination in the treatment of IBS. This association is currently weak, and further investigation is therefore needed.

Psychological Therapies

Cognitive behavioral therapy has been studied as a treatment for IBS. Techniques used by therapists may include psychotherapy, guided imagery, progressive muscle relaxation, and gut-directed hypnotherapy. A meta-analysis of psychological therapies in the treatment of adults with IBS showed a robust positive effect on symptoms [92]. However, as pointed out by the authors, the studies included in the analysis were highly subject to bias as none were well blinded, and true placebo groups were not incorporated into the study designs. A pediatric-focused Cochrane systematic review of psychosocial interventions (based on cognitive behavioral therapy) for recurrent abdominal pain and IBS concludes that there is some weak evidence for the efficacy of psychological therapies to treat IBS [93].

Physical Therapies

Although massage therapy, acupuncture, and reflexology have been proposed as potential treatments for IBS, there is only limited evidence to support their use.

Summary

Irritable bowel syndrome (IBS) is a commonly encountered functional gastrointestinal disorder seen in general pediatric as well as subspecialty practice. Given widely varying clinical presentations, multiple mechanisms likely contribute to the development of IBS. Current hypotheses regarding the pathophysiology of IBS involve visceral hypersensitivity, altered gastrointestinal microbiota, mucosal immune activation, psychiatric disorders and cerebral activation, and altered gastrointestinal motility. Prior to the advent of clinical criteria that culminated in the Rome III guidelines, IBS was considered a diagnosis of exclusion obliging extensive, often times low-yield medical testing in many patients. With clinical guidelines in place, the diagnosis of IBS can be usually made in a timely and efficient manner. There are myriad therapeutic options for the treatment of IBS involving medications, dietary manipulations, and behavioral and physical therapies. However, there is little strong evidence to support any one particular approach. An effective strategy is often multifaceted and should be individually tailored and symptom directed. Previous studies have demonstrated a particularly high placebo rate for the treatment of IBS [94], suggesting that with a strong physician-patient-family relationship, patients will improve regardless of the treatment approach. Future research in IBS will be focused on the pathophysiology of this disorder in the hopes of discovering more targeted therapies.

References

1. Rasquin A, Di Lorenzo C, Forbes D, et al. Childhood functional gastrointestinal disorders: child/adolescent. Gastroenterology. 2006;130(5):1527–37.
2. Anand KJ, Runeson B, Jacobson B. Gastric suction at birth associated with long-term risk for functional intestinal disorders in later life. J Pediatr. 2004;144(4):449–54.
3. Camilleri M, McKinzie S, Busciglio I, et al. Prospective study of motor, sensory, psychologic, and autonomic functions in patients with irritable bowel syndrome. Clin Gastroenterol Hepatol. 2008;6(7):772–81.
4. Van Ginkel R, Voskuijl WP, Benninga MA, Taminiau JA, Boeckxstaens GE. Alterations in rectal sensitivity and motility in childhood irritable bowel syndrome. Gastroenterology. 2001;120(1):31–8.
5. Adam B, Liebregts T, Holtmann G. Mechanisms of disease: genetics of functional gastrointestinal disorders–searching the genes that matter. Nat Clin Pract Gastroenterol Hepatol. 2007;4(2):102–10.
6. Hotoleanu C, Popp R, Trifa AP, Nedelcu L, Dumitrascu DL. Genetic determination of irritable bowel syndrome. World J Gastroenterol. 2008;14(43):6636–40.
7. Faure C, Patey N, Gauthier C, Brooks EM, Mawe GM. Serotonin signaling is altered in irritable bowel syndrome with diarrhea but not in functional dyspepsia in pediatric age patients. Gastroenterology. 2010;139(1):249–58.
8. van der Veek PP, van den Berg M, de Kroon YE, Verspaget HW, Masclee AA. Role of tumor necrosis factor-alpha and interleukin-10 gene polymorphisms in irritable bowel syndrome. Am J Gastroenterol. 2005;100(11):2510–6.

9. Faure C, Wieckowska A. Somatic referral of visceral sensations and rectal sensory threshold for pain in children with functional gastrointestinal disorders. J Pediatr. 2007;150(1):66–71.
10. Di Lorenzo C, Youssef NN, Sigurdsson L, Scharff L, Griffiths J, Wald A. Visceral hyperalgesia in children with functional abdominal pain. J Pediatr. 2001;139(6):838–43.
11. Manabe N, Tanaka T, Hata J, Kusunoki H, Haruma K. Pathophysiology underlying irritable bowel syndrome–from the viewpoint of dysfunction of autonomic nervous system activity. J Smooth Muscle Res. 2009;45(1):15–23.
12. Verne GN, Himes NC, Robinson ME, et al. Central representation of visceral and cutaneous hypersensitivity in the irritable bowel syndrome. Pain. 2003;103(1–2):99–110.
13. Arebi N, Gurmany S, Bullas D, Hobson A, Stagg A, Kamm M. Review article: the psychoneuroimmunology of irritable bowel syndrome–an exploration of interactions between psychological, neurological and immunological observations. Aliment Pharmacol Ther. 2008;28(7):830–40.
14. Chadwick VS, Chen W, Shu D, et al. Activation of the mucosal immune system in irritable bowel syndrome. Gastroenterology. 2002;122(7):1778–83.
15. Barbara G, Wang B, Stanghellini V, et al. Mast cell-dependent excitation of visceral-nociceptive sensory neurons in irritable bowel syndrome. Gastroenterology. 2007;132(1):26–37.
16. Thabane M, Simunovic M, Akhtar-Danesh N, et al. An outbreak of acute bacterial gastroenteritis is associated with an increased incidence of irritable bowel syndrome in children. Am J Gastroenterol. 2010;105(4):933–9.
17. Saps M, Pensabene L, Di Martino L, et al. Post-infectious functional gastrointestinal disorders in children. J Pediatr. 2008;152(6):812–6. 816 e811.
18. Saps M, Pensabene L, Turco R, Staiano A, Cupuro D, Di Lorenzo C. Rotavirus gastroenteritis: precursor of functional gastrointestinal disorders? J Pediatr Gastroenterol Nutr. 2009;49(5):580–3.
19. Kassinen A, Krogius-Kurikka L, Makivuokko H, et al. The fecal microbiota of irritable bowel syndrome patients differs significantly from that of healthy subjects. Gastroenterology. 2007;133(1):24–33.
20. Pimentel M, Lezcano S. Irritable Bowel Syndrome: Bacterial Overgrowth–What's Known and What to Do. Curr Treat Options Gastroenterol. 2007;10(4):328–37.
21. Chatterjee S, Park S, Low K, Kong Y, Pimentel M. The degree of breath methane production in IBS correlates with the severity of constipation. Am J Gastroenterol. 2007;102(4):837–41.
22. Pimentel M, Park S, Mirocha J, Kane SV, Kong Y. The effect of a nonabsorbed oral antibiotic (rifaximin) on the symptoms of the irritable bowel syndrome: a randomized trial. Ann Intern Med. 2006;145(8):557–63.
23. O'Mahony L, McCarthy J, Kelly P, et al. Lactobacillus and bifidobacterium in irritable bowel syndrome: symptom responses and relationship to cytokine profiles. Gastroenterology. 2005;128(3):541–51.
24. Hyams JS, Burke G, Davis PM, Rzepski B, Andrulonis PA. Abdominal pain and irritable bowel syndrome in adolescents: a community-based study. J Pediatr. 1996;129(2):220–6.
25. Teitelbaum JE, Sinha P, Micale M, Yeung S, Jaeger J. Obesity is related to multiple functional abdominal diseases. J Pediatr. 2009;154(3):444–6.
26. Longstreth GF, Wilson A, Knight K, et al. Irritable bowel syndrome, health care use, and costs: a U.S. managed care perspective. Am J Gastroenterol. 2003;98(3):600–7.
27. Wilson A, Longstreth GF, Knight K, et al. Quality of life in managed care patients with irritable bowel syndrome. Manag Care Interface. 2004;17(2):24–28, 34.
28. Manning AP, Thompson WG, Heaton KW, Morris AF. Towards positive diagnosis of the irritable bowel. Br Med J. 1978;2(6138):653–4.
29. Longstreth GF, Thompson WG, Chey WD, Houghton LA, Mearin F, Spiller RC. Functional bowel disorders. Gastroenterology. 2006;130(5):1480–91.
30. Whorwell PJ, McCallum M, Creed FH, Roberts CT. Non-colonic features of irritable bowel syndrome. Gut. 1986;27(1):37–40.
31. Mein SM, Ladabaum U. Serological testing for coeliac disease in patients with symptoms of irritable bowel syndrome: a cost-effectiveness analysis. Aliment Pharmacol Ther. 2004;19(11):1199–210.
32. Evans KE, Leeds JS, Morley S, Sanders DS. Pancreatic insufficiency in adult celiac disease: do patients require long-term enzyme supplementation? Dig Dis Sci. 2010;55(10):2999–3004.
33. Poynard T, Regimbeau C, Benhamou Y. Meta-analysis of smooth muscle relaxants in the treatment of irritable bowel syndrome. Aliment Pharmacol Ther. 2001;15(3):355–61.
34. Lesbros-Pantoflickova D, Michetti P, Fried M, Beglinger C, Blum AL. Meta-analysis: The treatment of irritable bowel syndrome. Aliment Pharmacol Ther. 2004;20(11–12):1253–69.
35. Cappello G, Spezzaferro M, Grossi L, Manzoli L, Marzio L. Peppermint oil (Mintoil) in the treatment of irritable bowel syndrome: a prospective double blind placebo-controlled randomized trial. Dig Liver Dis. 2007;39(6):530–6.
36. Merat S, Khalili S, Mostajabi P, Ghorbani A, Ansari R, Malekzadeh R. The effect of enteric-coated, delayed-release peppermint oil on irritable bowel syndrome. Dig Dis Sci. 2010;55(5):1385–90.
37. Liu JH, Chen GH, Yeh HZ, Huang CK, Poon SK. Enteric-coated peppermint-oil capsules in the treatment of irritable bowel syndrome: a prospective, randomized trial. J Gastroenterol. 1997;32(6):765–8.
38. Ford AC, Talley NJ, Spiegel BM, et al. Effect of fibre, antispasmodics, and peppermint oil in the treatment of irritable bowel syndrome: systematic review and meta-analysis. BMJ. 2008;337:a2313.
39. Kline RM, Kline JJ, Di Palma J, Barbero GJ. Enteric-coated, pH-dependent peppermint oil capsules for the treatment of irritable bowel syndrome in children. J Pediatr. 2001;138(1):125–8.

40. Pittler MH, Ernst E. Peppermint oil for irritable bowel syndrome: a critical review and metaanalysis. Am J Gastroenterol. 1998;93(7):1131–5.
41. Kilkens TO, Honig A, Rozendaal N, Van Nieuwenhoven MA, Brummer RJ. Systematic review: serotonergic modulators in the treatment of irritable bowel syndrome–influence on psychiatric and gastrointestinal symptoms. Aliment Pharmacol Ther. 2003;17(1):43–51.
42. Pasricha PJ. "Kapping" visceral pain in patients with irritable bowel syndrome: does it work? Gastroenterology. 1996;111(2):531–3.
43. Morgan V, Pickens D, Gautam S, Kessler R, Mertz H. Amitriptyline reduces rectal pain related activation of the anterior cingulate cortex in patients with irritable bowel syndrome. Gut. 2005;54(5):601–7.
44. Crowell MD. Role of serotonin in the pathophysiology of the irritable bowel syndrome. Br J Pharmacol. 2004;141(8):1285–93.
45. Jackson JL, O'Malley PG, Tomkins G, Balden E, Santoro J, Kroenke K. Treatment of functional gastrointestinal disorders with antidepressant medications: a meta-analysis. Am J Med. 2000;108(1):65–72.
46. Clouse RE, Lustman PJ, Geisman RA, Alpers DH. Antidepressant therapy in 138 patients with irritable bowel syndrome: a five-year clinical experience. Aliment Pharmacol Ther. 1994;8(4):409–16.
47. Bahar RJ, Collins BS, Steinmetz B, Ament ME. Double-blind placebo-controlled trial of amitriptyline for the treatment of irritable bowel syndrome in adolescents. J Pediatr. 2008;152(5):685–9.
48. Saps M, Youssef N, Miranda A, et al. Multicenter, randomized, placebo-controlled trial of amitriptyline in children with functional gastrointestinal disorders. Gastroenterology. 2009;137(4):1261–9.
49. Gorard DA, Libby GW, Farthing MJ. Influence of antidepressants on whole gut and orocaecal transit times in health and irritable bowel syndrome. Aliment Pharmacol Ther. 1994;8(2):159–66.
50. Tabas G, Beaves M, Wang J, Friday P, Mardini H, Arnold G. Paroxetine to treat irritable bowel syndrome not responding to high-fiber diet: a double-blind, placebo-controlled trial. Am J Gastroenterol. 2004;99(5):914–20.
51. Fan YJ, Chen SJ, Yu YC, Si JM, Liu B. A probiotic treatment containing Lactobacillus, Bifidobacterium and Enterococcus improves IBS symptoms in an open label trial. J Zhejiang Univ Sci B. 2006;7(12):987–91.
52. Whorwell PJ, Altringer L, Morel J, et al. Efficacy of an encapsulated probiotic Bifidobacterium infantis 35624 in women with irritable bowel syndrome. Am J Gastroenterol. 2006;101(7):1581–90.
53. Hong KS, Kang HW, Im JP, et al. Effect of probiotics on symptoms in korean adults with irritable bowel syndrome. Gut Liver. 2009;3(2):101–7.
54. Williams E, Stimpson J, Wang D, et al. Clinical trial: a multistrain probiotic preparation significantly reduces symptoms of irritable bowel syndrome in a double-blind placebo-controlled study. Aliment Pharmacol Ther. 2009;29(1):97–103.
55. Ligaarden SC, Axelsson L, Naterstad K, Lydersen S, Farup PG. A candidate probiotic with unfavourable effects in subjects with irritable bowel syndrome: a randomised controlled trial. BMC Gastroenterol. 2010;10:16.
56. Simren M, Ohman L, Olsson J, et al. Clinical trial: the effects of a fermented milk containing three probiotic bacteria in patients with irritable bowel syndrome—a randomized, double-blind, controlled study. Aliment Pharmacol Ther. 2010;31(2):218–27.
57. Niv E, Naftali T, Hallak R, Vaisman N. The efficacy of Lactobacillus reuteri ATCC 55730 in the treatment of patients with irritable bowel syndrome–a double blind, placebo-controlled, randomized study. Clin Nutr. 2005;24(6):925–31.
58. Francavilla R, Miniello V, Magista AM, et al. A randomized controlled trial of Lactobacillus GG in children with functional abdominal pain. Pediatrics. 2010;126(6):e1445–52.
59. Gawronska A, Dziechciarz P, Horvath A, Szajewska H. A randomized double-blind placebo-controlled trial of Lactobacillus GG for abdominal pain disorders in chil dren. Aliment Pharmacol Ther. 2007;25(2):177–84.
60. Bausserman M, Michail S. The use of Lactobacillus GG in irritable bowel syndrome in children: a double-blind randomized control trial. J Pediatr. 2005;147(2):197–201.
61. Morken MH, Valeur J, Norin E, Midtvedt T, Nysaeter G, Berstad A. Antibiotic or bacterial therapy in post-giardiasis irritable bowel syndrome. Scand J Gastroenterol. 2009;44(11):1296–303.
62. Pimentel M. Review of rifaximin as treatment for SIBO and IBS. Expert Opin Investig Drugs. 2009;18(3):349–58.
63. Fumi AL, Trexler K. Rifaximin treatment for symptoms of irritable bowel syndrome. Ann Pharmacother. 2008;42(3):408–12.
64. Radwan P, Skrzydlo-Radomanska B, Radwan-Kwiatek K, Burak-Czapiuk B, Strzemecka J. Is melatonin involved in the irritable bowel syndrome? J Physiol Pharmacol. 2009;60 Suppl 3:67–70.
65. Lu WZ, Song GH, Gwee KA, Ho KY. The effects of melatonin on colonic transit time in normal controls and IBS patients. Dig Dis Sci. 2009;54(5):1087–93.
66. Thor PJ, Krolczyk G, Gil K, Zurowski D, Nowak L. Melatonin and serotonin effects on gastrointestinal motility. J Physiol Pharmacol. 2007;58 Suppl 6:97–103.
67. Song GH, Leng PH, Gwee KA, Moochhala SM, Ho KY. Melatonin improves abdominal pain in irritable bowel syndrome patients who have sleep disturbances: a randomised, double blind, placebo controlled study. Gut. 2005;54(10):1402–7.
68. Saha L, Malhotra S, Rana S, Bhasin D, Pandhi P. A preliminary study of melatonin in irritable bowel syndrome. J Clin Gastroenterol. 2007;41(1):29–32.
69. Lu WZ, Gwee KA, Moochhalla S, Ho KY. Melatonin improves bowel symptoms in female patients with irritable bowel syndrome: a double-blind placebo-controlled study. Aliment Pharmacol Ther. 2005;22(10):927–34.

70. Drossman DA, Chey WD, Johanson JF, et al. Clinical trial: lubiprostone in patients with constipation-associated irritable bowel syndrome–results of two randomized, placebo-controlled studies. Aliment Pharmacol Ther. 2009;29(3):329–41.
71. Ford AC, Brandt LJ, Young C, Chey WD, Foxx-Orenstein AE, Moayyedi P. Efficacy of 5-HT3 antagonists and 5-HT4 agonists in irritable bowel syndrome: systematic review and meta-analysis. Am J Gastroenterol. 2009;104(7):1831–43. quiz 1844.
72. Nyhlin H, Bang C, Elsborg L, et al. A double-blind, placebo-controlled, randomized study to evaluate the efficacy, safety and tolerability of tegaserod in patients with irritable bowel syndrome. Scand J Gastroenterol. 2004;39(2):119–26.
73. Chang L, Ameen VZ, Dukes GE, McSorley DJ, Carter EG, Mayer EA. A dose-ranging, phase II study of the efficacy and safety of alosetron in men with diarrhea-predominant IBS. Am J Gastroenterol. 2005;100(1): 115–23.
74. Mayer EA, Bradesi S. Alosetron and irritable bowel syndrome. Expert Opin Pharmacother. 2003;4(11): 2089–98.
75. Eutamene H, Bradesi S, Larauche M, et al. Guanylate cyclase C-mediated antinociceptive effects of linaclotide in rodent models of visceral pain. Neurogastroenterol Motil. 2010;22(3):312–e384.
76. Lembo AJ, Kurtz CB, Macdougall JE, et al. Efficacy of linaclotide for patients with chronic constipation. Gastroenterology. 2010;138(3):886–95. e881.
77. Johnston JM, Kurtz CB, Drossman DA, et al. Pilot study on the effect of linaclotide in patients with chronic constipation. Am J Gastroenterol. 2009;104(1): 125–32.
78. Andresen V, Camilleri M, Busciglio IA, et al. Effect of 5 days linaclotide on transit and bowel function in females with constipation-predominant irritable bowel syndrome. Gastroenterology. 2007;133(3):761–8.
79. Bijkerk CJ, de Wit NJ, Stalman WA, Knottnerus JA, Hoes AW, Muris JW. Irritable bowel syndrome in primary care: the patients' and doctors' views on symptoms, etiology and management. Can J Gastroenterol. 2003;17(6):363–8. quiz 405–366.
80. Parisi GC, Zilli M, Miani MP, et al. High-fiber diet supplementation in patients with irritable bowel syndrome (IBS): a multicenter, randomized, open trial comparison between wheat bran diet and partially hydrolyzed guar gum (PHGG). Dig Dis Sci. 2002; 47(8):1697–704.
81. Akehurst R, Kaltenthaler E. Treatment of irritable bowel syndrome: a review of randomised controlled trials. Gut. 2001;48(2):272–82.
82. Francis CY, Whorwell PJ. Bran and irritable bowel syndrome: time for reappraisal. Lancet. 1994; 344(8914):39–40.
83. Lucey MR, Clark ML, Lowndes J, Dawson AM. Is bran efficacious in irritable bowel syndrome? A double blind placebo controlled crossover study. Gut. 1987;28(2):221–5.
84. Feldman W, McGrath P, Hodgson C, Ritter H, Shipman RT. The use of dietary fiber in the management of simple, childhood, idiopathic, recurrent, abdominal pain. Results in a prospective, double-blind, randomized, controlled trial. Am J Dis Child. 1985;139(12):1216–8.
85. Humphreys PA, Gevirtz RN. Treatment of recurrent abdominal pain: components analysis of four treatment protocols. J Pediatr Gastroenterol Nutr. 2000; 31(1):47–51.
86. Simren M, Mansson A, Langkilde AM, et al. Food-related gastrointestinal symptoms in the irritable bowel syndrome. Digestion. 2001;63(2):108–15.
87. Ragnarsson G, Bodemar G. Pain is temporally related to eating but not to defaecation in the irritable bowel syndrome (IBS). Patients' description of diarrhea, constipation and symptom variation during a prospective 6-week study. Eur J Gastroenterol Hepatol. 1998; 10(5):415–21.
88. Niec AM, Frankum B, Talley NJ. Are adverse food reactions linked to irritable bowel syndrome? Am J Gastroenterol. 1998;93(11):2184–90.
89. Atkinson W, Sheldon TA, Shaath N, Whorwell PJ. Food elimination based on IgG antibodies in irritable bowel syndrome: a randomised controlled trial. Gut. 2004;53(10):1459–64.
90. Zar S, Mincher L, Benson MJ, Kumar D. Food-specific IgG4 antibody-guided exclusion diet improves symptoms and rectal compliance in irritable bowel syndrome. Scand J Gastroenterol. 2005;40(7):800–7.
91. Jun DW, Lee OY, Yoon HJ, et al. Food intolerance and skin prick test in treated and untreated irritable bowel syndrome. World J Gastroenterol. 2006;12(15): 2382–7.
92. Spanier JA, Howden CW, Jones MP. A systematic review of alternative therapies in the irritable bowel syndrome. Arch Intern Med. 2003;163(3):265–74.
93. Huertas-Ceballos A, Logan S, Bennett C, Macarthur C. Psychosocial interventions for recurrent abdominal pain (RAP) and irritable bowel syndrome (IBS) in childhood. Cochrane Database Syst Rev. 2008; 23(1): CD003014.
94. Benninga MA, Mayer EA. The power of placebo in pediatric functional gastrointestinal disease. Gastroenterology. 2009;137(4):1207–10.

Functional Abdominal Pain

35

Manu R. Sood

Introduction

Functional gastrointestinal disorders (FGIDs) encompass a cluster of symptoms resulting from disorders of gastrointestinal (GI) function or central processing of information originating from the GI tract. Abdominal pain is one of the most common symptoms associated with FGIDs in children such as functional dyspepsia, irritable bowel syndrome, abdominal migraine, and functional abdominal pain (FAP). Although Rome criteria have differentiated pain-associated FGIDs into distinct categories, a degree of overlap exists. It is therefore not unusual for patients to fulfill symptom-based criteria for two or more FGIDs. Further confusion can occur when we label these disorders "functional," as some people may not understand what "functional" means. In the past, poorly descriptive terms such as idiopathic, chronic, and recurrent abdominal pain have been used to describe children with FAP. Since "recurrent abdominal pain" can be caused by many disparate conditions and does not necessarily reflect the functional nature of abdominal pain, experts in the field have recommended that this term should not be used to describe children with FAP. In this chapter, FAP implies children who fulfill the Rome criteria for FAP and, as per definition, have no identifiable cause for the pain. The term includes subjects and studies which have referred to this disorder as recurrent abdominal pain in the past.

M.R. Sood, M.D., F.R.C.P.C.H. (✉)
Chief Pediatric Gastroenterology Division, Medical College of Wisconsin, Medical Director of Pediatric Gastroenterology, Children's Hospital of Wisconsin, Milwaukee, WI 53226, USA
e-mail: MSood@mcw.edu

Definition

The Rome diagnostic criteria are widely used in research studies and are now being adapted for use in clinical practice. According to the Rome III criteria, childhood FAP is classified as abdominal pain which occurs at least once per week for at least 2 months, it can be episodic or continuous, and there are insufficient criteria for other FGIDs. There should be no evidence of an inflammatory, anatomic, metabolic, or neoplastic process that can explain the subject's symptoms [1]. Children with abdominal pain at least 25% of the time with loss of daily functioning or somatic symptoms such as headaches, limb pain, and/or difficulty sleeping should be classified under childhood functional abdominal pain syndrome [1]. This definition is a description of symptoms, and critics think it is too general, and there are very few studies which have attempted to validate the accuracy of the Rome criteria in clinical settings.

Since, the Rome criteria require the clinician to exclude inflammatory, anatomical, and metabolic disease process before diagnosing FAP, some diagnostic testing is inevitable. Alarm

C. Faure et al. (eds.), *Pediatric Neurogastroenterology: Gastrointestinal Motility and Functional Disorders in Children*, Clinical Gastroenterology,
DOI 10.1007/978-1-60761-709-9_35, © Springer Science+Business Media New York 2013

Table 35.1 Alarm symptoms suggestive of an organic disease in children with chronic abdominal pain

Symptoms
Involuntary weight loss
Vomiting especially bile or blood
GI blood loss
Unexplained fever
Persistent right upper or lower quadrant pain
Delayed puberty
Family history of IBD
Nocturnal symptoms waking the child from sleep
Dysuria, hematuria, or flank pain
Examination
Scleral icterus, pale conjunctivae
Rebound, guarding, or organomegaly
Perianal disease (skin tags, fissure, fistulae)
Occult or gross blood in the stool

symptoms which are more likely to occur in the presence of an organic disease have been proposed to circumvent this issue, but there is little clinical data regarding their accuracy (Table 35.1). Proponents of the biopsychosocial model recommend that in the absence of alarm symptoms, a presumptive diagnosis based on symptoms can be made and help avoid a diagnostic workup which is invariably negative in FAP. Recent studies suggest that the introduction of the Rome criteria has not altered physician practice behavior and diagnostic testing is still common in children with FAP [2, 3]. There are no evidence-based guidelines regarding which organic disease must be excluded or which tests are helpful before diagnosing FAP. A recent survey study suggested that the vast majority of gastroenterologists do not feel that the Rome criteria are very useful in clinical practice, and further work to refine and validate the Rome criteria is needed [4].

Epidemiology

In Apley's original survey of 1,000 primary and secondary school children, 10.8% of the children were found to have recurrent abdominal pain [5]. Subsequent studies have reported a prevalence of 0.3–25% in school-aged children [6]. The wide variability in estimated prevalence is likely to be due to different definitions and diagnostic criteria used to define FAP in these studies. Functional abdominal pain accounts for approximately 2–4% of pediatric clinic visits and almost 25% of the referrals to tertiary gastroenterology clinics [7]. Most studies evaluating symptoms in groups of children suggest there are two peaks in prevalence of FAP: one between 4 and 6 years of age and the second between 7 and 12 years of age [8, 9]. In contrast, Perquin et al. demonstrated a progressive rise in symptoms of RAP in children below 12–15 years of age [10].

The original study by Apley reported a slight female predominance with a female-to-male ratio of 1.3:1 [5]. Subsequent studies which included children and adolescents reported a female-to-male prevalence ratio of 1.4:1 [6]. Gender differences in the prevalence of FAP are not obvious in children younger than 8 years of age. In boys the prevalence in 5–10-year-olds is 10–12%, after which there is a slight decline followed by a later peak around 14 years of age. In girls there appears to be a sharp increase in reported incidence of abdominal pain after the age of 8 years [6, 10]. One study of adolescents in a suburban town in USA reported no significant difference in prevalence rates among males and females, although strict criteria for FAP were not applied [11].

Pathophysiology

Functional abdominal pain is thought to be a multifactorial disorder resulting from a complex interaction between psychosocial factors, familial genetic vulnerability, environmental factors, and earlier life experiences through the brain-gut axis (Fig. 35.1). The bidirectional brain-gut interaction in functional GI illness is well recognized. The brain receives a constant stream of input from the GI tract and integrates this with other interoceptive information from the body and the environment. It then sends an integrated response back to various target cells within the GI tract [12]. In healthy subjects, the majority of the interoceptive information reaching the brain is not consciously perceived but serves primarily as input to autonomic reflex pathways (see Fig. 35.1).

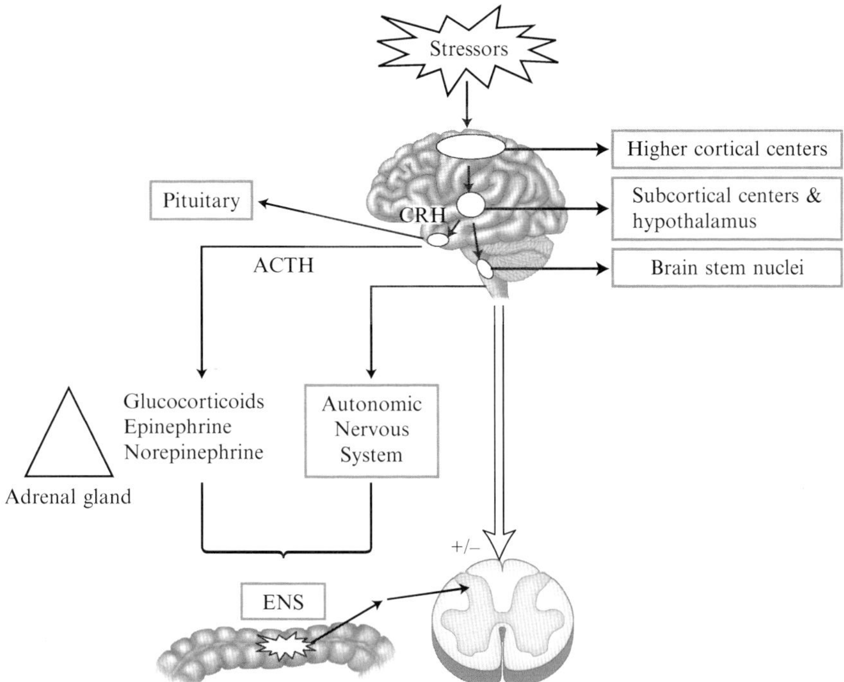

Fig. 35.1 Schematic representation of interaction between the sensory neuronal pathways and stress-related activation of the hypothalamic-pituitary-adrenal axis. The GI afferent stimulus perception is modulated by these interactions. Following activation of cortical and subcortical brain regions, increased quantities of corticotropin-releasing hormone (CRH) induces the release of adrenocorticotropin (ACTH) from the anterior pituitary. This in turn stimulates the release of glucocorticoids from the adrenal glands. In response to ANS activation, cells of the adrenal medulla produce catecholamines such as adrenaline and noradrenaline. These have potential to modulate activity of the sensory neuronal pathways and cause visceral hypersensitivity. The cortical and subcortical brain centers can facilitate or inhibit the activation of second-order spinal neurons in response to visceral afferent stimulus (adapted from Knowles and Aziz [20])

In children with FAP, the conscious perception of the interceptive information or recall of interoceptive memories of such an input can result in constant or recurrent pain. The model which incorporates peripheral and central abnormalities in patients with FAP is plausible, but the majority of the data this model is based upon are extrapolated from animal and adult human studies.

An afferent signal originating in the GI tract activates the nerve endings in the bowel wall and travels along the first-order spinal afferents which synapse with the second-order neurons in the dorsal horn of the spinal cord. The second-order neurons project to the brain through the spinoreticular, spinomesencephalic, spinohypothalamic, and spinothalamic tracts. While the first three tracts mainly activate unconscious and autonomic responses to visceral sensory input including changes in emotion and behavior, the latter transmits conscious sensation by its projections to the somatosensory cortex, anterior cingulate cortex, and the insula. The spinothalamic pathway is mainly responsible for pain localization and assessment of pain intensity, and the other three pathways modulate affective pain behavior with stimulation of important autonomic and descending inhibitory pathways (see Fig. 35.1). In animal models, the anterior cingulate cortex and its projections to the amygdala and periaqueductal gray matter of the midbrain and the rostral ventromedial medulla and the dorsolateral pontine tegmentum can selectively modulate nociceptive transmission. Stimulation of these sites inhibits responses of spinal neurons to noxious stimuli and can have an analgesic effect [13]. Therefore, second-order spinal neurons are activated by afferent input from the first-order neurons conveying messages from the bowel and inhibitory input from the brain. Disruption in this balance can result in hypersensitivity.

Peripheral sensitization represents a form of stimulus-evoked nociceptor plasticity in which more prolonged stimulation, especially in the context of inflammation or injury, leads to change in the chemical milieu that permits nociceptor firing at a lower level. The main sensitizers implicated in primary sensitization include bradykinin, histamine, serotonin, proteases, and cytokines [14]. Persistent abdominal pain following a gastrointestinal infection, surgery during infancy [15], or an inflammatory disorder such as gastroenteritis, Henoch-Schonlein purpura, and cow's milk intolerance can alter pain perception, and visceral hypersensitivity is thought to be one of the mechanisms responsible for this change [16–18].

Under physiological states, spinal afferents respond only to noxious stimuli, but under conditions of injury and inflammation of peripheral nerve endings or repetitive noxious stimulation, they can respond to lower-intensity afferent signal, a phenomenon called central sensitization [12]. Central sensitization can also affect adjacent neurons, leading to the recruitment of previously "silent" nociceptors and hyperalgesia in regions (somatic and visceral) remote to the site of peripheral sensitization. This is also termed secondary hyperalgesia. In animal models, this facilitation is triggered by presynaptic release of neurotransmitters and increased intracellular calcium which lead to phosphorylation of *N*-methyl-D-aspartate (NMDA) receptors and resultant changes in receptor kinetics. Substance P and other tachykinins play a crucial role in central sensitization [14]. Descending projections from the brain stem nuclei to the spinal cord enhance or reduce the excitability of dorsal horn neurons, which receive afferent input from the viscera, in part through the opioidergic and adrenergic descending pain inhibitory pathways. Using the water-drinking test and barostat studies, altered sensory gastric perception and visceral hypersensitivity have been reported in children with FAP [19–21].

Upregulation of central stress and arousal circuits through the hypothalamic-pituitary-adrenal axis can induce visceral hyperalgesia. Anxiety and depressive symptoms have been associated with FAP [22–25]. Children with FAP appear to be temperamentally anxious and suffer from emotional difficulties. Such temperamental traits have been associated with pessimistic worry, fear of uncertainty, harm avoidance, and a lowered response threshold to environmental challenges [23, 26]. Children with FAP also demonstrate a subliminal attention bias toward pain-related and social threat-related words, suggesting a heightened sensitivity to both internal and external threats [27]. Functional brain imaging studies in adults have shown that selectively focusing attention on visceral stimulus results in amplification of innocuous sensory events and increased activation of brain regions associated with sensory perception, attention, and motivation [13, 22]. These emotional responses are thought to play a role in the persistence and amplification of pain [22].

Early life stress can also influence illness behavior and emotional response to pain [28]. Work in animal models suggests that severe, prolonged, or repetitive pain can trigger neurobiological changes that can permanently modify pain pathways [29]. These changes are likely to be mediated through the hypothalamic-pituitary-adrenal axis [30–32]. A higher incidence of FGIDs and psychiatric comorbidities has been reported in adults who were abused as children [33, 34]. What constitutes a painful or a potential sensitizing event is not clear. Painful experiences in neonatal life have been related to altered pain processing and hypersensitivity in later life [35, 36]. A stressful life event such as marital turmoil in the family, school bullying, and being involved in an accident can predate the onset of FAP. Therefore, stressful life events both in early and later on in life seem to be a common in children with FAP. Corticotropin-releasing factor is an important hormone involved in stress response and can alter GI motility and visceral sensitivity [37].

Parenting style can influence a child's ability to cope with pain [38]. Children of parents who have IBS report more bothersome gastrointestinal symptoms compare to control children [38]. They also have more school absences and physician visits for gastrointestinal symptoms [39]. Twin studies have shown that the presence of IBS in the respondent's parents made a larger contribution to the risk of having IBS than did the presence of IBS in one's twin, suggesting social learning is more important than the environmental factors in determining illness behavior [40]. Further support for social learning in determining illness behavior comes from research showing a relationship between parental responses and children's behavior [6]. Higher levels of parental solicitousness in response to their child illness behaviors are related to higher levels of children's symptoms and disability as measured by school absences. Factors associated with solicitous behavior include non-Caucasian race, lower educational status, single mother or no partner, and parental perception of severity of their child's condition [6, 8].

Clinical Presentation and Evaluation

Functional abdominal pain is typically periumbilical and usually not associated with vomiting, weight loss, diarrhea, nocturnal symptoms, or growth deceleration. Organic abnormalities have been reported in 25–88% of children with recurrent abdominal pain [41–43]. However, the causal relationship of some of the reported abnormalities with abdominal pain is not clear. A good example is the relationship of *H. pylori* infection with abdominal pain; four studies assessed this and none found a positive association [38, 44–46]. Therefore, studies reporting positive yield of upper endoscopy in children with abdominal pain may overestimate the positive yield of upper endoscopy if they include *H. pylori* infection as an association with abdominal pain.

The majority of the GI disease which presents with abdominal pain as a symptom can be differentiated from FAP by a careful history and clinical examination (Table 35.2). Prandial or postprandial pain may be associated with pancreatobiliary disease and carbohydrate intolerance. Postprandial release of cholecystokinin stimulates gallbladder contractions and pancreatic secretions. These physiological events can induce pain in subjects with biliary tract obstruction and pancreatitis. Children with constipation and rectal fecal impaction can also present with postprandial pain [43]. The gastrocolonic reflex after the meal can result in cramping pain in the presence of hard stool in the rectum producing outlet obstruction. Intolerance to lactose or sucrose or from excess fructose or sorbitol ingestion in fruit juice can also cause pain, bloating, and diarrhea

Table 35.2 Differential diagnosis of functional abdominal pain

GI tract
Gastroesophageal reflux disease
Peptic ulcer disease
Esophagitis (peptic, eosinophilic, or infectious)
Celiac disease
Carbohydrate intolerance
Parasitic infestation
Inflammatory bowel disease
Malrotation and volvulus
Intussusception
Meckel diverticulum
Chronic appendicitis
Epiploic appendagitis
Gall bladder, liver, and pancreas
Cholelithiasis
Choledochal cyst
Hepatitis
Liver abscess
Recurrent pancreatitis
Genitourinary
Urinary tract infection
Hydronephrosis
Urolithiasis
Dysmenorrhea
Pelvic inflammatory disease
Endometriosis
Other
Gilbert's disease
Familial Mediterranean fever
Malignancies
Porphyria
Hereditary angioedema
Sickle-cell crisis
Lead poisoning
Vasculitis (e.g., Henoch-Schonlein purpura)

[47–49]. A detailed dietary history can help to identify dietary triggers and food intolerance which can present with abdominal pain. The "ritual" of this process provides important information and further assures the patient that the physician takes their complaints seriously and is seeking a cause.

Identification of troublesome symptoms, possible triggers, environmental stressors, social or emotional disturbances, impaired daily functioning, and underlying psychiatric conditions is helpful in excluding other diagnosis and comorbid conditions. It also helps to develop a patient-specific management plan. Older children and adolescent should be interviewed without their parents and assured of complete confidentiality. Physical and sexually abused children often present with functional GI symptoms.

Children with periumbilical abdominal pain and no alarm features usually do not require investigations. If the symptoms do not improve with empiric therapy or there is a high suspicion of an organic disease process investigations including a complete blood count, erythrocyte sedimentation rate, C-reactive protein, urine analysis, and culture are justified [1, 3, 50]. Other investigations such as biochemical profiles (liver and kidney), stool culture and examination for ova and parasites, and breath hydrogen testing for sugar malabsorption can be performed at the discretion of the clinician. The decision to perform these investigations is based on the child's predominant symptoms, degree of functional impairment, and parental anxiety. Plain abdominal X-ray is not a reliable investigation to diagnose constipation, except when a rectal fecal mass is suspected. Repeated negative laboratory and imaging studies can provoke anxiety, and the child may start thinking that the physician is unable to find a cause for the symptoms and a rare and unusual disease process is being missed.

In one prospective study, three trajectories based on symptom severity, psychological evaluation, functioning, and self-worth evaluation were identified [51]. Almost 70% of the subjects with low levels of symptoms and functional impairment improved within 2 months and had no recurrence at 1- and 5-year follow-up. All had low levels of anxiety and depression and scored better on self-worth compared to children in the other groups. The second trajectory classified as the short-term risk group had highest level of symptoms and functional impairment, but less severe depressive and anxiety symptoms. Symptoms in most of these patients improved in a few months, and they had no relapse in symptoms at 5-year follow-up. The third trajectory, classified as the long-term risk group, included children (14%) with high levels of symptoms and functional impairment. All had high levels of anxiety and depressive symptoms, more negative life events, and lower perceived self-worth. Children in this group had persistent symptoms during the 5-year study period. It appears that children in the short-term and long-term group would benefit from referral to a specialist center which has access to a multidisciplinary team, which includes a gastroenterologist with an interest in pain-associated FGIDs and a pain psychologist.

Management

When evaluating children with FAP, it is important to allocate sufficient time for the consult in order to allow the child and family to share their concerns. This assures them that the physician is listening and their complaints are being taken seriously. It is important to explain the pathophysiology of visceral hypersensitivity in a simple and child-friendly language. Establishing reasonable goals for improvement enables the physician to provide positive feedback and helps to maintain trust in the physician-patient relationship. Patients with prolonged or severe symptoms and a complex behavioral overlay that interfere with participation in a treatment plan may require early referral to a specialist center.

Psychological Therapy

Cognitive behavioral therapy (CBT) is based on the belief that our thoughts, behaviors, and feelings interact and aims to reduce or eliminate physical symptoms through cognitive and behavioral changes. Cognitive behavioral therapy guides patients to modify or change cognitive distortions or irrational, negative thinking to improve mood and functioning. Parental response to pain reports and beliefs about the significance of pain and levels of psychological distress in the child can affect the severity of GI symptoms and disability. Cognitive behavioral therapy would guide a patient who believes that his or her pain is a symptom of undiagnosed terminal illness to challenge this belief and consider substituting a more realistic thought, such as that the pain is likely to subside and does not represent a terminal illness. Several randomized controlled trials to test the effectiveness of pain interventions in children, using a self-management approach that includes components of CBT and involvement of parents in treatment, yielded encouraging results (Table 35.3) [52–55]. However, methodological limitations in some of these studies have made interpretation of results difficult. A recent Cochrane review thought CBT is worth considering for some children with functional abdominal pain, but better quality studies to show the efficacy of CBT are needed [56]. The American Academy of Pediatrics also rates CBT as efficacious in the treatment of FAP [57].

Relaxation treatments guide patients to reduce psychological distress by achieving a physiological state that is the opposite of how the body reacts under stress. Common relaxation techniques include abdominal breathing, progressive muscle relaxation, guided imagery, hypnotherapy, and biofeedback. Guided imagery directs patients to imagine themselves in a peaceful scene to create an experience that is incompatible with stress and anxiety. The peaceful scene is individualized for each patient and is visualized with sufficient sensory detail to absorb the patient's attention. Biofeedback is an approach that uses instruments to detect and amplify specific physical states in the body and help bring them under one's voluntary control. The mechanism of pain relief is based on specific physiological changes caused by the biofeedback. Selected physiological functions are measured such as heart rate, skin temperature, galvanic skin response, or electromyogram. Hypnotherapy includes three sequential elements: hypnotic induction, deep relaxation, and suggestion. Hypnotic induction is produced usually by eye fixation, and this sets the stage for the relaxation and deepening phases, which may incorporate the deep breathing, visualization, and muscle relaxation strategies. Once a state of deep relaxation is achieved, hypnotic suggestions are made, such as the pain is leaving your body. Most of the studies evaluating the role of relaxation therapy in FAP have reported beneficial effects [58–62]. Cognitive behavioral and relaxation therapies are emerging as the first-line treatment for children with FAP; larger and better designed studies in the future will help to confirm their beneficial effect in FAP.

Diet

Food triggers such as caffeine, fatty or large meals, carbonated soft drinks, and lactose, which exacerbate pain or gastrointestinal symptoms, should be identified, with an attempt to modify them. Lactose and fructose elimination may be useful in a small subset of patients [48, 49]. Dietary fibers may be helpful in some patients [63, 64]. Supplementing fiber can cause bloating, which may be distressing for some patients. A Cochrane review reported that there is a lack of high-quality evidence on the effectiveness of dietary interventions in children with recurrent abdominal pain. The authors also recommended that there was no evidence that fiber supplements, lactose-free diets, or Lactobacillus supplementation are effective in the management of children with RAP [65].

Pharmacotherapy

Antisecretory drugs are commonly used to treat children with abdominal pain, but their efficacy has not been evaluated. A double-blind placebo crossover trial evaluated the improvement in pain and global assessment scores in 25 children with abdominal pain. There was improvement in global assessment scores, but not in abdominal pain scores in children treated with famotidine compared to placebo [66].

Tricyclic antidepressants act primarily through noradrenergic and serotonergic pathways. They also have antimuscarinic and antihistaminic

Table 35.3 Studies using psychological therapy to treat FAP in children since 1990s. We have only included studies evaluating 10 or more children

Article	Population and study design	Intervention/control	Outcome
Levy et al. (2010)	*n*=200, 7–17 years RCS	CBT: • Relaxation training • Modify family response to illness • Cognitive restructuring Control group: • Educational support • 3 sessions each group • FU: 6-month posttreatment	Greater decrease in pain and GI symptoms in CBT group Less parental solicitous responses in CBT group
Duarte et al. (2006)	*n*=32, 5–13 years RCS	CBT: • Psycho-education • Cognitive and behavioral strategies • Self-monitoring Control group: SMC 4 monthly sessions FU: 4 months	CBT had higher reduction in pain scores compared to controls (86.6 vs. 33.3%) No significant difference in pressure pain threshold
Hicks et al. (2006)	*n*=47, 9–16 years RCS Recurrent headaches and abdominal pain	CBT: • Relaxation • Cognitive strategies (self-talk) Control: SMC Online and telephone sessions FU: 3 months	CBT group had significant improvement in pain scores compared to controls (72 vs. 14%) at 3-month follow-up
Robins et al. (2005)	*n*=69, 6–16 years RCS	CBT: • Psycho-education • Relaxation • Coping strategies Control : SMC Five 50-min sessions FU: 1 year	Significantly less abdominal pain in the CBT group compared to controls. Benefit maintained at 1-year FU No significant difference in functional disability
Sanders et al. (1994)	*n*=44, 6–12years RCS	CBT: • Parent contingency management • Relaxation training • Cognitive (self-talk) Control: wait list Six 50-min sessions	Both groups reported significant decrease in pain CBT group had lower relapse rate and higher rate of complete pain relief

van Tilburg et al. (2009)	$n=34$, 6–15 years RCS	Home-based guided imagery SMC 2 months treatment FU: 6 months	Treatment responders more in GI group compared to SMC (63.1 vs. 26.7%) 61.5% of SMC patients responded to GI Treatment benefit was maintained for 6 months
Vlieger et al. (2007)	$n=53$, 8–18 years RCS	Relaxation/hypnotherapy • General relaxation • Gut-directed hypnotherapy • Ego-strengthening suggestions Control: SMC Six 50-min sessions for 3 months FU: 1 year	Both groups had significant decrease in pain intensity and frequency Decrease was more marked in hypnotherapy group compared to controls (85 vs. 25%)
Weydert et al. (2006)	$N=22$, 5–18 years RCS	Guided imagery with progressive muscle relaxation Control: breathing exercises Four weekly 60-min sessions FU: 3 months	Significantly greater decrease in pain frequency and missed activities in GI group compare to controls (82 vs. 45%) at 2-month follow-up
Ball et al. (2003)	$n=11$, 5–18 years	Relaxation • Abdominal breathing • Progressive muscle relaxation • Visualization Control: wait list Four sessions	Significant decrease in pain episodes. All patients randomized to wait list withdrew from the study
Humphreys and Gervitz (2000)	$n=64$, 4–18 years RCS	Comparison between 4 randomized conditions: Fiber alone Fiber and relaxation Fiber, relaxation, and CBT Fiber, relaxation, CBT, and parent training Eight-session duration not stated	All groups reported reduction in pain. Fiber alone has 79% reduction in pain reports, and fiber and relaxation have 100% reduction in pain reports Addition of CBT and parent training has no additional benefit Three psychological treatments had greater benefit compared to fiber alone (70.6 vs. 38.1%)

properties. Tricyclic antidepressants with sedative properties can help children with sleep disruption and FAP. But their role in treatment of FAP is controversial. A multicenter placebo-controlled study of 90 children with FAP, irritable bowel syndrome, and functional dyspepsia compared the effect of 4-week amitriptyline therapy with placebo [67]. A total of 63% of patients reported feeling better in the amitriptyline group compared with 57.5% in the placebo group. None of the outcome variables were significantly different between the two groups. A fixed dose for a relatively short period of time was used in this trial. Future studies evaluating the effect of an escalating dosage schedule for a relatively longer period of time would help to clarify the role of tricyclic antidepressants in the treatment of FAP.

Another study evaluated citalopram, a selective serotonin reuptake inhibitor, in 25 children with FAP aged 7–18 years. In this flexible-dose, open-label trial, the initial daily dose of citalopram was 10 mg for a week, increasing to 20 mg at week 2 and then 40 mg at week 4 if there was no clinical response and the medication was well tolerated. Total duration of treatment was 12 weeks [68]. The primary outcome measure was Clinical Global Impression Scale-Improvement. Secondary outcome measures included self- and parental reports of abdominal pain, anxiety, depression, somatic symptoms, and functional impairment. Eighty-four percent of patients were classified as responders in whom the abdominal pain rating, anxiety, depression, and functional impairment all improved significantly. It is not clear if the primary beneficial effect of selective serotonin reuptake inhibitor therapy in FAP is through modulation of brain regions involved in visceral sensation or due to their effect on psychiatric comorbid symptoms.

Low-grade bowel inflammation and immune alteration have been reported in adults with IBS and are associated with changes in the gut flora. In post-infectious IBS patients, probiotics can help to restore the qualitative and quantitative changes in indigenous gut flora and improve symptoms [9]. Lactobacillus GG therapy for 4 weeks was compared to placebo in 104 children with FAP, functional dyspepsia, or irritable bowel syndrome [69]. Twenty-five percent of children in the Lactobacillus GG group compared to 9.6% in the placebo group had improvement in abdominal pain. In this study, children with irritable bowel syndrome were more likely to respond to Lactobacillus GG therapy compared to children with FAP. Another study compared 8-week *Lactobacillus rhamnosus* GG therapy in 141 children with irritable bowel syndrome and FAP with placebo [70]. At week 12, improvement in abdominal pain was achieved in 72% subjects in the probiotics group compared to 53% in the placebo group. Probiotics may be helpful in treating children with pain-associated FGIDs, but their mechanisms of action are not well understood. Modulation of gastrointestinal lumen toward an anti-inflammatory state and conversion of undigested carbohydrates into short-chain fatty acids may help to improve gut function.

Outcome

The relationship between FAP and FGIDs in adult life is controversial. A weak association between FAP in childhood and headaches and IBS in adult life has been suggested [71]. A recent meta-analysis of 18 studies that included 1,331 children with FAP who were followed for a median of 5 years, 29.1% continued to report abdominal pain at follow-up [72]. Chitkara et al. reported that 18–61% of children with FAP continue to report symptom of abdominal pain 5–30 years later [6]. The risk factors associated with poor prognosis include onset of symptoms before 6 years of age, duration of symptoms more than 6 months, family history of pain-related FGIDs, multiple surgical procedures, low educational level, and socioeconomic status [73, 74]. Mulvaney et al. identified higher levels of anxiety, depression, lower self-worth perception, and more negative life events in subjects who had poor outcome at 5-year follow-up [51].

Summary

Functional abdominal pain is one of the most common FGIDs of childhood. Since there are no identifiable structural abnormalities of the GI tract and no diagnostic tests to evaluate alterations in GI function in FAP, it is primarily a clinical diagnosis. Development of symptom-based criteria has helped in clinical decision making; however, further work is required to validate their accuracy in a clinical setting. Psychological comorbidities, functional disability, and parental perception of the severity of their child's illness have important bearing on treatment outcome. Recent data suggest that psychological therapy is effective in the vast majority of children and is likely to emerge as the first-line treatment for FAP in the coming years. Medication and dietary alterations serve as useful adjuncts to psychological treatment.

References

1. Rasquin A, Di Lorenzo C, Forbes D, Guiraldes E, Hyams JS, Staiano A, Walker LS. Childhood functional gastrointestinal disorders: child/adolescent. Gastroenterology. 2006;130:1527–37.
2. Schurman JV, Hunter HL, Friesen CA. Conceptualization and treatment of chronic abdominal pain in pediatric gastroenterology practice. J Pediatr Gastroenterol Nutr. 2010;50:32–7.
3. Dhroove G, Chogle A, Saps M. A million-dollar work-up for abdominal pain: is it worth it? J Pediatr Gastroenterol Nutr. 2010;51:579–83.
4. Sood MR, Di Lorenzo C, Hyams J, et al. Beliefs and Attitudes of General Pediatricians and Pediatric Gastroenterologists Regarding Functional Gastrointestinal Disorders—A Survey Study. Clin Pediatr. 2011;50(10):891–6.
5. Apley J, Naish N. Recurrent abdominal pains: a field survey of 1,000 school children. Arch Dis Child. 1958;33:165–70.
6. Chitkara DK, Rawat DJ, Talley NJ. The epidemiology of childhood recurrent abdominal pain in Western countries: a systematic review. Am J Gastroenterol. 2005;100:1868–75.
7. Starfield B, Hoekelman RA, McCormick M, Benson P, Mendenhall RC, Moynihan C, Radecki S. Who provides health care to children and adolescents in the United States? Pediatrics. 1984;74:991–7.
8. Alfven G. The covariation of common psychosomatic symptoms among children from socio-economically differing residential areas. An epidemiological study. Acta Paediatr. 1993;82:484–7.
9. Petersen S, Bergstrom E, Brulin C. High prevalence of tiredness and pain in young schoolchildren. Scand J Public Health. 2003;31:367–74.
10. Perquin CW, Hazebroek-Kampschreur AA, Hunfeld JA, Bohnen AM, van Suijlekom-Smit LW, Passchier J, van der Wouden JC. Pain in children and adolescents: a common experience. Pain. 2000;87:51–8.
11. Hyams JS, Burke G, Davis PM, Rzepski B, Andrulonis PA. Abdominal pain and irritable bowel syndrome in adolescents: a community-based study. J Pediatr. 1996;129:220–6.
12. Mayer EA, Tillisch K. The brain-gut axis in abdominal pain syndromes. Annu Rev Med. 2011;62:381–96.
13. Farmer AD, Aziz Q. Visceral pain hypersensitivity in functional gastrointestinal disorders. Br Med Bull. 2009;91:123–36.
14. Wood JD. Functional abdominal pain: the basic science. J Pediatr Gastroenterol Nutr. 2008;47:688–93.
15. Bonilla S, Saps M. Early Life Events: Infants with Pyloric Stenosis Have a Higher Risk of Developing Chronic Abdominal Pain in Childhood. J Pediatr. 2011;159(4):551–4.
16. Saps M, Pensabene L, Turco R, Staiano A, Cupuro D, Di Lorenzo C. Rotavirus gastroenteritis: precursor of functional gastrointestinal disorders? J Pediatr Gastroenterol Nutr. 2009;49:580–3.
17. Saps M, Dhroove G, Chogle A. Henoch-Schonlein Purpura Leads to Functional Gastrointestinal Disorders. Dig Dis Sci. 2011;56(6):1789–93.
18. Saps M, Lu P, Bonilla S. Cow's-milk allergy is a risk factor for the development of FGIDs in children. J Pediatr Gastroenterol Nutr. 2011;52:166–9.
19. Walker LS, Williams SE, Smith CA, Garber J, Van Slyke DA, Lipani T, Greene JW, Mertz H, Naliboff BD. Validation of a symptom provocation test for laboratory studies of abdominal pain and discomfort in children and adolescents. J Pediatr Psychol. 2006;31:703–13.
20. Di Lorenzo C, Youssef NN, Sigurdsson L, Scharff L, Griffiths J, Wald A. Visceral hyperalgesia in children with functional abdominal pain. J Pediatr. 2001;139:838–43.
21. Halac U, Noble A, Faure C. Rectal sensory threshold for pain is a diagnostic marker of irritable bowel syndrome and functional abdominal pain in children. J Pediatr. 2010;156:60–65. e1.
22. Knowles CH, Aziz Q. Basic and clinical aspects of gastrointestinal pain. Pain. 2009;141:191–209.
23. Campo JV, Bridge J, Ehmann M, Altman S, Lucas A, Birmaher B, Di Lorenzo C, Iyengar S, Brent DA. Recurrent abdominal pain, anxiety, and depression in primary care. Pediatrics. 2004;113:817–24.
24. Walker LS, Garber J, Greene JW. Psychosocial correlates of recurrent childhood pain: a comparison of pediatric patients with recurrent abdominal pain, organic illness, and psychiatric disorders. J Abnorm Psychol. 1993;102:248–58.
25. Hodges K, Kline JJ, Barbero G, Woodruff C. Anxiety in children with recurrent abdominal pain and their parents. Psychosomatics. 1985;26(859):862–6.
26. Davison IS, Faull C, Nicol AR. Research note: temperament and behaviour in six-year-olds with recurrent abdominal pain: a follow up. J Child Psychol Psychiatry. 1986;27:539–44.
27. Boyer MC, Compas BE, Stanger C, Colletti RB, Konik BS, Morrow SB, Thomsen AH. Attentional biases to pain and social threat in children with recurrent abdominal pain. J Pediatr Psychol. 2006; 31:209–20.

28. Miranda A. Early life events and the development of visceral hyperalgesia. J Pediatr Gastroenterol Nutr. 2008;47:682–4.
29. Miranda A, Peles S, Shaker R, Rudolph C, Sengupta JN. Neonatal nociceptive somatic stimulation differentially modifies the activity of spinal neurons in rats and results in altered somatic and visceral sensation. J Physiol. 2006;572:775–87.
30. Greenwood-Van Meerveld B, Johnson AC, Cochrane S, Schulkin J, Myers DA. Corticotropin-releasing factor 1 receptor-mediated mechanisms inhibit colonic hypersensitivity in rats. Neurogastroenterol Motil. 2005;17:415–22.
31. Miranda A, Peles S, Rudolph C, Shaker R, Sengupta JN. Altered visceral sensation in response to somatic pain in the rat. Gastroenterology. 2004;126:1082–9.
32. Miranda A. Early life stress and pain: an important link to functional bowel disorders. Pediatr Ann. 2009;38:279–82.
33. Whitehead WE, Crowell MD, Davidoff AL, Palsson OS, Schuster MM. Pain from rectal distension in women with irritable bowel syndrome: relationship to sexual abuse. Dig Dis Sci. 1997;42:796–804.
34. Ringel Y, Whitehead WE, Toner BB, Diamant NE, Hu Y, Jia H, Bangdiwala SI, Drossman DA. Sexual and physical abuse are not associated with rectal hypersensitivity in patients with irritable bowel syndrome. Gut. 2004;53:838–42.
35. Peters JW, Schouw R, Anand KJ, van Dijk M, Duivenvoorden HJ, Tibboel D. Does neonatal surgery lead to increased pain sensitivity in later childhood? Pain. 2005;114:444–54.
36. Andrews KA, Desai D, Dhillon HK, Wilcox DT, Fitzgerald M. Abdominal sensitivity in the first year of life: comparison of infants with and without prenatally diagnosed unilateral hydronephrosis. Pain. 2002; 100:35–46.
37. Nozu T, Okumura T. Visceral sensation and irritable bowel syndrome; with special reference to comparison with functional abdominal pain syndrome. J Gastroenterol Hepatol. 2011;26 Suppl 3:122–7.
38. Bode G, Brenner H, Adler G, Rothenbacher D. Recurrent abdominal pain in children: evidence from a population-based study that social and familial factors play a major role but not Helicobacter pylori infection. J Psychosom Res. 2003;54:417–21.
39. Campo JV, Bridge J, Lucas A, Savorelli S, Walker L, Di Lorenzo C, Iyengar S, Brent DA. Physical and emotional health of mothers of youth with functional abdominal pain. Arch Pediatr Adolesc Med. 2007; 161:131–7.
40. Levy RL, Jones KR, Whitehead WE, Feld SI, Talley NJ, Corey LA. Irritable bowel syndrome in twins: heredity and social learning both contribute to etiology. Gastroenterology. 2001;121:799–804.
41. Alfven G. One hundred cases of recurrent abdominal pain in children: diagnostic procedures and criteria for a psychosomatic diagnosis. Acta Paediatr. 2003; 92:43–9.
42. Croffie JM, Fitzgerald JF, Chong SK. Recurrent abdominal pain in children–a retrospective study of outcome in a group referred to a pediatric gastroenterology practice. Clin Pediatr (Phila). 2000;39:267–74.
43. Gijsbers C, Benninga M, Buller H. Clinical and laboratory findings in 220 children with recurrent abdominal pain. Acta Paediatr. 2011;100(7):1028–32.
44. O'Donohoe JM, Sullivan PB, Scott R, Rogers T, Brueton MJ, Barltrop D. Recurrent abdominal pain and Helicobacter pylori in a community-based sample of London children. Acta Paediatr. 1996;85:961–4.
45. De Giacomo C, Valdambrini V, Lizzoli F, Gissi A, Palestra M, Tinelli C, Zagari M, Bazzoli F. A population-based survey on gastrointestinal tract symptoms and Helicobacter pylori infection in children and adolescents. Helicobacter. 2002;7:356–63.
46. Kokkonen J, Haapalahti M, Tikkanen S, Karttunen R, Savilahti E. Gastrointestinal complaints and diagnosis in children: a population-based study. Acta Paediatr. 2004;93:880–6.
47. Lebenthal E, Rossi TM, Nord KS, Branski D. Recurrent abdominal pain and lactose absorption in children. Pediatrics. 1981;67:828–32.
48. Huertas-Ceballos A, Macarthur C, Logan S. Dietary interventions for recurrent abdominal pain (RAP) in childhood. Cochrane Database Syst Rev 2002:CD003019
49. Gomara RE, Halata MS, Newman LJ, Bostwick HE, Berezin SH, Cukaj L, See MC, Medow MS. Fructose intolerance in children presenting with abdominal pain. J Pediatr Gastroenterol Nutr. 2008;47:303–8.
50. Dodge JA. Recurrent abdominal pain in children. Br Med J. 1976;1:385–7.
51. Mulvaney S, Lambert EW, Garber J, Walker LS. Trajectories of symptoms and impairment for pediatric patients with functional abdominal pain: a 5-year longitudinal study. J Am Acad Child Adolesc Psychiatry. 2006;45:737–44.
52. Duarte MA, Penna FJ, Andrade EM, Cancela CS, Neto JC, Barbosa TF. Treatment of nonorganic recurrent abdominal pain: cognitive-behavioral family intervention. J Pediatr Gastroenterol Nutr. 2006;43:59–64.
53. Robins PM, Smith SM, Glutting JJ, Bishop CT. A randomized controlled trial of a cognitive-behavioral family intervention for pediatric recurrent abdominal pain. J Pediatr Psychol. 2005;30:397–408.
54. Sanders MR, Rebgetz M, Morrison M, Bor W, Gordon A, Dadds M, Shepherd R. Cognitive-behavioral treatment of recurrent nonspecific abdominal pain in children: an analysis of generalization, maintenance, and side effects. J Consult Clin Psychol. 1989;57:294–300.
55. Sanders MR, Shepherd RW, Cleghorn G, Woolford H. The treatment of recurrent abdominal pain in children: a controlled comparison of cognitive-behavioral family intervention and standard pediatric care. J Consult Clin Psychol. 1994;62:306–14.
56. Huertas-Ceballos AA, Logan S, Bennett C, Macarthur C. Psychological interventions for recurrent abdominal pain (RAP) and irritable bowel syndrome (IBS) in childhood. Cochrane Database Syst Rev 2009.

57. Chronic abdominal pain in children. Pediatrics 2005;115(3):812–5.
58. Vlieger AM, Menko-Frankenhuis C, Wolfkamp SC, Tromp E, Benninga MA. Hypnotherapy for children with functional abdominal pain or irritable bowel syndrome: a randomized controlled trial. Gastroenterology. 2007;133:1430–6.
59. Weydert JA, Shapiro DE, Acra SA, Monheim CJ, Chambers AS, Ball TM. Evaluation of guided imagery as treatment for recurrent abdominal pain in children: a randomized controlled trial. BMC Pediatr. 2006;6:29.
60. Ball TM, Shapiro DE, Monheim CJ, Weydert JA. A pilot study of the use of guided imagery for the treatment of recurrent abdominal pain in children. Clin Pediatr (Phila). 2003;42:527–32.
61. Anbar RD. Self-hypnosis for the treatment of functional abdominal pain in childhood. Clin Pediatr (Phila). 2001;40:447–51.
62. van Tilburg MA, Chitkara DK, Palsson OS, Turner M, Blois-Martin N, Ulshen M, Whitehead WE. Audio-recorded guided imagery treatment reduces functional abdominal pain in children: a pilot study. Pediatrics. 2009;124:e890–7.
63. Humphreys PA, Gevirtz RN. Treatment of recurrent abdominal pain: components analysis of four treatment protocols. J Pediatr Gastroenterol Nutr. 2000;31:47–51.
64. Feldman W, McGrath P, Hodgson C, Ritter H, Shipman RT. The use of dietary fiber in the management of simple, childhood, idiopathic, recurrent, abdominal pain. Results in a prospective, double-blind, randomized, controlled trial. Am J Dis Child. 1985;139:1216–8.
65. Huertas-Ceballos AA, Logan S, Bennett C, Macarthur C. Dietary interventions for recurrent abdominal pain (RAP) and irritable bowel syndrome (IBS) in childhood. Cochrane Database Syst Rev 2009:CD003019.
66. See MC, Birnbaum AH, Schechter CB, Goldenberg MM, Benkov KJ. Double-blind, placebo-controlled trial of famotidine in children with abdominal pain and dyspepsia: global and quantitative assessment. Dig Dis Sci. 2001;46:985–92.
67. Saps M, Youssef N, Miranda A, Nurko S, Hyman P, Cocjin J, Di Lorenzo C. Multicenter, randomized, placebo-controlled trial of amitriptyline in children with functional gastrointestinal disorders. Gastroenterology. 2009;137:1261–9.
68. Campo JV, Perel J, Lucas A, Bridge J, Ehmann M, Kalas C, Monk K, Axelson D, Birmaher B, Ryan N, Di Lorenzo C, Brent DA. Citalopram treatment of pediatric recurrent abdominal pain and comorbid internalizing disorders: an exploratory study. J Am Acad Child Adolesc Psychiatry. 2004;43:1234–42.
69. Gawronska A, Dziechciarz P, Horvath A, Szajewska H. A randomized double-blind placebo-controlled trial of Lactobacillus GG for abdominal pain disorders in children. Aliment Pharmacol Ther. 2007;25:177–84.
70. Francavilla R, Miniello V, Magista AM, De Canio A, Bucci N, Gagliardi F, Lionetti E, Castellaneta S, Polimeno L, Peccarisi L, Indrio F, Cavallo L. A randomized controlled trial of Lactobacillus GG in children with functional abdominal pain. Pediatrics. 2010;126:e1445–52.
71. Chitkara DK, Talley NJ, Schleck C, Zinsmeister AR, Shah ND, Locke 3rd GR. Recollection of childhood abdominal pain in adults with functional gastrointestinal disorders. Scand J Gastroenterol. 2009;44:301–7.
72. Gieteling MJ, Bierma-Zeinstra SM, Passchier J, Berger MY. Prognosis of chronic or recurrent abdominal pain in children. J Pediatr Gastroenterol Nutr. 2008;47:316–26.
73. Apley J, Hale B. Children with recurrent abdominal pain: how do they grow up? Br Med J. 1973;3:7–9.
74. Magni G, Pierri M, Donzelli F. Recurrent abdominal pain in children: a long term follow-up. Eur J Pediatr. 1987;146:72–4.

Cyclic Vomiting Syndrome: Comorbidities and Treatment

36

Bhanu Sunku and B.U.K. Li

Despite improved characterization, recognition, and understanding of cyclic vomiting syndrome (CVS) in the past two decades, without a delineated pathophysiologic cascade, it remains classified as a functional gastrointestinal disorder (Table 36.1). Although originally perceived to be a pediatric disorder, the past decade has been witness to a dramatic rise in diagnosed adults. In both children and adults, the hallmark symptoms described by Samuel Gee in 1882 remain applicable today and include stereotypical, severe episodes of vomiting punctuating symptom-free periods, or baseline health [1]. Recent work has begun to expand the list of comorbidities and clinical subphenotypes and identify pathophysiologic pathways and new therapeutic avenues.

Definition

Earlier clinical diagnosis has been facilitated by the recently defined consensus diagnostic criteria by NASPGHAN (2008) and Rome III (2006) criteria, the former being quantitatively more rigorous, i.e., requiring 3–5 vs. 2 total episodes [2] (Table 36.2).

B. Sunku, M.D. (✉)
Mount Kisco Medical Group,
110 South Bedford Rd Mount, Kisco, NY 10549, USA
e-mail: bsunku@MKMG.com

B.U.K. Li, M.D.
Division of Gastroenterology, Hepatology & Nutrition,
Pediatrics Department, Medical College of Wisconsin,
Milwaukee, WI, USA

There is common confusion over the nomenclature as the older classification is "abdominal migraine" and the newer term since the 1990s is "cyclic vomiting syndrome" or "cyclical vomiting syndrome" (UK). Today, from an operational standpoint, the predominant and most consistent symptom during episodes defines the illness, i.e., abdominal pain is termed abdominal migraine, and conversely vomiting is denoted CVS. However, there is considerable clinical overlap because ~50% of those diagnosed with abdominal migraine also vomit, and 80% of those with CVS also have abdominal pain.

The continuum between CVS and migraine was suggested by Whitney in 1898 and corroborated by other authors including us in 1998 [3, 4]. In a cross-sectional school survey in Scotland, Abu-Arafeh described a developmental progression from CVS to abdominal migraine and migraine headaches, median ages 5, 9, and 11 years with prevalences of 1.9%, 4%, and 11%, respectively [5]. This suggests a natural history that begins with CVS and ends with migraines. Although some experience all three phases, the largest group trades CVS for migraines by age 10. We estimate 75% will develop migraine headaches by age 18 years (Li, unpublished data).

The lack of a specific ICD 9 code and the use of persistent vomiting (536.2) render it difficult to establish the true prevalence of CVS. Typical misdiagnoses, including gastroenteritis, gastroesophageal reflux, food poisoning, and eating disorders, often delay accurate diagnosis by a median 2.5 years. At our GI clinic, CVS was

C. Faure et al. (eds.), *Pediatric Neurogastroenterology: Gastrointestinal Motility and Functional Disorders in Children*, Clinical Gastroenterology,
DOI 10.1007/978-1-60761-709-9_36, © Springer Science+Business Media New York 2013

Table 36.1 Functional nausea and vomiting disorders

Functional dyspepsia
Chronic idiopathic nausea (adult Rome III criteria)
Functional vomiting
Cyclic vomiting syndrome
Rumination syndrome
Aerophagia

Table 36.2 NASPGHAN and Rome III diagnostic criteria

NASPGHAN
1. At least five attacks in any interval or a minimum of three attacks during a 6-month period
2. Episodic attacks of intense nausea and vomiting lasting 1 h to 10 days and occurring at least 1 week apart
3. Stereotypical pattern and symptoms in the individual patient
4. Vomiting during attacks occurs at least 4 times/h for at least 1 h
5. Return to baseline health between episodes
6. Not attributed to another disorder
Rome III
1. Two or more periods of intense nausea and unremitting vomiting or retching lasting hours to days
2. Return to usual state of health lasting weeks to months

All respective criteria must be met to meet consensus definitions for both NASPGHAN and Rome III

Table 36.3 Epidemiology and demographics [8]

Features	
Age of onset	4.8 years
Delay in diagnosis	2.5 years
Prevalence	2%
Incidence	3.15/100,000
Female/male	57:43
Migraine association	39–87%

Adapted from Li BUK, Balint J. Cyclic vomiting syndrome: evolution in our understanding of a brain–gut disorder. In: Advances in Pediatrics. Mosby, 2000: 117–160

second only to gastroesophageal reflux as a cause of recurrent vomiting [6]. Two school-based surveys (not clinical exam) estimated the frequency to be 2% in Scottish and Turkish children (Table 36.3) [5, 7], and the incidence of new cases of CVS was reported to be 3.15 per 100,000 children per year in Irish children. In our series, the average age of onset of CVS is 4.8 years with a predominance in girls over boys (57:43).

Impact on QOL

CVS has a significant deleterious impact on the quality of life in affected children. Although well in between episodes approximately 90% of the time, 58% of affected children require intravenous fluids during episodes and average ten visits to the emergency department. School-age children miss an average of 24 days of school per year [8, 9]. Medical morbidity is reflected by the high average annualized cost of management of $17,000 in 1998 that includes doctor visits, emergency department visits, inpatient hospitalizations, missed work by parents, and biochemical, radiographic, and endoscopic testing [10]. A growing number of comorbid conditions such as anxiety and postural orthostatic tachycardia syndrome also contribute to functional disability. We have begun to document lower global quality of life scores than in healthy controls and those with functional GI disorders (irritable bowel syndrome) equivalent to organic GI diseases (e.g., inflammatory bowel disease, gastritis, fatty liver disease) (Tarbell S., unpublished data).

Pathophysiology

In the absence of a defined etiopathogenesis, CVS remains classified as an idiopathic disorder. Recent investigations support the contributory roles of mitochondrial DNA (mtDNA) mutations and dysfunction, heightened hypothalamic–pituitary–adrenal (HPA) axis activation, and autonomic nervous system (ANS) dysfunction. CVS is a functional brain–gut disorder perhaps mediated through altered brainstem modulation of effector signals.

Mitochondrial Dysfunction

In two series, a striking maternal inheritance pattern was recognized for migraines in 64% and 54% of probands with CVS [11, 12]. Evidence of mitochondrial dysfunction was first provided using NMR to establish decreased ATP production in peripheral muscle in migraineurs [13]. This mitochondrial pathogenesis gained substantial support following the recent identification of two tandem mtDNA polymorphisms, 16519T, and 3010A with impressive odds ratios of 17 and 15 in CVS and migraine in haplotype H, respectively [14]. Because the mutations are found in the control region rather than the enzyme sequence, the structure to function relationship is unclear. However, elevated lactates, ketones, and Krebs cycle intermediates during attacks are consistent with mitochondrial dysfunction. In addition, therapeutic trials show promising effects of mitochondrial supplements coenzyme Q10, L-carnitine, and riboflavin in the treatment of migraines and CVS [15, 16].

These two mtDNA mutations are also found in depression, chronic fatigue, and irritable bowel syndrome and may link these clinical comorbidities together to a common mitochondrial susceptibility factor.

HPA Axis Activation

Stressors, both psychological (excitement, panic) and physical (fever, lack of sleep), are common triggers of attacks of CVS. Activation of the HPA axis during episodes of CVS was first described by Wolfe, Adler, and later Sato, and they documented elevated levels of adrenocorticotropic hormone (ACTH), antidiuretic hormone, cortisol, catecholamines, and prostaglandin E2 and hypertension [17, 18]. Attenuation of CVS symptoms occurred after use of high-dose dexamethasone by Wolfe and Adler and indomethacin and clonidine by Sato et al. [19].

The role of corticotropin-releasing factor (CRF) as a brain–gut neuroendocrine mediator of foregut motility has been extensively described in animals by Taché et al. [20]. In response to stressors, released CRF from the hypothalamus stimulates inhibitory motor neurons in the dorsal motor nucleus of the vagus and causes delayed gastric emptying, independent of downstream effects of ACTH and cortisol secretion. In animals, like humans, psychological (water avoidance) and physical (cytokine IL-1β(beta)) stressors can impair foregut motility. Ongoing investigation of the pathophysiologic role of CRF in CVS may open a potential therapeutic avenue using CRF antagonists. Tricyclic antidepressants, which inhibit the promoter activity of the CRF gene, are the most efficacious agents in treating CVS.

Autonomic Dysfunction

Most of the prominent symptoms of CVS are expressed through the ANS. The peripheral vasoconstriction, hypersalivation, diaphoresis, tachycardia, and listlessness are in fact prominent manifestations of nausea that persist throughout the episode typically unrelieved by evacuation of the stomach. Autonomic dysfunction in the form of postural orthostatic tachycardia syndrome (POTS) in children with CVS was recently reported by Chelimsky [21]. They noted that treatment of the POTS appeared to help reduce the frequency of CVS episodes. We found an overall prevalence of 19% in our CVS patients, and when we limited the cohort to adolescents >11 years in whom POTS is known to be more common, the rate was 31%. Formal investigation of the ANS function in children and adults with CVS reveals a consistent pattern of heightened sympathetic tone and normal parasympathetic tone [21]. This imbalance is also described in migraines and other functional gastrointestinal disorders [22].

A Model

How these pathophysiologic pathways fit together in a comprehensive model remains to be delineated. mtDNA mutations impair cellular energy production when needs are increased during psychological or physical stress conditions. If the production cannot meet the heightened demands, autonomic neurons may be the target because of their high intrinsic energy demands. CRF may be the initiating signal triggered by psychological or physical stressors that inhibits the upper GI tract motility. The penultimate defect in CVS that allows the emetic motor program to feed forward and continue for hours even despite evacuation of all gastric contents has been hypothesized to be in the periaqueductal gray area [23]. This area modulates brain-to-peripheral ANS signals such as the emetic motor program mediated by the vagus.

Clinical Patterns

CVS has a distinctive on–off temporal pattern of vomiting that serves as an essential criterion for diagnosis. CVS is distinguished by the "on" pattern of discrete, recurrent, and singularly severe episodes of vomiting that are stereotypical within the individual as to time of onset (usually early morning), duration (hours or days), and symptomatology (pallor, listlessness). The "off" pattern is week- or month-long intervals when the child resumes completely normal or baseline health (e.g., if there is other chronic disease), although 5% may have interepisodic symptoms of nausea and mild vomiting [8]. During the episodes, the most common symptoms are listlessness (93%) and pallor (91%), and others include low grade fever or hypothermia, intermittent flushing, diaphoresis, drooling, diarrhea, and hypertension in the Sato variant. Although found in significantly higher frequency than in patients with GI disorders, fewer than half have migraine features of headache, photophobia, and phonophobia.

The duration of episodes generally ranges from hours to days with a median duration of 27 h. They can last as long as 10 days but are always self-limited. Half of patients have "cyclic" intervals most commonly 4 weeks, predictable within a week, and half have "sporadic," unpredictable attacks. The most common time of onset is early morning (2–4 a.m.) or upon awakening (6–8 a.m.) in 42%. Many have a remarkably rapid onset (1.5 h) and denouement (8 h) from the last emesis to the point of being able to eat and be playful. The 67% with a prodrome have the pre-emesis pallor, diaphoresis, abdominal pain, and headache but rarely visual disturbances of a classical migraine aura.

The vomiting in CVS is uniquely rapid fire and peaks at a median frequency of six times an hour and 15 times per episode (Table 36.3). The vomiting is typically projectile and contains bile, mucus, and occasionally blood, the latter usually the result of prolapse gastropathy. The intense nausea differs from that in gastroenteritis in that it persists even after complete evacuation of gastric contents as if independent of gastric feedback. In fact, many adolescents describe it as the most distressing symptom, only relieved during sleep. Due to the unrelenting nausea, during episodes, these children appear much more debilitated when compared to those with gastroenteritis, often curled into a fetal position, listless, and withdrawn to the point of being unable to walk or interact. Anorexia, nausea, midline abdominal pain, and retching are the most common gastrointestinal symptoms.

Certain unusual behaviors can be observed during CVS episodes that can raise questions about an underlying psychiatric disorder. There are children who drink compulsively and then vomit and describe that that maneuver dilutes the bitter bile and aids in evacuating it. Others take prolonged, scalding hot showers or baths until the hot water supply is exhausted. Nearly all turn their rooms into a darkened cave in order to avoid lights and sounds that trigger more nausea. Many are hyperesthetic to motion, odor, taste, and even parental touch and attempt to shut out the external environment.

Various recurring stressors are recognized to precipitate CVS episodes in 76% of patients. These include psychological (44%), infectious (31%), and physical triggers. The psychological stress is more often of an excitatory nature such as holidays, birthdays, outings, and vacations such as at Disney World. Episodes may be triggered by various infections including upper respiratory infections, sinusitis, strep throat, and flu. Dietary factors include aged-cheese, chocolate, monosodium glutamate, and fluctuating caffeine intake (23%). Lack of sleep from excess physical exhaustion from travel, sports, sleepovers or a sleep disorder (24%), and menses (catamenial CVS—22%) are also common inciting events. Environmental triggers include changes in barometric pressures in weather fronts. One subgroup with a precisely timed interval every 60 days (predictable within a week) with no identifiable triggers is especially refractory to therapy.

Comorbidities

The evolving clinical picture of CVS has included an increasing number of associated comorbidities. In Boles' series, 25% had coexisting neurological findings of developmental delay, seizures, hypotonia, and skeletal myopathy as well as cognitive and cranial nerve dysfunction [24]. These children classified as CVS+ were found to have an earlier age of onset for CVS and a three- to eightfold higher prevalence of dysautonomic (neurovascular dystrophy) and constitutional (growth retardation) manifestations than CVS patients without neurological findings. Other comorbidities in non-neurologically impaired children include anxiety (47%) and depression (14%) [25], irritable bowel syndrome in (67%) [26], GERD (39%), colonic dysmotility (20%) [24], postural orthostatic tachycardia syndrome (19%) (Li, unpublished), and chronic fatigue and complex regional pain syndrome (12%) [27]. Often, these contribute to the poor quality of life and have to be treated concomitantly to help restore the child to functionality.

Subgroups

There appear to be subphenotypes of CVS, some of which overlap and may be present in the same patient. The 83% that are migraine related (positive family or self history) tend to have significantly less severe episodes that are more responsive to antimigraine therapy [28]. It now appears that the majority has a matrilineal inheritance pattern (for migraine and other functional disorders) and may have mtDNA mutations and mitochondrial dysfunction [12]. Many appear to have predominantly sympathetic overtone and comorbid POTS in whom treatment of POTS helps reduce frequency of vomiting episodes. The Sato variant is associated with hypertension during episodes and an endocrine profile of heightened HPA axis activation. Those with long-interval calendar-timed episodes every 60+ days apart appear particularly difficult to treat. Boles has described a group with neurodevelopmental deficits in whom CVS begins early in life [24]. There are post-menarcheal girls with catamenial CVS who respond to low-estrogen birth control pills or ablation of menses.

There is a group of adolescents and adults with CVS who use marijuana to alleviate nausea and vomiting that instead may aggravate CVS symptoms and has been labeled as cannabis-induced hyperemesis. It is more likely cannabis-triggered CVS [29]. One series of nine patients reports termination of bouts of emesis after cessation of chronic use of marijuana. Another case series noted 7 out of 13 marijuana users experienced improvement of nausea and anxiety raising the possibility that marijuana may be aggravate in some and mitigate in others [30].

Evaluation

At present, there are no specific tests to diagnose CVS, and the diagnosis rests primarily upon fulfilling clinical criteria. The first step requires differentiating a cyclic pattern (high intensity, low frequency) of vomiting in which extraintestinal disorders including CVS are most common from a chronic vomiting (low intensity, high frequency) one in which upper GI tract disorders predominate [6]. Approximately 90% of children who fulfill the NASPGHAN consensus criteria (Table 36.2) are ultimately found to have CVS [2, 6]. Most of the testing in undiagnosed children who present with recurrent vomiting is directed toward identifying underlying gastrointestinal, neurologic, renal, metabolic, and endocrine causes that can be uncovered in the remaining 10%. The challenge to the clinician is to determine which and how much testing should be performed, as the traditional "shotgun" approach is costly, time-consuming, and invasive.

The recent NASPGHAN Consensus Statement (2008) guidelines recommend against the traditional shotgun approach and only for initial an upper gastrointestinal series to exclude malrota-

Table 36.4 Evaluation of cyclic vomiting

• Patient meets consensus criteria for CVS UGI series to evaluate for malrotation + serum electrolytes, BUN, creatinine and no warning signs or findings to suggest an organic disorder trial of empiric therapy to treat CVS
If warning signs are present:
• Severe abdominal pain, bilious, and/or hematemesis liver and pancreatic serum chemistries, abdominal ultrasound (or CT or MRI), esophagogastroduodenoscopy
• Fasting, high-protein meal, intercurrent illness precipitating episodes of vomiting serum and urine metabolic evaluation (lactate, ammonia, carnitine profile, amino acids, and organic acids) *prior to treatment during episode and metabolic consult*
• Abnormal neurological findings (altered mental status, papilledema) brain MRI, neurology consult

tion and anatomic obstructions and a basic metabolic profile (electrolytes, glucose, BUN, creatinine) [2]. Further testing beyond that should be based upon specific warning signs (Table 36.4). In those who present with bilious vomiting and abdominal tenderness, abdominal imaging should be performed to exclude hydronephrosis, pancreatitis, and cholecystitis. In those in whom episodes are triggered by intercurrent illnesses, fasting, or high-protein meals, screening should be performed for urea cycle, fatty acid oxidation, disorders of organic and amino acid metabolism, and mitochondrial disorders. This screening has a better diagnostic yield in the early part of an episode of CVS before intravenous glucose and fluids are administered. Those presenting with abnormal neurological findings including altered mental status, papilledema, ataxia, or seizure should have a neurological evaluation and brain MRI considered. Presentation of CVS under the age of 2 should also prompt further metabolic or neurological testing [2].

Treatment

Management of CVS is multifaceted and challenging. The goals of treatment are to reduce the frequency and severity of episodes, reduce school absenteeism and enhance functionality, improve quality of life, and establish a protocol for rescue therapy in home and hospital settings. Treatment of nausea and vomiting, abdominal pain, and dehydration during acute episodes requires a protocol for use at home, emergency departments, and hospital wards. Lifestyle modifications, similar to those in migraines, during the well phase can help prevent episodes and are discussed below. For those with more frequent or severe episodes (e.g., more than once a month), prophylactic therapy taken daily to prevent the next episode is best. In some with less frequent or severe episodes, abortive therapy taken only during the prodrome or at the onset of the episode is successful. The use of mitochondrial supplements to treat suspected underlying mitochondrial dysfunction is gaining evidence and acceptance.

At present, there are no controlled therapeutic trials. One formal randomized controlled trial on IV ondansetron was attempted by the authors and thwarted by an impressive 90% reduction in rate of episodes upon enrollment even without prophylactic therapy (Li, unpublished data). The NASPGHAN Consensus Statement recommendations on treatment are based upon therapeutic responses from case series and expert opinion of the task force [2]. The main recommendations include first-line prophylactic use of cyproheptadine and amitriptyline in children under age 5 years and 5 years or older, respectively, with propranolol as the second line. Sumatriptan was recommended as an abortive agent for those >12 years. For rescue therapy during acute episodes, IV rehydration with high-dose antiemetic ondansetron (0.3–0.4 mg/kg/dose) and sedation from diphenhydramine or lorazepam was recommended.

Rescue Approach

The rescue therapies are used when the vomiting is well established in an episode and fails to respond to abortive strategies. The goal is to correct fluid and electrolyte deficits and render the child more comfortable through antiemetic therapy, analgesics, and sedation for relief from intractable nausea and pain. The recommendation is for an IV bolus of saline for rapid correction of fluid deficits and 10% dextrose 0.45 normal saline at 1.5× maintenance rates to provide sufficient cellular energy to terminate ketosis. One may have to reduce IV rates and increase Na+ content when hyponatremia

Table 36.5 Abortive and rescue pharmacotherapy

Antimigraine
Sumatriptan 20 mg intranasal at episode onset and may repeat once or 25 mg po once. SE: chest and neck burning, coronary vasospasm, headache
Alternatives: *frovatriptan, rizatriptan, zolmitriptan*
Antiemetic
Ondansetron 0.3–0.4 mg/kg per dose q 4–6 h iv/po/rectal/topical. SE: headache, drowsiness, dry mouth
Alternatives: *granisetron*
Aprepitant 125, 80, 80 mg one q.d. prior to anticipated episode
Sedative
Lorazepam 0.05–0.1 mg/kg per dose q 6 h iv/po: useful adjunct to ondansetron. SE: sedation, respiratory depression
Chlorpromazine 0.5–1 mg/kg per dose q 6 h iv/po. SE: drowsiness, hypotension, seizures
Diphenhydramine 1.25 mg/kg per dose q 6 h iv/po: useful adjunct to chlorpromazine. SE: hypotension, sedation, dizziness
Analgesic
Ketorolac 0.5–1 mg/kg per dose q 6 h iv/po. SE: gastrointestinal bleeding, dyspepsia
Alternatives: opioids (hydromorphone)

From Sunku B. Cyclic vomiting syndrome, a disorder of all ages. Gastroenterol Hepatol (NY). 2009 July; 5(7):507–515. Reprinted with permission

and diminished urine output from elevated antidiuretic hormone release is present in Sato-variant CVS. Ondansetron has been the most widely used $5HT_3$ antagonist given safely at higher than standard doses (0.3–0.4 mg/kg/dose) [11]. Diphenhydramine, lorazepam, or chlorpromazine combined with diphenhydramine are used for sedation because for some sedation is the only means of providing relief from the unrelenting nausea and pain (Table 36.5). When the first-line analgesic ketorolac fails to alleviate pain, hydromorphone can be used and is occasionally required as a continuous patient-controlled analgesia.

Lifestyle Modifications

Lifestyle modifications are used during the interictal phase of CVS when the child is not in an episode in order to avoid exposure to known and potential precipitants of episodes. The lack of sleep resulting from disturbed sleep patterns, sleepovers, or travel sports tournaments are often cited as triggers of episodes. Good sleep hygiene (e.g., turning off all phones, computers, music, TV) with a regimented sleep time can help reduce the frequency of episodes. Providing at least maintenance volumes of fluids is widely used to treat migraines and postural orthostatic tachycardia syndrome. Providing energy sources before strenuous activity, preferably of low glycemic index and high-protein sources, may prevent an energy deficit. Routine exercise can help reverse the deconditioned state. Finally, avoiding identified triggers specific to the individual (e.g., lack of sleep) or generally found in migraines (monosodium glutamate and fluctuations in caffeine intake) may help reduce the frequency of episodes. Although there is limited evidence of efficacy, Fleisher reported that consultation and lifestyle modifications alone reduced the frequency of episode in 70% of patients without beginning prophylactic therapy [26].

Prophylactic therapy

Prophylactic therapy is administered during the interictal period in order to prevent future episodes. The NASPGHAN consensus recommendations for the initial treatment were for cyproheptadine for the younger (<5 years) and amitriptyline for the older children and adolescents (≥5 years) [2] (Table 36.6). Despite its pharmacokinetics, cyproheptadine (0.25–0.5 mg/kg) appears to be effective given as a single nighttime dose, rather than in two or three divided doses [31]. Amitriptyline causes side effects in 50%, the most common being morning sedation (like a hangover), and is stopped in 21% [32]. Beginning at a low dosage of 0.2–0.3 mg/kg at bedtime and titrating in 10 mg increments every week (unless too sedated) to the target dose of 1.0–1.5 mg/kg allows the child to adapt to the side effects. Switching to other tricyclic antidepressants such as nortriptyline and desipramine may circumvent intolerable side effects. An EKG for QTc interval is recommended before starting amitriptyline and after reaching the target dose to monitor for prolonged QTc interval [33]. Propranolol is second

Table 36.6 Prophylactic pharmacotherapy

Antimigraine
Amitriptyline start and 0.2–0.3 mg/kg and advance to 1–1.5 mg/kg/day q.h.s.: monitor EKG QTc interval prior to starting. First choice ≥ 5 yrs old. Side effects: sedation, anticholinergic
Propranolol 0.25–1 mg/kg/day divided b.i.d or t.i.d: monitor resting heart rate. SE: hypotension, bradycardia, fatigue
Cyproheptadine 0.25–0.5 mg/kg/day divided b.i.d. or q.h.s.: First choice <5 years old. SE: sedation, weight gain, anticholinergic
Alternatives: *nortriptyline, imipramine, desipramine*
Anticonvulsants
Topiramate increase to 1.5–2.0 mg/kg/day divided b.i.d.
Phenobarbital 2–3 mg/kg/day q.h.s. SE: sedation, cognitive impairment
Alternatives: *gabapentin, levetiracetam, zonisamide, valproate, carbamazepine*
Mitochondrial supplements
l-*Carnitine* 50–100 mg/kg ≤ 2 g/day divided b.i.d. SE: diarrhea, fishy body odor.
Coenzyme Q_{10} 10 mg/kg/ divided b.i.d. ≤400 mg/day
Riboflavin 10 mg/kg/day divided b.i.d. ≤400 mg/day

From Sunku B. Cyclic vomiting syndrome, a disorder of all ages. Gastroenterol Hepatol (NY). 2009 July; 5(7):507–515. Reprinted with permission

line and can be monitored for efficacy and toxicity by a drop in pulse rate of 15–20 beats per minute and below 55 bpm, respectively.

If standard prophylactic therapy fails, anticonvulsants and Ca^{2+}-channel antagonists have been used. Phenobarbital at low (2–3 mg/kg) nighttime doses has been reported to be effective [34]. In children, cognitive dysfunction is a well-known side effect and one that occurs with other anticonvulsants as well. Others used topiramate, zonisamide, and levetiracetam, with positive evidence in adults with migraine headaches and cyclic vomiting syndrome [35, 36]. Another group of agents includes Ca^{2+}-channel antagonists with the main side effect of hypotension.

Treatment by Subgroup

Treatment may be selected by clinical subgroup. Children with so-called migraine related with a positive family history or migraines themselves are much more likely to respond to antimigraine agents such as cyproheptadine, amitriptyline, and propranolol (79% vs. 36%) than those children without a migraine connection [28]. Post-menarcheal girls with catamenial CVS often respond to low-estrogen birth control pills (Loestrin, Lo/Ovral, Alesse, Seasonale) or Depo-Provera. Sato-variant CVS associated with intraepisode hypertension have been treated with tricyclic antidepressants in the USA and Depakote (divalproex sodium) in Japan [19].

Abortive Therapy

Abortive therapy is given during the prodrome or at the beginning of the vomiting episode in the hope of stopping it. The most specific abortive therapy includes antimigraine triptans. The nasal (sumatriptan or zolmitriptan) or subcutaneous (sumatriptan) forms appear more effective than oral forms that cannot effectively reach the duodenum due to repeated vomiting (Table 36.5) [2, 37]. The triptans appear to be either fully effective or not at all and more effective if administered early in episode and if the duration of episodes is less than 24 h (Li, unpublished data).

In a few children, ondansetron given alone aborts episodes in progress. Although the oral forms may not reach to duodenum, ondansetron can be reformulated by individual pharmacies into a rectal suppository or topical forms. Although not established, we use the same dose as the oral form. In a few adolescents with severe, disabling abdominal pain accompanying the vomiting, use of opioids such as hydromorphone can quickly abolish the pain and vomiting. The NK1 antagonist aprepitant may be given orally prior to the anticipated vomiting in a calendar-timed CVS episode.

Mitochondrial Supplements

The use of mitochondrial supplements as adjunctive prophylactic therapy in CVS is being used more and more based upon evidence in migraines. Their use in suspected mitochondrial dysfunction has been bolstered by the recent finding of two mitochondrial DNA mutations by Boles [15]. In some children, the accompanying chronic fatigue may respond to these supplements. These supplements have demonstrated efficacy in prevention of migraine headaches in adults (randomized controlled trial) and preliminary evidence of efficacy in pediatric migraine and CVS in children [38–40]. The doses used include riboflavin at 10 mg/kg divided b.i.d. to 400 mg/day, L-carnitine at 50–100 mg/kg up to 2 g/day divided b.i.d., and CoQ10 10 mg/kg up to 400 mg/day divided b.i.d. The dose and duration of therapy has not been established in children with CVS. Acupuncture using P6 point has also been used with variable efficacy [41].

Approach to the Refractory Patient

In tertiary and quaternary referral settings, a sizeable number of children with CVS do not respond to the therapies outlined above. There are several approaches we have used in such patients. The first is to reinvestigate the possibility of a specific precipitating factor(s) that can be addressed. In our experience the most common is a family- or school-related psychological stressor or intense anxiety in the child that requires a psychologist for diagnosis and treatment. Some have been diagnosed with intractable chronic sinusitis that fails to respond to standard antibiotic and decongestant therapy and requires otolaryngological intervention. The second is to reconsider the diagnosis of CVS and whether there is an alternate specific underlying cause. Identified surgical diagnoses found upon retesting in episodic vomiting include volvulus from malrotation, acute hydronephrosis, and subtentorial tumors (e.g., Chiari malformation).

If no specific trigger or cause can be identified and prophylactic monotherapy fails to reduce the frequency and severity of episodes, combination therapy has been anecdotally successful. Amitriptyline can be combined with either propranolol, topiramate, or phenobarbital in children refractory to single agent therapy.

In children with prolonged episodes longer than 5 days who continue to have severe and debilitating nausea and vomiting despite therapy, induced sleep may be the only rescue option. In fact, 72% of the children in our series report sleep as the harbinger of the end of the episode. We have observed that induced sleep will sometimes end the episode, seemingly as if the "vomiting center" in the brainstem has "rebooted" back to baseline in the off position. The consensus recommendation is either intravenous lorazepam or chlorpromazine with diphenhydramine [2]. However, if both fail to sedate and ameliorate the unrelenting nausea and vomiting, general anesthesia may be the last resort. In one case series, 18 h of dexmedetomidine-induced general anesthesia terminated prolonged, intractable episodes in three children [42]. Although this protocol required continuous monitoring in the PICU, it did not require intubation because of its lack of respiratory depression. We have also used this approach successfully in extreme cases.

References

1. Gee S. On fitful or recurrent vomiting. St Bartholemew Hosp Rev. 1882;18:1–6.
2. Li BUK, Lefevre F, Chelminsky GG, et al. North American Society for Pediatric Gastroenterology, Hepatology, and Nutrition Consensus Statement on the diagnosis and management of cyclic vomiting syndrome. J Pediatr Gastroenterol Nutr. 2008;47:379–93.
3. Whitney HB. Cyclic vomiting: a brief review of this affection as illustrated by a typical case. Arch Pediatr. 1898;15:839–45.
4. Li BUK. Cyclic vomiting syndrome and abdominal migraine. Int Semin Pediatr Gastroenterol. 2000;9:1–9.
5. Abu-Arafeh I, Russel G. Cyclic vomiting syndrome in children: a population based study. J Pediatr Gastroenterol Nutr. 1995;21:454–8.
6. Pfau BT, Li BUK, Murray RD, et al. Differentiating cyclic from chronic vomiting patterns in children: quantitative criteria and diagnostic implications. Pediatrics. 1996;97:364–8.
7. Ertekin V, Selimoglu MA, Altnkaynak S. Prevalence of cyclic vomiting syndrome in a sample of Turkish school children in an urban area. J Clin Gastroenterol. 2006;40:896–8.
8. Li BUK, Balint J. Cyclic vomiting syndrome: evolution in our understanding of a brain–gut disorder. In: Advances in pediatrics. Mosby; 2000. p. 117–160.
9. Venkatesan T, Tarbell S, Adams K. A survey of emergency department use in patients with cyclic vomiting syndrome. BMC Emerg Med. 2010;10:4.
10. Olson AD, Li BUK. The diagnostic evaluation of children with cyclic vomiting: a cost-effectiveness assessment. J Pediatr. 2002;141:724–8.

11. Li BUK, Fleisher DR. Cyclic vomiting syndrome: features to be explained by a pathophysiologic model. Dig Dis Sci. 1999;44:13S–8.
12. Boles RG, Adams K, Li BUK. Maternal Inheritance in cyclic vomiting syndrome. Am J Med Gen. 2005;133A:71–7.
13. Bresolin N, Martinelli P, Barbiroli B, et al. Muscle mitochondrial DNA deletion and 31P-NMR spectroscopy alterations in a migraine patient. J Neurol Sci. 1991;104(2):182–9.
14. Camilleri M, Carlson P, Zinsmeister AR, et al. Mitochondrial DNA and gastrointestinal motor and sensory functions in health and functional gastrointestinal disorders. Am J Physiol Gastrointest Liver Physiol. 2009;296(3):G510–6.
15. Boles RG. High degree of efficacy in the treatment of cyclic vomiting syndrome with combined co-enzyme Q10, L-carnitine and amitriptyline, a case series. BMC Neurol. 2011;11:102.
16. Boehnke C, Reuter U, Flach U, et al. High-dose riboflavin treatment is efficacious in migraine prophylaxis: an open study in a tertiary care centre. Eur J Neurol. 2004;11(7):475–7.
17. Wolfe SM, Adler R. A syndrome of periodic hypothalamic discharge. Am J Med. 1964;36:956–67.
18. Sato T, Uchigata Y, Uwadana N, et al. A syndrome of periodic adrenocorticotropin and vasopressin discharge. J Clin Endocrinol Metab. 1982;54:517–22.
19. Sato T, Igarashi M, Minami S, et al. Recurrent attacks of vomiting, hypertension, and psychotic depression: a syndrome of periodic catecholamine and prostaglandin discharge. Acta Endocrinol. 1988;117:189–97.
20. Taché Y, Martinez V, Million M, et al. Corticotropin-releasing factor and the brain-gut motor response to stress. Can J Gastroenterol. 1999;13(Suppl A):18A–25A.
21. Chelminsky TC, Chelminsky GG. Autonomic abnormalities in cyclic vomiting syndrome. J Pediatr Gastroenterol Nutr. 2007;44:326–30.
22. Rashed R, Abell TL, Familoni BO, et al. Autonomic function in cyclic vomiting syndrome and classic migraine. Dig Dis Sci. 1999;44:74S–8.
23. Welch KM. Scientific basis of migraine: speculation on the relationship to cyclic vomiting. Dig Dis Sci. 1999;44(8 Suppl):26S–30.
24. Boles RG, Powers AL, Adams K. Cyclic vomiting syndrome plus. J Child Neurol. 2006;21:182–8.
25. Tarbell S, Li BU. Psychiatric symptoms in children and adolescents with cyclic vomiting syndrome and their parents. Headache. 2008;48:259–66.
26. Fleisher DR. Cyclic vomiting. In: Hyman PE, DiLorenzo C, editors. Pediatric gastrointestinal motility disorders. New York: Academy Professional Information Services; 1994. p. 89–103.
27. Higashimoto T, Baldwin EE, Gold JI, Boles RG. Reflex sympathetic dystrophy: complex regional pain syndrome type I in children with mitochondrial disease and maternal inheritance. Arch Dis Child. 2008;93(5):390–7.
28. Li BUK, Murray RD, Heitlinger LA. Is cyclic vomiting syndrome related to migraine? J Pediatr. 1999;134:567–72.
29. Allen JH, De Moore GM, Heddle R, et al. Cannabinoid hyperemesis: cyclical hyperemesis in association with chronic cannabis abuse. Gut. 2004;53:1566–70.
30. Namin F, Patel J, Lin Z, et al. Clinical, psychiatric and manometric profile of cyclic vomiting syndrome in adults and response to tricyclic therapy. Neurogastroenterol Motil. 2007;19(3):196–202.
31. Andersen JM, Sugerman KS, Lockhart JR, Weinberg WA. Effective prophylactic therapy for cyclic vomiting syndrome in children using amitriptyline or cyproheptadine. Pediatrics. 1997;100(6):977–81.
32. Boles RG, Lovett-Barr MR, Preston A, et al. Treatment of cyclic vomiting syndrome with co-enzyme Q10 and amitriptyline, a retrospective study. BMC Neurol. 2010;10:10.
33. Prakash C, Clouse RE. Cyclic vomiting syndrome in adults: clinical features and response to tricyclic antidepressants. Am J Gastroenterol. 1999;94:2855–9.
34. Gokhale R, Huttenlocher PR, Brady L, et al. Use of barbiturates in the treatment of cyclic vomiting during childhood. J Pediatr Gastroenterol Nutr. 1997;25:64–7.
35. Olmez A, Köse G, Turanli G. Cyclic vomiting with generalized epileptiform discharges responsive to topiramate therapy. Pediatr Neurol. 2006;35(5):348–51.
36. Clouse RE, Sayuk GS, Lustman PH, Prakash C. Zonisamide or levetiracetam for adults with cyclic vomiting syndrome: a case series. Clin Gastroenterol Hepatol. 2007;5:44–8.
37. Benson JM, Zorn SL, Book LS. Sumatriptan in the treatment of cyclic vomiting. Ann Pharmacother. 1995;29(10):997–9.
38. Slater SK, Nelson TD, Kabbouche MA, et al. A randomized, double-blinded, placebo controlled, crossover, add-on study of CoEnzyme Q10 in the prevention of pediatric and adolescent migraine. Cephalalgia. 2011;31(8):897–905.
39. Schoenen J, Jacquy J, Lenaerts M. Effectiveness of high-dose riboflavin in migraine prophylaxis. A randomized controlled trial. Neurology. 1998;50(2):466–70.
40. Van Calcar SC, Harding CO, Wolff JA. L-Carnitine administration reduces number of episodes in cyclic vomiting syndrome. Clin Pediatr (Phila). 2002;41:171–4.
41. Miller AD. Central mechanisms of vomiting. Dig Dis Sci. 1999;44(8 Suppl):39S–43.
42. Khasawinah TA, Ramirez A, Berkenbosch JW, et al. Preliminary experience with dexmedetomidine in the treatment of cyclic vomiting syndrome. Am J Ther. 2003;10(4):303–7.

Aerophagia

37

Oren Koslowe and Denesh K. Chitkara

Introduction

Aerophagia is a functional gastrointestinal disorder recognized with relative frequency in the pediatric and adult population. The term "aerophagia" was applied in the late nineteenth century by Bouveret and quickly adopted by others [1, 2], although reports of the symptoms associated with aerophagia predate that description, perhaps by centuries. There is a report of a conscript who swallowed large quantities of air in order to develop tympany and escape military service in 1814 [3], but one could even imagine that those with *morbus ructuosus* (a term applied to sufferers of "wind"-related conditions) and the "pneumatists" (practitioners of such disorders), who often cared for them dating to the time of Hippocrates, were also exhibiting similar features of aerophagia [4]. Differentiating aerophagia as a unique functional and pathologic entity has been a challenge. It is characterized primarily in descriptive and symptomatic terms based on the Rome criteria which include air swallowing and belching [5], though some studies use more inclusive criteria [6, 7]. The Rome III committee defined aerophagia in children as including two or more of the following symptoms at least once per week for a minimum 2 months before diagnosis: (1) air swallowing, (2) abdominal distention because of intraluminal air, and (3) repetitive belching and/or increased flatus (Table 37.1) [5]. These criteria modified slightly the criteria established by the Rome II committee by decreasing the required duration of symptoms [8]. The symptom-based diagnostic criteria frequently overlap with other functional gastrointestinal disorders such as functional dyspepsia and irritable bowel syndrome. However, there are clinical clues and diagnostic techniques to help in the differentiation [9]. Although not required to make a diagnosis of aerophagia, an esophageal air sign (an abnormal air shadow over the proximal esophagus) on chest radiograph has been suggested as a specific diagnostic criterion for pathologic aerophagia [7]. The Rome III committee shortened the required presence of symptoms for diagnosis from 12 weeks over the preceding 12 months to once per week over the preceding 2 months to more closely approximate the clinical presentation and be more inclusive. While several reports have associated aerophagia with developmentally delayed children, many children with aerophagia are developmentally appropriate for age [6].

O. Koslowe, M.D.
Department of Pediatrics Gastroenterology and Nutrition, Goryeb Children's Hospital/Atlantic Health System, Morristown Memorial Hospital, 100 Madison Avenue, Morristown, NJ 07962, USA

D.K. Chitkara, M.D. (✉)
Department of Pediatrics Gastroenterology and Nutrition, Goryeb Children's Hospital, Atlantic Health, Morristown, NJ, USA
e-mail: dchitkara@pol.net

C. Faure et al. (eds.), *Pediatric Neurogastroenterology: Gastrointestinal Motility and Functional Disorders in Children*, Clinical Gastroenterology,
DOI 10.1007/978-1-60761-709-9_37,

Table 37.1 Rome III diagnostic criteria for children and adolescents with aerophagia two or more of the following occurring at least once per week for at least 2 months before diagnosis

Air swallowing
Abdominal distention because of intraluminal air
Repetitive belching and/or flatus

Adapted from Rasquin et al. [5]

Pathophysiology

The mechanism of air entry into the intestinal tract, which appears responsible for the symptoms of aerophagia, is not entirely clear. Certainly, there is a population of children who swallow excessively, whether volitionally or not, and in so doing increase intraluminal air resulting in increased eructation and/or flatus and symptoms of gastrointestinal distention. The swallowing rate for normal adults is approximately 818/24 h, and the rate of air swallowing is approximately 176/24 h [10]; however, the presence of increased air swallowing in the setting of aerophagia is debatable. Clinically apparent and excessive air swallowing alone may not be entirely responsible for the symptoms of aerophagia [6, 7]. The availability of impedance monitoring has allowed for better and more complete evaluations of swallows, and a recent study indeed showed an increase in air swallowing in adults with aerophagia, though not in swallowing overall [11].

To the extent that increased eructation is associated with aerophagia, there may be two primary mechanisms of action. The first, as stated above, is that excessive air is ingested. This results in proximal gastric distention which, aside from increasing intragastric pressure, promotes an increase in transient lower esophageal relaxations allowing for increased frequency of air expulsion [12, 13]. The second is that eructation does not represent expelled intragastric air, but rather supragastric air that accumulates in the esophagus either by negative intrathoracic pressure against the glottis or mechanical injection by muscular contraction [14, 15]. The latter population, with symptoms limited to frequent belching, may not truly belong to the category of aerophagia [15, 16]. Interestingly, it has been suggested that supragastric belching may be a response to esophageal discomfort associated with gastroesophageal reflux disease (GERD) [17].

The retained intraluminal gas and frequently associated flatus may also incorporate several mechanisms. We find it important to separate abdominal distention from increased intraluminal gas; while they may occur concomitantly (as they must, in order to meet Rome diagnostic criteria), they are often distinct entities [18, 19]. Again, intraluminal gas may arise simply from swallowing large quantities of air; however, gas is also endogenously produced, and several factors may aid in increasing endogenous gas production or delaying transit of intestinal gas. Small bowel bacterial overgrowth, high-fiber diets, sugar malabsorption, and caloric content of meals have all been shown to have an impact on intestinal gas production and/or transit [11, 18, 20, 21].

Treatment

Management of aerophagia depends on the severity of symptoms generated. Certainly there are infrequent reports of severe sequelae associated with aerophagia including massive distention, ileus, and volvulus [7, 22–25]. In such severe cases, a gastrostomy or other means of relief may have to be utilized [23, 26]. Most commonly, children with aerophagia are brought to the attention of care providers with complaints of abdominal pain and abdominal distention which are present in the majority of children at diagnosis [6, 7]. Notably, those symptoms are very nonspecific and are present in many other functional disorders and organic diseases; additionally, abdominal pain is not required for, and would not contribute to, the definition of aerophagia in children according to the Rome criteria. As an example of symptom overlap, GERD patients were shown to swallow air and belch more frequently than controls, although the increased air swallowing was not shown to increase acid reflux [10]. Once a diagnosis of aerophagia has been made, education, reassurance, and supportive techniques are the most often employed measures [6] and may represent the most effective intervention [5, 8]. Hypnosis has been suggested as a mode of therapy in a case report [27]. Where primary psychological disorders are present, they should be addressed [8, 15], although they do not appear to be present to any greater degree in aerophagia than other functional conditions [6]. A variety of behavioral and mechanical techniques that have incorporated biofeedback have been attempted, though only in small-scale trials and rarely with children, to promote self-awareness of swallowing and thereby limit its frequency [28–31]. The duration of response has come into question in most studies. One case report demonstrated sustained response at 18-month follow-up [32]. Pharmacologic therapy may play an extremely limited role for the treatment of pediatric patients with aerophagia due to the significant side effects of the medications that have been utilized. Anxiolytic therapies have been employed likely on the basis that mood or emotional state may impact swallowing rates [33, 34]. In one report in which aerophagia was the result of paroxysmal opening of the upper esophageal sphincter associated with reflex-induced swallowing, clonazepam was shown to be effective [26]. Some reports have suggested a benefit in relieving gas retention using neostigmine [35], but no controlled studies have shown benefit with prokinetic agents for relieving intraluminal air in aerophagia specifically.

There is a benefit in making a diagnosis of aerophagia in children primarily to the extent that one is able to exclude other organic disease entities. The classic features of aerophagia, i.e., those most readily identifiable as being related to excessive air swallowing, are included in the Rome criteria. Those same symptoms seem relatively unchanged in terms of description over the past several centuries and also appear to be generally benign in terms of impacting quality of life. Despite symptoms of aerophagia being reported by nearly one quarter of respondents in a household survey, only 13% of them sought medical care compared to roughly 60% of those with symptoms of functional dyspepsia [36]. A large pediatric study noted similarly that there was limited follow-up for children diagnosed with aerophagia despite the majority not receiving conventional therapy of any kind [6]. There may be some discrepancy in terms of symptom severity between adults and children. A recent phone survey identified what was termed "clinically relevant" belching/burping in 3% of adults [37]; a larger figure than one would expect in children in whom the prevalence of aerophagia in a Rome II validation study was noted to be 1.3% [38].

Conclusion

Symptom overlap and phenotypic variability make the diagnosis and management of aerophagia in children a challenge. While symptoms are generally benign and either resolve spontaneously or are amenable to therapy primarily involving education and reassurance, in some children they may be more severe with both physical and social impact. There have been great strides in recent years understanding and modeling the complex neuromuscular and neuroenteric relationships in a host of functional gastrointestinal disorders, and this comprehension should provide opportunities for improved pharmacologic and non-pharmacologic interventions for children with aerophagia in the future.

References

1. Bouveret L. Spasmes cliniques du pharynx. Revue de Médecine: Aérophagie hystérique; 1891.
2. Foy G. Aerophagia. Dublin J Med Sci (1872–1920). 1901;111(4):301–4.
3. Vanderhoof D. The clinical significance of aerophagia. In: Paper presented at: transactions of the 14th Annual Session of the Medical Society of Virginia, 5–8 Oct 1909, Roanoke, VA
4. Kantor JL. A study of atmospheric air in the upper digestive tract. Am J Med Sci. 1918;155(6):829–56.
5. Rasquin A, Di Lorenzo C, Forbes D, et al. Childhood functional gastrointestinal disorders: child/adolescent. Gastroenterology. 2006;130(5):1527–37.
6. Chitkara DK, Bredenoord AJ, Wang M, Rucker MJ, Talley NJ. Aerophagia in children: characterization of a functional gastrointestinal disorder. Neurogastroenterol Motil. 2005;17(4):518–22.
7. Hwang JB, Choi WJ, Kim JS, et al. Clinical features of pathologic childhood aerophagia: early recognition and essential diagnostic criteria. J Pediatr Gastroenterol Nutr. 2005;41(5):612–6.
8. Rasquin-Weber A, Hyman PE, Cucchiara S, et al. Childhood functional gastrointestinal disorders. Gut. 1999;45 Suppl 2:II60–8.
9. Chitkara DK, Delgado-Aros S, Bredenoord AJ, et al. Functional dyspepsia, upper gastrointestinal symptoms, and transit in children. J Pediatr. 2003;143(5): 609–13.

10. Bredenoord AJ, Weusten BL, Timmer R, Smout AJ. Air swallowing, belching, and reflux in patients with gastroesophageal reflux disease. Am J Gastroenterol. 2006;101(8):1721–6.
11. Hemmink GJ, Weusten BL, Bredenoord AJ, Timmer R, Smout AJ. Aerophagia: excessive air swallowing demonstrated by esophageal impedance monitoring. Clin Gastroenterol Hepatol. 2009;7(10):1127–9.
12. Penagini R, Carmagnola S, Cantu P, Allocca M, Bianchi PA. Mechanoreceptors of the proximal stomach: role in triggering transient lower esophageal sphincter relaxation. Gastroenterology. 2004;126(1):49–56.
13. Straathof JW, Ringers J, Lamers CB, Masclee AA. Provocation of transient lower esophageal sphincter relaxations by gastric distension with air. Am J Gastroenterol. 2001;96(8):2317–23.
14. Bredenoord AJ, Weusten BL, Sifrim D, Timmer R, Smout AJ. Aerophagia, gastric, and supragastric belching: a study using intraluminal electrical impedance monitoring. Gut. 2004;53(11):1561–5.
15. Bredenoord AJ, Smout AJ. Physiologic and pathologic belching. Clin Gastroenterol Hepatol. 2007; 5(7):772–5.
16. Bredenoord AJ. Excessive belching and aerophagia: two different disorders. Dis Esophagus. 2010; 23(4): 347–52.
17. Hemmink GJ, Bredenoord AJ, Weusten BL, Timmer R, Smout AJ. Supragastric belching in patients with reflux symptoms. Am J Gastroenterol. 2009;104(8):1992–7.
18. Maxton DG, Martin DF, Whorwell PJ, Godfrey M. Abdominal distension in female patients with irritable bowel syndrome: exploration of possible mechanisms. Gut. 1991;32(6):662–4.
19. Agrawal A, Whorwell PJ. Review article: abdominal bloating and distension in functional gastrointestinal disorders—epidemiology and exploration of possible mechanisms. Aliment Pharmacol Ther. 2008; 27(1):2–10.
20. Gonlachanvit S, Coleski R, Owyang C, Hasler W. Inhibitory actions of a high fibre diet on intestinal gas transit in healthy volunteers. Gut. 2004;53(11):1577–82.
21. Gonlachanvit S, Coleski R, Owyang C, Hasler WL. Nutrient modulation of intestinal gas dynamics in healthy humans: dependence on caloric content and meal consistency. Am J Physiol Gastrointest Liver Physiol. 2006;291(3):G389–95.
22. Komuro H, Matoba K, Kaneko M. Laparoscopic gastropexy for chronic gastric volvulus complicated by pathologic aerophagia in a boy. Pediatr Int. 2005;47(6): 701–3.
23. van der Kolk MB, Bender MH, Goris RJ. Acute abdomen in mentally retarded patients: role of aerophagia. Report of nine cases. Eur J Surg. 1999;165(5):507–11.
24. Frye RE, Hait EJ. Air swallowing caused recurrent ileus in Tourette's syndrome. Pediatrics. 2006;117(6): e1249–52.
25. Weil RS, Cavanna AE, Willoughby JM, Robertson MM. Air swallowing as a tic. J Psychosom Res. 2008;65(5):497–500.
26. Hwang JB, Kim JS, Ahn BH, Jung CH, Lee YH, Kam S. Clonazepam treatment of pathologic childhood aerophagia with psychological stresses. J Korean Med Sci. 2007;22(2):205–8.
27. Spiegel SB. Uses of hypnosis in the treatment of uncontrollable belching: a case report. Am J Clin Hypn. 1996;38(4):263–70.
28. Chiarioni G, Whitehead WE. The role of biofeedback in the treatment of gastrointestinal disorders. Nat Clin Pract Gastroenterol Hepatol. 2008;5(7):371–82.
29. Calloway SP, Fonagy P, Pounder RE, Morgan MJ. Behavioural techniques in the management of aerophagia in patients with hiatus hernia. J Psychosom Res. 1983;27(6):499–502.
30. Garcia D, Starin S, Churchill RM. Treating aerophagia with contingent physical guidance. J Appl Behav Anal. 2001;34(1):89–92.
31. Bassotti G, Whitehead WE. Biofeedback as a treatment approach to gastrointestinal tract disorders. Am J Gastroenterol. 1994;89(2):158–64.
32. Cigrang JA, Hunter CM, Peterson AL. Behavioral treatment of chronic belching due to aerophagia in a normal adult. Behav Modif. 2006;30(3):341–51.
33. Ritz T, Thons M. Affective modulation of swallowing rates: unpleasantness or arousal? J Psychosom Res. 2006;61(6):829–33.
34. Fonagy P, Calloway SP. The effect of emotional arousal on spontaneous swallowing rates. J Psychosom Res. 1986;30(2):183–8.
35. Caldarella MP, Serra J, Azpiroz F, Malagelada JR. Prokinetic effects in patients with intestinal gas retention. Gastroenterology. 2002;122(7):1748–55.
36. Drossman DA, Li Z, Andruzzi E, et al. U.S. householder survey of functional gastrointestinal disorders. Prevalence, sociodemography, and health impact. Dig Dis Sci. 1993;38(9):1569–80.
37. Camilleri M, Dubois D, Coulie B, et al. Prevalence and socioeconomic impact of upper gastrointestinal disorders in the United States: results of the US Upper Gastrointestinal Study. Clin Gastroenterol Hepatol. 2005;3(6):543–52.
38. Caplan A, Walker L, Rasquin A. Validation of the pediatric Rome II criteria for functional gastrointestinal disorders using the questionnaire on pediatric gastrointestinal symptoms. J Pediatr Gastroenterol Nutr. 2005;41(3):305–16.

38 Adolescent Rumination Syndrome

Anthony Alioto and Carlo Di Lorenzo

Introduction

Rumination is a phenomenon considered normal in ruminant animals, but its occurrence in humans is always pathologic. This condition had been reported in the past as being typical of emotionally deprived and often cognitively impaired infants and adults. More recently, there have been large case series describing it as occurring in adolescents and adults with intact cognitive abilities. Given the substantial differences in etiologic factors, phenotypic presentation, and treatment strategies between infantile and adolescent forms, the current chapter will focus solely on adolescent rumination syndrome.

Despite a recent increase in scientific publications on the subject, adolescent rumination syndrome remains poorly understood and rarely recognized, even by practitioners with a great deal of clinical experience. Its presentation is so characteristic that the high frequency of misdiagnoses is perplexing and likely related to the unfortunate convergence of several factors. First and foremost, there may be some degree of discomfort in making a diagnosis of a disorder that has a behavioral component. In this regard, rumination may be similar to functional dyspepsia or irritable bowel syndrome. In these conditions, physicians may feel more comfortable with a "medical" diagnosis such as gastritis, reflux disease, or colitis rather than embarking in a lengthy and at times antagonistic discussion with the family of the biopsychosocial components of a functional disorder. Second, there is no "test" to conclusively diagnose rumination syndrome. In Western culture, medicine (and patient expectations) often is based on the biomedical model which postulates that a symptom is due to a demonstrable anatomical, inflammatory, serologic, immune, or other system dysregulation. Without a test demonstrating positive symptoms, many practitioners and patients feel uncomfortable with the diagnosis. Third, the lack of a standard and relatively easy to implement therapy for rumination syndrome may give some providers a sense of futility when making such a diagnosis for which they have little therapeutic advise to offer. In order to guide the practitioner, we will discuss the most recent understanding of the epidemiology, pathophysiology, diagnosis, and therapy of adolescent rumination syndrome.

Epidemiology

There have been no population-based epidemiologic studies of the prevalence of rumination syndrome in children. Traditionally, this condition has

A. Alioto, Ph.D.
Division of Pediatric Gastroenterology, Department of Psychology, Nationwide Children's Hospital, The Ohio State University, Columbus, OH, USA

C. Di Lorenzo, M.D. (✉)
Department of Pediatrics, Nationwide Children's Hospital, The Ohio State University,
700 Children's Drive, Columbus, OH 43205, USA
e-mail: carlo.dilorenzo@nationwidechildrens.org

C. Faure et al. (eds.), *Pediatric Neurogastroenterology: Gastrointestinal Motility and Functional Disorders in Children*, Clinical Gastroenterology,
DOI 10.1007/978-1-60761-709-9_38, © Springer Science+Business Media New York 2013

been considered as having a low prevalence in adolescents [1]. As described earlier, the insufficient recognition of rumination syndrome as a diagnostic entity undermines efforts to understand its prevalence. Further complicating estimates, the symptoms of rumination syndrome overlap with symptoms of more readily recognized conditions such as gastroesophageal reflux disease, gastroparesis, pseudoobstruction, and eating disorders [2–6].

Due to these challenges, patients with rumination syndrome often are evaluated by multiple physicians over the course of several years prior to receiving the correct diagnosis [5]. In the interim, they undergo multiple fruitless and expensive medical evaluations and diagnostic testing. In one sample of adolescents [3], onset of rumination symptoms occurred around age 13 years, with the diagnosis of rumination syndrome ultimately given approximately 2 years later.

Available evidence suggests that rumination syndrome is found in females significantly more often than in males. Physical or psychological stressors often occur just before the onset of the symptoms in a sizable subset of subjects, and a substantial portion of diagnosed patients have associated physical illnesses or concomitant psychological disorders [3].

Pathophysiology

The precise etiology of rumination syndrome remains unknown at this time. Even so, many patients' histories are suggestive of a trigger at the onset of symptoms, such as a gastrointestinal mucosal disease or stressors involving emotional arousal. After the initial stressor has resolved, the vomiting behavior appears to remain in place, almost similar to a "tic."

Gastric motor and sensory abnormalities have been reported in rumination syndrome. Barostat and manometric studies have demonstrated gastric hypersensitivity with more frequent episodes of lower esophageal sphincter relaxation in response to gastric distension [7]. Some individuals have impaired postprandial gastric accommodation [7]. A mild degree of gastroparesis may be found in approximately 40 % of adolescents with rumination [3], although emptying studies are difficult to interpret in individuals who continuously regurgitate during the test. A poorly accommodating fundus and an impaired antral pump may lead to postprandial distress that the patient tends to relieve by expelling the food just ingested. As such, the behavior of regurgitating gastric contents serves to relieve epigastric discomfort and becomes a learned response to the ingestion of food or fluid. Upon ingestion of food (or even in anticipation of ingestion of food), a sequence of behaviors has been generated, including contraction of the abdominal wall, opening of the lower and upper esophageal sphincter, and subsequent expulsion of food [8].

Clinical Features

The main clinical characteristic of rumination is the timing of the act of vomiting. There are very few other medical gastrointestinal diseases associated with vomiting within seconds or minutes from food ingestion. Although the regurgitated gastric contents may be re-swallowed, in adolescents they frequently are expelled. Rumination persists up to an hour after eating and rarely occurs at night [3]. Table 38.1 shows some of the features differentiating rumination from other clinical entities. Weight loss is a common feature of the most severe forms of rumination syndrome and may lead to the need for tube feedings or even parenteral nutrition. Other symptoms, particularly abdominal pain, heartburn, and nausea are less frequently reported, but often serve as a "signal," allowing patients to recognize when rumination is about to occur.

Diagnosis

Rumination syndrome is a clinical diagnosis [6] and very minimal testing should be needed in the classic cases. A patient who satisfies the symptoms-based Rome III criteria for this condition (Table 38.2) should need no further investigation. Pointing out to the patients and to the parents how saliva is easily swallowed but even a sip of water causes symptoms is particularly enlightening with regard to the behavioral component of this disorder.

Table 38.1 Differential diagnosis of rumination syndrome from other conditions presenting with emesis in adolescents

	Vomiting	Esophagitis	Prokinetics	Fundoplication
Rumination	During or minutes after meal	No	Not helpful	Not helpful
Achalasia	Hours after meal	Often (from stasis)	Not helpful	Contraindicated
GERD	After large meals or when lying down	Often	Helpful	Helpful
Gastroparesis	Hours after meal	No	Helpful	Not helpful
Cyclic vomiting	Intermittent, unrelated to meal	During episodes	Not helpful	Not helpful

Table 38.2 Rome III criteria for adolescent rumination syndrome

1. At least a 2 month history of repeated painless regurgitation and re-chewing or expulsion of food
2. The behavior begins soon after ingestion of a meal
3. The behavior does not occur during sleep
4. There is no retching
5. Symptoms do not respond to standard treatment for gastroesophageal reflux
6. No evidence of an inflammatory, anatomic, metabolic, or neoplastic process considered likely to be an explanation for the subject's symptoms

Antroduodenal manometry is not always necessary to make the diagnosis, but it can be considered as the "big convincer" in cases when the referring physicians or the families are not yet confident with the diagnosis of rumination syndrome. Manometry may be used to clinch the diagnosis and rule out the presence of an underlying motility disorder, a common fear among family of patients with this disorder. In patients with rumination syndrome, antroduodenal manometry shows essentially normal fasting and postprandial motor patterns [6, 9]. The characteristic manometric abnormality is a synchronous increase in pressure ("r" waves) across both gastric and duodenal recording sites when the rumination occurs. The "r waves" are thought to represent the effect of an increase in intra-gastric or intra-abdominal pressure generated by the contraction of the skeletal abdominal muscles. Interestingly, under the pressure of being in a laboratory setting with constant attention being paid to their symptoms, adolescents with rumination are often able to eat the test meal during the manometry study without symptoms (Fig. 38.1).

Postprandial impedance-manometry monitoring allows distinction between rumination from postprandial belching and regurgitation. During rumination, esophageal liquid retrograde flow is first driven by an early small rise in intra-gastric pressure preceding the peak pressure observed during straining [10].

Treatment

As practitioners and researchers strive to understand the pathogenesis of this complex functional disorder, many have proposed mechanisms by which rumination is maintained (e.g., habit disorder, learned adaptation of the belch reflex, sympathetic nervous system arousal). Based on these postulates, several approaches to treatment have been put forward and demonstrated to be effective. Despite the variety of conceptualizations of rumination syndrome, similar treatment strategies appear to be utilized across studies and treatment centers and are categorized and described below.

Education and Reassurance

Several authors have discussed how accurate diagnosis and reassurance often provide considerable relief to families and patients [1, 11]. Education about rumination syndrome may allow for a reduction in anxiety, as patients are provided with a diagnosis and understand that no structural or intrinsic motility problems exist. In addition, accurate description of the disorder may allow patients to be a more active part in their own treatment.

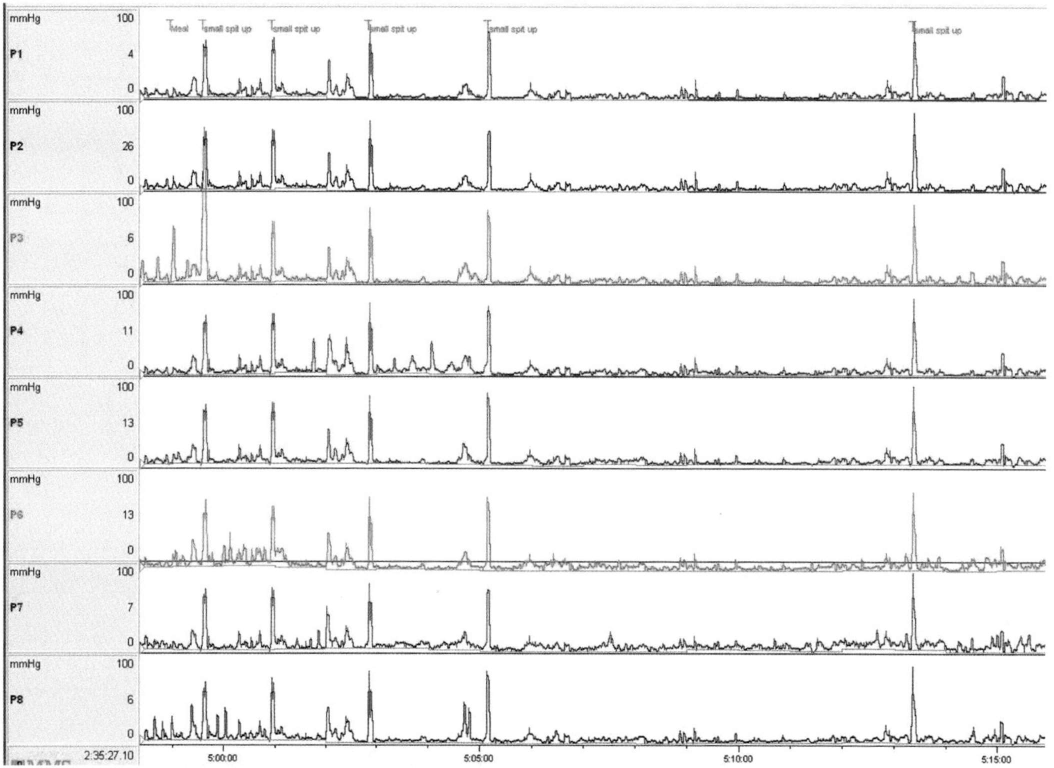

Fig. 38.1 An example of an antroduodenal tracing from an adolescent with rumination syndrome. The end of the meal is marked and almost immediately afterwards, the patient begins to have episodes of "small spit up," marked as such on the tracing. Those events are associated with a simultaneous increase in pressure in all recording sites (known as "r waves")

Presentation of rumination syndrome from a biopsychosocial perspective allows families to understand the interplay among physical, behavioral, emotional, and situational factors [12]. The educational intervention should include a discussion of how no further testing is needed, how rumination syndrome can be diagnosed by symptoms (and it is not simply a diagnosis of exclusion), and how the condition is treatable using behavioral interventions. In our experience, families who continue to seek further diagnostic testing and a "medical" explanation for the rumination tend to be less invested and less successful with treatment.

Behavioral Strategies

Many authors have conceptualized rumination syndrome in terms of a learned "habit," and therefore have utilized strategies that have been empirically supported in the treatment of habit disorders [8, 12–14]. Traditional components of habit reversal training (HRT) include increasing awareness of the behavior, introducing a competing response to the behavior, pairing an aversive stimulus to the behavior, encouraging relaxation, and providing social support. Applied to rumination syndrome, effective interventions include charting and monitoring rumination episodes ("waves") and at times the use of electromyographic biofeedback to elucidate the contraction of the abdominal wall during rumination (i.e., awareness), utilizing diaphragmatic breathing and deep inhalation in order to relax the abdominal wall (i.e., competing response), having the patient reswallow all emesis (i.e., aversive stimulus), diaphragmatic breathing and distraction (i.e., relaxation), and family involvement in therapy (i.e., social support).

Use of Self-regulation Strategies

Several authors have discussed the importance of providing strategies for improving self-control over the behavioral manifestation of rumination. As rumination involves contraction of the abdominal wall, diaphragmatic breathing has been utilized to provide abdominal muscle relaxation [15]. Other authors have utilized progressive muscle relaxation in order to achieve general relaxation [14].

Functional gastrointestinal disorders recently have been understood in terms of the multiple pathways that influence symptom presentation, with autonomic nervous system dysregulation playing an integral role [16]. The autonomic nervous system's reactivity and recovery has been shown to have an impact on symptom presentation in patients with functional gastrointestinal disorders such as irritable bowel syndrome [17]. It has also been demonstrated that biofeedback approaches (i.e., instruction on autonomic nervous system regulation) allows for increased vagal tone as well as symptom improvement in patients with functional abdominal pain [18]. Given the role of autonomic dysregulation in functional disorders, it is likely that similar mechanisms contribute to the challenges demonstrated by patients with rumination syndrome.

The use of biofeedback has been described by several authors as a beneficial intervention in patients with rumination syndrome [3, 13, 15, 19], often with minimal description of the specific biofeedback modality employed or the proposed mechanism by which the biofeedback allowed for improvement (e.g., as a "behavioral" intervention, to allow for general relaxation, targeted abdominal wall relaxation). It may be the case that biofeedback training plays a specific role in allowing the patient greater self-regulation of the autonomic nervous system and a reduction in sensitivity to gastric distension.

Gradual Refeeding

Many authors have discussed the importance of having patients slowly reintroduce food and fluid intake [20]. Gradual reintroduction of oral intake allows patients to practice and utilize their self-management skills while working with increasingly challenging quantities of food and tolerating the discomfort that arises with gastric distension. The use of frequent, small feeding trials seems to provide other benefits to patients. First, frequent, small eating/drinking trials allow for repeated re-exposure to a stressful stimulus (i.e., actual eating/drinking and/or anticipatory anxiety about eating/drinking). Second, smaller amounts of food and fluid are more manageable as patients focus on reswallowing their food and not expelling the emesis. Finally, this measured approach provides patients with a sense of self-efficacy as they make progress and have successful experiences with keeping food down.

Support Strategies

In the early stages of treatment, progress can be measured by the patient's ability to refrain from expelling emesis (i.e., reswallowing the emesis) and reducing the frequency of the rumination behavior itself. To support patients as they achieve these goals, many strategies are employed to reduce some of the barriers to success. Patients frequently are encouraged to engage in distraction activities. Distraction utilized includes listening to music, watching television, playing video games, or reading aloud. The goal of distraction is to direct attention away from the physical sensations that often prompt an episode of rumination (e.g., pain, pressure, nausea). Although medications alone have not been shown to be an effective treatment for rumination [2], several drugs may be beneficial in reducing many of the sensations that serve as a "signal" to ruminate. Amitriptyline, cyproheptadine, buspirone, ondansetron, acid suppression, and prokinetics act on different gastric and central nervous system targets and may provide benefit to individual patients undergoing treatment. Special means of alimentation with post-pyloric feedings, either through naso-jejunal or gastro-jejunal feeding catheters, may be used initially to maintain adequate nutritional status when weight loss is significant and should always be attempted prior to parenteral nutrition.

Address Accompanying Psychological Factors

A subset of patients with rumination syndrome also has comorbid emotional difficulties including depression, anxiety, histories of abuse, and life stressors [3, 21]. The relationship between emotional state, autonomic nervous system activation, and the experience of pain has been widely recognized [22, 23]. While these comorbid conditions likely are not the cause of the rumination, failure to identify and address these challenges will have a deleterious impact on treatment. Patients with comorbid emotional difficulties may experience greater discomfort during treatment, anticipatory anxiety, and experience greater emotional distress as a result of the discomfort.

Interdisciplinary Approaches

Several authors have discussed programmatic approaches to the treatment of rumination syndrome [3, 13]. Intensive treatment approaches allow multiple disciplines to address similar components of the patients' challenges in a complementary manner, while providing a more controlled environment in which treatment may take place. Treatment in an inpatient medical setting provides the additional benefit of close monitoring of associated medical difficulties (e.g., severe nausea, pain, transition from enteral feedings).

Conclusion

Rumination syndrome is a relatively easily diagnosed, but often misidentified condition that has a significant impact on patients' quality of life. Rumination has been shown to be responsive to behavioral interventions. While some cases may benefit from a simplified treatment protocol carried out as an outpatient [6], more disabled patients may benefit more from an intensive, programmatic approach. Regardless of the approach, several factors seem to have an impact on treatment success. Families who accept the diagnosis, have a solid understanding of the mechanisms that maintain rumination, and provide the patient with ongoing support tend to demonstrate better recovery. Further research will serve to elucidate patient and family variables that may be empirically predictive of treatment success.

References

1. Khan S, Hyman PE, Cocjin J, Di Lorenzo C. Rumination syndrome in adolescents. J Pediatr. 2000; 136:528–31.
2. Chitkara D, Bredenoord AJ, Talley N, Whitehead WE. Aerophagia and rumination: recognition and therapy. Curr Treat Options Gastroenterol. 2006;9: 305–13.
3. Chial H, Camilleri M, Williams DE, Litzinger K, Perrault J. Rumination syndrome in children and adolescents: diagnosis, treatment, and prognosis. Pediatrics. 2003;111:158–62.
4. Graff J, Surprise J, Sarosiek I, Twillman R, McCallum RW. Rumination syndrome: challenges with diagnosis and treatment. Am J Gastroenterol. 2002; 97(Suppl):S48.
5. Eckern M, Stevens W, Mitchell J. The relationship between rumination and eating disorders. Int J Eat Disord. 1999;26:414–9.
6. O'Brien M, Bruce B, Camilleri M. The rumination syndrome: clinical features rather than manometric diagnosis. Gastroenterology. 1995;108:1024–9.
7. Thumshirn M, Camilleri M, Hanson RB, Williams DE, Schei AJ, Kammer PP. New insights into the pathogenesis of rumination: what's coming up next. Am J Physiol Gastrointest Liver Physiol. 1998;275: 314–21.
8. Chitkara D, VanTilburg M, Whitehead WE, Talley NJ. Teaching diaphragmatic breathing for rumination syndrome. Am J Gastroenterol. 2006;101:2449–52.
9. Amarnath R, Abell T, Malagelada J. The rumination syndrome in adults: a characteristic manometric pattern. Ann Intern Med. 1986;105:513–8.
10. Rommel N, Tack J, Caenepeel P, Bisschops R, Sifrim D. Rumination or belching-regurgitation? Differential diagnosis using oesophageal impedance-manometry. Neurogastroenterol Motil. 2010;22:e97–104.
11. Banez GA, Gallagher HM. Recurrent abdominal pain. Behav Modif. 2006;30:50–71.
12. Dalton WT, Czyzewski D. Behavioral treatment of habitual rumination: case reports. Dig Dis Sci. 2009; 54:1804–7.
13. Green AD, Alioto A, Mousa H, Di Lorenzo C. Severe pediatric rumination syndrome: successful interdisciplinary inpatient management. J Pediatr Gastroenterol Nutr. 2011;52(4):414–8.
14. Wagaman J, Williams D, Camilleri M. Behavioral intervention for the treatment of rumination. J Pediatr Gastroenterol Nutr. 1998;27:596–8.

15. Shay SS, Johnson LF, Wong RK, et al. Rumination, heartburn, and daytime gastroesophageal reflux. J Clin Gastroenterol. 1986;8:115–26.
16. Cunningham CL, Banez GA. Theoretical and historical basis for a biopsychosocial approach to pediatric gastrointestinal disorders. In: Cunningham CL, Banez GA, editors. Pediatric gastrointestinal disorders. New York, NY: Springer; 2006. p. 13–30.
17. Aggarwal A, Cutts TF, Abell TL, et al. Predominant symptoms in irritable bowel syndrome correlate with specific autonomic nervous system abnormalities. Gastroenterology. 1994;106:945–50.
18. Sowder E, Gevirtz R, Shapiro W, Ebert C. Restoration of vagal tone: a possible mechanism for functional abdominal pain. Appl Psychophysiol Biofeedback. 2010;35:199–206.
19. Olden K. Rumination. Curr Treat Options Gastroenterol. 2001;4:351–8.
20. Chial HJ, Camilleri M. A twenty-one-year-old college student with postprandial regurgitation and weight loss. Clin Gastroenterol Hepatol. 2006;4:1314–7.
21. Soykan I, Chen J, Kendall BJ, McCallum R. The rumination syndrome: clinical and manometric profile, therapy, and long-term outcome. Dig Dis Sci. 1997;42:1866–72.
22. Fernandez S, Aspirot A, Kerzner B, Friedlander J, Di Lorenzo C. Do some adolescents with rumination syndrome have "supragastric vomiting"? J Pediatr Gastroenterol Nutr. 2010;50:103–5.
23. Beidel DC, Christ MG, Long PJ. Somatic complaints in anxious children. J Abnorm Child Psychol. 1991; 19:659–70.

Constipation

39

Vera Loening-Baucke and Alexander Swidsinski

Introduction

Many children experience constipation at one time or another [1]. Constipation is the most common digestive complaint in the general population, both in adults and children, and occurs worldwide [1]. Usually the problem persists for a short time; however, some children are chronically constipated suffering for months and even years. Three percent of infants suffered from constipation in the first and 10% in the second year of life in a primary care clinic in North America [2]. Issenman reported that 16% of 22 month olds were thought by their parents to be constipated [3]. Five percent of otherwise healthy 4–11-year-old British school-children had constipation lasting more than 6 months [4], 18% of 4–17-year-old children had functional constipation in a primary care clinic in USA [5], and 18–37% of Brazilian children suffered from constipation [6–8]. No significant difference in prevalence between boys and girls has been reported [1].

Chronic constipation is functional in more than 90% of the cases. Functional constipation is constipation not due to organic or anatomical causes or use of medication. Despite the functional nature of constipation, the health-related problems of affected children are extensive and their quality of life is reduced.

Pathophysiology

Like many pediatric gastrointestinal disorders, the etiology and course of functional constipation are increasingly conceptualized within a broad biopsychosocial perspective that assumes that a child's condition is a function of multiple interacting determinants, such as genetic predisposition, environmental factors, life stress, psychological state, coping, social support, and interactions between physiologic and psychological factors via the central nervous and enteric nervous system.

Infants and Toddlers

In 90% of normal newborns the first bowel movement occurs within the first 24 h after birth and in 98% within 48 h. The first bowel movement may happen much later in the premature infant. A number of studies have revealed a decline in stool

V. Loening-Baucke, M.D. (✉)
Pediatrics Department, General Pediatric Division, University of Iowa, Beldon Avenue, Iowa City, IA 52246, USA

Medizinische Klinik und Poliklinik, Gastroenterologie, Hepatologie and Endokrinologie, Charité Universitätsmedizin, Berlin, Germany
e-mail: vera-loening-baucke@uiowa.edu

A. Swidsinski, M.D., Ph.D
Medizinische Klinik und Poliklinik, Gastroenterologie, Hepatologie and Endokrinologie, Charité Universitätsmedizin, Berlin, Germany
e-mail: alexander.swidsinski@charite.de

C. Faure et al. (eds.), *Pediatric Neurogastroenterology: Gastrointestinal Motility and Functional Disorders in Children*, Clinical Gastroenterology,
DOI 10.1007/978-1-60761-709-9_39, © Springer Science+Business Media New York 2013

frequency from more than four stools per day during the first week of life to 1.2 per day at 4 years of age with a corresponding increase in stool size. Fontana et al. [9] showed that in the first 3 years of life, 97% of healthy children had at least one bowel movement every other day.

The Rome III Committee suggested these mostly symptom-based diagnostic criteria for functional constipation in infants and toddlers up to 4 years of age [10]. At least two of the following symptoms must occur for at least 1 month.

- ≤2 defecations per week
- ≥1 episode per week of incontinence after the acquisition of toileting skills
- History of excessive stool retention
- History of painful or hard bowel movements
- Presence of a large fecal mass in the rectum
- History of large-diameter stools that may obstruct the toilet

Constipation in early life is a special situation because of the possibility of serious congenital disorders. If meconium passage is delayed for more than 24 h, several rare diseases need to be considered. Evaluation for Hirschsprung's disease may include a barium enema, anorectal manometry, and rectal suction biopsy. The barium enema most often shows a transition zone, but the transition zone can be absent in the newborn period. The anorectal manometry shows an absent anorectal (recto-sphincteric) reflex. The diagnosis is confirmed by the absence of ganglion cells in the submucosal and myenteric plexus in the rectal biopsy. Defects of the spinal cord (such as myelomeningocele), or anomalies of the anorectum (such as anal atresia and anal stenosis), must be ruled out by examination and, if necessary, by appropriate imaging studies. Meconium plugs may cause neonatal constipation, and may be associated with either Hirschsprung's disease or cystic fibrosis. Other organic causes of constipation include endocrine, metabolic, and neuromuscular diseases.

There are two periods in which the infant and toddler are prone to develop constipation. The first occurs during the change from breast milk to commercial formula or introduction of solids, the second during toilet training. The most common cause of constipation in infants and toddlers is an acquired behavior after experiencing painful bowel movements. This notion is supported by 93% of parents of infants and toddlers with functional constipation reporting hard to rock-hard stools, 27% reported having seen blood around their child's stool, and 42% of children were crying and screaming when passing stools [2]. Then the fear of defecation leads to voluntary withholding of stool, called retentive posturing. Instead of relaxing the pelvic floor for defecation, the retentive infant will contract the pelvic floor and gluteal muscles in an attempt to avoid defecation. Infants will often grunt, arch back, and stiffen their legs. Toddlers often rise on their toes and rock back and forth while squeezing the buttocks together and stiffening their legs, or assume other unusual postures. These maneuvers are often misinterpreted by the parents as straining for defecation. Forty-five percent of our constipated infants and toddlers exhibited stool withholding behavior [2]. Only 10% had an abdominal fecal mass present, and 53% of those with a rectal examination had a rectal impaction [2]. Incontinence may be mistaken for diarrhea by some parents. Other accompanying symptoms may include irritability, decreased appetite, and/or early satiety. These accompanying symptoms disappear immediately following passage of a large stool.

The second period in which the toddler is prone to develop constipation is during toilet training. In order to master toileting, the toddler must develop the ability and interest in retaining a bowel movement until it can be deposited into the toilet. The attempt to retain stool leads to less frequent bowel movements and sometimes to hard and painful bowel movements. A power struggle may develop if toilet training is forced on the toddler by the parent, potentially leading to constipation. Parents should avoid pushing for early toilet training, but rather wait till the child shows signs of readiness for toilet training. These signs include signs of physiologic maturation, such as the ability to sit, walk, dress and undress, the child understands and responds to instruction, has the desire to imitate and identify with the parent, has self-determination, and shows signs of independence.

The physical examination should be complete with special attention to the size of the rectal fecal mass during abdominal examination and, if none is felt, during the rectal examination.

Infant dyschezia and infrequent bowel movements in breastfed infants, both accompanied by soft to loose stools, are often misinterpreted as constipation. Infant dyschezia is the term used for otherwise healthy infants in the first few months of life who appear to have significant discomfort and excessive straining associated with defecation and crying for over 10 min, followed by successful passage of soft to liquid stools. It is speculated that this disorder occurs when neonates fail to coordinate increased intra-abdominal pressure with relaxation of the pelvic floor. Symptoms resolve without intervention in most cases. Breastfed infants may defecate after each feeding and other exclusively breastfed infants may have infrequent soft bowel movements. In our review of 4,157 infants and toddlers, we found that 18 well-nourished exclusively breastfed infants had long intervals between soft to loose bowel movements (2–14 days, mean 5.4±3.0 days) [2]. This bowel pattern is considered normal for breastfed infants.

Children and Adolescents

The Rome III Committee recommended symptom-based diagnostic criteria for functional constipation in children and adolescents [11]. Symptom must occur at least once per week for at least 2 months and include 2 or more of the following in a child with a developmental age of ≥4 years with insufficient criteria for a diagnosis of irritable bowel syndrome.

- Two or fewer defecations in the toilet per week
- At least 1 episode of fecal incontinence per week
- History of retentive posturing or excessive volitional stool retention
- History of painful or hard bowel movements
- Presence of a large fecal mass in the rectum
- History of large diameter stools that may obstruct the toilet

A positive family history has been found in 28–50% of constipated children, and a higher incidence has been reported in monozygotic than dizygotic twins [12]. Often the onset of functional constipation in children ≥4 years of age occurs when a child begins to attend school, when toilet use is reserved to special times and toilets may not be clean and private. Children who have been constipated for years may have had withholding behavior long before the visit to the physician, and by the time they are evaluated, the rectum has become dilated and has accommodated to the point that withholding is no longer necessary in order to delay the passage of stools. The term excessive volitional stool retention is used to describe older children who still withhold their stools without necessarily displaying retentive posturing. Many parents of constipated children give a history of passage of enormous stools, obstruction of the toilet by the stool, retentive posturing, abdominal pain and irritability, anal or rectal pain, anorexia, and unusual behaviors, such as a nonchalant attitude regarding the fecal incontinence, hiding their dirty underwear, and lack of awareness of an incontinence episode. Most symptoms disappear dramatically following the passage of a huge stool.

Complications of Constipation

Fecal Incontinence

Fecal incontinence, also known as encopresis or fecal soiling, is the most obvious complication of constipation. Fecal incontinence is the involuntary loss of formed, semi-formed, or liquid stool into the child's underwear and is considered a problem after the child has reached a developmental age of 4 years. Fecal incontinence in children is most often associated with functional constipation. Loening-Baucke [5] showed a 4% prevalence rate for functional fecal incontinence in a retrospective review in 482 children, 4–17 years of age, attending a primary care clinic in the USA. In this study fecal incontinence was associated with constipation in 95% of the children [5].

Seventy-nine percent of children with functional constipation and fecal incontinence were reported to have a history of retentive posturing [13]. When stool withholding is successful, greater amounts of stool accumulate in the rectum with longer exposure to its drying action, and a vicious cycle is started. When stool retention remains untreated for a prolonged period of time, the rectal wall stretches and a megarectum develops. The intervals between bowel movements become increasingly longer and the rectum becomes so large that the stored stool can be felt as an abdominal mass that sometimes reaches up to the umbilicus, above the umbilicus, and occasionally up to the sternum. The progressive fecal accumulation eventually leads to pelvic floor muscle fatigue and poor anal sphincter competence, leading to leakage of stools. Usually, the consistency of stool found in the underwear is loose or clay-like. Sometimes the core of the impaction breaks off and is found as a firm stool in the underwear. Occasionally, what appears to be a full bowel movement is passed into the underwear. A period free of fecal incontinence may occur after a huge bowel movement is passed and fecal incontinence will resume only after several days of stool retention. The social stigma which goes along with increased flatulence and the odor of fecal incontinence can be devastating to the child's self-esteem and his/her acceptance by siblings, parents, peers, and teachers.

Abdominal Pain

Abdominal pain and anal and rectal pain are reported by approximately half of the constipated children. Severe attacks of abdominal pain can occur either just before a bowel movement, for several days prior to a large bowel movement, or daily. Many children suffer from vague chronic abdominal pain. Some patients with large stool masses throughout the entire colon may not experience any abdominal pain. A chart review at the University of Iowa in a primary care setting revealed that 9% of 962 children ≥4 years of age had a visit for acute abdominal pain and 12.7% for chronic abdominal pain. Acute and chronic constipation were the most frequent causes of abdominal pain [14, 15].

Urinary Complications

Anorectal and lower urinary tract function are interrelated. As a result, constipation is often associated with urinary symptoms such as daytime and/or nighttime urinary incontinence and urinary tract infections. Daytime urinary incontinence occurred in 29%, bed wetting in 34%, and one or more urinary tract infections in 33% of girls and 3% of boys of our constipated and fecal incontinent children [16]. Other less common urinary complications are vesicoureteral reflux, urinary retention, megacystis, and ureteral obstruction.

Behavioral Problems

Behavioral problems are common in children with functional constipation and in children who have fecal incontinence [17, 18]. Children with constipation and fecal incontinence score above the means but not in the abnormal range on all behavior subscales when compared to sex- and age-matched controls [19]. Behavior problems can be the cause or the consequence of constipation with or without fecal incontinence. Several intervention studies have shown an association between successful treatment and the reduction of behavior problems, suggesting that behavior problems are secondary to the clinical problem of constipation, in particular when fecal incontinence is also present.

Quality of Life

It has been shown that functional constipation has a great impact on the child's emotional well-being. Children with constipation report a lower quality of life than a healthy control group, children with inflammatory bowel disease or children with gastroesophageal reflux [20].

Diagnosis

History

The history should include information regarding the general health of the child and the presenting signs and symptoms. A careful history needs to elicit the intervals, amount, diameter, and consistency of bowel movements deposited into the toilet and of stools deposited into the underwear.

The amount, intervals, diameter, and consistency of bowel movements are important because some children may have daily bowel movements but evacuate incompletely, as evidenced by periodic passage of very large amounts of stool of hard to loose consistency. Do the stools clog the toilet? Is or was stool withholding/retentive behavior present? What was the age at onset of constipation? Was there a problem with the timing of passage of meconium? The character of the stools is reviewed from birth for consistency, caliber, and frequency. Is abdominal pain present? Is urinary incontinence or urinary tract infection present? What are the dietary habits?

Physical Examination

The physical examination should be thorough in order to rule out an underlying disorder and often includes a rectal examination. Weight and height should be plotted. An abdominal fecal mass can be palpated in many constipated children during abdominal examination. Sometimes the mass extends throughout the entire colon, but more commonly the mass is felt suprapubically and midline, sometimes filling the left or the right lower quadrant. The anal size and location need to be assessed. A low anal pressure during digital rectal examination suggests either fecal retention with inhibition of the anal resting pressure or a disease involving the external or internal anal sphincter or both. The neurological examination should include perineal sensation testing in cooperative children using a Q-tip. Loss of perianal skin sensation can be associated with various neurologic diseases of the spinal cord.

In most cases, a carefully performed rectal examination causes a minimal degree of physical or emotional trauma to the child. Often the rectum is packed with stool, either of hard consistency or, more commonly, the outside of the fecal impaction feels like clay and the core of the fecal retention is rock hard. No rectal fecal impaction is felt in children with a recent large bowel movement. Occasionally, the rectal examination will reveal an organic cause for the constipation, such as a large anal fissure, anal stenosis, anal atresia with perineal fistula or a tight rectal ampulla, suggestive of Hirschsprung's disease. Rarely, a sacral tumor obstructing the rectum has been found. Failure to appreciate the degree of fecal retention in these children, can lead to erroneous treatments, can further delay effective treatment or lead to misdirected psychotherapy.

Laboratory Investigation

Most children with functional constipation need no or minimal laboratory testing. Laboratory and radiologic testing should be selected based upon the history and physical examination and should be pursued only if the child fails to respond to the treatment program and in patients with signs and symptoms suggestive of an organic cause. Rarely, serologic studies (deficiency or excess of thyroid or adrenal hormones, electrolyte imbalances, and calcium level, celiac antibodies), urine culture, X-ray studies, anorectal manometric studies, or rectal biopsy will be necessary.

Occult Blood Testing

It is recommended that stool is tested for occult blood in all infants with constipation as well as in any child who has abdominal pain, failure to thrive, intermittent diarrhea, or a family history of colon cancer or colonic polyps.

Abdominal Radiographs

Radiologic studies usually are not indicated in uncomplicated functional constipation. A plain abdominal film can be useful in assessing the presence or absence of retained stool, its extent, and whether or not the lower spine is normal. It should be pursued in children with symptoms suggestive of constipation and absence of a fecal mass on abdominal and rectal examination, in children who vehemently refuse the rectal examination, in children who are markedly obese, and in children who are still symptomatic while on laxatives.

Barium Enema Study

A barium enema is unnecessary in uncomplicated cases of functional constipation.

Colonic Transit Study

A colonic transit study provides an objective measure of presence and the severity of constipation in children, but is unnecessary in most children with functional constipation. It does not influence the initial decision how to treat the child. It may be helpful to differentiate children with nonretentive fecal incontinence from those with functional constipation with overflow fecal incontinence.

Anorectal Manometry

Anorectal manometry is unnecessary in children with functional constipation with or without functional fecal incontinence. The main clinical role of anorectal manometry is in the evaluation of infants and children with severe constipation, where the diagnosis of Hirschsprung's disease needs to be excluded. It may also be helpful in evaluating other conditions, such as spinal defects and anal achalasia. We have performed numerous manometric studies in children with functional constipation with fecal incontinence and have documented many abnormalities, including increased threshold to rectal distention and decreased rectal contractility as compared to controls [17]. After 3 years of therapy, many children will show persistent abnormalities of anorectal function, leaving them at risk for recurrent problems [19, 21]. Another abnormality often reported is the contraction of the external anal sphincter and pelvic floor muscles instead of relaxation of these muscles during defecation attempts (a pattern characteristic of dyssynergic defecation) [17, 22, 23].

Colonic Manometry

Colonic manometry study is unnecessary in most children with functional constipation. A colonic motility study may be helpful in children with suspected dysmotility of the colon or the total gastrointestinal tract.

Treatment in Infants and Toddlers

After assessment of the constipated infant/toddler, all parents should receive education, including explanation that passing hard stools and experiencing painful defecation are the primary precipitants of constipation and withholding behavior during infancy and the toddler years [2, 24–26].

Disimpaction

Most fecal impactions at this age can be resolved with a few days of laxative treatment. Occasionally, a glycerin suppository is necessary and if unsuccessful, a 6 mL/kg bodyweight phosphate enema can be used.

Diet and fiber

Acute, simple constipation in infants and toddlers frequently resolves with ingestion of non-digestible, osmotically active carbohydrates, including sorbitol-containing juices, such as prune, pear, and apple juice; addition of pureed fruits and vegetables; or medications with high sugar content (barley malt extract or corn syrup). Several studies have claimed a causal relationship between cow's milk exposure and constipation in children [27–32], but this could not be confirmed by Simeone et al. [33], Loening-Baucke [2], and Benninga et al. [34].

Laxative

If despite dietary changes, the stool is still hard and painful to evacuate, then osmotic laxatives are given, such as polyethylene glycol, lactulose, sorbitol, or milk of magnesia (see Table 39.1). The key to effective maintenance is assuring painless

Table 39.1 Suggested medications and dosages for maintenance therapy of constipation in infants and toddlers

Medication	Age (month)	Dose
Polyethylene glycol 3350	>1	0.7 g/kg body weight/day [24, 35]
Lactulose or sorbitol	>1	1–3 mL/kg body weight/day, divide in 1–2 doses
Milk of magnesia	>1	1–3 mL/kg body weight/day, divide in 1–2 doses
Mineral oil	>12	1–3 mL/kg body weight/day, divided in 1–2 doses

defecation. Parents are counseled on how to adjust the laxative dose according to the clinical response every 3 days until the infant or toddler has 1–2 soft bowel movements per day. Laxatives should be continued until the child is comfortable or acquisition of toilet learning is complete.

Toilet training

Toilet training should be postponed till defecation is pain free, the fear of painful bowel movements has resolved and rectal awareness is restored. Behavior modification using rewards for successes in toilet learning is helpful.

Treatment in Children and Adolescents

Most children with functional constipation benefit from a detailed, well-organized plan. The treatment is comprehensive and has four phases: education, disimpaction, prevention of re-accumulation of stools, and withdrawal of treatment.

Education

Effective education is an important first step in the treatment and includes developmentally appropriate description to parents and child about the anatomy and physiology of defecation and its associated disorders and explanation of the prevalence of constipation. If fecal incontinence is present then a discussion of the related shame, embarrassment, and social issues is necessary. Parents must understand that the fecal incontinence is due to overflow incontinence and does not constitute willful or defiant behavior of the child. The physician must make clear to the family that the rock-hard stools are difficult and painful for the child to pass. The child therefore associates bowel movements with pain, which leads to stool withholding, which in turn leads to rock-hard stools. Thus, a vicious cycle is started that leads to chronic fecal retention and eventually to overflow fecal incontinence. The child and parent are told that many children are troubled with this condition. The parents need to understand that there is no quick solution for this condition and that months to years of treatment will be necessary, until the stretched rectal muscles and the impaired rectal perception readjusts, and the child has learned to properly coordinate the muscles for defecation. A caring and trustworthy relationship between medical provider and family needs to be established, because the treatment of functional constipation is a long-term process and without the family's and the child's compliance, the recommended therapy will not be successful.

Disimpaction

When the evaluation shows that a large fecal mass is present, then the impaction needs to be removed using oral or rectal interventions. Suggested medications and dosages for disimpaction are given in Table 39.2. Disimpaction can be achieved without the use of enemas with oral laxatives, such as polyethylene glycol-without electrolytes [36, 37] and with electrolytes [38, 39]. A study by Youssef et al. [36] demonstrated that 1.5 g/kg body weight/

Table 39.2 Suggested medications for fecal disimpaction in children and adolescents

Medication	Age	Dose
Slow oral disimpaction		
PEG without electrolytes (for 3 days) [36]		1.5 g/kg body weight/day
PEG with electrolytes (for 6 days) [38, 39]	2–4-year olds	52 g/day
	5–11-year olds	78 g/day
Milk of magnesia (for 7 days)		2 mL/kg body weight twice/day
Mineral oil (for 7 days)		3 mL/kg body weight twice/day
Lactulose or sorbitol (7 days)		2 mL/kg body weight twice/day
Rapid rectal disimpaction		
Phosphate enema	>6 months	6 mL/kg body weight, up to 135 mL 1–2 times

PEG polyethylene glycol 3350

day of electrolyte-free polyethylene glycol for 3 days was efficient in removing the rectal fecal impaction. In a study by Candy et al. [37], 92% of the children were disimpacted using an escalating dose of up to 78 g of polyethylene glycol 3350 plus electrolytes for 6 days. The fecal impaction can also be softened and liquefied with large quantities of oral mineral oil or other osmotic laxatives with the oral administration continued daily until the fecal mass is passed. Fecal incontinence, abdominal pain, and cramping may increase during oral disimpaction.

Enemas and polyethylene glycol were equally effective in treating rectal fecal impaction in children [40]. Enemas are invasive and can cause psychological harm to an occasional child, but are more rapidly effective, may be a powerful motivator for toilet sitting, and can rapidly relieve the severe pain being present in some children due to stool retention. Hypertonic phosphate enemas are often used and can be repeated twice if necessary. Severe vomiting with hypernatremia, hyperphosphatemia, hypocalcemia, hypokalemia, dehydration, seizures, coma, and death have been reported after the first phosphate enema in a few children with functional constipation less than 5 years of age [41]. Therefore, the first hypertonic enema may be given in the clinic or doctor's office to those children who have never received a phosphate enema before. Enemas are nowadays rarely necessary and can be combined with oral medication. The use of tap water, soapsuds, or Epsom salt enemas is not recommended. Manual disimpaction is performed rarely, and if necessary, should be done under anesthesia.

Prevention of Re-accumulation of Stools (Maintenance Therapy)

Behavior Modification

The child needs to be reconditioned to normal bowel habits by regular toilet use. The child is encouraged to sit on the toilet for up to 5 min, three to four times a day, following meals. The gastrocolic reflex, which goes into effect during and shortly after a meal, should be used to his or her advantage. The children and their parents need to be instructed to keep a daily record of bowel movements and medication use. This helps to monitor compliance and allows parents and physician to make appropriate adjustments in the treatment. If necessary positive reinforcement and rewards for compliant behavior are given for effort and later for success, using star charts, little presents, or television viewing time and computer game time as rewards.

Fiber

The modern diet has been cited as a chief suspect in the etiology of childhood constipation. Dietary fiber increases water retention, provides substrate for bacterial growth with increase of colonic motility and gas production during colonic fermentation of fiber. Several studies have reported that the fiber intake is lower [42, 43] or similar [44] in constipated children as compared to controls. Unlike past generations, children today consume large amounts of highly processed food items at the expense of fruit and vegetables. It is commonly believed that functional constipation

Table 39.3 Suggested medications and dosages for maintenance therapy of constipation for children and adolescents

Medication	Dose
For long-term treatment (years)	
Polyethylene glycol	
3350 (MiraLax®)	0.7 g/kg body weight/day [13, 24] or 0.4 g/kg body weight/day [52]
3350 + electrolytes (Movicol®)	13.8–40 g/day [38, 39]
4000 (Forlax®)	0.5 g/kg body weight/day [37]
Lactulose or sorbitol	1–3 mL/kg body weight/day, divide in 1–2 doses
Milk of magnesia	1–3 mL/kg body weight/day, divide in 1–2 doses
Mineral oil	1–3 mL/kg body weight/day, divided in 1–2 doses
For short-term treatment (months)	
Senna (Senokot®) syrup/tablets	5–10 mL with breakfast, max. 15 mL daily or 1–2 tablets with breakfast, maximum 3 tablets daily
Bisacodyl suppositories	10 mg daily
Phosphate enema	135 mL daily
Glycerin enema	20–30 mL/day (1/2 glycerin and 1/2 normal saline)

can be improved by providing appropriate amounts of fiber and fluids. The dietary recommendation for children older than 2 years of age is to consume an amount of dietary fiber equivalent to age in years plus 5 g/day [45]. Recommended are several servings daily from a variety of fiber-rich foods such as whole grain breads and cereals, fruits, vegetables, and legumes. Synthetic preparations are available, such as guar gum and pectin fiber, glucomannan [46, 47], cocoa husk [48], or a yogurt drink with a fiber mixture [49]. Treatment with fiber or fiber supplementation alone for functional constipation that is severe enough to come to medical attention is inadequate.

Laxatives

In most constipated patients, daily defecation is maintained by the daily administration of laxatives. Suggested dosages of commonly used laxatives are given in Table 39.3. There is no evidence that tolerance develops to osmotic laxatives. Polyethylene glycol (PEG) without added electrolytes (PEG 3350, MiraLax®, Braintree Laboratories, Inc., Braintree, MA, PEG 4000, Forlax®, Ipsen, Paris, France) and polyethylene glycol 3350 with electrolytes (Movicol®, Norgine Pharmaceuticals Ltd., UK) have been developed and have now been tested for long-term daily use in infants, toddlers, and older children [24, 37–39, 50–54]. PEG without electrolytes is tasteless, odorless, colorless, and has no grit when stirred in juice, Kool-aid, or water for several minutes. PEG is not degraded by bacteria, is not readily absorbed and thus, acts as an excellent osmotic agent, and is safe [13, 39, 50, 54]. Preparations of PEG *with* electrolytes are available outside the USA. The addition of electrolytes alters the taste and therefore these medications are more often refused by children then PEG without electrolytes. Polyethylene glycol 3350 has become the first-line drug to use for pediatric constipation [55].

Lactulose and sorbitol are nonabsorbable carbohydrates. They cause increased water content by the osmotic effects of lactulose, sorbitol, and their metabolites. They are fermented by colonic bacteria, thereby producing gas and sometimes causing abdominal discomfort. Both are easily taken by the children when mixed in soft drinks. The mechanism of action of milk of magnesia is the relative nonabsorption of magnesium and the resultant increase in luminal osmolality. Mineral oil is converted into hydroxy fatty acids, which induce fluid and electrolyte accumulation. Mineral oil should never be force-fed or given to patients with dysphagia or vomiting because of the danger of aspiration pneumonia.

Senna has an effect on intestinal motility as well as on fluid and electrolyte transport and stimulates defecation. We use senna when liquid stools produced by osmotic laxatives are retained and in children with fecal incontinence and constipation due to organic or anatomic causes. The North American Society for Pediatric Gastroenterology, Hepatology and Nutrition recommended senna products for short-term therapy [56]. There is very little evidence that tolerance develops to stimulant laxatives [57]. Occasionally, the use of a 10-mg bisacodyl suppository or either a phosphate or a glycerin enema daily is advised as initial treatment for several months in an older constipated child who would like immediate control of his/her fecal incontinence.

Laxatives should be used according to body weight and severity of constipation. The choice of medication for functional constipation does not seem as important as the children's and parents' compliance with the treatment regimen. There is no set dosage for any laxative. There is only a starting dosage for each child (Table 39.3) that must be adjusted to induce one to two bowel movements per day that are loose enough to ensure complete daily emptying of the lower bowel and to prevent fecal incontinence and abdominal pain. Parents and children should be warned that some leakage or incontinence may continue at first, especially if the child continues to resist the use of the toilet.

Psychological Treatment

Functional constipation and particularly fecal incontinence affect the lives of these children and families in several areas: physically, psychologically, educationally, socially, and in terms of self-esteem. If coexisting behavior problems are secondary to functional fecal incontinence and/or constipation, then they will improve with treatment. The presence of coexisting behavioral problems often is associated with poor treatment outcome. Children who do not improve should be referred for further evaluation, because continued problems can be due to noncompliance or control issues by the child and/or the parent.

Follow-Up Visits and Weaning from Medication

Since the treatment of functional constipation requires months to years of considerable patience and effort on the part of the child and parents, it is important to provide necessary support and encouragement through regularly scheduled office visits. Progress should be initially assessed monthly, later less frequently by reviewing the stool records and repeating the abdominal and possibly the rectal examination to assure that the problem is adequately managed. If necessary, dosage adjustment is made and the child and parents are encouraged to continue with the regimen. After regular bowel habits are established, the frequency of toilet sitting is reduced and the medication dosage is gradually decreased to a dosage that maintains one bowel movement daily and prevents the abdominal pain and the fecal incontinence. Once the child feels the urge to defecate and initiates toilet use on his/her own the scheduled toilet times are discontinued. After 6–12 months, reduction with discontinuation of the medication is attempted. Treatment (laxatives and/or toilet sitting) needs to resume if constipation, fecal incontinence, or abdominal pain recur.

Treatment Failure

Errors by physician, parents, and children may lead to treatment failures. More common mistakes by physicians are treating with stool softeners and laxatives but not removing the fecal impaction, removing the fecal impaction but failing to start maintenance therapy, recommending a laxative dose that is too low, not controlling the adequacy and success of therapy with enough follow-up visits, stopping the laxative too soon, and not providing education, anticipatory guidance, continuing support and regular follow-up. Frequent mistakes by parents and children include not insisting that the child uses the toilet at regular times for defecation trials, not giving the medication daily or discontinuing the laxatives as soon as symptoms have improved, and not restarting the laxative after the child had a relapse. Sometimes the fault lies with the child who refuses to take medications or to sit on the toilet. Issues may also arise in school. The teacher needs to permit the child to use the bathroom without having to draw attention to his/her need. A change of clothing should be available in school, so that the parent does not have to bring a change of clothing or have to take the child home, should an incontinence episode occur.

Outcome in Infants and Toddlers

Improvement can be expected in virtually every infant and toddler whose parents cooperate with the treatment plan. Complete recovery is often seen. Dietary changes resolved all symptoms of constipation in 25% of constipated infants [2]. Ninety-two percent of constipated infants and toddlers responded to laxative treatment [2]. Several retrospective chart reviews have shown that PEG can be effective, safe, and well tolerated in children younger than 2 years of age [2, 24, 35]. The length of treatment with PEG varied between 1 and 37 months [24] and 3 weeks to 21 months [35]. The individual effective dose varied between 0.3 and 2.1 g/kg bodyweight per day [2, 24, 35], but the mean effective dose was 0.8–1.0 g/kg body weight per day in all studies. The results of laboratory evaluations during long-term PEG use were within normal limits [24, 54].

Outcome in Children and Adolescents

The goal of treatment is to accomplish one soft stool per day. Weeks, months, and sometimes years of treatment may be necessary before this goal is achieved. Improvement can be achieved in most patients, but complete recovery is less often seen. Outcome in most publications of functional constipated children (≥4 years of age) with or without fecal incontinence has been assessed by rates of "successful treatment" and "recovery." The constipation has been rated as successfully treated if the child had in the previous month ≥3 bowel movements per week, ≤2 fecal incontinence episodes per month, and suffered no abdominal pain, independent of laxative use [16, 58]. Recovery has been defined by the same criteria, except that the child needs to have been off laxatives for at least 1 month [17, 19, 21, 22, 59–61].

Behavior modification: The only study to examine behavior modification as single therapy for children with functional constipation and fecal incontinence was by Nolan et al. [60] from Australia. In this randomized study, they found that 1 year after start of behavior modification, 36% had recovered but more children had recovered with behavior modification and, 51%, additional laxative treatment.

Fiber: Three randomized double-blind controlled studies to evaluate fiber in constipated children have been published [47–49]. Glucomannan, 100 mg/kg body weight daily (maximal 5 g/day) with 50 mL fluid/500 mg and placebo for 4 weeks each was evaluated in 31 constipated children, using a crossover design [47]. While on additional fiber, significantly fewer children complained of abdominal pain as compared to placebo (10 vs. 42%) and significantly more children were relieved from constipation (45 vs. 13%). In another study, a significantly higher number of parents and children reported subjective improvement in stool consistency while on cocoa husk [48]. Kokke et al. [49] reported that a mixture of dietary fiber was similar to lactulose in an 8-week trial in regards to stool frequency, frequency of fecal incontinence, and presence of abdominal pain and flatulence.

Laxatives and Behavior Modification

Short-term outcome: A double-blinded, placebo-controlled trial of PEG 3350 without electrolytes showed that a significantly higher proportion of constipated children responded to treatment compared to placebo in the second week of treatment [52]. PEG plus electrolytes was significantly more effective than placebo in a 2-week treatment trial [62]. PEG 3350 was similarly effective as lactulose in improving stool frequency, stool consistency, and ease of stool passage [63].

Table 39.4 1-year recovery rates in constipated children with or without fecal incontinence

Author	Subject number	Laxative	Recovery rate (%)
Constipation with or without fecal incontinence			
Abrahamian et al. [64]	68	Multiple laxatives	47
Staiano et al. [65]	31	Lactulose	47
van Ginket et al. [59]	212	Lactulose	31
van Ginket et al. [58]	399	Lactulose	59
Constipation with fecal incontinence			
Levine et al. [66]	110	Mineral oil	51
Loening-Baucke [17]	97	Milk of magnesia	43
Nolan et al. [60]	83	Multiple laxatives	51
Loening-Baucke [67]	181	Milk of magnesia	39
Loening-Baucke et al. [13]	39	Polyethylene glycol 3350	33
Overall 6–12 months recovery rates [68]			40

1-year outcome: At least 9 well-designed studies have evaluated 1-year outcome (Table 39.4). Laxative treatment with behavior modification dramatically improved constipation, abdominal pain, and functional fecal incontinence. Four of these studies evaluated children who had constipation with or without functional fecal incontinence [58, 59, 64, 65]. They showed that 47% of these children in the USA [68], 47% in Italy [65], and 31–59% in the Netherlands [58, 59], had recovered 1 year after start of treatment (Table 39.4).

Five of the nine studies evaluated children with functional constipation with fecal incontinence. The 1-year recovery rates ranged from 33 to 51% [13, 17, 60, 66, 67]. They showed that 33–51% of the children in the USA [13, 17, 66, 67] and 51% of children in Australia [60] had recovered 1 year after start of therapy with milk of magnesia, lactulose, or polyethylene glycol. Pijpers et al. [68] summarized the outcome of 14 publications of prospective follow-up studies. They found that 6–12 months after start of treatment, 40% of constipated children had recovered and 61% were successfully treated. All studies suggest that constipation is not a problem that all children will eventually outgrow.

Long-term outcome: Long-term outcome studies (4–10 year follow-up) report recovery rates between 48 and 69% (Table 39.5) [58, 65, 69–72]. One study specifically targeted younger children (<4 years) to examine whether early intervention might improve outcome [69]. Of 90 children who were followed for a mean of 7 years after beginning treatment, 63% had recovered. Staiano et al. [65] found that early age of onset of constipation and family history of constipation were predictive of persistence of constipation [65]. The largest follow-up study is by van Ginkel et al. [58]. They initially enrolled 418 children with functional constipation, 2/3 with and 1/3 without fecal incontinence. All were older than 5 years of age at initiation of therapy. Some of the children were followed for as long as 8 years, with a median follow-up of 5 years. Fifty-nine percent had recovered at the 1-year follow-up. Three-year data showed a decline in the recovery rate to about 50%, as some children relapsed and were not restarted on laxative therapy and others recovered. The recovery rate of 193 children was 63% after 5 years, 69% of 120 children had recovered after 7 years, and 68% of 48 children had recovered after 8 years [58]. However, 50% of recovered children had at least one relapse and approximately 30% of children, who had reached adolescence, were still having problems with constipation or fecal incontinence.

Other Treatments

Probiotics: One rational for the use of probiotics for the treatment of constipation in children is that dysbiosis has been reported in the intestinal flora of these children [73]. The dysbiosis consisted of a change in the selected bacterial species. A high clostridia count in comparison to

Table 39.5 Long-term recovery rates in children with constipation only, constipation with and without fecal incontinence, and constipation with fecal incontinence

Author	Subject number	Age (years)	Laxative	Years of follow-up	Recovery rate (%)
Constipation only					
Loening-Baucke [69]	90	1–4	Milk of magnesia	Mean 7 year	63
Michaud et al. [72]	45	0.5–14	Lactulose	10 year	54
Constipation with and without fecal incontinence					
Staiano et al. [65]	62	1–11	Lactulose	5 year	48
van Ginket et al. [58]	193	>5	Lactulose	5 year	69
Constipation with fecal incontinence					
Loening-Baucke [70]	129	>4	Milk of magnesia	Mean 4 year	53
Procter et al. [71]	76	0.3–16	Laxative	6 year	64

From Loening-Baucke V. "Constipation and fecal incontinence." In: Pediatric Gastrointestinal and Liver Disease, 4th edition. Wyllie R, Hyams JS, Kay M., Elsevier Ltd., Philadelphia 2011, pp 127–135. Reprinted with permission from Elsevier

Bacteroides and *Escherichia coli* was seen and a substantial presence of clostridia and enterobacteriaceae species were observed, bacteria which are rarely isolated in healthy children [73]. A randomized controlled trial concluded that 10^9 colony forming units of *Lactobacillus GG* given twice daily was not an effective adjunct to lactulose [74]. *Lactobacillus casei rhamnosus* 8×10^8 colony forming units given twice daily has shown a benefit in regards to increased stool frequency, in comparison to placebo, but showed similar results to magnesium oxide [75]. Both studies are short-term treatment trials of 12 weeks. So far, only limited evidence is available from controlled trials and no long-term studies are available to evaluate the benefit of probiotics.

Biofeedback treatment as adjunct therapy: Previous research showed that 25–56% of constipated children abnormally contracted the external anal sphincter and pelvic floor muscles during attempted defecation [17, 19, 21–23]. The concept of applying biofeedback to optimize anorectal function is logical because anorectal function is regulated by physiologic processes, some of which are under cortical influence, such as the ability to sense rectal distention and impending defecation and the ability to relax and contract the striated muscles of the pelvic floor. Patients can be taught these functions. One small randomized study showed a statistically significant benefit of additional biofeedback treatment [76]; however, four other randomized studies have found no statistically significant benefit of additional biofeedback treatment in children when compared to conventional treatment alone, in 6-month, 1-year, and long-term follow-up studies [23, 61, 70, 77].

References

1. van den Berg MM, Benninga MA, DiLorenzo C. Epidemiology of childhood constipation: a systemic review. Am J Gastroenterol. 2006;101:2401–9.
2. Loening-Baucke V. Prevalence, symptoms and outcome of constipation in infants and toddlers. J Pediatr. 2005;146:359–63.
3. Issenman RM, Hewson S, Pirhonen D, et al. Are chronic digestive complaints the result of abnormal dietary patterns? Am J Dis Child. 1987;141:679–82.
4. Yong D, Beattie RM. Normal bowel habit and prevalence of constipation in primary school children. Amb Child Health. 1998;4:277–82.
5. Loening-Baucke V. Prevalence rates for constipation and faecal and urinary incontinence in children. Arch Dis Child. 2007;92:486–9.
6. de Araújo Sant'Anna AM, Calçado AC. Constipation in school-aged children at public schools in Rio de Janeiro, Brazil. J Pediatr Gastroenterol Nutr. 1999;29:190–3.
7. Zaslavsky C, Ávila EL, Araújo MA, et al. Constipação intestinal da infância—um estudo de prevalência. Rev AMRIGS. 1988;32:100–2.
8. Maffei HVL, Moreira FL, Oliveira WM, et al. Constipação intestinal em escolare. J Pediatr. 1997;73:340–4.

9. Fontana M, Bianchi C, Cataldo F, et al. Bowel frequency in healthy children. Acta Paediatr Scand. 1989;78:682–4.
10. Hyman PE, Milla PJ, Benninga MA, et al. Childhood functional gastrointestinal disorders: neonate/toddler. Gastroenterology. 2006;130:1519–26.
11. Rasquin A, Di Lorenzo C, Forber D, et al. Childhood functional gastrointestinal disorders: child/adolescent. Gastroenterology. 2006;130:1527–37.
12. Morris-Yates A, Talley NJ, Boyce PM, et al. Evidence of a genetic contribution to functional bowel disorder. Am J Gastroenterol. 1998;93:1311–7.
13. Loening-Baucke V, Pashankar DS. A randomized, prospective, comparison study of polyethylene glycol 3350 without electrolytes and milk of magnesia in children with constipation and fecal incontinence. Pediatrics. 2006;118:528–35.
14. Loening-Baucke V, Swidsinski A. Constipation as cause of acute abdominal pain in children. J Pediatr. 2007;151:666–9.
15. Loening-Baucke V. Functional constipation is the most frequent cause of functional abdominal pain in children. Open Pediatr Med J. 2008;2:7–10.
16. Loening-Baucke V. Urinary incontinence and urinary tract infection and their resolution with treatment of chronic constipation of childhood. Pediatrics. 1997;100:228–32.
17. Loening-Baucke V. Factors determining outcome in children with chronic constipation and faecal. Gut. 1989;30:999–1006.
18. van Dijk M, Benninga MA, Grootenhuis MA, et al. Prevalence and associated clinical characteristics of behavior problems in constipated children. Pediatrics. 2010;125:e309–17. Assessed March 23, 2010.
19. Loening-Baucke V, Cruikshank B, Savage C. Evaluation of defecation dynamics and behavior profiles in encopretic children. Pediatrics. 1987;80:672–9.
20. Youssef N, Langseder A, Verga B, et al. Chronic childhood constipation is associated with impaired quality of life: a case-controlled study. J Pediatr Gastroenterol Nutr. 2005;41:56–60.
21. Loening-Baucke V. Factors responsible for persistence of childhood constipation. J Pediatr Gastroenterol Nutr. 1987;6:915–22.
22. Loening-Baucke V. Abnormal defecation dynamics in chronically constipated children with functional fecal incontinence. J Pediatr. 1996;128:336–40.
23. Wald A, Chandra R, Gabel S, et al. Evaluation of biofeedback in childhood functional fecal incontinence. J Pediatr Gastroenterol Nutr. 1987;6:554–8.
24. Loening-Baucke V, Krishna R, Pashankar DS. Polyethylene glycol 3350 without electrolytes for the treatment of functional constipation in infants and toddlers. J Pediatr Gastroenterol Nutr. 2004;39:536–9.
25. Partin JC, Hamill SK, Fischel JE, et al. Painful defecation and fecal incontinence in children. Pediatrics. 1992;89:1007–9.
26. Borowitz SM, Cox DJ, Tam A, et al. Precipitants of constipation during early childhood. J Am Board Fam Pract. 2003;16:213–8.
27. Iacono G, Cavataio F, Montalto G, et al. Intolerance of cow's milk and chronic constipation in children. N Engl J Med. 1998;339:1100–4.
28. Shah N, Lindley K, Milla P. Cow's milk and chronic constipation in children. N Engl J Med. 1999;340:891–2.
29. Daher S, Tahan S, Solé D, et al. Cow's milk protein intolerance and chronic constipation in children. Pediatr Allergy Immunol. 2001;12:339–42.
30. Vanderhoof JA, Perry D, Hanner TL, et al. Allergic constipation: association with infantile milk allergy. Clin Pediatr. 2001;40:399–402.
31. Turunen S, Karttunen TJ, Kokkonen J. Lymphoid hyperplasia and cow's milk hypersensitivity in children with chronic constipation. J Pediatr. 2004;145:606–11.
32. El-Hodhod MA, Younis NT, Zaitoun YA, et al. Cow's milk allergy related pediatric constipation: appropriate time of milk tolerance. Pediatr Allergy Immunol. 2009;DOI: 10.1111/j.1399-3038.2009.00898.x Assessed March 23, 2010
33. Simeone D, Miele E, Boccia G, et al. Prevalence of atopy in children with chronic constipation. Arch Dis Child. 2008;93:1044–7.
34. Benninga MA, Voskuijl WP, Taminiau AJM. Childhood constipation: is there new light in the tunnel? J Pediatr Gastroenterol Nutr. 2004;39:448–64.
35. Michail S, Gendy E, Preud'Homme D, et al. Polyethylene glycol for constipation in children younger than eighteen months old. J Pediatr Gastroenterol Nutr. 2004;39:197–9.
36. Youssef NN, Peters JM, Henderson W, et al. Dose responses of PEG 3350 for the treatment of childhood fecal impaction. J Pediatr. 2002;141:410–4.
37. Dupont C, Leluyer B, Amar F, et al. A dose determination study of polyethylene glycol 4000 in constipated children; factors influencing the maintenance dose. J Pediatr Gastroenterol Nutr. 2006;42:178–85.
38. Candy D, Belsey J. Macrogol (polyethylene glycol) laxatives in children with functional constipation and faecal impaction: a systemic review. Arch Dis Child. 2009;94:156–60.
39. Candy DC, Edwards D, Geraint M. Treatment of faecal impaction with polyethylene glycol plus electrolytes (PEG + E) followed by a double-blind comparison of PEG + E versus lactulose as maintenance therapy. J Pediatr Gastroenterol Nutr. 2006;43:65–70.
40. Bekkali NL, van den Berg MM, Dijkgraaf MG, et al. Rectal fecal impaction treatment in childhood constipation: enemas versus high doses oral PEG. Pediatrics. 2009;124:e1108–15. Accessed March 23, 2010.
41. Harrington L, Schuh S. Complications of Fleet® enema administration and suggested guidelines for use in the pediatric emergency department. Pediatr Emergency Care. 1997;13:225–6.

42. Roma E, Adamidis D, Nikolara R, et al. Diet and chronic constipation in children: the role of fiber. J Ped Gastroenterol Nutr. 1999;28:169–74.
43. Morais MB, Vitolo MR, Aquirre ANC, et al. Measurement of low dietary fiber intake as a risk factor for chronic constipation in children. J Ped Gastroenterol Nutr. 1999;29:132–5.
44. Zaslavsky C, Reverbel da Silveira T, Maguilnik I. Total and segmental colonic transit time with radio-opaque markers in adolescents with functional constipation. J Ped Gastroenterol Nutr. 1998;27:138–42.
45. Williams CL, Bollella M, Wynder EL. A new recommendation for dietary fiber in childhood. Pediatrics. 1995;96:985–8.
46. Staiano A, Simeone D, Del Giudice E, et al. Effect of the dietary fiber glucomannan on chronic constipation in neurologically impaired children. J Pediatr. 2000;136:41–5.
47. Loening-Baucke V, Miele E, Staiano A. Fiber (glucomannan) is beneficial in the treatment of childhood constipation. Pediatrics. 2004;113:e259–64. Assessed March 23, 2010.
48. Castillejo G, Bullo M, Anguera A, et al. A controlled, randomized, double-blind trial to evaluate the effect of supplement of cocoa husk that is rich in fiber on colonic transit in constipated pediatric patients. Pediatrics. 2006;118:641–8.
49. Kokke FTM, Scholtens PAMJ, et al. A dietary fiber mixture versus lactulose in the treatment of childhood constipation: a double-blind randomized controlled trial. J Pediatr Gastroenterol Nutr. 2008; 47:592–7.
50. Loening-Baucke V. Polyethylene glycol without electrolytes for children with constipation and functional fecal incontinence. J Pediatr Gastroenterol Nutr. 2002;34:372–7.
51. Pashankar DS, Bishop WP. Efficacy and optimal dose of daily polyethylene glycol 3350 for treatment of constipation and functional fecal incontinence in children. J Pediatr. 2001;139:428–32.
52. Nurko S, Youssef NN, Sabri M, et al. PEG3350 in the treatment of childhood constipation: a multicenter, double-blinded, placebo-controlled trial. J Pediatr. 2008;153:254–61.
53. Pashankar DS, Bishop WP, Loening-Baucke V. Long-term efficacy of polyethylene glycol 3350 for the treatment of chronic constipation in children with and without functional fecal incontinence. Clin Pediatr. 2003;42:815–9.
54. Pashankar DS, Loening-Baucke V, Bishop WP. Safety of polyethylene glycol 3350 for the treatment of chronic constipation in children. Arch Pediatr Adolesc Med. 2003;157:661–4.
55. Baker S, Liptak G, Colletti R, et al. Evaluation and treatment of constipation in children: summary of updated recommendations of the North American Society for Pediatric Gastroenterology, Hepatology and Nutrition. J Pediatr Gastroenterol Nutr. 2006;43:405–7.
56. Baker SS, Liptak GS, Colletti RB, et al. Constipation in infants and children: evaluation and treatment. J Pediatr Gastroenterol Nutr. 1999;29:612–26.
57. Müller-Lissner SA, Kamm MA, Scarpignato C, et al. Myths and misconceptions about chronic constipation. Am J Gastroenterol. 2005;100:232–42.
58. van Ginkel R, Reitsma JB, Büller HA, et al. Childhood constipation: longitudinal follow-up beyond puberty. Gastroenterology. 2003;125:357–63.
59. van Ginkel R, Bueller HA, Boeckxstaens GE, et al. The effect of anorectal manometry on the outcome of treatment in severe childhood constipation: a randomized, controlled trial. Pediatrics. 2001;108:E9. \.
60. Nolan TM, Debelle G, Oberklaid F, et al. Randomised trial of laxatives in treatment of childhood functional fecal incontinence. Lancet. 1991;338(8766):523–7.
61. Nolan T, Catto-Smith T, Coffey C, et al. Randomised controlled trial of biofeedback training in persistent functional fecal incontinence with anismus. Arch Dis Child. 1998;79:131–5.
62. Thomson MA, Jenkins HR, Bisset WM, et al. Polyethylene glycol 3350 plus electrolytes for chronic constipation in children: a double blind, placebo controlled, crossover study. Arch Dis Child. 2008;92:996–1000.
63. Gremse DA, Hixon J, Crutchfield A. Comparison of polyethylene glycol 3350 and lactulose for treatment of chronic constipation in children. Clin Pediatr. 2002;41:225–9.
64. Abrahamian FP, Lloyd-Still JD. Chronic constipation in childhood: a longitudinal study of 186 patients. J Pediatr Gastroenterol Nutr. 1984;3:460–7.
65. Staiano A, Andreotti MR, Greco L, et al. Long-term follow-up of children with chronic idiopathic constipation. Dig Dis Sci. 1994;39:561–4.
66. Levine MD, Bakow H. Children with functional fecal incontinence: a study of treatment outcome. Pediatrics. 1976;58:845–52.
67. Loening-Baucke V. Functional fecal retention with functional fecal incontinence in childhood. J Pediatr Gastroenterol Nutr. 2004;38:79–84.
68. Pijpers M, Bongers M, Benninga M, et al. Functional constipation in children: a systemic review on prognosis and predictive factors. J Pediatr Gastroenterol Nutr. 2010;50:256–68.
69. Loening-Baucke V. Constipation in early childhood: patient characteristics, treatment, and longterm follow up. Gut. 1993;34:1400–4.
70. Loening-Baucke V. Biofeedback treatment for chronic constipation and functional fecal incontinence in childhood: long-term outcome. Pediatrics. 1995;96:105–10.
71. Procter E, Loader P. A 6 year follow-up study of chronic constipation and soiling in a specialist paediatric service. Childcare Health Dev. 2003;29:203–9.
72. Michaud L, Lamblin M-D, Mairesse S, et al. Outcome of functional constipation in childhood: a 10-year follow-up study. Clin Pediatr. 2009;48:26–31.
73. Zoppi G, Cinquetti M, Luciano A, et al. The intestinal ecosystem in functional constipation. Acta Paediatr. 1998;87:836–41.

74. Banaszkiewicz A, Szajewska H. Ineffectiveness of Lactobacillus GG as an adjunct to lactulose for the treatment of constipation in children: a double-blind, placebo-controlled randomized trial. J Pediatr. 2005;146:364–9.
75. Bu LN, Chang MH, Ni YH, et al. Lactobacillus casei rhamnosus Lcr35 in children with chronic constipation. Pediatr Int. 2007;49:485–90.
76. Loening-Baucke V. Modulation of abnormal defecation dynamics by biofeedback treatment in chronically constipated children with functional fecal incontinence. J Pediatr. 1990;116:214–22.
77. van der Plas RN, Benninga MA, Büller HA, et al. Biofeedback training in treatment of childhood constipation: A randomised controlled study. Lancet. 1996;348(9030):776–80.

Functional Fecal Incontinence

40

Rosa Burgers and Marc A. Benninga

Introduction

Fecal incontinence (FI) is defined as defecation into places inappropriate to the social context, at least once per month, for a minimum period of 2 months. It represents one of the most upsetting and psychologically distressing problems of childhood. These children leak stools into their underwear, smell bad, and are rejected by their peers. It has a great impact on the development, social interactions, and education of the affected children.

The amount of feces lost in the underwear was the basis for the differentiation of FI in two definitions; *encopresis* encompassed expulsion of a normal bowel moment in inappropriate places and *soiling* the leakage of small amounts of stool. In the literature, fecal incontinence in children is frequently described by the terms "encopresis" and "fecal soiling," but given the different meanings that these terms have across different cultures and different nations, Rome III have adopted the term "functional fecal incontinence" which will be used in this chapter [1]. The accompanying symptoms should be evaluated to find out whether FI exists in the presence or absence of constipation and to unravel possible different pathophysiological mechanisms [2, 3].

Functional fecal incontinence in children can also be categorized as either primary, in those children that have never been toilet trained, or secondary, in those in which the incontinence comes back after successful toilet training. It has been proposed that the occurrence of secondary incontinence is associated with better response to treatment.

Prevalence

The exact prevalence of functional fecal incontinence associated with constipation varies depending on the population being studied and changes with age. Bellman, in her landmark study, reported incidence rates for FI in Stockholm school children in 1963, of 2.8% in 4 year olds and 1.5% in 7–8 year olds [4]. Recently van de Wal et al. showed a prevalence of fecal incontinence of 4.1% in a 5- to 6-year-old age group and 1.6% in an 11-to 12-year-old age group in the Netherlands, with a 1.5-fold higher prevalence in boys [5]. In a retrospective review in 482 children of 4–7 years of age attending a primary care clinic in the USA a prevalence rate for fecal incontinence of 4.4% was reported [6]. In this study fecal incontinence was coupled with constipation in 95% of the children. A recent study evaluating the applicability of the new Rome III criteria, reported fecal incontinence in 9% of the patients referred to a tertiary Italian hospital with complaints of chronic constipation

R. Burgers, M.D. • M.A. Benninga, M.D., Ph.D. (✉)
Department of Pediatric Gastroenterology, Emma Children's Hospital/Academic Medical Centre, H7-Meibergdreef 9, 1105 AZ, Amsterdam, The Netherlands
e-mail: m.a.benninga@amc.nl

C. Faure et al. (eds.), *Pediatric Neurogastroenterology: Gastrointestinal Motility and Functional Disorders in Children*, Clinical Gastroenterology,
DOI 10.1007/978-1-60761-709-9_40, © Springer Science+Business Media New York 2013

of at least 2 months duration [7]. An epidemiologic study in Sri Lanka showed that fecal incontinence was present in 2% of the general population. Approximately 82% had constipation-associated FI and 18.2% had nonretentive FI [8]. The highest prevalence was found in children aged 10 (5.4%). FI was significantly higher in boys (boys 3.2%, girls 0.9%), those exposed to recent school- and family-related stressful life events, and those from lower social classes ($P<0.05$). Inconsistent data exist about the prevalence of fecal incontinence in obese children, varying from 21 to 33% [9, 10]. Also FI without constipation, functional non-retentive fecal incontinence (FNRFI), is more common in boys with male to female ratio's ranging from 3:1 to 6:1[2, 3, 11, 12].

Causes

Four main groups of children present with fecal incontinence: (1) children who have functional constipation with overflow incontinence, (2) children with functional non-retentive fecal incontinence, (3) children with anorectal malformations, and (4) children with spinal problems [3]. In approximately 95% of the children, no organic cause can be identified and these children are considered to have a functional defecation disorder. In approximately 90% of the children with a functional defecation disorder the loss of feces in the underwear is the result of constipation and treatment with laxatives is recommended. The remaining 10% have fecal incontinence with no other symptoms or signs of constipation, these children are classified as functional non-retentive fecal incontinence (FNRFI). Figure 40.1 presents an overview of the different causes of fecal incontinence in children [1–3, 6, 13, 14].

Epidemiology, diagnosis and treatment of fecal incontinence as result of either anorectal malformations or spinal problems will not be further discussed in this chapter.

Functional Constipation

In children with constipation, fecal incontinence is the consequence of overflow in an already impacted rectum. FI is reported in approximately 80% of children with functional constipation, whereas a defecation frequency below three times per week is found in up to 88% of children with chronic functional constipation [15, 16]. A painful defecation is reported by half of the children. The involuntary loss of stool can occur at any time during the day, whenever the child tries to expel gas or the muscles used to withhold the rectal contents become fatigued. Children suffering from extreme fecal impaction may have fecal incontinence episodes even during the night [17]. Furthermore, accumulation of feces in the rectum causes decreased motility in the foregut, resulting in loss of appetite, irritability, and abdominal distension [16].

An association between constipation and urinary tract dysfunction (i.e., urine incontinence and recurrent urinary tract infections) is well established [2, 3, 18–20]. A higher frequency of daytime and nighttime urinary incontinence in children without constipation (around 45%) was found by van Ginkel, while daytime and nighttime incontinence was found in 25–29% of those with constipation [3, 21–23]. A high prevalence of urine incontinence in children with FI without constipation, suggests an overall delay in the achievement of toilet training or the neglect of normal physiological stimuli to go to the toilet [11, 21].

Functional Non-retentive Fecal Incontinence

Apart from the FI episodes, children with FNRFI present with a normal defecation pattern, without other symptoms or signs of constipation or organic malfunctioning. They have daily bowel movements of normal size and on physical examination they have no palpable abdominal or rectal fecal mass. According to the Rome III classification, the definition for FNRFI in a child with a developmental age of at least 4 years is a history of defecation into places inappropriate to the social context at least once per month with no evidence of an inflammatory, anatomic, metabolic, or neoplastic process and no evidence of fecal retention for at least 2 months prior to diagnosis [1].

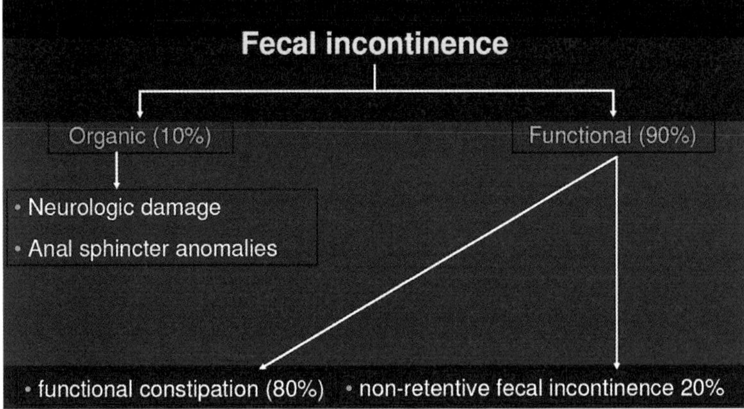

Fig. 40.1 Organic and functional causes of fecal incontinence in children

The underlying mechanism of FNRFI is largely unknown. The pathophysiology seems to be complex and is considered to be multifactorial. Historically, FI was seen as a manifestation of emotional disturbance, although the association between FI and stress has not been well documented. In the mid-1990s it was suggested that children with FNRFI deny or neglect their normal physiological stimuli to defecate and contract the external anal sphincter to retain stool in the rectum [2]. This hypothesis is supported by the normal anorectal sensorimotor function, anorectal manometry, and rectal barostat testing but abnormal defecation dynamics and high rates of urinary incontinence [2, 24]. This is possibly due to an abnormal interpretation of rectal sensation or disturbed rectoanal coordination. Further research is indicated to explore disruptions in the rectum or the anal sphincter complex in this condition.

Patients presenting with FNRFI undergo less therapy before intake (5.5 months vs. 15 months), visit the outpatient clinic at a higher age (age of 9.2 years vs. 6.5 years) and are more likely to have a positive family history (20% vs. 13%) compared to children with constipation [11, 23]. It is unknown why patients visit the outpatient clinic at a higher age. Parents might postpone a visit to the doctor because of shame that they are not capable in getting their child properly toilet trained before the age of 4 years.

Quality of Life and Behavioral Problems

Quality of life scores of children with constipation and fecal incontinence are significantly reduced [25, 26]. Children with functional defecation disorders and their parents report impaired quality of life in relation to physical complaints and long duration of symptoms [25]. Moreover, parent-reported quality of life in children with constipation was even lower than that reported by their children. Although, young adults with constipation, which already started in childhood, report a good quality of life, persistence of childhood constipation into adulthood is associated with impaired HRQoL at adult age. It is noteworthy that symptoms affect social contacts in a fifth of adults with unsuccessful clinical outcome [26].

Behavioral problems are more common in children with FI (40%), with and without constipation compared to their healthy controls. These behavioral problems might be a reflection of the impact of defecation disorders on the normal development of children [11, 12, 27, 28]. A study by van der Plas et al. showed that successful treatment of children with FNRFI normalized scores for behavioral problems [12]. This implies that FI is an important factor in the occurrence and maintenance of behavioral problems in these children. The question whether fecal incontinence results in behavior problems or vice versa is an important issue and still under debate.

Clinical Presentation

A timely and correct diagnosis is essential for the appropriate treatment of FI. Medical history and a thorough physical examination are often sufficient for an adequate assessment regarding the underlying cause. Only in rare cases, additional tests might be useful.

History

A careful history needs to elicit the specific symptoms related to the FI episodes. The amount of feces (leakage of small amounts or normal stools), the frequency, the time of the day when FI accidents occur and the age the problem started are all relevant. The majority of FNRFI children have FI accidents after school during the late afternoon and before bedtime [2]. To be able to differentiate between the separate causes underlying FI, additional more detailed information about the bowel habits and any accompanying symptoms has to be obtained. It is important to ask about the defecation frequency, stool characteristics (consistency, caliber, and volume), pain at defecation, abdominal pain, and stool withholding behavior. Also urinary problems and neurologic deficits have to be evaluated.

Physical Examination

Physical examination is important to establish or rule out constipation. Furthermore it is essential to look for signs of other underlying causes for FI symptoms. A thorough physical and neurological examination should be performed including perianal inspection and anorectal digital examination. To exclude signs of spinal dysraphism it is important to inspect the perineum and perianal area. Physicians should consider the possibility of sexual abuse, especially if anal fissures and scars are found. Only recently, gluteal cleft deviation was found to be an important sign of lumbosacral spine abnormalities in children with either functional constipation or FNRFI [29].

The Constipation Guideline Committee of the North American Society for Pediatric Gastroenterology, Hepatology and Nutrition (NASPGHAN) recommended performing a rectal examination at least once in children presenting with FI [30]. Both in children and adults digital rectal examination has been shown to provide useful information regarding anal sphincter function in patients with constipation and fecal incontinence [31, 32]. Furthermore it is done to assess the presence of a fecal lump in the rectal ampulla. However, a recent study showed that there is a lack of emphasis on the use of digital rectal examination during medical school [33]. Moreover, it is either not performed or inadequately used in clinical practice in the evaluation of children with functional anorectal disorders. Interestingly, the vast majority (85%) of primary care physicians do not perform digital rectal examination in their patients, resulting in missed diagnoses and treatment [34]. Based on their study in 128 children referred for functional constipation, Gold et al. stated that digital examination can help to differentiate functional constipation from an organic process and may alter the course of therapy [35].

Diagnostic Tests

Functional defecation disorders accompanied by fecal incontinence are clinical diagnoses that can be made in most cases on the basis of a medical history and an essentially normal physical examination. In these cases, it is not necessary to perform diagnostic tests before treatment is started. The marker test to evaluate colonic transit time (described below) has been proven useful in differentiating between children with constipation and children with FNRFI. In atypical cases or when conventional treatment fails, additional diagnostic tests can be performed to diagnose an underlying organic cause [11].

Abdominal Radiography

Insufficient evidence exists for a diagnostic association between clinical symptoms of constipation and fecal loading on abdominal radiographs, colonic transit time, and rectal diameter on ultrasonography in children [30, 36–38]. However, in case of doubt about the presence of a fecal mass, in a child who is obese or when rectal examination is not possible when a child refuses or when it is considered traumatic, an abdominal X-ray in combination with radio-opaque markers might be useful. As described above, in our center we use the colonic transit test to discriminate between functional constipation and FNRFI. Based on the results of this test we decide to either start with laxatives or a strict regime of education and toilet training in the case of children with FNRFI.

Colonic Transit Time

Colonic transit time (CTT) can be assessed by performing one or more abdominal X-rays after the ingestion of radio-opaque markers [39–41]. With this technique both overall colonic transit and segmental transit can be determined to distinguish different transit patterns: (1) normal colonic transit time: normal transit through all colonic segments, (2) outlet obstruction: delayed transit through the anorectal region, and (3) slow transit constipation: prolonged transit through the entire colon [16]. Normal CTT for children is based on the upper limit (mean + 2 SD, hours) in healthy controls. Based on the CTT data in healthy children by Arhan et al., colonic transit time is considered delayed when the total CTT exceeds 62 h [39]. In approximately 50% of constipated children CTT is delayed [15, 16, 42]. In the majority of these children the delay of transit is found in the anorectal region [15]. In children and adults a good correlation is found between symptoms of constipation such as defecation frequency and fecal incontinence frequency and colonic transit time [15]. A delay of colonic transit <100 h is not predictive for treatment outcome. Only those patients with CTT > 100 h have a less favorable outcome at 1-year follow-up. In contrast to children with constipation a normal CTT is found in more than 90% of the children with FNRFI. Thus, a normal CTT in combination with a normal defecation frequency and no rectal mass indicates FNRFI [2].

MRI

MRI is not required to assess lumbosacral spine abnormalities in the standard workup of children with intractable constipation or non-retentive fecal incontinence. We recommend only performing an MRI in those children presenting with alarming neurological signs including motor and sensory dysfunction of the lower extremities and abnormal reflexes, or abnormal anorectal sensation, gluteal cleft deviation, and anal wink suggestive of spinal cord abnormalities [29, 43].

Manometry and Barostat

Several techniques can be used to assess anorectal function. Anorectal manometry measures, through volume-controlled distension, pressures in the anorectal region and is useful to assess sphincter function and contraction patterns. Barostat measurements, using pressure-controlled distension, give valuable information about rectal sensitivity and contractility. At this moment, there is no indication for routinely performing anorectal manometry or barostat in children with constipation and fecal incontinence, as findings have no clinical implications. Therefore these techniques will not be discussed in detail here [44–46].

Colonic manometry is a diagnostic test performed in specialized motility centers to differentiate between normal colonic motor function and colonic neuromuscular disorders in the evaluation of children with intractable constipation and in children with rare organic causes such as intestinal pseudo-obstruction [47]. Manometry can also help predict whether antegrade enema treatment through a Malone stoma or cecostomy will be successful [48].

Abdominal Ultrasound

Pelvic ultrasound can show the impression of the rectum behind the urinary bladder. With this noninvasive technique, which does not involve radiation, urologists are able to measure the transverse rectal diameter. Some studies show that measuring rectal diameter correlates with the results of digital rectal examination and therewith seems to assess fecal impaction [49, 50]. However, as for now, there is insufficient evidence that the transverse diameter can be used as a predictor of constipation and fecal impaction.

Treatment

The lack of randomized controlled studies in children has made the treatment of constipation and fecal incontinence largely based on clinical experience rather than on evidence-based controlled clinical trials [11, 51]. Acute simple constipation is traditionally treated with a high-fiber diet and sufficient fluid intake, filling out a bowel diary and toilet training. The NASPGHAN recommendations include four important phases in the treatment of chronic constipation: (1) education, (2) disimpaction, (3) prevention of re-accumulation of feces, and (4) follow-up [30]. In contrast to children with constipation, no laxatives should be used in children with functional non-retentive fecal incontinence [11, 52]. Treatment in these children consists of education, toilet training, a daily bowel diary with rewarding system, and loperamide [53]. The role of enemas in these children is still unclear but should be investigated in a large randomized controlled trial.

The ultimate treatment goals in children with FI are preventing stool accidents and have regular bowel movements. How to achieve this depends on the underlying pathophysiology, with different approaches and prognoses for the different causes. Treatment can be directed towards the stool itself (consistency, volume), stool transit, rectosigmoid/anorectal function, and the child's behavior. An essential first step is educating both the child and the parents about the gastrointestinal tract with specific attention to the rectum, defecation, and FI. It is also important to explain that FI is a common disorder in childhood and that the child may not always be aware of fecal accidents. Drawings, illustrating the pathophysiological mechanisms are often helpful. The myths and fears should be addressed, a positive atmosphere towards the treatment approach is essential. The child and the parents should be prepared for a long-lasting treatment process with many "ups and downs" [1, 3, 11].

Functional Constipation

Education and behavior modification (no withholding with urge to defecate), toilet training, a bowel diary, and medical treatment are the cornerstones of the treatment of children with functional constipation. The toilet training program consists of trying to defecate for 5 min after each meal. Defecation frequency, episodes of FI, abdominal pain, the use of laxatives, and compliance with toilet training are registered daily in the diary. Besides these behavior changes, oral and sometimes rectal laxatives are necessary in almost all constipated children. A recent trial showed that enemas and PEG are equally effective in treating severe rectal fecal impaction [54]. Stool softeners are preferred to stimulant laxatives for maintenance therapy [51]. Bongers et al. showed that enemas as maintenance therapy had no additional effect compared to oral laxatives alone for severely and chronically constipated children between 8 and 18 years treated in a tertiary center [55]. The duration of maintenance therapy is unclear, but is usually necessary for at least 3 months [30]. Only when the child has been having regular bowel movements without difficulty is discontinuation considered. Health carers and families should be aware that relapses are common and that difficulty with bowel movements may continue into adulthood [56, 57].

Functional Non-retentive Fecal Incontinence

Education, strict toilet training, and positive motivation are the cornerstones of treating children with FNRFI. An additional reward system (praise and small gifts) can enhance motivation as well in these cases [11, 52]. After this demystifying process, we emphasize to patients and parents that treatment is often long-lasting and that progress is often irregular and marked by periods of improvement alternating with deterioration. Not surprisingly, FNRFI patients do not benefit from laxatives. Van Ginkel and colleagues showed that indeed laxatives soften stool and have a positive effect on gastrointestinal motility, but they subsequently lead to an increase of urge to defecate, which finally results in an increase in the number of fecal incontinence episodes [21]. In contrast, beneficial effects were reported with the use of loperamide in a father and son with long-lasting fecal incontinence. These effects can be explained by increasing the basal internal anal sphincter pressure and by decreasing rectal contractions [53]. A large randomized control is warranted confirming these observations. Biofeedback training includes feedback about the voluntary controlled muscles such as the external anal sphincter, the muscularis puborectalis, and pelvic floor and aims to enhance rectal sensation. After a training session, which lasts approximately 25 min, the therapist impresses upon the children that they should immediately go to their home toilet the moment they feel the same sensation that they learned during biofeedback training. However, a randomized controlled trial comparing conventional therapy (dietary and toilet advice in combination with oral laxatives) with conventional therapy alone with 5 biofeedback sessions in 71 children with FNRFI showed that 50% of children in each group was successfully treated at the end of 12- and 18-month treatment period suggesting no additional effect of biofeedback training in these children [12].

Treatment of FNRFI is challenging, as symptoms often persist for years and relapses are frequent. No prognostic factors for success were found so far [23]. After 2 years of intensive medical and behavioral treatment, only 29% of children were treated successfully. This result is in contrast to earlier findings in a long-term follow-up study in 403 children with chronic constipation, which reported that 52% of these children were treated successfully after 2 years [55]. After 5 years of follow-up almost similar success rates were observed in children with constipation and patients with FNRFI—70% and 65%, respectively. Thereafter, success further increased to 90% in patients with FNRFI, whereas the percentage remained at 70% in children with constipation [23, 58].

Conclusions

Fecal incontinence is a common and frustrating symptom in children and requires much effort and patience from their parents. In the majority of patients a functional disorder, such as functional constipation or functional non-retentive fecal incontinence, is the underlying condition. FNRFI as a separate clinical disorder is often not recognized by medical professionals. This often causes a delay in referral and frequently leads to inadequate treatment, which negatively influences long-term outcomes. Although 40% of these children have behavior scores within the clinical range, children with FNRFI can be characterized as having only mild psychiatric problems, suggesting that these children should be treated primarily in a pediatric setting and not in a psychiatric outpatient clinic. A thorough clinical history and a physical examination are essential to discriminate between the different underlying entities. An intensive, positive and long-lasting approach is required for successful treatment of fecal incontinence in children.

References

1. Rasquin A, Di Lorenzo C, Forbes D, Guiraldes E, Hyams JS, et al. Childhood functional gastrointestinal disorders: child/adolescent. Gastroenterology. 2006;130:1527–37.
2. Benninga MA, B ller HA, Heymans HS, Tytgat GN, Taminiau JA. Is encopresis always the result of constipation? Arch Dis Child. 1994;71:186–93.
3. Di Lorenzo C, Benninga MA. Pathophysiology of pediatric fecal incontinence. Gastroenterology. 2004;126(Suppl):33–40.
4. Bellman M. Studies on encopresis. Acta Paediatr Scand. 1966;Suppl 170:1+.
5. van der Wal MF, Benninga MA, Hirasing RA. The prevalence of encopresis in a multicultural population. J Pediatr Gastroenterol Nutr. 2005;40:345–8.
6. Loening-Baucke V. Prevalence rates for constipation and faecal and urinary incontinence. Arch Dis Child. 2007;92:486–9.

7. Boccia G, Manguso F, Coccorullo P, Masi P, Pensabene L, Staiano A. Functional defecation disorders in children: PACCT criteria versus Rome II criteria. J Pediatr. 2007;151:394–8.
8. Rajindrajith S, Devanarayana NM, Benninga MA. Constipation-associated and nonretentive fecal incontinence in children and adolescents: an epidemiological survey in Sri Lanka. J Pediatr Gastroenterol Nutr. 2010;51:472–6.
9. Fishman L, Lenders C, Fortunato C, Noonan C, Nurko S. Increased prevalence of constipation and fecal soiling in a population of obese children. J Pediatr. 2004;145:253–4.
10. vd Baan-Slootweg OH, Liem O, Bekkali N, van Aalderen WMC, Pels Rijcken TH, Benninga MA. Constipation and colonic transit times in morbidly obese children. J Pediatr Gastroenterol Nutr. 2011; 52:442–5.
11. Bongers ME, Tabbers MM, Benninga MA. Functional nonretentive fecal incontinence in children. J Pediatr Gastroenterol Nutr. 2007;44:5–13.
12. van der Plas RN, Benninga MA, Redekop WK, Taminiau JA, B ller HA. Randomised trial of biofeedback training for encopresis. Arch Dis Child. 1996;75:367–74.
13. Di Lorenzo C. Pediatric anorectal disorders. Gastroenterol Clin North Am. 2001;30:269–87.
14. Voskuijl WP, Heijmans J, Heijmans HS, Taminiau JA, Benninga MA. Use of Rome II criteria in childhood defecation disorders: applicability in clinical and research practice. J Pediatr. 2004;145:213–7.
15. de Lorijn F, van Wijk MP, Reitsma JB, van Ginkel R, Taminiau JA, Benninga MA. Prognosis of constipation: clinical factors and colonic transit time. Arch Dis Child. 2004;89:723–7.
16. Benninga MA, Voskuijl WP, Taminiau JA. Childhood constipation: is there new light in the tunnel? J Pediatr Gastroenterol Nutr. 2004;39:448–64.
17. Benninga MA, Büller HA, Tytgat GNJ, Akkermans LMA, Bossuyt PM, et al. Colonic transit time in constipated children; does pediatric slow transit constipation exist? J Pediatr Gastroenterol Nutr. 1996; 23:241–51.
18. Dohil R, Roberts E, Jones KV, Jenkins HR. Constipation and reversible urinary tract abnormalities. Arch Dis Child. 1994;70:56–7.
19. Burgers R, Liem O, Canon S, Mousa H, Benninga MA, et al. Effect of rectal distention on lower urinary tract function in children. J Urol. 2010;184(4 Suppl):1680–5.
20. Yazbeck S, Schick E, O'Regan S. Relevance of constipation to enuresis, urinary tract infection and reflux. A review. Eur Urol. 1987;13:318–21.
21. van Ginkel R, Benninga MA, Blommaart PJ, van der Plas RN, Boeckxstaens GE, et al. Lack of benefit of laxatives as adjunctive therapy for functional nonretentive fecal soiling in children. J Pediatr. 2000;137:808–13.
22. van der Plas RN, Benninga MA, Büller HA, Bossuyt PM, Akkermans LMA, et al. Biofeedback training in treatment of childhood constipation: a randomised controlled study. Lancet. 1996;348:776–80.
23. Voskuijl WP, Reitsma JB, van Ginkel R, Büller HA, Taminiau JA, Benninga MA. Longitudinal follow-up of children with functional nonretentive fecal incontinence. Clin Gastroenterol Hepatol. 2006;4:67–72.
24. Voskuijl WP, van Ginkel R, Benninga MA, Hart GA, Taminiau JAJM, Boeckxstaens GE. New insight into rectal function in pediatric defecation disorders: disturbed rectal compliance is an essential mechanism in pediatric constipation. J Pediatr. 2006;148:62–7.
25. Youssef NN, Langseder AL, Verga BJ, Mones RL, Rosh JR. Chronic childhood constipation is associated with impaired quality of life: a case-controlled study. J Pediatr Gastroenterol Nutr. 2005;41:56–60.
26. Bongers ME, van Dijk M, Benninga MA, Grootenhuis MA. Health related quality of life in children with constipation-associated fecal incontinence. J Pediatr. 2009;154(5):749–53.
27. Benninga MA, Voskuijl WP, Akkerhuis GW, Taminiau JA, B ller HA. Colonic transit times and behaviour profiles in children with defecation disorders. Arch Dis Child. 2004;89:13–6.
28. Loening-Baucke V, Cruikshank B, Savage C. Defecation dynamics and behavior profiles in encopretic children. Pediatrics. 1987;80:672–9.
29. Bekkali NL, Hagebeuk EE, Bongers ME, van Rijn RR, Wijk PM, et al. Magnetic resonance imaging of the lumbosacral spine in children with chronic constipation or non-retentive fecal incontinence: a prospective study. J Pediatr. 2010;156:461–5.
30. Constipation Guideline Committee of the North American Society for Pediatric Gastroenterology, Hepatology and Nutrition. Evaluation and treatment of constipation in children: summary of updated recommendations of the North American Society for Pediatric Gastroenterology, Hepatology and Nutrition. J Pediatr Gastroenterol Nutr. 2006;43:e1–13.
31. Hill J, Corson RJ, Brandon H. History and examination in the assessment of patients with idiopathic fecal incontinence. Dis Colon Rectum. 1994;37:473–7.
32. Tantiphlachiva K, Rao P, Attaluri A, Rao SS. Digital rectal examination is a useful tool for identifying patients with dyssynergia. Clin Gastroenterol Hepatol. 2010;8:955–60.
33. Lawrentschuk N, Bolton DM. Experience and attitudes of final-year medical students to digital rectal examination. Med J Aust. 2004;181:323–5.
34. Safder S, Rewalt M, Elitsur Y. Digital rectal examination and the primary care physicians: a lost art? Clin Pediatr (Phila). 2006;45:411–4.
35. Gold DM, Levine J, Weinstein TA, Kessler BH, Pettei MJ. Frequency of digital rectal examination in children with chronic constipation. Arch Pediatr Adolesc Med. 1999;153:377–9.
36. Reuchlin-Vroklage LM, Bierma-Zeinstra S, Benninga MA, Berger MY. Diagnostic value of abdominal radiography in constipated children: a systematic review. Arch Pediatr Adolesc Med. 2005;159:671–8.
37. Bongers ME, Voskuijl WP, van Rijn RR, Benninga MA. The value of the abdominal radiograph in children with functional gastrointestinal disorders. Eur J Radiol. 2006;59:8–13.

38. Pensabene L, Buonomo C, Fishman L, Chitkara D, Nurko S. Lack of utility of abdominal x-rays in the evaluation of children with constipation: comparison of different scoring methods. J Pediatr Gastroenterol Nutr. 2010;51:155–9.
39. Arhan P, Devroede G, Jehannin B, Lanza M, Faverdin C, et al. Segmental colonic transit time. Dis Colon Rectum. 1981;24:625–9.
40. Metcalf AM, Phillips SF, Zinsmeister AR, MacCarty RL, Beart RW, Wolff BG. Simplified assessment of segmental colonic transit. Gastroenterology. 1987; 92:40–7.
41. Bouchoucha M, Devroede G, Arhan P, Strom B, Weber J, et al. What is the meaning of colorectal transit time measurement? Dis Colon Rectum. 1992;35:773–82.
42. Papadopoulou A, Clayden GS, Booth IW. The clinical value of solid marker transit studies in childhood constipation and soiling. Eur J Pediatr. 1994;153:560–4.
43. Rosen R, Buonomo C, Andrade R, Nurko S. Incidence of spinal cord lesions in patients with intractable constipation. J Pediatr. 2004;145:409–11.
44. Nurko S. Gastrointestinal manometry, methodology and indications. In: Walker W, Durie PR, Hamilton JR, Walker-Smith J, Watkins JB, editors. Pediatric gastrointestinal disease. Philadelphia, PA: Hamilton; 2000. p. 1485–510.
45. van den Berg MM, Bongers ME, Voskuijl WP, Benninga MA. No role for increased rectal compliance in pediatric functional constipation. Gastroenterology. 2009;137:1963–9.
46. van den Berg MM, Di Lorenzo C, van Ginkel R, Mousa HM, Benninga MA. Barostat testing in children with functional gastrointestinal disorders. Curr Gastroenterol Rep. 2006;8:224–9.
47. Dinning PG, Benninga MA, Southwell BR, Scott SM. Paediatric and adult colonic manometry: a tool to help unravel the pathophysiology of constipation. World J Gastroenterol. 2010;16:5162–72.
48. van den Berg MM, Hogan M, Caniano DA, Di Lorenzo C, Benninga MA, Mousa HM. Colonic manometry as predictor of cecostomy success in children with defecation disorders. J Pediatr Surg. 2006;41:730–6.
49. Klijn AJ, Asselman M, Vijverberg MA, Dik P, de Jong TP. The diameter of the rectum on ultrasonography as a diagnostic tool for constipation in children with dysfunctional voiding. J Urol. 2004; 172:1986–8.
50. Singh SJ, Gibbonsa NJ, Vincenta MV, Sitholeb J, Nwokomaa NJ, Alagarswami KV. Use of pelvic ultrasound in the diagnosis of megarectum in children with constipation. J Pediatr Surg. 2005;40:1941–4.
51. Pijpers MA, Tabbers M, Benninga MA, Berger MY. Currently recommended treatments of childhood constipation are not evidence based. A systematic literature review on the effect of laxative treatment and dietary measures. Arch Dis Child. 2009;94:117–31.
52. Pensabene L, Nurko S. Management of fecal incontinence in children without functional fecal retention. Curr Treat Options Gastroenterol. 2004;7:381–90.
53. Voskuijl WP, van Ginkel R, Taminiau JA, Boeckxstaens GE, Benninga MA. Loperamide suppositories in an adolescent with childhood-onset functional nonretentive fecal soiling. J Pediatr Gastroenterol Nutr. 2003;37:198–200.
54. Bekkali NL, van den Berg MM, Dijkgraaf MG, van Wijk MP, Bongers ME, Liem O, Benninga MA. Rectal fecal impaction treatment in childhood constipation: enemas versus high doses oral PEG. Pediatrics. 2009;124:e1108–15.
55. Bongers ME, van den Berg MM, Reitsma JB, Voskuijl WP, Benninga MA. A randomized controlled trial of enemas in combination with oral laxative therapy for children with chronic constipation. Clin Gastroenterol Hepatol. 2009;7:1069–74.
56. Bongers ME, van Wijk MP, Reitsma JB, Benninga MA. Long-term prognosis for childhood constipation: clinical outcomes in adulthood. Pediatrics. 2010; 126:e156–62.
57. Pijpers M, Bongers M, Benninga M, Berger M. Functional constipation in children: a systematic review on prognosis and predictive factors. J Pediatr Gastroenterol Nutr. 2010;50:256–68.
58. Van Ginkel R, Reitsma JB, Buller HA, Van Wijk MP, Taminiau JA, Benninga MA. Childhood constipation: longitudinal follow-up beyond puberty. Gastroenterology. 2003;125:357–63.

Part VI

Treatments

41 Drugs Acting on the Gut: Prokinetics, Antispasmodics, Laxatives

Aileen F. Har and Joseph M.B. Croffie

Introduction

Disorders of gastrointestinal motility result from abnormal contractions of the smooth muscles of the gastrointestinal tract. This may result in diarrhea and bloating or constipation with or without accompanying abdominal pain. Drugs that act on the gastrointestinal tract may be categorized into three groups: (1) agents that enhance smooth muscle contractions, referred to as prokinetic agents; (2) agents that inhibit contractions, which may be agents that retard normal peristalsis referred to as antimotility agents (opiates and opiate receptor agonists) or agents that reduce abnormally elevated gastrointestinal smooth muscle tone, referred to as antispasmodics (anticholinergics, direct smooth muscle relaxers, and calcium channel blockers); (3) agents that act to promote evacuation of stool, referred to as laxatives. This chapter discusses prokinetics, antimotility agents, and antispasmodics, as well as laxatives commonly used in clinical practice.

A.F. Har, M.B., B.Ch • J.M.B. Croffie, M.D., M.P.H. (✉)
Division of Gastroenterology, Pediatrics Department, James Whitcomb Riley Hospital for Children, 702 Barnhill Dr, ROC 4210, Indianapolis, IN 46202, USA
e-mail: jcroffie@iupui.edu

Prokinetic Agents

Available prokinetic medications generally fall under three groups of drugs: dopamine receptor antagonists, motilin receptor agonists, and 5-hydroxytryptamine-4 ($5HT_4$) receptor agonists.

Dopamine-2 (D2) Receptor Antagonists

Domperidone

Domperidone is a peripheral dopamine-2 (D2) receptor antagonist that is used to treat gastroesophageal reflux, gastroparesis, functional dyspepsia, nausea, and vomiting. While it is available in over 50 countries worldwide, it is only available in the USA as an investigational drug. D2 receptors are located both within the brain and in the peripheral nervous system, however since domperidone has poor penetration of the blood–brain barrier, most of its effects are derived from peripheral receptors. Domperidone has the ability to cross the placenta and small amounts are excreted in breast milk (2 ng/mL when dosed at 10 mg PO TID) [1]. It is rapidly metabolized in the liver and has a half-life of 7.5 h [2, 3]. In the gastrointestinal tract, D2 receptor stimulation leads to inhibition of gastric motility, therefore D2 receptor antagonists decrease the symptoms of bloating, premature satiety, nausea, and vomiting by accelerating gastric emptying, increasing antroduodenal contractions, and promoting

C. Faure et al. (eds.), *Pediatric Neurogastroenterology: Gastrointestinal Motility and Functional Disorders in Children*, Clinical Gastroenterology,
DOI 10.1007/978-1-60761-709-9_41, © Springer Science+Business Media New York 2013

esophageal motility [4]. Domperidone also exerts an antiemetic effect on the chemoreceptor trigger zone, which is not protected by the blood–brain barrier. One of the side effects of domperidone is hyperprolactinemia and it has been used off-label to increase milk production for mothers of preterm infants.

Safety and efficacy has not been adequately established for the pediatric population. In children admitted to the hospital for vomiting, compared to placebo and metaclopramide (10 mg) the symptoms of nausea and vomiting were significantly lower using domperidone (30 mg), however this study was conducted for a 24 h period only [5]. Using domperidone to treat gastroesophageal reflux in children, a double-blind placebo-controlled trial was done on 17 patients [6]; after 4 weeks of therapy there was a significant decrease in the number of measured postprandial reflux episodes but no decrease in reported symptoms. The most commonly reported adverse event was diarrhea. Two systematic reviews of pediatric GERD treatments did not recommend the use of domperidone in this patient population due to lack of data showing its efficacy [7, 8]. Oral domperidone in neonates is associated with prolonged QTc interval in patients ≥32 weeks of gestation [9]. Mean QTc prolongation was 14 ms with increasing gestational age and serum potassium at the upper limit of normal being independent risk factors.

A systematic review of qualified studies in adults found that approximately 64% of studies showed that domperidone was effective in improving symptoms of diabetic gastroparesis and 60% showed efficacy in improving gastric emptying [10]. In cases of GERD without evidence of gastric dysmotility, domperidone does not provide increased benefit to adult patients in comparison to acid suppression alone [11]. For adult treatment of functional dyspepsia, a meta-analysis revealed that there was significant improvement in the patient's global assessment with an OR of 7 (95% CI 3.6–16), however there was not enough data to support measured improvement in gastric emptying [12]. Patients with postoperative nausea as well as nausea from cytotoxic medications have improvement of their symptoms compared to placebo; however domperidone was given in the IV form which is no longer available [13–16].

Due to poor CNS penetration, domperidone does not have the neurologic side effects seen with metoclopramide, which is also a D2 receptor antagonist. Domperidone is a CYP3A4 inhibitor and should be avoided in combination with other CYP3A4 inhibitors. There is the potential for prolongation of the QT interval leading to arrhythmias as it acts similar to class III antiarrhythmic agents. Arrhythmia and sudden cardiac death have been associated with patients given intravenous domperidone in the setting of hypokalemia and as a result the IV formulation is no longer available [17, 18]. Risk of cardiac events associated with oral domperidone use compared to PPI use and nonuse of either medication was evaluated in a large-scale nested case–control study [19]. 83,212 patients were exposed to oral domperidone, PPI, or both and within this group there were 49 confirmed cases of serious ventricular arrhythmia and 1,559 confirmed cases of sudden cardiac death. Up to four controls were matched to each case and the adjusted odds ratio for serious ventricular arrhythmia and sudden cardiac death with current use of domperidone was 1.59 (95% CI: 1.28–1.98) compared to nonuse of PPI and 1.44 (95% CI: 1.12–1.86) compared to current use of PPI. Past use of domperidone was not associated with increased risk of cardiac events. Risk may also be increased in patients older than 60 years, males, and those without diabetes.

Domperidone is available in oral tablet, oral suspension, and rectal formulations. The recommended dosing is 10–20 mg two to four times daily 15–30 min before meals. Pediatric dosing is 0.3 mg/kg/dose two to four times daily, not exceeding adult dose. Tablets may be crushed and given through gastrostomy, nasogastric, or jejunostomy tubes.

Metoclopramide

Metoclopramide is a dopamine (D2) receptor antagonist that stimulates the stomach and duodenum by causing efferent myenteric cholinergic neurons to release acetylcholine. There is also an increase in the lower esophageal sphincter tone [20, 21]. Metoclopramide's antiemetic properties are due to its effects on the central nervous system D2 receptors in the chemoreceptor trigger zone.

However, due to its ability to cross the blood–brain barrier it also has the potential to cause acute extrapyramidal reactions [22, 23] and tardive dyskinesia with long-term or high-dose use [24, 25]. Metoclopramide is used to treat gastroesophageal reflux, chemotherapy-induced nausea, postoperative nausea and vomiting, and gastroparesis. Evidence for use in pediatric gastroesophageal reflux is conflicting as some studies show that there is no significant improvement in symptoms and esophageal pH measurements compared to placebo, while others show significant improvement [26, 27]. Metoclopramide is used frequently to treat postoperative nausea and vomiting, and in the setting of strabismus surgery where, a review determined that there was significant improvement in symptoms for the early postoperative period compared to that of placebo [28].

Metoclopramide is available in the PO, SC, IM, IV forms. The adult dose is 10 mg three to four times daily. The pediatric dose is 0.4–0.8 mg/kg/day divided 4 times a day not to exceed adult dosage. A black box warning issued by the United States Food and Drug Administration cautions that cumulative use greater than 12 weeks in duration, increases risk of tardive dyskinesia, which may be irreversible. Extrapyramidal symptoms occur more commonly within 24–48 h of initiation of therapy and children are at increased risk especially with higher dosing. Pseudoparkinsonism has also been reported and is usually reversible. Other side effects include sedation and hyperprolactinemia. The half life in children is around 4 h with 85% being eliminated in the urine; therefore, dosing should be adjusted in cases of renal dysfunction. Metoclopramide does cross the placenta and is excreted in breast milk. Onset of action is 15–30 min after oral dosing and 1–3 min after intravenous administration [29].

Motilin Agonists

Erythromycin

Erythromycin is a macrolide antibiotic, and it also acts as a motilin agonist and its primary prokinetic use is for the treatment of gastroparesis. Motilin is a peptide hormone secreted by the small intestine from the enterochromaffin cells [30]. The receptors for motilin are found mainly in the smooth muscle and cholinergic neurons of the stomach antrum and proximal duodenum [31]. The effect of motilin pertains to stimulation of phase 3 MMCs in the interdigestive state [31]. Janssens et al. first studied the effect of erythromycin on gastric motility in 10 adult diabetic patients with gastroparesis in 1990 [32]. Compared with placebo, an IV dose of 200 mg significantly improved gastric emptying from a 120 min mean retention of 63 ± 9–$4 \pm 1\%$. This preliminary study also showed an improvement in gastric emptying in the same 10 patients after 4 weeks of 250 mg, PO, TID, but to a lesser degree.

Erythromycin may be given through both oral and intravenous routes. Adult dosing ranges from 50 to 250 mg, three or four times a day and pediatric dosing is typically 5 mg/kg/dose. Different motor patterns are elicited from varying erythromycin dosages [33]. Low dose erythromycin (1–3 mg/kg IV) stimulates the neural motilin receptors leading to augmentation of phase 3 MMCs [33, 34]. A higher dose of the drug stimulates the smooth muscle motilin receptors leading to sustained contractions in the antrum and antroduodenal coordination [33–35]. Long-term therapy appears to be safe; however, decreased efficacy is seen after prolonged treatment due to downregulation of motilin receptors. There has been no evidence that erythromycin has any prokinetic effect on the colon as shown by administration of the drug during colonic manometry studies [36, 37].

Commonly reported side effects include nausea, vomiting, and abdominal pain. There have been reports of erythromycin being associated with serious cardiac arrhythmias and prolonged QTc [38–40]. Erythromycin should not be used concurrently with medications metabolized by cytochrome P450 3A4 (CYP3A4) such as cisapride, terfenadine, pimozide, or astemizole as it is a CYP3A4 inhibitor. Caution must be used in young infants as there is an eight- to tenfold increased risk of developing hypertrophic pyloric stenosis in term or near-term infants when used within the first 2 weeks of life and when the treatment course is >14 days [41]. There is insufficient data in the preterm infant population as to whether there is increased risk of pyloric stenosis and a recent review did not show increased incidence for this particular population for treatment of dysmotility due to immaturity of the gastrointestinal tract [42]. Erythromycin is excreted in breast milk at levels ranging from 50 to 100% of maternal serum levels [43] and should be taken into consideration when treating nursing mothers.

Cholinergics

Bethanechol

Bethanechol is a cholinergic medication, which acts as a muscarinic receptor agonist leading to stimulation of esophageal peristalsis and increased antral contractility. It is also used to treat urinary retention secondary to neurogenic bladder. It causes decreased episodes of esophageal reflux by increasing lower esophageal sphincter (LES) pressure and increasing esophageal clearance [44–47]. Bethanechol's effect on the amplitude and duration of esophageal contractions are more pronounced in the distal esophagus and there is less effect on upper esophageal motility [48]. In patients with normal lower esophageal sphincter tone and normal esophageal motility, it is questionable if bethanechol is useful in the treatment of uncomplicated gastroesophageal reflux and acid suppression may better serve this population [49, 50]. Patients with known esophageal dysmotility and abnormal LES tone, such as those post-tracheoesophageal fistula or esophageal atresia repair, may benefit from bethanechol [51]. It improves smooth muscle function in patients with ineffective esophageal motility documented by esophageal manometry [52].

Bethanechol is available by oral and subcutaneous administration only and the onset of action is 30–90 min. It should not be used in combination with anticholinesterase inhibitors. The mechanism of metabolism and excretion is unclear. Pediatric dosing is 0.1–0.2 mg/kg/dose before meals up to four times a day and the adult dose is 10–50 mg two to four times a day. Side effects to note include bronchial constriction and it should be used with caution in asthmatics. Bethanechol does produce other cholinergic effects including urinary frequency, miosis, lacrimation, and flushing.

Neostigmine

Neostigmine is a synthetic, reversible acetylcholinesterase inhibitor. It is used in the treatment of myasthenia gravis and for reversing nondepolarizing muscle relaxants. Neostigmine has also been used to treat patients with acute colonic pseudo-obstruction (ACPO), known as Ogilvie's Syndrome. Its use as a promotility agent has not been well studied in pediatric patients. The first reported case of successful treatment of a pediatric patient with ACPO was in a 4-year-old male with spastic quadriplegia who was 10 days postoperative for bilateral femoral varus derotational osteotomies and botulinum toxin injections of the gastrocnemius muscles [53]. Neostigmine was administered intravenously at a total dose of 0.05 mg/kg over 5 h [53]. In a group of 10 pediatric patients with hematologic malignancies who experienced ACPO, 8 responded to doses of neostigmine at 0.01 mg/kg/dose administered subcutaneously, given twice a day for no more than 5 doses [54]. One patient reported diplopia and one reported abdominal pain [54]. In another case report, a 9-year-old boy with cerebellar medulloblastoma, on chemotherapy, was successfully treated for ACPO with the same subcutaneous dosage after 3 injections [55]. In a third case report, a 3-year-old girl with sickle cell disease with acute colonic pseudo-obstruction had resolution after 2 doses of neostigmine at 10 mcg/kg [56]. The patient was in vaso-occlusive crisis and had a colon measuring 6.5 cm in diameter and no mechanical obstruction found on gastrograffin enema. She started passing stool within 6 h of neostigmine injection.

5-Hydroxytryptamine-4 Receptor Agonists

Cisapride

Cisapride is a $5HT_4$ receptor agonist which acts on the myenteric plexus of the bowel wall to stimulate smooth muscle contraction by release of acetylcholine. $5HT_4$ receptors are found throughout the gastrointestinal tract and stimulation causes increased peristalsis as well as intraluminal fluid secretion. Stimulation of the stomach smooth muscle leads to accelerated gastric emptying. Amplitude of esophageal peristalsis as well as resting lower esophageal sphincter tone is increased [57]. Cisapride also decreases mouth to cecum time and colonic transit time [58].

While cisapride has never been approved for children under the age of 12, it has historically been used extensively in this population. The consensus statements issued by NASPGHAN and ESPGHAN in 2000 states that cisapride is recommended for pediatric GERD when non-pharmacologic treatment fails, but that the medication does require close monitoring, and specific precautions should be taken [59, 60]. However, more recently the 2010 Cochrane Review did not show any difference in symptom improvement or weight gain when cisapride is compared to placebo [61]. Nine studies comparing cisapride with placebo or no treatment, that met inclusion criteria, were included in the meta-analysis [62–69]. The authors reviewed five studies comparing results of esophageal pH probe in patients being treated with cisapride vs. placebo and while there was improvement in the reflux index, there was no significant improvement in the number of reflux episodes and episodes lasting longer than 5 min. Histologic examination of the esophagus was performed in three studies and in 2 ($n-6$, $n=20$) studies there was no statistical difference between cisapride and placebo [63, 67], however 1 study ($n=17$) did have histologic improvement from baseline. Further large-scale studies are needed to assess the utility of cisapride for GERD, though due to limited access, it is unlikely this information will be obtained. Although cisapride may be efficacious in treating constipation, it is not recommended for treatment of standard constipation as the risks do not outweigh the benefits [70].

Availability of cisapride is restricted due to risk of prolonged QTc interval and serious cardiac arrhythmias and it is only available in most countries through limited-access programs. Multiple studies have shown increase in QTc interval in neonates, infants and children, however in many of these cases the medication was dosed above the recommended dosing and some were taking a macrolide antibiotic concurrently [71–75]. Arrhythmias have also been reported ranging from notched t waves to torsades de points [71, 74, 76]. In a multicenter, double-blind placebo-controlled trial of 49 children (age 6 months–4 years), however, a dose of 0.2 mg/kg given three times a day in patients without cardiac risk factors, for a treatment duration of at least 6 weeks, did not show a statistically significant increase in QTc interval and no subjects experienced cardiac events [62].

Cisapride is metabolized in the liver by cytochrome P450 into norcisapride. It is eliminated in urine and feces and its half-life is 7–10 h. Adult dosing should start at 10 mg PO two to four times a day 15 min before meals; dose may be increased to 20 mg for efficacy. Pediatric dosing is 0.8 mg/kg/day divided into 3–4 doses and not exceeding adult dose. 50% of the recommended dose should be started in the case of renal or hepatic failure. It is contraindicated in combination with macrolide antibiotics, azole antifungals, and any drug that prolongs the QT interval. It should be avoided while CYP3A4 inhibitors are being used. Also grapefruit juice should be avoided as it can increase cisapride serum concentrations. Caution must be taken in infants who are breastfed as mothers may excrete medications in their breast milk that are contraindicated while using cisapride. Patients with known history of prolonged QTc should not be prescribed cisapride and patients with other known arrhythmias need careful monitoring. Electrolyte imbalance, especially hypokalemia, increases the risk of serious cardiac side effects.

Tegaserod

Tegaserod is a $5HT_4$ receptor partial agonist. It was previously approved for treatment of females ≤55 years of age with constipation-predominant IBS or for chronic idiopathic constipation; however, it has subsequently been withdrawn from the US market due to an increased risk of cardiovascular events. In an open label study, 22 adult patients with symptoms of upper intestinal dysmotility underwent a 24 h antrodoudenal motility study comparing the effects of tegaserod (12 mg

PO) and erythromycin (125 mg IV) [77]. Both medications showed significantly increased motility in the antrum, duodenum, and jejunum. There were differences in the timing and where the two medications exerted their prokinetic effects—tegaserod had higher motor responses in the duodenum and jejunum, which occurred 2–3 h after administration, whereas erythromycin had stronger motor effects on the antrum that occurred within 30 min. Both tegaserod and erythromycin induced phase III migrating motor complexes (MMCs) in 55 and 36% of patients, respectively.

While tegaserod was never approved for pediatric use, it was widely used off label in many practices. A report on a single center's experience in pediatric patients reviewed 72 patients with a median age of 10 (1.1–18.3) [78]; most of these children were treated for functional constipation and the mean follow-up time was 11.3 months (2.3–45.2). Patients reported a statistically significant improvement in bowel frequency and fecal continence. The most common adverse events were diarrhea (20%), abdominal pain (8%), and headache (4%). No cardiovascular events were reported.

Adult dosing is 6 mg, PO, BID before meals and the tablets come in 2 and 6 mg forms. Bioavailability is 11% and decreased by up to 65% when taken with food [79, 80]. It is metabolized in the liver and 66% is excreted unchanged in stool and 33% as metabolites in urine. Use is contraindicated in severe hepatic or renal impairment. Adverse reactions include diarrhea, abdominal pain, nausea, flatulence, headache, and back pain.

Prucalopride

Prucalopride is a highly selective, high affinity 5-HT$_4$ receptor agonist, which increases colonic motility by stimulating serotonin release leading to giant migrating contractions [81]. Gastro-pyloro-duodenal motility as well as gastric emptying is also enhanced in the canine model [82]. Prucalopride is structurally different from previously available 5-HT$_4$ receptor agonist and due to its selectivity; the cardiac side effects seen with cisapride and tegaserod have not been reported. Use of prucalopride has mostly been in adult patients with chronic constipation. No pediatric studies have been published. Evaluation of prucalopride in healthy volunteers showed accelerated orocecal transit, colonic transit, and total gastrointestinal transit time [83–85]. Treatment of patients with chronic constipation showed similar improvements in transit times [86–89] and significant increases in spontaneous complete bowel movements, stool consistency, urge to defecate, and quality of life compared to placebo [86, 88–92]. No significant increase in QTc interval has been reported and the most common complaints have been abdominal pain, abdominal distension, diarrhea, nausea, flatulence, back pain, headache, and dizziness [89–91, 93].

Prucalopride is approved in Europe for use in women with chronic constipation that is not relieved by laxatives. Recommended adult dose is 2 mg, PO, daily. The half life is 24–30 h, it is minimally metabolized, and excreted mainly by the kidneys [94]. Dosing for geriatrics and patients with severe renal or hepatic dysfunction should start at 50% of the recommended dose.

Velusetrag (TD-5108)

Velusetrag is a highly selective 5HT$_4$ receptor agonist. A phase 2 study has investigated the effect of velusetrag on colonic transit, colonic filling and emptying, and gastric emptying in healthy volunteers and patients with chronic constipation [95]. In this double-blind placebo-controlled study, healthy subjects were given 5, 15, 30, and 50 mg of Velusetrag or placebo. Gastric emptying was not affected after a single dose, however there was a significant increase in emptying after 6 days of consecutive treatment for the 15, 30, and 50 mg dosing. Small bowel transit as measured by colonic filling at 6 h was significantly increased after a single dose at 30 and 50 mg, but there was no statistical significance after multiple day dosing. Colonic transit as measured by $t_{1/2}$ of ascending colon emptying, and colonic geometric center at 24 h was increased for the 30 and 50 mg doses after a single dose; however, there was no significant increase in colonic transit compared to placebo after multiple doses. Patients with chronic constipation were age- and sex-matched to the control group and given a single oral dose of 15 mg. There was no significant difference in pharmacokinetics between the control and constipation groups. The two study groups reported similar stool consistency, time to first bowel movement, and number of bowel movements in the 24 h after administration. There was an increase in heart rate by 10 bpm at 4 h after ingestion, but no change in blood pressure or EKG tracings. Subjects reported nausea, diarrhea, and headache as the most common adverse events, which was dose related. A single subject on 30 mg experienced palpitations and one patient on 50 mg developed asymptomatic junctional escape rhythm.

Other Prokinetic Agents

Octreotide

Octreotide is a synthetic cyclic tetradecapeptide that is a long acting somatostatin analogue used to treat many disease processes including gastrointestinal bleeding, pancreatitis, secretory diarrhea, chylous leakage, hypoglycemia, and gastrointestinal dysmotility. For the purposes of this section, only the use of octreotide in gastrointestinal dysmotility will be discussed. Somatostatin, studied in patients with normal gastrointestinal motility as well as the canine model, causes inhibition of gastric activity and stimulation of small intestinal phase 3 migrating motor complexes (MMCs) beginning in the duodenum [96, 97]. It is commercially available for SC, IV, and IM use. Subcutaneous absorption is rapid and IM is released slowly in a depot formulation. Metabolism is through the liver with 32% unmetabolized excretion through the urine [98]. Half-life is 1.7–1.9 h, but it is 3.7 h in patients with cirrhosis and 3.1 h in patients with renal impairment [79].

Octreotide has been studied in adult patients with scleroderma and pseudo obstruction; subcutaneous octreotide increased the frequency of intestinal migrating complexes in this group of patients [99]. After 3 weeks of treatment patients had a reduction in bacterial overgrowth as measured by hydrogen breath testing and had reported decrease in bloating, nausea, vomiting, and abdominal pain [99]. A single case report described a 12-year-old girl with chronic idiopathic pseudo obstruction who was successfully treated using 50 mcg of subcutaneous octreotide daily [100].

Methylnaltrexone

Methylnaltrexone is a peripheral μ-opiate antagonist that has been used to treat patients in the setting of opiate-induced constipation [101]. It is a quaternary ammonium derivative of naltrexone which, due to its low polarity, has reduced penetration of the blood–brain barrier [102, 103]. μ-Receptors are found throughout the gastrointestinal tract [106] and their stimulation leads to delayed transit and non-propulsive activity [107]. Decreased intestinal secretion as well as increased absorption in the small bowel and colon also contributes to the constipating effect of opioid medications [108]. Opioid-induced constipation is reversed, without inducing withdrawal symptoms or decreasing analgesic effect, by methylnaltrexone [101, 104, 105].

In the treatment of adult patients receiving chronic opioids for nonmalignant pain doses of 12 mg every day and every other day have been used; both regimens significantly decreased the time to rescue-free bowel movement as well as increased the number of weekly bowel movements compared to placebo [109]. In the treatment of adults with advanced illness and opioid-induced constipation using doses of 0.15 and 0.3 mg/kg, subjects had significantly increased rates of rescue-free bowel movements within 4 h of administration compared to placebo [104, 105].

A single case report of the use of methylnaltrexone to treat postoperative ileus in a neonate demonstrated success in restoring bowel motility 15 min after a 0.15 mg/kg IV infusion [110]. The infant had undergone two separate exploratory laparoscopies for necrotizing enterocolitis and was on a fentanyl drip for pain control. Five doses were given in total on POD 8–12.

Methylnaltrexone is available in subcutaneous form with onset of action between 30 min to 4 h and a half life of 8–9 h [109, 111, 112]. It is administered every other day with dosing based on body weight. Excretion is through both urine and feces, primarily as unchanged drug [112]. Side effects include flatulence, abdominal pain, nausea, dizziness, excessive sweating, and diarrhea. Intestinal perforation has been reported with use and it should be used with caution in patients with diminished gastrointestinal wall integrity. Patients with severe renal impairment (creatinine clearance <30 mL/min) should be dosed at 50% of recommended dosing Table 41.1.

Antimotility Agents

The commonly used agents are the opioid receptor agonists loperamide and diphenoxylate.

Loperamide

Loperamide is a synthetic opioid receptor agonist acting on the μ opioid receptors in the myenteric plexus of the large intestine [113]. It is a peripherally acting agent and does not cross the blood–brain barrier. It has been shown in meta-analysis of randomized controlled trials to be safe and effective in treating acute diarrhea in adults and children [114, 115]. In children serious side effects were reported more often in those younger than 3 years old [115]. Loperamide has also been shown in clinical trials to be effective in reducing stool frequency and urgency in patients with diarrhea-predominant irritable bowel syndrome [116]. It is available in tablet and liquid suspension. The side effects include abdominal pain and bloating, constipation, sedation, dry mouth and, rarely, paralytic ileus. This medication should not be used in the setting of acute diarrhea caused by enteric bacterial pathogens such as salmonella and Shigella and in acute ulcerative colitis as it can precipitate toxic megacolon. It should also not be used in children less than 2 years old; indeed deaths have been reported in young children given loperamide to treat acute diarrhea [117].

Diphenoxylate

Diphenoxylate is a synthetic opioid receptor agonist related to meperidine and fentanyl [113]. Like loperamide it inhibits gastrointestinal propulsion and has been shown to be effective in treating acute diarrhea. Unlike loperamide however, diphenoxylate crosses the blood–brain barrier and therefore can be habit forming. Atropine is reportedly added to the preparation to reduce the abuse potential [118, 119]. Side effects include sedation, euphoria, lethargy, confusion, respiratory depression, restlessness, hyperthermia, tachycardia, nausea, vomiting, paralytic ileus, and toxic megacolon. Like loperamide, diphenoxylate should not be used in the setting of acute diarrhea caused by enteric bacterial pathogens and acute ulcerative colitis because of potential to precipitate toxic megacolon. Diphenoxylate should not be used in children less than 2 years old; opiate and atropine toxicity from diphenoxylate-atropine overdosage leading to death has been reported in children less than 2 years old [120].

Antispasmodics

Antimuscarinics

Antimuscarinics are a class of drugs that work by blocking the action of acetylcholine at postganglionic parasympathetic receptors in the intestinal smooth muscle. They are the most frequently prescribed antispasmodics in the USA. Meta-analysis of placebo-controlled trials of drugs used to treat irritable bowel syndrome confirm the therapeutic benefit of this class of drugs in adults, although many of the trials were reportedly of low quality [121]. Similar studies in children are lacking. The antimuscarinics currently available in clinical practice are derivatives of belladonna, a naturally occurring plant alkaloid, and include drugs such as hyoscyamine, dicyclomine, cimetropium, scopolamine, clidinium, and trimebutine.

Hyoscyamine is the levorotatory Isomer of atropine. It is available as oral tablets, extended

Table 41.1 Prokinetics

Medication	Dosing	Notes
Domperidone	0.3 mg/kg/dose two to four times daily[a] (PO, PR)	Adult dose 10–20 mg two to four times daily
Metoclopramide	0.4–0.8 mg/kg/day divided four times daily[a] (PO, SC, IM, IV)	Adult dose 10 mg three to four times daily
Erythromycin	1–3 mg/kg/dose (IV); 5 mg/kg/dose (PO) up to four times a day	Adult dose 50–250 mg three or four times a day
Bethanechol	0.1–0.2 mg/kg/dose up to four times a day[a] (PO,SC)	Adult dose 10–50 mg 2–4 times a day
Neostigmine	0.01 mg/kg/dose (IV, SC)	Oral formulation is available, but absorption is poor and not studied for treatment of acute colonic pseudo-obstruction
Cisapride	0.8 mg/kg/day divided three to four times daily[a] (PO)	Adult dose 10–20 mg two to four times a day
Tegaserod	Not determined in children	Adult dose 6 mg PO twice a day
Prucalopride	Not determined in children	Adult dose 2 mg, PO, daily
Octreotide	1–10 mcg/kg every 12 h (SC, IV, IM)	Adult dose 50 mcg up to three times a day. IM route is delayed release
Methylnaltrexone	<38 kg—0.15 mg/kg/dose 38 to ≤62 kg—8 mg 62–114 kg—12 mg >114 kg—0.15 mg/kg/dose	Round to nearest 0.1 mL Administered every other day

[a]Not to exceed maximum adult dose

release tablets, sublingual tablets, oral solutions, elixirs, and drops. It has been used to treat symptoms of colic and irritable bowel syndrome [122, 123]. Although commonly used, there are no randomized controlled trials establishing the safety and efficacy of this medication in treating gastrointestinal disorders, particularly in children. Anticholinergic poisoning has been reported in some colicky infants treated with hyoscyamine [122].

Dicyclomine is an m1-specific muscarinic antagonist which has been used to treat symptoms of colic, irritable bowel syndrome and diverticulitis. It has been shown in many double-blind studies to be effective in the treatment of infantile colic [124, 125]; however, 5% of treated infants had side effects [126]. Although commonly used to treat irritable bowel syndrome, there are no randomized controlled trials establishing the safety and efficacy of the drug in treating irritable bowel syndrome in children. It has been shown in only one study to reduce symptoms of irritable bowel syndrome including pain and fecal urgency in adults [127].

Scopolamine (hyoscine) is another m1-specific muscarinic antagonist which has been used to treat various gastrointestinal disorders including irritable bowel syndrome and motion sickness [128]. Methscopolamine and butylscopolamine are derivatives of scopolamine which have also been used to treat irritable bowel syndrome. Scopolamine was found in a meta-analysis study to offer benefit in the treatment of irritable bowel syndrome in adults [129] however, there are no published randomized controlled studies establishing its effectiveness in treating this condition in children.

Cimetropium is a synthetic derivative of scopolamine which has both antimuscarinic and direct myolytic activity [130]. It has been shown to be more effective than placebo in reducing the duration of crying in children with infantile colic [130] and a double-blind placebo-controlled study in adults showed that it is effective in relieving pain in patients with irritable bowel syndrome [131].

Clidinium is a rarely used muscarinic antagonist which is marketed in combination with chlordiazepoxide as a treatment for irritable bowel syndrome, although there are no randomized controlled trials showing its safety or efficacy in treating this condition.

Trimebutine is an antimuscarinic drug which also has some opioid agonistic effects; it accelerates gastric emptying and induces premature phase III of the migrating motor complex in the small bowel, but it inhibits colonic motility through its antimuscarinic activity [132]. This drug has been found to be efficacious in the treatment of recurrent abdominal pain and irritable bowel syndrome in children and adults. It was found in a meta-analysis study to be effective in the treatment of irritable bowel syndrome in adults [129].

Common side effects of antimuscarinic agents include dry mouth, urinary retention, blurred vision, constipation, sedation, and palpitations.

Direct Smooth Muscle Relaxers

Mebeverine and related drugs including alverine, otilonium, and drotaverine [133–135] are not available in the USA but are available in many countries. They are antispasmodics which are believed to be mostly musculotropic. These drugs exert their antispasmodic effect by acting directly at the cellular level of the gastrointestinal smooth muscle. They have been used to treat irritable bowel syndrome. A systematic review of several studies in adults found these agents to be efficacious in improving the symptoms of abdominal pain in adult patients with irritable bowel syndrome [136, 137].

OnabotulinumtoxinA (Botox®)

Onabotulinumtoxin A is the drug name for botulinum toxin A—it is used commonly in cosmetic procedures, but is also used to treat strabismus, blepharospasm, muscle spasticity, cervical dystonia, and hyperhidrosis. It has been used off-label to treat esophageal achalasia, gastroparesis, anal fissure, and anal achalasia. Botulinum toxin A is one of seven serotypes of botulinum neurotoxins produced by the aneorobic bacteria *Clostridium*

Botulinum [138]. The neurotoxin targets the neuromuscular junction and blocks acetylcholine release causing flaccid paralysis.

In a single center report, postoperative follow-up of adult patients treated for esophageal achalasia revealed recurrent or persistent symptoms in 71.4% ($n=7$) of patients treated with endoscopic botulinum injection [139] compared to recurrent/persistent symptoms in 50% of patients who underwent endoscopic balloon dilation ($n=30$) and recurrent/persistent symptoms in 30% of patients who underwent surgical myotomy ($n=20$). Thus in this report, patients who underwent surgical myotomy had the most reliable outcome. Treatment with Botox injections has an initial success rate of 70%, however the effect usually lasts 6–12 months and repeated injections are required [140]. There have been conflicting reports on whether prior injection with Botox decreases the effectiveness of a later Heller myotomy or whether it impacts the ease of the procedure [141–144]. A single center reviewed their experience with pediatric patients diagnosed with esophageal achalasia; out of their 33 patients, 7 were treated with Botox [145]. They used 100 U of Botox per session with 25 U injected into each quadrant of the lower esophageal sphincter. Six of the seven required 2–3 repeated injections and the longest duration of symptom-free period postinjection was 10 months. Four eventually had a Heller myotomy. One case report also reported response for 8 months postinjection in an 11-year-old boy [146]. A single case report of the use of Botox to treat a diabetic, obese adult with esophageal achalasia was complicated by mediastinitis [147]. The development of a sinus tract between the esophagus and gastric fundus has been reported in a 10-year-old girl following her fifth Botox injection for esophageal achalasia [148].

In two studies, pediatric patients treated with Botox injections for anal outlet obstruction (post-surgical repair of Hirschsprung Disease and primary internal anal sphincter achalasia) had variable outcomes [149, 150]. The dosage used was 3–6 U/kg/session to a maximum of 100 U. 31–53% of patients had good long-term outcome and 62–89% had initial clinical improvement after a single injection. About 75% required more than one session. Complications included pain following the injection and fecal incontinence.

Botox injections have also been used to treat chronic anal fissures. At one center, 13 children (age 1–10 years) were given Botox injections in the external anal sphincter under light sedation to treat chronic anal fissures [151]; patients under age 2 were injected with 1.25 U ×2 doses and patients over age 2 were injected with 2.5 U×2 doses. 11 of the 13 patients had resolution of their symptoms within 1 week of treatment and no adverse events were reported. In a systematic review of nonsurgical therapies for chronic anal fissures, Botox was found to be equivalent to topical nitroglycerin in efficacy; however, nitroglycerin itself was only marginally better than placebo [152].

There is a paucity of data on the usefulness of intrapyloric injections of Botox for treatment of gastroparesis. One randomized controlled crossover study of 23 adult patients with gastroparesis showed no benefit of Botox injection (25 U/quadrant; 100 U total) compared to placebo [153] and no pediatric studies have been published.

Topical Nitrates

Topical nitrates have been used to treat painful anal conditions. There are three formulations available—mono, di, and trinitrates—all act to relax smooth muscle by stimulating production of cGMP, irrespective of autonomic innervations [154]. The only topical formulation available in the USA is nitroglycerin, which is a trinitrate. Its most common use in gastroenterology is for treatment of chronic anal fissures.

In children with anal fissures, 0.2% glyceryl trinitrate (GTN) applied topically to the distal anal canal twice a day resulted in improvement of symptoms by day 10 of treatment and higher rates of complete resolution after 8 weeks compared to placebo and topical lidocaine [155, 156]. However, one study comparing GTN plus oral senna and lactulose with placebo plus oral senna and lactulose, found similar response rates, with 84% healing overall [157]. Concentrations of 0.05 and 0.1% ointments were also found to be effective for fissure healing after 8 weeks of treatment [158]. Results at 8 weeks of treatment were similar to results using a eutectic mixture of 5% prilocaine and 5% lidocaine (EMLA) [156].

Long-term treatment of chronic anal fissure in 31 children using 0.2% GTN resulted in a 32% relapse 1 year after treatment and no relapses for 4 years following initial treatment in 68% [159].

Glycerine trinitrate has also been used to treat proctalgia fugax, which mainly occurs in patients aged 30–60 years [160, 161].

Calcium Channel Blockers

It has been suggested that calcium channel blockers may be effective in the treatment of some gastrointestinal motility disorders because of their ability to relax smooth muscles. Nifedipine and verapamil have been shown to inhibit sigmoid colon myoelectric response to eating in healthy adult volunteers [162] and reduce internal anal sphincter pressures in patients and controls with high resting anal sphincter pressures [163].

Nifedipine has been used to treat disorders of esophageal hyper motility such as nutcracker esophagus and achalasia in children and adults [164–167]. Diltiazem has been used anecdotally to treat diffuse esophageal spasm in adolescents [168]. Verapamil has anecdotally been used to treat antral spasms in children [169]. Pinaverium is a calcium channel blocker which acts selectively on the gastrointestinal tract; it has been found to reduce the duration of abdominal pain in randomized, placebo-controlled studies of adult patients with irritable bowel syndrome [170, 171]. Peppermint oil is believed to be a calcium channel blocker which has been found to relax the lower esophageal sphincter, and reduce colonic spasms in patients undergoing colonoscopy [172, 173]. It has been found in double-blind randomized controlled studies to be effective in treating children and adults with irritable bowel syndrome [174, 175] and in meta-analysis studies of published trials, it was found to be effective in the treatment of both adults and children with irritable bowel syndrome [176, 177]. Side effects of calcium channel blockers include headaches, lightheadedness, and constipation.

Meta-analysis studies of controlled trials of antispasmodics in the treatment of irritable bowel syndrome have found them to be superior to placebo, at least for the short term, in the management of irritable bowel syndrome in both adults and children [121, 129, 178, 179].

Other Antispamodic Agents

Oral Nitrates have been used in adults to treat spastic disorders of the esophagus, although there are no randomized controlled studies supporting their effectiveness [167]. Sildenafil, a Phosphodiesterase inhibitor, has been found in a double-blind placebo-controlled study to reduce lower esophageal sphincter pressure [167]. No studies of nitrates or sildenafil for these purposes have been reported in children Table 41.2.

Laxatives

Laxatives can be divided into osmotic/lubricant laxatives and stimulant laxatives (see Table 41.3). First-line treatment for constipation starts with osmotic/lubricant laxatives followed by stimulants for cases that are poorly responsive.

Osmotic and Lubricant Laxatives

Lactulose

Lactulose (1-4-beta-galactosidofructose) is a semi-synthetic disaccharide created through the isomerization of lactose [180]. Lactulose increases osmotic load as well as decreases the stool pH thereby increasing colonic propulsion [181]. It passes through the small intestine intact without degradation by dissacharidases and is broken down by bacteria in the colon to produce lactic and acetic acid [182]. Systemic absorption is minimal with majority of excretion through the stool and <3% excretion in urine. Formulations contain both lactose and galactose so use is contraindicated in patients with galactosemia. Onset

Table 41.2 Antimotility and antispasmodic agents

Medication	Dosing	Notes
Loperamide	Acute Diarrhea (first 24 h) – 2–5 years (13–20 kg): 1 mg three times a day – 6–8 years (21–30 kg): 2 mg twice a day – 9–12 years (>30 kg): 2 mg three times a day—After first 24 h–0.1 mg/kg doses after each loose stool not exceeding initial dose Chronic diarrhea—0.08–0.24 mg/kg/day divided 2–3 times a day, maximum: 2 mg/dose(PO)	Adult dose acute and chronic diarrhea—first dose 4 mg, then 2 mg after each loose stool, maximum 16 mg daily
Diphenoxylate	– 2–5 years—2 mg three times a day – 5–8 years—2 mg four times a day – 8–12 years—2 mg five times a day (PO)	Adult dose 5 mg four times a day
Hyoscyamine	2–12 years—0.0625–0.125 mg every 4 h as needed—maximum daily dose 0.75 mg (PO, SL)	Adult dose—0.125–0.25 mg every 4 h as needed—maximum daily dose 1.5 mg (PO, SL) Adult dose—0.25–0.5 mg every 4 h for 1–4 doses only (IV, IM)
Dicyclomine	>6 months old—5 mg, three to four times a day Children—10 mg, three to four times a day (PO)	Adult dose 20 mg, four times a day—may increase to 40 mg, four times a day (PO) Adult IM dose 20 mg, four times a day
Scopolamine	Antiemetic – 6 mcg/kg/dose (maximum 0.3 mg per dose) every 6–8 h (PO, IV, SC)	Adult dose for antiemetic 0.3–0.65 mg/dose every 6–8 h (PO, IV, SC) Adult dose and children >12 years—for motion sickness 10–20 mg every 8 h as needed (PO) Adult dose for transdermal patch—1 patch behind the ear every 72 h as needed
Trimebutine	Children >12 years—100–200 mg three times a day (PO)	Adult dose 100–200 mg three times a day (PO)
Mebeverine	Children >10 years—100 mg three times a day (PO)	Adult dose 100–135 mg three times a day (PO) OR 200 mg twice a day (PO modified release)
Onabotulinumtoxin A	Esophageal achalasia – 20–25 U into each quadrant (80–100 U total per treatment) Anal outlet obstruction – 3–6 U/kg/session to a maximum of 100 U divided into 4 quadrants Chronic anal fissure 1.25–2.5units ×2 per session	Adult gastroparesis – 25 U into each quadrant (100 U total per treatment)
Glyceryl trinitrate (0.2%)	Apply ointment to the distal anal canal twice a day	
Nifedipine		Adult dose 10–20 mg before meals (PO, SL)

Table 41.3 Laxatives

Therapy	Dosage
Osmotic agents	
Lactulose	– 1–3 mL/kg/day in divided doses
Magnesium citrate	– May use divided doses – <6 years—1–3 mL/kg/day – 6–12 years—100–150 mL/day – >12 years—150–300 mL/day
Magnesium hydroxide	– May use divided doses – 1–3 mL/kg/day of 400 mg/5 mL solution
Polyethylene glycol	– 1 g/kg/day
Sorbitol	– 1–3 mL/kg/day in divided doses
Lubricants	
Mineral oil	– 1–3 mL/kg/day
Stimulants	
Bisacodyl	– 3–12 years—5 mg/day – >12 years—5–15 mg/day
Senna	– 2–5 years—2.5–7.5 mL at bedtime – 6–12 years—5–15 mL at bedtime
Lubiprostone (adult dosing only)	– Chronic idiopathic constipation—24 mcg BID – Female IBS with constipation—8 mcg BID

From Har AF, Croffie JM. Encopresis. Ped in Rev 2010;31(9):368–374. Reprinted with permission from American Academy of Pediatrics

of action is 24–48 h and side effects include cramping, abdominal distension, flatulence, diarrhea, nausea, vomiting, and electrolyte imbalances. Long-term use is safe with few reported adverse events [70].

Magnesium Salts

Magnesium salts are available commercially as magnesium citrate and magnesium hydroxide. All magnesium salts promote bowel evacuation by osmotic fluid retention. Absorption is 15–30% and excretion is in the urine. Use is contraindicated in patients with renal failure and renal insufficiency as hypermagnesemia is a significant risk. Caution should be used even in patients who do not have renal dysfunction as excessive ingestion can lead to severe hypermagnesemia in otherwise healthy children [183, 184]. Other side effects include diarrhea, abdominal cramps, flatulence, hypotension, and respiratory depression. There are few studies evaluating the efficacy of magnesium salts in treatment of constipation, however compared to a bulk laxative, it may produce more frequent bowel movements [185]. Palatability of magnesium may decrease compliance. When compared to PEG solution over a 12-month period, 95% of children using PEG were compliant vs. 65% using magnesium hydroxide [186].

Polyethylene Glycol

Polyethylene glycol (PEG) is a high molecular weight, non-soluble polymer that acts as an osmotic laxative. Hydrogen bonds are formed between PEG and water, which prevents reabsorption of water in the colon. With increased water retention, stool is thereby softened and its bulk is increased. The onset of action is 24–96 h; excretion is 93% through feces with minimal systemic absorption and a bioavailability of 0.2% [187]. Contraindications to PEG include hypersensitivity, ileus, bowel perforation or obstruction, and toxic megacolon.

PEG is available with or without electrolytes added. In general PEG with electrolytes is used for colonoscopy preparation or disimpaction. PEG without electrolytes is more commonly used for daily management of chronic constipation, but has been used in children for colonoscopy preparation as well [188, 189]. High-dose PEG without electrolytes can be as successful as rectal enemas for disimpaction in the pediatric population [190] with highest success for doses of 1–1.5 g/kg/day [191]. PEG is safe and well tolerated for long-term treatment of chronic constipation with few noted side effects [186, 192–195].

Sorbitol

Sorbitol is a polyalcoholic sugar and acts as a hyperosmotic laxative. Absorption is minimal and it is metabolized in the liver mainly into fructose. There is a paucity of studies evaluating the efficacy of sorbitol for treatment of constipation. Compared to lactulose it has similar safety and efficacy in the geriatric population [196]. Excessive ingestion of sorbitol in non-constipated pediatric patients is known to cause loose stool and diarrhea [197, 198]. Side effects include diarrhea, nausea, vomiting, lactic acidosis, and electrolyte imbalances.

Mineral Oil

Mineral oil is a lubricant laxative with minimal systemic absorption and primary elimination in the feces. It is a mixture of hydrocarbons derived from petroleum. The oil lubricates the colon, but it also decreases water reabsorption and softens the stool. It should not be used in infants and patients with swallowing dysfunction since there is a risk for lipid pneumonitis with aspiration [199–201]. Other adverse effects include diarrhea, nausea, vomiting, anal itching, and anal seepage. Chronic use could theoretically decrease absorption of fat soluble vitamins; however, there is no published evidence to support this [202, 203]. One study showed a reduction in beta-carotene levels after just 1 month of treatment [203].

Stimulant Laxatives

Bisacodyl

Bisacodyl is a diphenolic laxative that stimulates intestinal fluid secretion and motor activity. It induces intestinal fluid secretion by direct action on the enterocyte, activating adenylate cyclase and causing an increase in production of cyclic-AMP [204, 205]. Chloride and bicarbonate ions are actively secreted, while sodium and potassium are passively effluxed into the bowel. Sodium and chloride are then inhibited from reabsorption back into the enterocyte. Contraction of the colonic smooth muscle is caused by increasing the myoelectrical activity through direct irritation of the bowel wall [206, 207]. Systemic absorption is <5% with onset of action between 4 and 6 h for oral administration and 0.25–1 h for rectal administration [207, 208]. The small fraction that is absorbed is conjugated by the liver and excreted in urine. Most formulations are enteric coated and should not be administered within 1 h of antacids. Side effects include nausea, vomiting, diarrhea, abdominal cramping, proctitis, and electrolyte imbalance.

Bisacodyl and other stimulant laxatives should be used as second line agents for patients who are refractory to osmotic/lubricant laxatives [70]. There is no data on safety and efficacy of bisacodyl for treatment of constipation, particularly in the pediatric population [209]; however, there is clear evidence that it does increase colonic transit and stimulates colonic motor activity [210–212]. Chronic and prolonged use of stimulant laxatives may lead to loss of haustra and anatomic changes in the colon, possibly due to muscular or neuronal injury [213, 214]; it is unclear, however, if this is a true risk of long-term usage of bisacodyl [215].

Senna

The mechanism of action of senna as a stimulant laxative is unclear; however, it may increase production of cyclic-AMP in the colon leading to increased ion secretion and increased peristalsis, by direct irritation of the colon [216]. Senna is derived from the plant *Senna alexandrina* and has been used for centuries. Absorption is minimal and onset is 6–12 h after ingestion. Senna is metabolized in the liver and excreted through feces and urine. Reported adverse events include hepatitis, hypertrophic osteoarthropathy, analgesic nephropathy, and melanosis coli, which is reversible. There is poor evidence for development of cathartic colon with long-term use of senna [217]. As with other stimulant laxatives, it is a second-line agent and is used in constipated patients failing first-line treatment. Although it is commonly used, there is a paucity of studies evaluating its efficacy in treatment of constipation [209].

Lubiprostone

Lubiprostone is a prostone that acts locally on the gastrointestinal tract by activation of type-2 chloride channels (CIC-2) [218]. It is approved for use in adults with chronic idiopathic constipation and females older than 18 years of age with constipation-predominant irritable bowel syndrome. Prostones are bicyclic fatty acids derived from prostaglandin E_1 that do not significantly act on prostaglandin E or F receptors or cause smooth muscle contractions [219]. Activation of the chloride channels increases intestinal fluid chloride concentration and fluid secretion, leading to increased stool passage without causing significant change in serum electrolyte levels [218]. Lubiprostone decreases gastric emptying while increasing small bowel and colonic transit time in normal adult volunteers [220]. There are currently no published studies of its use in the pediatric population. Adult dosing is 24 mcg PO BID for chronic idiopathic constipation and 8 mcg PO BID for constipation-predominant IBS.

Lubiprostone is distributed mainly in the gastrointestinal tract with minimal systemic absorption; it is rapidly metabolized in the stomach and jejunum by carbonyl reductase into the active metabolite M3. 60% is excreted in the urine and 30% through the feces. Most common reported side effects include nausea, diarrhea, and headache [221]. There have been no studies on patients with hepatic or renal insufficiency and caution is recommended in these populations. No teratogenic effects have been reported; however, there has been increased fetal loss in the guinea pig model and therefore female patients should have a negative pregnancy test prior to initiation of therapy and be advised on contraception [219].

Linaclotide (MD-1100)

Linaclotide is a new guanylate cyclase-C (GC-C) agonist [222] that is currently undergoing phase III trials for the treatment of IBS-C and chronic constipation. Activation of GC-C leads to activation of the cystic fibrosis transmembrane conductance regulator causing secretion of chloride and bicarbonate into the small intestinal lumen [223]. Visceral hypersensitivity is suppressed by cGMP acting on submucosal afferent pain fibers to decrease nerve reactivity [224] and a decrease in abdominal pain compared to baseline and to placebo has been reported [225]. Doses ranging from 75 to 600 mcg improved bowel habits in men and women >18 years of age with IBS-C [225]. In adult women with IBS-C, colonic transit was improved over a 5-day treatment period with 1,000 mcg of linaclotide [226]. For adult patients with chronic constipation, bowel movement frequency, stool consistency, and straining as well as overall quality of life were improved on trials of linaclotide [227, 228] (Table 41.3).

References

1. Hofmeyr GJ, Van Iddekinge B, Blott JA. Domperidone: secretion in breast milk and effect on puerperal prolactin levels. Br J Obstet Gynaecol. 1985;92(2):141–4.
2. Champion MC, Hartnett M, Yen M. Domperidone, a new dopamine antagonist. CMA J. 1986; 135(5):457–61.
3. Heykants J, Hendriks R, Meuldermans W, Michiels M, Scheygrond H, Reyntjens H. On the pharmacokinetics of domperidone in animals and man. IV. The pharmacokinetics of intravenous domperidone and its bioavailability in man following intramuscular, oral and rectal administration. Eur J Drug Metab Pharmacokinet. 1981;6(1):61–70.
4. Reddymasu SC, Soykan I, McCallum RW. Domperidone: review of pharmacology and clinical applications in gastroenterology. Am J Gastroenterol. 2007;102(9):2036–45.
5. Van Eygen M, Dhondt F, Heck E, Ameryckx L, Van Ravensteyn H. A double-blind comparison of domperidone and metoclopramide suppositories in the treatment of nausea and vomiting in children. Postgrad Med J. 1979;55 Suppl 1:36–9.
6. Bines JE, Quinlan JE, Treves S, Kleinman RE, Winter HS. Efficacy of domperidone in infants and children with gastroesophageal reflux. J Pediatr Gastroenterol Nutr. 1992;14(4):400–5.
7. Tighe MP, Afzal NA, Bevan A, Beattie RM. Current pharmacological management of gastro-esophageal reflux in children: an evidence-based systematic review. Paediatr Drugs. 2009;11(3):185–202.
8. Pritchard DS, Baber N, Stephenson T. Should domperidone be used for the treatment of gastro-oesophageal reflux in children? Systematic review of randomized controlled trials in children aged 1

month to 11 years old. Br J Clin Pharmacol. 2005;59(6):725–9.
9. Djeddi D, Kongolo G, Lefaix C, Mounard J, Leke A. Effect of domperidone on QT interval in neonates. J Pediatr. 2008;153(5):663–6.
10. Sugumar A, Singh A, Pasricha PJ. A systematic review of the efficacy of domperidone for the treatment of diabetic gastroparesis. Clin Gastroenterol Hepatol. 2008;6(7):726–33.
11. Maton PN. Profile and assessment of GERD pharmacotherapy. Cleve Clin J Med. 2003;70 Suppl 5:S51–70.
12. Veldhuyzen van Zanten SJ, Jones MJ, Verlinden M, Talley NJ. Efficacy of cisapride and domperidone in functional (nonulcer) dyspepsia: a meta-analysis. Am J Gastroenterol. 2001;96(3):689–96.
13. Hamers J. Cytostatic therapy-induced vomiting inhibited by domperidone. A double-blind crossover study. Biomedicine. 1978;29(7):242–4.
14. Huys J. Cytostatic-associated vomiting effectively inhibited by domperidone (R 33 812). Cancer Chemother Pharmacol. 1978;1(4):215–8.
15. Zegveld C, Knape H, Smits J, et al. Domperidone in the treatment of postoperative vomiting: a double-blind multicenter study. Anesth Analg. 1978;57(6):700–3.
16. van Leeuwen L, Helmers JH. The efficacy of Domperidone (R 33812) in the treatment of postoperative vomiting. A double-blind study with a placebo. Anaesthesist. 1980;29(9):490–3.
17. Osborne RJ, Slevin ML, Hunter RW, Hamer J. Cardiotoxicity of intravenous domperidone. Lancet. 1985;2(8451):385.
18. Roussak JB, Carey P, Parry H. Cardiac arrest after treatment with intravenous domperidone. Br Med J (Clin Res Ed). 1984;289(6458):1579.
19. Johannes CB, Varas-Lorenzo C, McQuay LJ, Midkiff KD, Fife D. Risk of serious ventricular arrhythmia and sudden cardiac death in a cohort of users of domperidone: a nested case–control study. Pharmacoepidemiol Drug Saf. 2010;19(9):881–8.
20. Brock-Utne JG, Dimopoulos GE, Downing JW, Moshal MG. Effect of metoclopramide given before atropine sulphate on lower oesophageal sphincter tone. S Afr Med J. 1982;61(13):465–7.
21. McCallum RW, Kline MM, Curry N, Sturdevant RA. Comparative effects of metoclopramide and bethanechol on lower esophageal sphincter pressure in reflux patients. Gastroenterology. 1975;68(5 Pt 1):1114–8.
22. Yis U, Ozdemir D, Duman M, Unal N. Metoclopramide induced dystonia in children: two case reports. Eur J Emerg Med. 2005;12(3):117–9.
23. Hyams JS, Leichtner AM, Zamett LO, Walters JK. Effect of metoclopramide on prolonged intraesophageal pH testing in infants with gastroesophageal reflux. J Pediatr Gastroenterol Nutr. 1986;5(5):716–20.
24. Putnam PE, Orenstein SR, Wessel HB, Stowe RM. Tardive dyskinesia associated with use of metoclopramide in a child. J Pediatr. 1992;121(6):983–5.
25. Mejia NI, Jankovic J. Metoclopramide-induced tardive dyskinesia in an infant. Mov Disord. 2005;20(1):86–9.
26. Chicella MF, Batres LA, Heesters MS, Dice JE. Prokinetic drug therapy in children: a review of current options. Ann Pharmacother. 2005; 39(4):706–11.
27. Craig WR, Hanlon-Dearman A, Sinclair C, Taback S, Moffatt M. Metoclopramide, thickened feedings, and positioning for gastro-oesophageal reflux in children under two years. Cochrane Database Syst Rev. 2004(4):CD003502.
28. Henzi I, Walder B, Tramer MR. Metoclopramide in the prevention of postoperative nausea and vomiting: a quantitative systematic review of randomized, placebo-controlled studies. Br J Anaesth. 1999; 83(5):761–71.
29. Ponte CD, Nappi JM. Review of a new gastrointestinal drug–metoclopramide. Am J Hosp Pharm. 1981;38(6):829–33.
30. Brown JC, Cook MA, Dryburgh JR. Motilin, a gastric motor activity-stimulating polypeptide: final purification, amino acid composition, and C-terminal residues. Gastroenterology. 1972;62(3):401–4.
31. Peeters TL, Bormans V, Vantrappen G. Comparison of motilin binding to crude homogenates of human and canine gastrointestinal smooth muscle tissue. Regul Pept. 1988;23(2):171–82.
32. Janssens J, Peeters TL, Vantrappen G, et al. Improvement of gastric emptying in diabetic gastroparesis by erythromycin. Preliminary studies. N Engl J Med. 1990;322(15):1028–31.
33. Tack J, Janssens J, Vantrappen G, et al. Effect of erythromycin on gastric motility in controls and in diabetic gastroparesis. Gastroenterology. 1992;103(1):72–9.
34. Coulie B, Tack J, Peeters T, Janssens J. Involvement of two different pathways in the motor effects of erythromycin on the gastric antrum in humans. Gut. 1998;43(3):395–400.
35. Annese V, Janssens J, Vantrappen G, et al. Erythromycin accelerates gastric emptying by inducing antral contractions and improved gastroduodenal coordination. Gastroenterology. 1992;102(3):823–8.
36. Venkatasubramani N, Rudolph CD, Sood MR. Erythromycin lacks colon prokinetic effect in children with functional gastrointestinal disorders: a retrospective study. BMC Gastroenterol. 2008;8:38.
37. Dranove J, Horn D, Reddy SN, Croffie J. Effect of intravenous erythromycin on the colonic motility of children and young adults during colonic manometry. J Pediatr Surg. 2010;45(4):777–83.
38. Ray WA, Murray KT, Meredith S, Narasimhulu SS, Hall K, Stein CM. Oral erythromycin and the risk of sudden death from cardiac causes. N Engl J Med. 2004;351(11):1089–96.
39. Milberg P, Eckardt L, Bruns HJ, et al. Divergent proarrhythmic potential of macrolide antibiotics despite similar QT prolongation: fast phase 3 repolarization prevents early afterdepolarizations and torsade de pointes. J Pharmacol Exp Ther. 2002;303(1):218–25.

40. Wisialowski T, Crimin K, Engtrakul J, O'Donnell J, Fermini B, Fossa AA. Differentiation of arrhythmia risk of the antibacterials moxifloxacin, erythromycin, and telithromycin based on analysis of monophasic action potential duration alternans and cardiac instability. J Pharmacol Exp Ther. 2006;318(1):352–9.
41. Maheshwai N. Are young infants treated with erythromycin at risk for developing hypertrophic pyloric stenosis? Arch Dis Child. 2007;92(3):271–3.
42. Ng PC. Use of oral erythromycin for the treatment of gastrointestinal dysmotility in preterm infants. Neonatology. 2009;95(2):97–104.
43. Briggs GG. Drugs in pregnancy and lactation a reference guide to fetal and neonatal risk on CD-ROM. Philadelphia, Pa.: Lippincott, Williams & Wilkins; 1999: http://www.loc.gov/catdir/enhancements/fy0730/2002565226-d.html.
44. Euler AR. Use of bethanechol for the treatment of gastroesophageal reflux. J Pediatr. 1980; 96(2):321–4.
45. Strickland AD, Chang JH. Results of treatment of gastroesophageal reflux with bethanechol. J Pediatr. 1983;103(2):311–5.
46. Farrell RL, Roling GT, Castell DO. Cholinergic therapy of chronic heartburn. A controlled trial. Ann Intern Med. 1974;80(5):573–6.
47. Blonski W, Vela MF, Freeman J, Sharma N, Castell DO. The effect of oral buspirone, pyridostigmine, and bethanechol on esophageal function evaluated with combined multichannel esophageal impedance-manometry in healthy volunteers. J Clin Gastroenterol. 2009;43(3):253–60.
48. Sondheimer JM, Arnold GL. Early effects of bethanechol on the esophageal motor function of infants with gastroesophageal reflux. J Pediatr Gastroenterol Nutr. 1986;5(1):47–51.
49. Orenstein SR, Lofton SW, Orenstein DM. Bethanechol for pediatric gastroesophageal reflux: a prospective, blind, controlled study. J Pediatr Gastroenterol Nutr. 1986;5(4):549–55.
50. Levi P, Marmo F, Saluzzo C, et al. Bethanechol versus antiacids in the treatment of gastroesophageal reflux. Helv Paediatr Acta. 1985;40(5):349–59.
51. Shermeta DW, Whitington PF, Seto DS, Haller JA. Lower esophageal sphincter dysfunction in esophageal atresia: nocturnal regurgitation and aspiration pneumonia. J Pediatr Surg. 1977;12(6):871–6.
52. Agrawal A, Hila A, Tutuian R, Mainie I, Castell DO. Bethanechol improves smooth muscle function in patients with severe ineffective esophageal motility. J Clin Gastroenterol. 2007;41(4):366–70.
53. Lee JW, Bang KW, Jang PS, et al. Neostigmine for the treatment of acute colonic pseudo-obstruction (ACPO) in pediatric hematologic malignancies. Korean J Hematol. 2010;45(1):62–5.
54. Kim TS, Lee JW, Kim MJ, et al. Acute colonic pseudo-obstruction in postchemotherapy complication of brain tumor treated with neostigmine. J Pediatr Hematol Oncol. 2007;29(6):420–2.
55. Gmora S, Poenaru D, Tsai E. Neostigmine for the treatment of pediatric acute colonic pseudo-obstruction. J Pediatr Surg. 2002;37(10):E28.
56. Khosla A, Ponsky TA. Acute colonic pseudoobstruction in a child with sickle cell disease treated with neostigmine. J Pediatr Surg. 2008;43(12):2281–4.
57. Corazziari E, Bontempo I, Anzini F. Effects of cisapride on distal esophageal motility in humans. Dig Dis Sci. 1989;34(10):1600–5.
58. Veysey MJ, Malcolm P, Mallet AI, et al. Effects of cisapride on gall bladder emptying, intestinal transit, and serum deoxycholate: a prospective, randomised, double blind, placebo controlled trial. Gut. 2001;49(6):828–34.
59. Shulman RJ, Boyle JT, Colletti RB, et al. The use of cisapride in children. The North American Society for Pediatric Gastroenterology and Nutrition. J Pediatr Gastroenterol Nutr. 1999;28(5):529–33.
60. Vandenplas Y. Current pediatric indications for cisapride. J Pediatr Gastroenterol Nutr. 2000;31(5):480–9.
61. Maclennan S, Augood C, Cash-Gibson L, Logan S, Gilbert RE. Cisapride treatment for gastro-oesophageal reflux in children. Cochrane Database Syst Rev. 2010;4:CD002300.
62. Levy J, Hayes C, Kern J, et al. Does cisapride influence cardiac rhythm? Results of a United States multicenter, double-blind, placebo-controlled pediatric study. J Pediatr Gastroenterol Nutr. 2001;32(4):458–63.
63. Cohen RC, O'Loughlin EV, Davidson GP, Moore DJ, Lawrence DM. Cisapride in the control of symptoms in infants with gastroesophageal reflux: A randomized, double-blind, placebo-controlled trial. J Pediatr. 1999;134(3):287–92.
64. Cucchiara S, Staiano A, Capozzi C, Di Lorenzo C, Boccieri A, Auricchio S. Cisapride for gastro-oesophageal reflux and peptic oesophagitis. Arch Dis Child. 1987;62(5):454–7.
65. Escobar Castro HBFG, Suarez Cortina L, Camarero Salces C, Lima M. Efficacy of cisapride in the treatment of gastroesophageal reflux (GER) in children. Evaluation of a double blind study [Efectividad del Cisapride en el tratamiento del reflujo gastroesofagico (R.G.E.) en ninos. Valoracion de un estudio a doble ciego]. An Esp Pediatr. 1994;40(1):5–8.
66. Moya M. JM, Cortes E, Auxina A, Ortiz L. Clinical evaluation of the different therapeutic possibilities in the treatment of infant regurgitation. [Valoracion clinica de las distintas posibilidades terapeuticas en el manejo de las regurgitaciones del lactante]. Rev Esp Pediatr. 1999;55(3):219–23.
67. Scott RB, Ferreira C, Smith L, et al. Cisapride in pediatric gastroesophageal reflux. J Pediatr Gastroenterol Nutr. 1997;25(5):499–506.
68. Van Eygen M, Van Ravensteyn H. Effect of cisapride on excessive regurgitation in infants. Clin Ther. 1989;11(5):669–77.
69. Vandenplas Y, de Roy C, Sacre L. Cisapride decreases prolonged episodes of reflux in infants. J Pediatr Gastroenterol Nutr. 1991;12(1):44–7.

70. Baker SS, Liptak GS, Colletti RB, Croffie JM, DiLorenzo C, Ector W, Nurko S. Constipation Guideline Committee of the North American Society for Paediatric Gastroenterology, Hepatology and Nutrition. J Pediatr Gastroenterol Nutr 2006;43(3): e1–13.
71. Khongphatthanayothin A, Lane J, Thomas D, Yen L, Chang D, Bubolz B. Effects of cisapride on QT interval in children. J Pediatr. 1998;133(1):51–6.
72. Benatar A, Feenstra A, Decraene T, Vandenplas Y. Cisapride plasma levels and corrected QT interval in infants undergoing routine polysomnography. J Pediatr Gastroenterol Nutr. 2001;33(1):41–6.
73. Bernardini S, Semama DS, Huet F, Sgro C, Gouyon JB. Effects of cisapride on QTc interval in neonates. Arch Dis Child Fetal Neonatal Ed. 1997;77(3):F241–3.
74. Lupoglazoff JM, Bedu A, Faure C, et al. Long QT syndrome under cisapride in neonates and infants. Arch Pediatr. 1997;4(6):509–14.
75. Zamora SA, Belli DC, Friedli B, Jaeggi E. 24-hour electrocardiogram before and during cisapride treatment in neonates and infants. Biol Neonate. 2004;85(4):229–36.
76. Ward RM, Lemons JA, Molteni RA. Cisapride: a survey of the frequency of use and adverse events in premature newborns. Pediatrics. 1999;103(2):469–72.
77. Nasr I, Rao SS, Attaluri A, Hashmi SM, Summers R. Effects of tegaserod and erythromycin in upper gut dysmotility: a comparative study. Indian J Gastroenterol. 2009;28(4):136–42.
78. Liem O, Mousa HM, Benninga MA, Di Lorenzo C. Tegaserod use in children: a single-center experience. J Pediatr Gastroenterol Nutr. 2008;46(1):54–8.
79. Zhou HH, Khalilieh S, Lau H, et al. Effect of meal timing not critical for the pharmacokinetics of tegaserod (HTF 919). J Clin Pharmacol. 1999;39(9):911–9.
80. Appel S, Kumle A, Hubert M, Duvauchelle T. First pharmacokinetic-pharmacodynamic study in humans with a selective 5-hydroxytryptamine(4) receptor agonist. J Clin Pharmacol. 1997;37(3):229–37.
81. Briejer MR, Akkermans LM, Schuurkes JA. Gastrointestinal prokinetic benzamides: the pharmacology underlying stimulation of motility. Pharmacol Rev. 1995;47(4):631–51.
82. Briejer MR, Prins NH, Schuurkes JA. Effects of the enterokinetic prucalopride (R093877) on colonic motility in fasted dogs. Neurogastroenterol Motil. 2001;13(5):465–72.
83. Emmanuel AV, Kamm MA, Roy AJ, Antonelli K. Effect of a novel prokinetic drug, R093877, on gastrointestinal transit in healthy volunteers. Gut. 1998;42(4):511–6.
84. Bouras EP, Camilleri M, Burton DD, McKinzie S. Selective stimulation of colonic transit by the benzofuran 5HT4 agonist, prucalopride, in healthy humans. Gut. 1999;44(5):682–6.
85. Poen AC, Felt-Bersma RJ, Van Dongen PA, Meuwissen SG. Effect of prucalopride, a new enterokinetic agent, on gastrointestinal transit and anorectal function in healthy volunteers. Aliment Pharmacol Ther. 1999;13(11):1493–7.
86. Emmanuel AV, Roy AJ, Nicholls TJ, Kamm MA. Prucalopride, a systemic enterokinetic, for the treatment of constipation. Aliment Pharmacol Ther. 2002;16(7):1347–56.
87. Bouras EP, Camilleri M, Burton DD, Thomforde G, McKinzie S, Zinsmeister AR. Prucalopride accelerates gastrointestinal and colonic transit in patients with constipation without a rectal evacuation disorder. Gastroenterology. 2001;120(2):354–60.
88. Camilleri M, Kerstens R, Rykx A, Vandeplassche L. A placebo-controlled trial of prucalopride for severe chronic constipation. N Engl J Med. 2008;358(22):2344–54.
89. Quigley EM, Vandeplassche L, Kerstens R, Ausma J. Clinical trial: the efficacy, impact on quality of life, and safety and tolerability of prucalopride in severe chronic constipation a 12-week, randomized, double-blind, placebo-controlled study. Aliment Pharmacol Ther. 2009;29(3):315–28.
90. Muller-Lissner S, Rykx A, Kerstens R, Vandeplassche L. A double-blind, placebo-controlled study of prucalopride in elderly patients with chronic constipation. Neurogastroenterol Motil. 2010;22(9):991–98, e255.
91. Tack J, van Outryve M, Beyens G, Kerstens R, Vandeplassche L. Prucalopride (Resolor) in the treatment of severe chronic constipation in patients dissatisfied with laxatives. Gut. 2009;58(3):357–65.
92. Sloots CE, Poen AC, Kerstens R, et al. Effects of prucalopride on colonic transit, anorectal function and bowel habits in patients with chronic constipation. Aliment Pharmacol Ther. 2002;16(4): 759–67.
93. Camilleri M, Beyens G, Kerstens R, Robinson P, Vandeplassche L. Safety assessment of prucalopride in elderly patients with constipation: a double-blind, placebo-controlled study. Neurogastroenterol Motil. 2009;21(12):1256–e1117.
94. Van de Velde VAJ, Vandeplassche L. Pharmacokinetics of prucalorpide (Resolor) in man [abstract no. P0891]. Gut. 2008;21(57 Suppl I):A282.
95. Manini ML, Camilleri M, Goldberg M, et al. Effects of Velusetrag (TD-5108) on gastrointestinal transit and bowel function in health and pharmacokinetics in health and constipation. Neurogastroenterol Motil. 2010;22(1):42–9. e47–48.
96. Peeters TL, Janssens J, Vantrappen GR. Somatostatin and the interdigestive migrating motor complex in man. Regul Pept. 1983;5(3):209–17.
97. Peeters TL, Romanski KW, Janssens J, Vantrappen G. Effect of the long-acting somatostatin analogue SMS 201–995 on small-intestinal interdigestive motility in the dog. Scand J Gastroenterol. 1988;23(7):769–74.

98. Novartis. Sandostatin LAR® Depot (octreotide acetate for injectable suspension) prescribing information. East Hanover, NJ2006.
99. Soudah HC, Hasler WL, Owyang C. Effect of octreotide on intestinal motility and bacterial overgrowth in scleroderma. N Engl J Med. 1991;325(21):1461–7.
100. Dalgic B, Sari S, Dogan I, Unal S. Chronic intestinal pseudoobstruction: report of four pediatric patients. Turk J Gastroenterol. 2005;16(2):93–7.
101. Portenoy RK, Thomas J, Moehl Boatwright ML, et al. Subcutaneous methylnaltrexone for the treatment of opioid-induced constipation in patients with advanced illness: a double-blind, randomized, parallel group, dose-ranging study. J Pain Symptom Manage. 2008;35(5):458–68.
102. Russell J, Bass P, Goldberg LI, Schuster CR, Merz H. Antagonism of gut, but not central effects of morphine with quaternary narcotic antagonists. Eur J Pharmacol. 1982;78(3):255–61.
103. Brown DR, Goldberg LI. The use of quaternary narcotic antagonists in opiate research. Neuropharmacology. 1985;24(3):181–91.
104. Slatkin N, Thomas J, Lipman AG, et al. Methylnaltrexone for treatment of opioid-induced constipation in advanced illness patients. J Support Oncol. 2009;7(1):39–46.
105. Thomas J, Karver S, Cooney GA, et al. Methylnaltrexone for opioid-induced constipation in advanced illness. N Engl J Med. 2008;358(22):2332–43.
106. Bagnol D, Mansour A, Akil H, Watson SJ. Cellular localization and distribution of the cloned mu and kappa opioid receptors in rat gastrointestinal tract. Neuroscience. 1997;81(2):579–91.
107. Churchill GA, Airey DC, Allayee H, et al. The Collaborative Cross, a community resource for the genetic analysis of complex traits. Nat Genet. 2004;36(11):1133–7.
108. Deschepper CF, Olson JL, Otis M, Gallo-Payet N. Characterization of blood pressure and morphological traits in cardiovascular-related organs in 13 different inbred mouse strains. J Appl Physiol. 2004;97(1):369–76.
109. Michna E, Blonsky ER, Schulman S, et al. Subcutaneous Methylnaltrexone for Treatment of Opioid-Induced Constipation in Patients with Chronic, Nonmalignant Pain: A Randomized Controlled Study. J Pain. 2011;12(5):554–62.
110. Garten L, Degenhardt P, Buhrer C. Resolution of opioid-induced postoperative ileus in a newborn infant after methylnaltrexone. J Pediatr Surg. 2011;46(3):e13–5.
111. Yuan CS. Methylnaltrexone mechanisms of action and effects on opioid bowel dysfunction and other opioid adverse effects. Ann Pharmacother. 2007;41(6):984–93.
112. Rotshteyn Y, Boyd TA, Yuan CS. Methylnaltrexone bromide: research update of pharmacokinetics following parenteral administration. Expert Opin Drug Metab Toxicol. 2011;7(2):227–35.
113. Awouters F, Niemegeers CJ, Janssen PA. Pharmacology of antidiarrheal drugs. Annu Rev Pharmacol Toxicol. 1983;23:279–301.
114. Ericsson CD, Johnson PC. Safety and efficacy of loperamide. Am J Med. 1990;88(6A):10S–4.
115. Li ST, Grossman DC, Cummings P. Loperamide therapy for acute diarrhea in children: systematic review and meta-analysis. PLoS Med. 2007;4(3):e98.
116. Cann PA, Read NW, Holdsworth CD, Barends D. Role of loperamide and placebo in management of irritable bowel syndrome (IBS). Dig Dis Sci. 1984;29(3):239–47.
117. Bhutta TI, Tahir KI. Loperamide poisoning in children. Lancet. 1990;335(8685):363.
118. Thomas TJ, Pauze D, Love JN. Are one or two dangerous? Diphenoxylate-atropine exposure in toddlers. J Emerg Med. 2008;34(1):71–5.
119. Firoozabadi A, Mowla A, Farashbandi H, Gorman JM. Diphenoxylate hydrochloride dependency. J Psychiatr Pract. 2007;13(4):278–80.
120. McCarron MM, Challoner KR, Thompson GA. Diphenoxylate-atropine (Lomotil) overdose in children: an update (report of eight cases and review of the literature). Pediatrics. 1991;87(5):694–700.
121. Quartero AO, Meineche-Schmidt V, Muris J, Rubin G, de Wit N. Bulking agents, antispasmodic and antidepressant medication for the treatment of irritable bowel syndrome. Cochrane Database Syst Rev. 2005(2):CD003460.
122. Myers JH, Moro-Sutherland D, Shook JE. Anticholinergic poisoning in colicky infants treated with hyoscyamine sulfate. Am J Emerg Med. 1997;15(5):532–5.
123. Hammerle CW, Surawicz CM. Updates on treatment of irritable bowel syndrome. World J Gastroenterol. 2008;14(17):2639–49.
124. Lehtonen LA, Rautava PT. Infantile colic: natural history and treatment. Curr Probl Pediatr. 1996;26(3):79–85.
125. Hwang CP, Danielsson B. Dicyclomine hydrochloride in infantile colic. Br Med J (Clin Res Ed). 1985;291(6501):1014.
126. Lucassen PL, Assendelft WJ, Gubbels JW, van Eijk JT, van Geldrop WJ, Neven AK. Effectiveness of treatments for infantile colic: systematic review. BMJ. 1998;316(7144):1563–9.
127. Page JG, Dirnberger GM. Treatment of the irritable bowel syndrome with Bentyl (dicyclomine hydrochloride). J Clin Gastroenterol. 1981;3(2):153–6.
128. Hasler WL. Pharmacotherapy for intestinal motor and sensory disorders. Gastroenterol Clin North Am. 2003;32(2):707–32, viii–ix.
129. Poynard T, Regimbeau C, Benhamou Y. Meta-analysis of smooth muscle relaxants in the treatment of irritable bowel syndrome. Aliment Pharmacol Ther. 2001;15(3):355–61.

130. Savino F, Brondello C, Cresi F, Oggero R, Silvestro L. Cimetropium bromide in the treatment of crisis in infantile colic. J Pediatr Gastroenterol Nutr. 2002;34(4):417–9.
131. Dobrilla G, Imbimbo BP, Piazzi L, Bensi G. Longterm treatment of irritable bowel syndrome with cimetropium bromide: a double blind placebo controlled clinical trial. Gut. 1990;31(3):355–8.
132. Delvaux M, Wingate D. Trimebutine: mechanism of action, effects on gastrointestinal function and clinical results. J Int Med Res. 1997;25(5):225–46.
133. Wittmann T, Paradowski L, Ducrotte P, Bueno L, Andro Delestrain MC. Clinical trial: the efficacy of alverine citrate/simeticone combination on abdominal pain/discomfort in irritable bowel syndrome–a randomized, double-blind, placebo-controlled study. Aliment Pharmacol Ther. 2010;31(6):615–24.
134. Lindqvist S, Hernon J, Sharp P, et al. The colon-selective spasmolytic otilonium bromide inhibits muscarinic M(3) receptor-coupled calcium signals in isolated human colonic crypts. Br J Pharmacol. 2002;137(7):1134–42.
135. Evangelista S. Quaternary ammonium derivatives as spasmolytics for irritable bowel syndrome. Curr Pharm Des. 2004;10(28):3561–8.
136. Jailwala J, Imperiale TF, Kroenke K. Pharmacologic treatment of the irritable bowel syndrome: a systematic review of randomized, controlled trials. Ann Intern Med. 2000;133(2):136–47.
137. Darvish-Damavandi M, Nikfar S, Abdollahi M. A systematic review of efficacy and tolerability of mebeverine in irritable bowel syndrome. World J Gastroenterol. 2010;16(5):547–53.
138. Caleo M, Antonucci F, Restani L, Mazzocchio R. A reappraisal of the central effects of botulinum neurotoxin type A: by what mechanism? J Neurochem. 2009;109(1):15–24.
139. Gutschow CA, Tox U, Leers J, Schafer H, Prenzel KL, Holscher AH. Botox, dilation, or myotomy? Clinical outcome of interventional and surgical therapies for achalasia. Langenbecks Arch Surg. 2010;395(8):1093–9.
140. Pehlivanov N, Pasricha PJ. Achalasia: botox, dilatation or laparoscopic surgery in 2006. Neurogastroenterol Motil. 2006;18(9):799–804.
141. Horgan S, Hudda K, Eubanks T, McAllister J, Pellegrini CA. Does botulinum toxin injection make esophagomyotomy a more difficult operation? Surg Endosc. 1999;13(6):576–9.
142. Cowgill SM, Villadolid DV, Al-Saadi S, Rosemurgy AS. Difficult myotomy is not determined by preoperative therapy and does not impact outcome. JSLS. 2007;11(3):336–43.
143. Smith CD, Stival A, Howell DL, Swafford V. Endoscopic therapy for achalasia before Heller myotomy results in worse outcomes than heller myotomy alone. Ann Surg. 2006;243(5):579–84. discussion 584–576.
144. Peracchia A, Bonavina L. Achalasia: dilation, injection or surgery? Can J Gastroenterol. 2000;14(5):441–3.
145. Hussain SZ, Thomas R, Tolia V. A review of achalasia in 33 children. Dig Dis Sci. 2002;47(11):2538–43.
146. Walton JM, Tougas G. Botulinum toxin use in pediatric esophageal achalasia: a case report. J Pediatr Surg. 1997;32(6):916–7.
147. MacIver R, Liptay M, Johnson Y. A case of mediastinitis following botulinum toxin type A treatment for achalasia. Nat Clin Pract Gastroenterol Hepatol. 2007;4(10):579–82.
148. Fitzgerald JF, Troncone R, Sukerek H, Tolia V. Clinical quiz. Sinus tract between esophagus and fundus. J Pediatr Gastroenterol Nutr. 2002;35(1):38, 98.
149. Koivusalo AI, Pakarinen MP, Rintala RJ. Botox injection treatment for anal outlet obstruction in patients with internal anal sphincter achalasia and Hirschsprung's disease. Pediatr Surg Int. 2009;25(10):873–6.
150. Chumpitazi BP, Fishman SJ, Nurko S. Long-term clinical outcome after botulinum toxin injection in children with nonrelaxing internal anal sphincter. Am J Gastroenterol. 2009;104(4):976–83.
151. Husberg B, Malmborg P, Strigard K. Treatment with botulinum toxin in children with chronic anal fissure. Eur J Pediatr Surg. 2009;19(5):290–2.
152. Nelson R. Non surgical therapy for anal fissure. Cochrane Database Syst Rev. 2006(4):CD003431.
153. Arts J, Holvoet L, Caenepeel P, et al. Clinical trial: a randomized-controlled crossover study of intrapyloric injection of botulinum toxin in gastroparesis. Aliment Pharmacol Ther. 2007;26(9):1251–8.
154. McEvoy G. Nitrates and Nitrites General Statement. In: Pharmacists ASoH-S, ed. AHFS drug information 2004. Bethesda, MD2004:1679–1684.
155. Tander B, Guven A, Demirbag S, Ozkan Y, Ozturk H, Cetinkursun S. A prospective, randomized, double-blind, placebo-controlled trial of glyceryl-trinitrate ointment in the treatment of children with anal fissure. J Pediatr Surg. 1999;34(12):1810–2.
156. Sonmez K, Demirogullari B, Ekingen G, et al. Randomized, placebo-controlled treatment of anal fissure by lidocaine, EMLA, and GTN in children. J Pediatr Surg. 2002;37(9):1313–6.
157. Kenny SE, Irvine T, Driver CP, et al. Double blind randomised controlled trial of topical glyceryl trinitrate in anal fissure. Arch Dis Child. 2001;85(5):404–7.
158. Simpson J, Lund JN, Thompson RJ, Kapila L, Scholefield JH. The use of glyceryl trinitrate (GTN) in the treatment of chronic anal fissure in children. Med Sci Monit. 2003;9(10):PI123–6.
159. Demirbag S, Tander B, Atabek C, Surer I, Ozturk H, Cetinkursun S. Long-term results of topical glyceryl trinitrate ointment in children with anal fissure. Ann Trop Paediatr. 2005;25(2):135–7.

160. Bharucha AE, Trabuco E. Functional and chronic anorectal and pelvic pain disorders. Gastroenterol Clin North Am. 2008;37(3):685–696, ix.
161. Jeyarajah S, Chow A, Ziprin P, Tilney H, Purkayastha S. Proctalgia fugax, an evidence-based management pathway. Int J Colorectal Dis. 2010;25(9):1037–46.
162. Bassotti G, Calcara C, Annese V, Fiorella S, Roselli P, Morelli A. Nifedipine and verapamil inhibit the sigmoid colon myoelectric response to eating in healthy volunteers. Dis Colon Rectum. 1998;41(3):377–80.
163. Chrysos E, Xynos E, Tzovaras G, Zoras OJ, Tsiaoussis J, Vassilakis SJ. Effect of nifedipine on rectoanal motility. Dis Colon Rectum. 1996;39(2):212–6.
164. Glassman MS, Medow MS, Berezin S, Newman LJ. Spectrum of esophageal disorders in children with chest pain. Dig Dis Sci. 1992;37(5):663–6.
165. Richter JE, Dalton CB, Buice RG, Castell DO. Nifedipine: a potent inhibitor of contractions in the body of the human esophagus. Studies in healthy volunteers and patients with the nutcracker esophagus. Gastroenterology. 1985;89(3):549–54.
166. Maksimak M, Perlmutter DH, Winter HS. The use of nifedipine for the treatment of achalasia in children. J Pediatr Gastroenterol Nutr. 1986;5(6):883–6.
167. Lacy BE, Weiser K. Esophageal motility disorders: medical therapy. J Clin Gastroenterol. 2008;42(5):652–8.
168. Milov DE, Cynamon HA, Andres JM. Chest pain and dysphagia in adolescents caused by diffuse esophageal spasm. J Pediatr Gastroenterol Nutr. 1989;9(4):450–3.
169. Freeman L, Mazur LJ. Verapamil therapy for persistent antral spasms in a child. South Med J. 1996;89(5):529–30.
170. Awad R, Dibildox M, Ortiz F. Irritable bowel syndrome treatment using pinaverium bromide as a calcium channel blocker. A randomized double-blind placebo-controlled trial. Acta Gastroenterol Latinoam. 1995;25(3):137–44.
171. Lu CL, Chen CY, Chang FY, et al. Effect of a calcium channel blocker and antispasmodic in diarrhoea-predominant irritable bowel syndrome. J Gastroenterol Hepatol. 2000;15(8):925–30.
172. Grigoleit HG, Grigoleit P. Gastrointestinal clinical pharmacology of peppermint oil. Phytomedicine. 2005;12(8):607–11.
173. Asao T, Mochiki E, Suzuki H, et al. An easy method for the intraluminal administration of peppermint oil before colonoscopy and its effectiveness in reducing colonic spasm. Gastrointest Endosc. 2001;53(2):172–7.
174. Kline RM, Kline JJ, Di Palma J, Barbero GJ. Enteric-coated, pH-dependent peppermint oil capsules for the treatment of irritable bowel syndrome in children. J Pediatr. 2001;138(1):125–8.
175. Liu JH, Chen GH, Yeh HZ, Huang CK, Poon SK. Enteric-coated peppermint-oil capsules in the treatment of irritable bowel syndrome: a prospective, randomized trial. J Gastroenterol. 1997;32(6):765–8.
176. Pittler MH, Ernst E. Peppermint oil for irritable bowel syndrome: a critical review and metaanalysis. Am J Gastroenterol. 1998;93(7):1131–5.
177. Weydert JA, Ball TM, Davis MF. Systematic review of treatments for recurrent abdominal pain. Pediatrics. 2003;111(1):e1–11.
178. Huertas-Ceballos AA, Logan S, Bennett C, Macarthur C. Dietary interventions for recurrent abdominal pain (RAP) and irritable bowel syndrome (IBS) in childhood. Cochrane Database Syst Rev. 2009(1):CD003019.
179. Brandt LJ, Chey WD, Foxx-Orenstein AE, et al. An evidence-based position statement on the management of irritable bowel syndrome. Am J Gastroenterol. 2009;104 Suppl 1:S1–35.
180. Schumann C. Medical, nutritional and technological properties of lactulose. An update. Eur J Nutr. 2002;41(Suppl):I17–25. 1.
181. Bennett A, Eley KG. Intestinal pH and propulsion: an explanation of diarrhoea in lactase deficiency and laxation by lactulose. J Pharm Pharmacol. 1976;28(3):192–5.
182. Bown RL, Gibson JA, Sladen GE, Hicks B, Dawson AM. Effects of lactulose and other laxatives on ileal and colonic pH as measured by a radiotelemetry device. Gut. 1974;15(12):999–1004.
183. Kutsal E, Aydemir C, Eldes N, et al. Severe hypermagnesemia as a result of excessive cathartic ingestion in a child without renal failure. Pediatr Emerg Care. 2007;23(8):570–2.
184. McGuire JK, Kulkarni MS, Baden HP. Fatal hypermagnesemia in a child treated with megavitamin/megamineral therapy. Pediatrics. 2000;105(2):E18.
185. Kinnunen O, Salokannel J. Constipation in elderly long-stay patients: its treatment by magnesium hydroxide and bulk-laxative. Ann Clin Res. 1987;19(5):321–3.
186. Loening-Baucke V, Pashankar DS. A randomized, prospective, comparison study of polyethylene glycol 3350 without electrolytes and milk of magnesia for children with constipation and fecal incontinence. Pediatrics. 2006;118(2):528–35.
187. Pelham RW, Nix LC, Chavira RE, Cleveland MV, Stetson P. Clinical trial: single- and multiple-dose pharmacokinetics of polyethylene glycol (PEG-3350) in healthy young and elderly subjects. Aliment Pharmacol Ther. 2008;28(2):256–65.
188. Adamiak T, Altaf M, Jensen MK, et al. One-day bowel preparation with polyethylene glycol 3350: an effective regimen for colonoscopy in children. Gastrointest Endosc. 2010;71(3):573–7.
189. Pashankar DS, Uc A, Bishop WP. Polyethylene glycol 3350 without electrolytes: a new safe, effective, and palatable bowel preparation for colonoscopy in children. J Pediatr. 2004;144(3):358–62.

190. Bekkali NL, van den Berg MM, Dijkgraaf MG, et al. Rectal fecal impaction treatment in childhood constipation: enemas versus high doses oral PEG. Pediatrics. 2009;124(6):e1108–15.
191. Youssef NN, Peters JM, Henderson W, Shultz-Peters S, Lockhart DK, Di Lorenzo C. Dose response of PEG 3350 for the treatment of childhood fecal impaction. J Pediatr. 2002;141(3):410–4.
192. Michail S, Gendy E, Preud'Homme D, Mezoff A. Polyethylene glycol for constipation in children younger than eighteen months old. J Pediatr Gastroenterol Nutr. 2004;39(2):197–9.
193. Dupont C, Leluyer B, Maamri N, et al. Double-blind randomized evaluation of clinical and biological tolerance of polyethylene glycol 4000 versus lactulose in constipated children. J Pediatr Gastroenterol Nutr. 2005;41(5):625–33.
194. Loening-Baucke V, Krishna R, Pashankar DS. Polyethylene glycol 3350 without electrolytes for the treatment of functional constipation in infants and toddlers. J Pediatr Gastroenterol Nutr. 2004;39(5):536–9.
195. Pashankar DS, Bishop WP, Loening-Baucke V. Long-term efficacy of polyethylene glycol 3350 for the treatment of chronic constipation in children with and without encopresis. Clin Pediatr (Phila). 2003;42(9):815–9.
196. Lederle FA, Busch DL, Mattox KM, West MJ, Aske DM. Cost-effective treatment of constipation in the elderly: a randomized double-blind comparison of sorbitol and lactulose. Am J Med. 1990;89(5):597–601.
197. Ament ME. Malabsorption of apple juice and pear nectar in infants and children: clinical implications. J Am Coll Nutr. 1996;15(5 Suppl):26S–9.
198. Smith MM, Davis M, Chasalow FI, Lifshitz F. Carbohydrate absorption from fruit juice in young children. Pediatrics. 1995;95(3):340–4.
199. Sias SM, Ferreira AS, Daltro PA, Caetano RL, Moreira Jda S, Quirico-Santos T. Evolution of exogenous lipoid pneumonia in children: clinical aspects, radiological aspects and the role of bronchoalveolar lavage. J Bras Pneumol. 2009;35(9):839–45.
200. Bandla HP, Davis SH, Hopkins NE. Lipoid pneumonia: a silent complication of mineral oil aspiration. Pediatrics. 1999;103(2):E19.
201. Ciravegna B, Sacco O, Moroni C, et al. Mineral oil lipoid pneumonia in a child with anoxic encephalopathy: treatment by whole lung lavage. Pediatr Pulmonol. 1997;23(3):233–7.
202. Gal-Ezer S, Shaoul R. The safety of mineral oil in the treatment of constipation–a lesson from prolonged overdose. Clin Pediatr (Phila). 2006;45(9):856–8.
203. Clark JH, Russell GJ, Fitzgerald JF, Nagamori KE. Serum beta-carotene, retinol, and alpha-tocopherol levels during mineral oil therapy for constipation. Am J Dis Child. 1987;141(11):1210–2.
204. Beubler E, Schirgi-Degen A. Stimulation of enterocyte protein kinase C by laxatives in-vitro. J Pharm Pharmacol. 1993;45(1):59–62.
205. Ratnaike RN, Jones TE. Mechanisms of drug-induced diarrhoea in the elderly. Drugs Aging. 1998;13(3):245–53.
206. Taylor I, Duthie HL, Smallwood R, Brown BH, Linkens D. The effect of stimulation on the myoelectrical activity of the rectosigmoid in man. Gut. 1974;15(8):599–607.
207. Flig E, Hermann TW, Zabel M. Is bisacodyl absorbed at all from suppositories in man? Int J Pharm. 2000;196(1):11–20.
208. Roth W, Beschke K. Pharmacokinetics and laxative effect of bisacodyl following administration of various dosage forms. Arzneimittelforschung. 1988;38(4):570–4.
209. Ramkumar D, Rao SS. Efficacy and safety of traditional medical therapies for chronic constipation: systematic review. Am J Gastroenterol. 2005;100(4):936–71.
210. Manabe N, Cremonini F, Camilleri M, Sandborn WJ, Burton DD. Effects of bisacodyl on ascending colon emptying and overall colonic transit in healthy volunteers. Aliment Pharmacol Ther. 2009;30(9):930–6.
211. Herve S, Savoye G, Behbahani A, Leroi AM, Denis P, Ducrotte P. Results of 24-h manometric recording of colonic motor activity with endoluminal instillation of bisacodyl in patients with severe chronic slow transit constipation. Neurogastroenterol Motil. 2004;16(4):397–402.
212. De Schryver AM, Samsom M, Smout AI. Effects of a meal and bisacodyl on colonic motility in healthy volunteers and patients with slow-transit constipation. Dig Dis Sci. 2003;48(7):1206–12.
213. Joo JS, Ehrenpreis ED, Gonzalez L, et al. Alterations in colonic anatomy induced by chronic stimulant laxatives: the cathartic colon revisited. J Clin Gastroenterol. 1998;26(4):283–6.
214. Rawson MD. Cathartic colon. Lancet. 1966;1(7447):1121–4.
215. Muller-Lissner S. What has happened to the cathartic colon? Gut. 1996;39(3):486–8.
216. McEvoy G, ed AHFS drug information Bethesda, MD: American Society of Health-System Pharmacists; 2007. Anthraquinones.
217. Morales MA, Hernandez D, Bustamante S, Bachiller I, Rojas A. Is senna laxative use associated to cathartic colon, genotoxicity, or carcinogenicity? J Toxicol. 2009;2009:287247.
218. Cuppoletti J, Malinowska DH, Tewari KP, et al. SPI-0211 activates T84 cell chloride transport and recombinant human ClC-2 chloride currents. Am J Physiol Cell Physiol. 2004;287(5):C1173–83.
219. Ambizas EM, Ginzburg R. Lubiprostone: a chloride channel activator for treatment of chronic constipation. Ann Pharmacother. 2007;41(6):957–64.

220. Camilleri M, Bharucha AE, Ueno R, et al. Effect of a selective chloride channel activator, lubiprostone, on gastrointestinal transit, gastric sensory, and motor functions in healthy volunteers. Am J Physiol Gastrointest Liver Physiol. 2006;290(5):G942–7.
221. Johanson JF, Ueno R. Lubiprostone, a locally acting chloride channel activator, in adult patients with chronic constipation: a double-blind, placebo-controlled, dose-ranging study to evaluate efficacy and safety. Aliment Pharmacol Ther. 2007;25(11):1351–61.
222. Currie MG, Fok KF, Kato J, et al. Guanylin: an endogenous activator of intestinal guanylate cyclase. Proc Natl Acad Sci USA. 1992;89(3):947–51.
223. Forte Jr LR. Uroguanylin and guanylin peptides: pharmacology and experimental therapeutics. Pharmacol Ther. 2004;104(2):137–62.
224. Eutamene H, Bradesi S, Larauche M, et al. Guanylate cyclase C-mediated antinociceptive effects of linaclotide in rodent models of visceral pain. Neurogastroenterol Motil. 2010;22(3):312–e384.
225. Johnston JM, Kurtz CB, Macdougall JE, et al. Linaclotide improves abdominal pain and bowel habits in a phase IIb study of patients with irritable bowel syndrome with constipation. Gastroenterology. 2010;139(6):1877–86, e1872.
226. Andresen V, Camilleri M, Busciglio IA, et al. Effect of 5 days linaclotide on transit and bowel function in females with constipation-predominant irritable bowel syndrome. Gastroenterology. 2007;133(3):761–8.
227. Johnston JM, Kurtz CB, Drossman DA, et al. Pilot study on the effect of linaclotide in patients with chronic constipation. Am J Gastroenterol. 2009;104(1):125–32.
228. Lembo AJ, Kurtz CB, Macdougall JE, et al. Efficacy of linaclotide for patients with chronic constipation. Gastroenterology. 2010;138(3):886–95, e881.

Gastric Electrical Stimulation

42

Carlo Di Lorenzo, Hayat Mousa, and Steven Teich

Introduction

It may be successfully argued that the pharmacological armamentarium available to the gastroenterologist who specializes in the care of patients with motility disorders has shrunk in the past several years. After the withdrawal from the market of cisapride, tegaserod, and alosetron, there are very few prokinetic drugs currently available, and their efficacy in treating severe motility disorders is modest at best. Surgery rarely provides significant symptom relief in patients with generalized gut dysmotility. Thus, alternative interventions have been actively explored. Gastroparesis and severe dyspepsia represent two conditions that affect quality of life, are associated with high medical cost [1, 2], and are often refractory to dietary and pharmacological interventions. In order to improve gastric emptying and decrease nausea and vomiting, electrical stimulation of the stomach began to be used in human subjects in the 1990s [3, 4] and eventually led to the approval by the Food and Drug Administration of the Enterra™ Therapy System (Medtronic Inc., Minneapolis, MN) as a humanitarian device for drug-refractory gastroparesis in 2000. Humanitarian Device Exemption (HDE) is a terminology used for devices which provide treatment to uncommon conditions (<4,000 implantations/year) for which no less invasive, equally effective therapy is available. Marketing of the system is allowed under restricted conditions, and its use requires approval by Institutional Review Boards. Since that time, gastric electrical stimulation (GES) has been performed in hundreds of adults with gastroparesis and in few patients with more generalized motility disorders. Use in pediatrics is more recent, and there are probably <100 children who have received GES placement so far.

Although it is now clear that GES improves nausea and vomiting, the mechanism behind its effects remains unclear. The low-energy electrical stimulation provided by GES has not been shown to directly induce muscle contraction. Proposed mechanisms have included modulation of enteric or afferent neural activity that influences symptom perception, enhanced vagal activity, acceleration of gastric emptying, alterations in CNS control mechanisms of nausea and vomiting, and improved gastric accommodation [5].

C. Di Lorenzo, M.D. (✉)
Division of Pediatric Gastroenterology, Department of Pediatrics, Nationwide Children's Hospital, The Ohio State University, 700 Children's Drive, Columbus, OH 43205, USA
e-mail: Carlo.DiLorenzo@nationwidechildrens.org

H. Mousa, M.D.
Division of Pediatric Gastroenterology, Hepatology and Nutrition, Department of Pediatrics, Nationwide Children Hospital, Ohio State University, Columbus, OH, USA

S. Teich, M.D.
Pediatric Surgery, Nationwide Children's Hospital, The Ohio State University, Columbus, OH, USA

C. Faure et al. (eds.), *Pediatric Neurogastroenterology: Gastrointestinal Motility and Functional Disorders in Children*, Clinical Gastroenterology,
DOI 10.1007/978-1-60761-709-9_42, © Springer Science+Business Media New York 2013

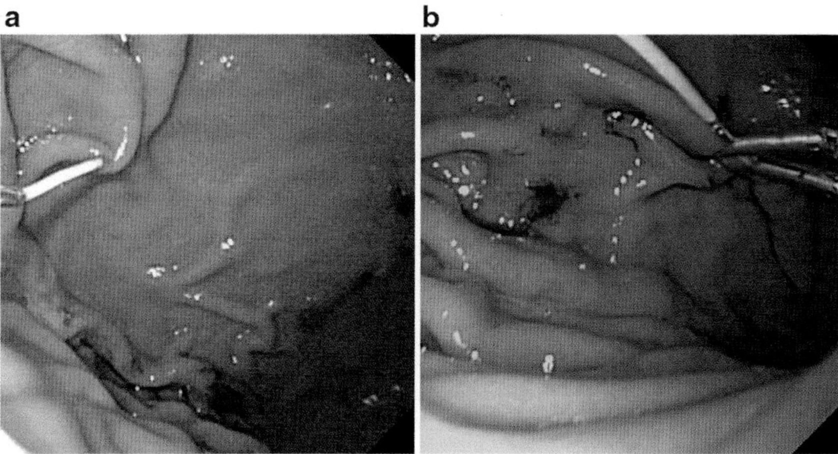

Fig. 42.1 Endoscopic pictures of temporary GES placement. The lead is screwed clockwise into the gastric mucosa (**a**). Clips are placed endoscopically to anchor the lead to the mucosa between the gastric body and antrum (**b**)

There seems to be little correlation between changes in gastric emptying time or electrogastrographic patterns and symptomatic improvement. Symptomatic improvement has been observed after GES therapy in patients with normal baseline gastric emptying. GES does not appear to negatively impact adjacent organs, likely because the stomach already contains natural pacemakers.

Temporary Gastric Stimulation

In some patients, temporary GES is used to predict whether a patient will respond to GES [6]. A temporary GES electrode can be introduced through a previously created gastrostomy site. If there is no gastrostomy, then a temporary GES electrode is placed through the mouth or the nose by endoscopy. A standard pediatric endoscope is utilized for the placement of the temporary GES electrode. The endoscope is inserted into the stomach, and a cardiac pacing lead with a corkscrew tip (model 6414–200; Medtronic, Inc.) is advanced through the biopsy channel and screwed into the gastric mucosa with a clockwise motion at the junction of the body and antrum of the stomach (Fig. 42.1a). This temporary lead has an inner bipolar electrode pacing lead and an outer covering sheath. The endoscope is then withdrawn while advancing the pacing lead so that the tip remains in position with an extra length of approximately 10 cm left in the stomach. The endoscope is reinserted into the stomach and an endoscopic clipping device is passed through the biopsy channel. Two to four clips are applied to hold the lead in place, with at least one clip placed near the distal metallic part of the lead (Fig. 42.1b). The endoscope is again withdrawn and the lead is brought out through the nares and connected to the external GES device that is placed in a cardiac telemetry pouch.

When placing the temporary GES lead via a gastrostomy site a shorter temporary lead (model 6416–100; Medtronic, Inc.) is passed through the gastrostomy and screwed into the gastric mucosa at the junction of the body and antrum of the stomach. Again, the lead is secured in place using an endoscopic clipping device but is then brought out through the gastrostomy site and connected to the external GES device. The gastrostomy tube is then replaced.

After placement of the temporary GES electrode, the lead is connected to the external GES pulse generator and the impedance is determined (desirable 400–1,500 Ω). The pulse generator is initially programmed at relatively high settings (voltage, 5 V; pulse width, 450 μs; frequency ~28 Hz; time on 1.0 s; time off 4.0 s), so that the patient response to temporary GES can be ascertained within 2–3 days. In general, the lead remains in place for 7–10 days before dislodgement. The temporary electrode is easily removed by rotating it counterclockwise and applying gentle traction.

Permanent Gastric Stimulation

The electrodes for the permanent gastric electrical stimulator can be placed laparoscopically or via laparotomy. However, most patients with a previously placed gastrostomy require a laparotomy for lead placement.

Using laparoscopy, abdominal access is obtained at the umbilicus and pneumoperitoneum is established. Two 5 mm ports are placed in the umbilicus and on the right side at the level of the umbilicus, while a 12 mm port is placed in the left axillary line superior to the umbilicus. Two electrodes (model 4351; Medtronic, Inc.) are passed through the 12 mm port into the abdomen. In adults, a point 10 cm proximal to the pylorus along the greater curvature of the stomach is marked. This corresponds to the junction between the antrum and body of the stomach. In children, the site on the gastric wall for placement of the electrodes is determined with the aid of an endoscopist who, during the initial phases of the surgery, identifies the junction of the body and antrum of the stomach with the surgeon marking the point on the external gastric surface along the greater curvature. Starting adjacent to the greater curvature, the needle of the first electrode enters and traverses the seromuscular layer of the gastric wall for at least 2 cm and then exits (Fig. 42.2a). The second electrode is placed parallel to the first electrode 1 cm away (Fig. 42.2b). The electrodes are placed under direct endoscopic visualization to ensure that they do not pass full thickness through the gastric wall. If this occurs, the needle is withdrawn from the gastric wall and repositioned. The electrodes are secured to the gastric wall and the needles are removed. The distal ends of the electrodes are extracted from the abdomen through the 12 mm port.

Traditional laparotomy is usually required for placement of the permanent GES electrodes in patients with a previously placed gastrostomy since the site for placement of the electrodes is often very close to the gastrostomy site. The location for lead placement on the stomach wall is determined in the same manner as with the laparoscopic placement and the leads are again placed under direct endoscopic visualization.

The two permanent GES leads are then connected to the GES pulse generator (Fig. 42.2c), a superficial abdominal pocket is created, and the generator is placed within the pocket (Fig. 42.2d). Using the external programming device the impedance is determined (desirable 400–800 Ω) and the GES pulse generator is initially programmed (voltage, 5 V; pulse width, 330 μs; frequency ~14 Hz; time on 1.0 s; time off 4.0 s). Postoperatively, in patients who have not had satisfactory symptom relief, the GES parameters can be modified. However, there is no agreed upon algorithm for adjustment of the settings. In general, we initiate gastric stimulation at a voltage of 5 V (current ~10 mA; assuming an impedance of ~500 Ω). We usually leave the voltage unchanged and increase the pulse width and frequency. We have had greater success with this strategy rather than with increasing the current while leaving the other parameters unchanged. Theoretically, increasing pulse width and frequency is a quicker way to build up energy in a nerve and reach an action potential than simply increasing current. Adjustments are usually performed every few weeks to months, as indicated.

Outcome

According to most reports, GES is associated with long-term success in adults with gastroparesis. McCallum et al. recently showed overall improvement in symptoms and nutritional status and decreased medication use during an average 56-month follow-up after placement of the GES in adults [7]. Lin et al. reported the outcome of 63 adults diagnosed with gastroparesis and treated with GES [8]. After at least 1 year follow-up, the severity of each symptom (abdominal pain, bloating/distention, nausea, vomiting, early satiety) was significantly reduced although the 4-h gastric emptying did not accelerate

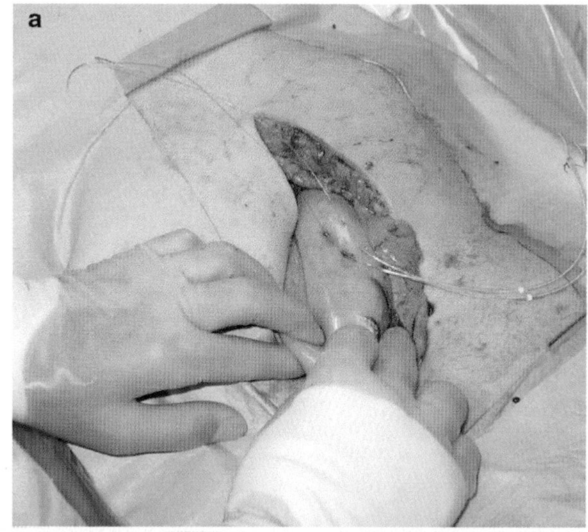

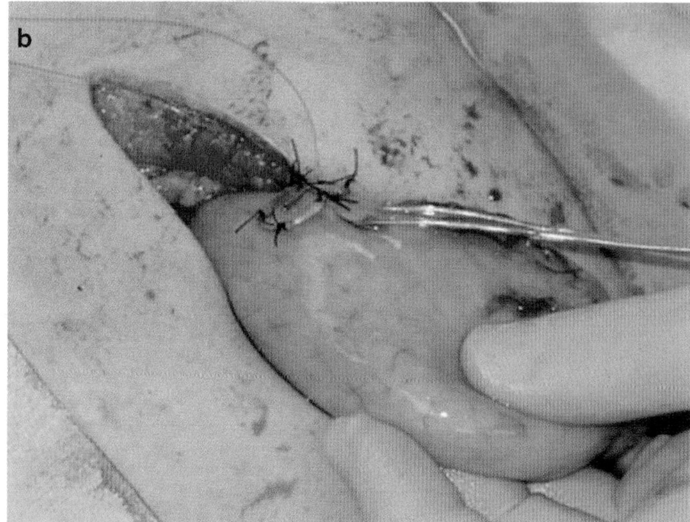

Fig. 42.2 Surgical placement of a GES via laparotomy. Gastric stimulator leads placed parallel to each other in the gastric wall along the greater curvature (**a**). The leads are sutured to the gastric wall (**b**). The leads are attached to the pulse generator (**c**). The pulse generator is sutured into the superficial pocket (**d**)

significantly, confirming the lack of correlation between symptoms and scintigraphic data. The group did not report significant adverse events.

There is some evidence that patients with more generalized motility disturbances may also benefit from the use of GES, probably due to its effects on afferent nerves. In a case series of adult patients with intestinal pseudoobstruction, vomiting improved just as much as it did in patients with gastroparesis and the authors concluded that GES may be considered as a viable therapy both for idiopathic pseudoobstruction and for non-idiopathic cases and its use should be considered irrespective of whether gastric emptying is normal or delayed [9]. Electrical stimulation of the jejunal limb has also been described as a potential effective treatment for Roux stasis syndrome [10]. In general, GES has been found to be safe. However, Becker et al. described the case of a 37-year-old woman who suffered gastric wall perforation from device leads years after placement [11].

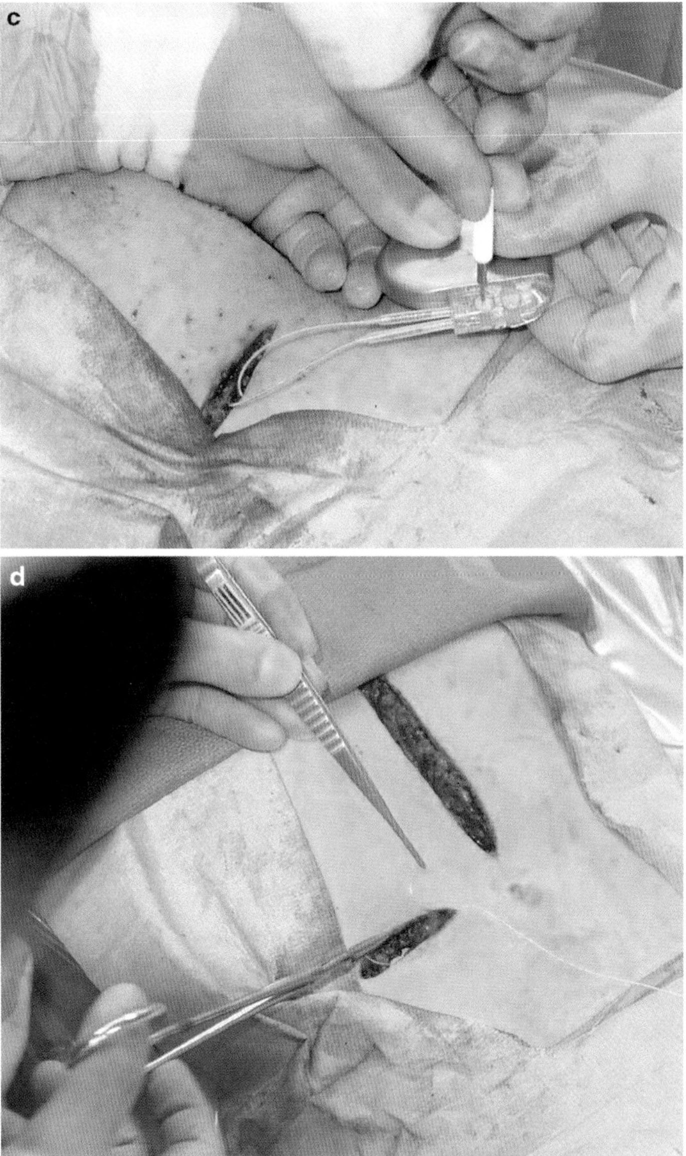

Fig 42.2 (continued)

Islam et al. first reported on the use of GES in pediatrics by describing nine adolescents with chronic nausea and vomiting [12]. With temporary stimulation, the group reported significant improvement of both symptoms. After permanent stimulation improvement persisted, although two subjects experienced adverse events. Symptoms recurred in one child who later needed enteral nutrition support and another patient had the device removed due to tissue deterioration at the implantation site. The remaining participants were able to return to normal diet and activity levels. Elfvin et al. published their experience with GES implantation in three children under the age of 3 years [13]. All three patients responded positively to GES therapy, demonstrating 50 % improvement in symptom frequency. These results indicate that this therapy in the pediatric population seems to be safe. Our own, yet unpublished data, in more the 25 children who have received temporary and permanent GES go along with the results of the previously published studies, showing very encouraging results in a heterogeneous group of children presenting mostly with nausea and vomiting. Pediatric patients who have received implantation of a GES pose significantly more challenges than adults, due to their active lifestyle that may make them more prone to the risk of abdominal traumas that might damage the pacemaker. The effect of growth on the connection between the pacemaker and the stomach has not been evaluated and long-term follow-up of pediatric GES patients has not been reported yet.

References

1. Dudekula A, O'Connell M, Bielefeldt K. Hospitalizations and testing in gastroparesis. J Gastroenterol Hepatol. 2011;26:1275–82.
2. Aro P, Talley NJ, Agréus L, Johansson SE, Bolling-Sternevald E, Storskrubb T, Ronkainen J. Functional dyspepsia impairs quality of life in the adult population. Aliment Pharmacol Ther. 2011;33:1215–24.
3. Familoni BO, Abell TL, Voeller G, Salem A, Gaber O. Electrical stimulation at a frequency higher than basal rate in human stomach. Dig Dis Sci. 1997;42:885–91.
4. McCallum RW, Chen JD, Lin Z, Schirmer BD, Williams RD, Ross RA. Gastric pacing improves emptying and symptoms in patients with gastroparesis. Gastroenterology. 1998;114:456–61.
5. Soffer E, Abell T, Lin Z, Lorincz A, McCallum R, Parkman H, Policker S, Ordog T. Review article: gastric electrical stimulation for gastroparesis—physiological foundations, technical aspects and clinical implications. Aliment Pharmacol Ther. 2009;30:681–94.
6. Ayinala S, Batista O, Goyal A. Temporary gastric electrical stimulation with orally or PEG-placed electrodes in patients with drug refractory gastroparesis. Gastrointest Endosc. 2005;61:455–61.
7. McCallum RW, Lin Z, Forster J, Roeser K, Hou Q, Sarosiek I. Gastric electrical stimulation improves outcomes of patients with gastroparesis for up to 10 years. Clin Gastroenterol Hepatol. 2011;9:314–9.
8. Lin Z, Hou Q, Sarosiek I, Forster J, McCallum RW. Association between changes in symptoms and gastric emptying in gastroparetic patients treated with gastric electrical stimulation. Neurogastroenterol Motil. 2007;20:464–70.
9. Andersson S, Lönroth H, Simrén M, Ringström G, Elfvin A, Abrahamsson H. Gastric electrical stimulation for intractable vomiting in patients with chronic intestinal pseudoobstruction. Neurogastroenterol Motil. 2006;18:823–30.
10. Daram SR, Tang SJ, Vick K, Aru G, Lahr C, Amin O, Taylor M, Sheehan JJ, Abell TL. Novel application of GI electrical stimulation in Roux stasis syndrome (with video). Gastrointest Endosc. 2011;74:683–6.
11. Becker JC, Dietl KH, Konturek JW, Domschke W, Pohle T. Gastric wall perforation: a rare complication of gastric electrical stimulation. Gastrointest Endosc. 2004;59:584–6.
12. Islam S, Vick LR, Runnels MJ, Gosche JR, Abell T. Gastric electrical stimulation for children with intractable nausea and gastroparesis. J Pediatr Surg. 2008;43:437–42.
13. Elfvin A, Gothberg G, Lönroth H, Saalman R, Abrahamsson H. Temporary percutaneous and permanent gastric electrical stimulation in children younger than 3 years with chronic vomiting. J Pediatr Surg. 2011;46:655–61.

Cognitive Behavioral Therapy for Children with Functional Abdominal Pain

43

Nader N. Youssef and Miranda A.L. van Tilburg

Background

Over the past decades it has increasingly become evident that functional gastrointestinal disorders (FGIDs) are explained by dysregulation of the brain–gut axis. FGID symptoms are not only caused and maintained by gut processes but may also be modified by extraintestinal components such as those related to cognition, emotions, and behavior. Currently, therapies for FGIDs can be divided into two main categories: those directed to the predominant symptom (or-end organ therapy) and treatment aimed at psychosocial aspects of the disorder with a focus on providing patients with adequate tools for modifying disease perception and responses to pain.

Among the various psychosocial interventions available, cognitive behavioral therapy (CBT) has recently gained more popularity as a modality in the treatment for FGIDs. This is not surprising, as CBT has a large evidence base in many conditions that have a psychosomatic component. These include traditional behaviorally based conditions which have some biological base, such as mood, anxiety, personality, and eating disorders, and also established organic disorders, such as inflammatory bowel disease, diabetes, and cardiovascular disease [1–8] which conversely have been found to have a significant psychosocial component. When considering evidence-based treatment, where specific treatments for symptom-based diagnoses are utilized, CBT has been recommended over other psychosocial approaches.

Within childhood FGIDs, CBT is being used to treat various conditions, and data for its effectiveness exists for fecal incontinence [4], rumination [6], aerophagia [7], and cyclic vomiting [9]. But the most evidence for the effectiveness of CBT is in treating functional abdominal pain (FAP) in childhood [10–12]. Therefore, in the remaining part of this chapter, we will discuss the use of CBT in the treatment of FAP. First, we will explore the common components of CBT for the treatment of FAP and show the versatility of the approach to many different situations such as the application of CBT in school, family, and at home. Last, we will discuss the literature on mechanisms that may be responsible for the positive effect seen with CBT [13–15].

It is equally important that the role of parent/family of the affected child be acknowledged when planning a successful intervention for children with FAP and utilizing CBT [11, 12]. Human behavior is routinely motivated and rewarded by positive reinforcement. Many well-meaning

N.N. Youssef, M.D., F.A.A.P., F.A.C.G. (✉)
Digestive Health Care Center, 511 Courtyard Drive, Hillsborough, NJ 08844, USA
e-mail: naderyoussefmd@gmail.com

M.A.L. van Tilburg, Ph.D.
Division of Gastroenterology and Hepatology, Department of Medicine, University of North Carolina at Chapel Hill, Chapel Hill, NC, USA

C. Faure et al. (eds.), *Pediatric Neurogastroenterology: Gastrointestinal Motility and Functional Disorders in Children*, Clinical Gastroenterology,
DOI 10.1007/978-1-60761-709-9_43, © Springer Science+Business Media New York 2013

parents show empathy and sympathy for their child's pain and may give extra attention, gifts, or excuse the child from chores, a behavior which unintentionally reinforces pain complaints and disability. Teaching parents to withhold reinforcement of their child's pain and replacing it with other techniques such as distraction can improve symptoms in children [16].

Aims of Cognitive Behavioral Therapy

As the name implies, cognitive behavioral therapy combines cognitive and behavioral treatment approaches with the aim to provide the child with the skills to promote pain relief and feelings of well-being [17]. Within a course of 3–12 weekly treatment sessions, the therapist generally uses *cognitive* techniques to help patients overcome distorted and negative thinking patterns that amplify physical symptoms, and *behavioral* techniques to change dysfunctional responses to pain. Under the guidance of a trained therapist, the child learns how to reduce pain and distress and gradually these techniques become self-administered. For children, CBT can also include changing the thoughts and behaviors of the caregivers. There is no generic model for CBT, in fact CBT refers to a set of behavioral and cognitive interventions which can be used in many different combinations. It is therefore highly adaptable to the disease or disorder and individual to maximize therapeutic benefit [18–24]. This also means that the content of CBT can be very different across therapists, disorders, age range, and other individual or situational characteristics.

Therapeutic Delivery Techniques

The particular therapeutic techniques vary within CBT, but commonly may include questioning and testing cognitions, assumptions, evaluations, and beliefs that might be unhelpful and unrealistic; gradually facing activities which may have been avoided; trying out new ways of behaving and reacting, and keeping a diary of significant events and associated feelings, thoughts, and behaviors [17–23]. Relaxation, mindfulness, guided imagery, and distraction techniques are usually also included.

Major Components to Cognitive Behavioral Therapy

Education. An explanation of the prevalence and nature of FAP, including the role of the brain–gut axis forms the foundation of therapy. It is important for the family to understand and "buy" into the role of stress and maladaptive thoughts in symptom initiation and maintenance. It is generally preferable to shift the focus from monitoring of symptoms to participation in daily activities (e.g., school attendance, social activities) to emphasize treatment success. The child and caregiver are often reminded of the ultimate goal of returning to a normal routine.

Cognitive techniques. Once the foundation has been laid with education that the primary goal of CBT is to examine, identify, and correct irrational beliefs and automatic thoughts, the therapist guides the patient in discovering his or her cognitive distortions that contribute to the etiology or maintenance of abdominal pain and/or disability. Several techniques are used to counter these distortions. For example, children are taught to identify and replace negative self-talk (e.g., "This pain will never go away") with more adaptive cognitions (e.g., "I have handled pain like this before, so I can handle it again"). Or children may be asked to test the validity of their beliefs by defending his or her thoughts. If the patient cannot produce objective evidence supporting his or her assumptions, the invalidity, or faulty nature, is exposed (e.g., "When I'm bloated nobody wants to be my friend" in a child that has a rich social life).

Behavioral techniques. The therapist has a large arsenal of behavioral techniques to induce relaxation, improve coping, and extinct unwanted behaviors. Some of the most commonly used strategies are guided imagery and relaxation training:

Guided imagery. This is a form of relaxed, focused concentration similar to hypnosis. The therapist uses verbal guidance to help the patient experience specific detailed vivid imagery that has beneficial effects on the patient behavior, cognitions, emotions, or physiology. With input from a therapist, children develop and imagine a vivid scene such as going to a favorite place, and focus on the elements and sensations of the scene. This imagery makes children calm and relaxed while they also achieve a state of focused attention not unlike playing imaginary games or watching a movie and feeling you are part of a story. During this focused state of attention, children are more open to therapist suggestions for pain reduction and increased well-being.

Relaxation training. Two commonly used relaxation techniques are deep breathing exercises and progressive muscle relaxation; in deep breathing exercises, children are taught diaphragmatic breathing which is deep abdominal breathing, by flexing the diaphragm, rather than shallow breathing by raising the rib cage. Children may learn this by pretending to blow up and deflate a balloon in their stomachs or by lying on the ground trying to keep a book or hand placed on one's chest from moving, while raising a book/hand on one's stomach with each breath. In progressive muscle relaxation, children are taught to systematically tense and relax various muscle groups. Age-appropriate explanations are employed to assist children with this task (e.g., young children are asked to pretend to be a "robot" and then a "rag doll").

Mindfulness training. Mindfulness training involves learning to attend to present moment experiences without evaluating them based on past or future fixations. For example, children may be instructed to observe and describe unwanted thoughts and feelings as they come and go, rather than suppressing them. This process increases children's ability to know their sensations better and ultimately to reduce the suffering associated with pain.

Homework. In order to encourage self-discovery and reinforce techniques learned in therapy, the therapist usually asks the patient to do homework assignments. These may include practicing newly learned skills or journaling of symptoms, unwanted thoughts, or difficult situations.

The techniques described above are some of the most used approaches in CBT but this list is not exhaustive. Therapists can draw on many more cognitive and behavioral techniques to help their patients, modify unwanted thoughts and behaviors that impact symptoms and disability. In addition, these techniques are simple to learn and safe, without any major side-effects, making them an ideal treatment option for children and adolescents at a vulnerable age of development.

Who Benefits from CBT?

In the early management of children with FGID, it is of paramount importance to identify from both patient and their families the "willingness or acceptance" of psychosocial therapies including CBT [20, 21]. Once established, children are highly responsive to many CBT techniques due to their natural ability to use imagination, high suggestibility, and sense of play. However, CBT requires children to be willing participants with a relatively long attention span and fairly good concentration. In addition, cognitive strategies within CBT have the most appeal to children who have developed meta-cognition. This means that children need to have an awareness of their own thinking, an ability to understand how to control and manipulate their thinking, and being able to evaluate success of making changes to their thinking. In short, cognitive strategies appeal the most to children who can *think about their thinking*. Therefore, CBT usually is suggested for children age 8 and up but developmental level should be taken into account in all children before recommending and starting CBT [22–24]. In practice, young children can master some of these concepts and may become more proficient at using them over time. Children under the age of 8 can benefit from behavioral approaches and some simple cognitive strategies (such as imagery or positive self-talk) under the guidance of a coach, usually the parent, who prompts and helps the child to implement strategies at home.

Physicians, parents, and patients can often be unintentional obstacles to the early initiation of CBT. They feel CBT is only warranted when significant psychiatric overlap such as anxiety and depression is present. Therefore, few children are referred for CBT who do not have comorbid psychiatric problems. Although CBT is well suited to treat children with these comorbid conditions, it can also be effective in children who do not have any obvious mental health problems but still struggle with significant symptoms and disability.

Effective CBT for Chronic Pain

Investigators from Oregon and others have recently published an updated metanalytical review of randomized controlled trials of psychological therapies for management of chronic pain in children and adolescents [23, 24]. The purpose of this meta-analytic review was to quantify the effects of psychological therapies for the management of chronic pain in youth [23]. Specifically, systematic reviews of randomized controlled trials by including new trials, and by adding disability and emotional functioning to pain as treatment outcomes were assessed. Twenty-five trials including 1,247 young people met inclusion criteria and were included in the meta-analysis. Meta-analytic findings demonstrated a large positive effect of psychological intervention on pain reduction at immediate post-treatment and follow-up in youth with headache, abdominal pain, and fibromyalgia. Small and non-significant effects were found for improvements in disability and emotional functioning, although there were limited data on these outcomes. All cognitive behavioral therapy, relaxation therapy, and biofeedback produced significant and positive effects on pain reduction. Studies directly comparing the effects of self-administered versus therapist-administered interventions found similar effects on pain reduction.

CBT for Abdominal Pain

A number of randomized controlled trials to test the effectiveness of pain interventions on children and their families using a self-management approach that includes components of cognitive behavior therapy have been conducted, yielding encouraging findings for this approach [10–12]. The following techniques are a sample of novel approaches utilized by investigators recently showing that CBT is efficacious in treating FAP and can be delivered in ways to increase access and feasibility.

Therapeutic Delivery Techniques

Family Intervention

Increasingly, parents are recognized as critical partners in CBT programs. Success often depends on the parent's willingness to encourage the child to practice, including practicing with him or her, and using positive reinforcement for cooperation and successful outcomes. Acceptance by parents of a biopsychosocial model of illness is important for the resolution of FAP in children [11, 12]. Discussing these issues in clinical practice is difficult as parents often feel misunderstood and blamed for their child's pain. Discussing parents' fears and worries about their children's chronic abdominal pain may facilitate discussions of social learning of gastrointestinal illness behavior.

In a randomized controlled trial [11], investigators tested the efficacy of an intervention designed to improve outcomes in idiopathic childhood abdominal pain by altering parental responses to pain and children's ways of coping and thinking about their symptoms. Two-hundred children with persistent FAP and their parents were randomly assigned to one of two conditions: a three-session intervention of cognitive behavioral treatment targeting parents' responses to their children's pain complaints and children's coping responses, or a three-session educational intervention that controlled for time and attention. Children in the cognitive behavioral condition showed greater baseline to follow-up decreases in pain and gastrointestinal symptom severity (as reported by parents) than children in the comparison condition. Also, parents in the cognitive behavioral condition reported greater decreases in solicitous responses to their child's symptoms compared with parents in the comparison condition. Investigators concluded that an intervention aimed at reducing protective parental responses and increasing child coping skills is effective in reducing children's pain and symptom levels compared with an educational control condition.

Community-School Based Intervention

Because assessment of FAP is frequently made at the school nurse level, schools may represent an excellent opportunity for intervention [25]. A questionnaire was sent to 425 school nurses to evaluate perceptions about FAP. Questions seeking to address perceived causes and treatment needs for children with chronic abdominal pain revealed that school nurses are unclear about epidemiologic and etiologic features of FAP and have negative views that may inadvertently contribute to the anxiety felt by affected children. Investigators concluded that increased education of school nurses and communication from physicians may advance strategies designed to reduce the fiscal and social costs associated with FAP.

In order to help school nurses in the community, the same investigators utilized a novel approach to deliver guided imagery directly to children presenting with FAP at school. In a pilot study, the feasibility and efficacy of a school nurse administered guided imagery program was assessed [26]. Nurses recruited children with FAP and no other distress symptoms such as weight loss, fever, or change in bowel habits. Children were randomized to six sessions of Guided Imagery (GIM) or Rest and Relaxation (RR) over 1 week. Initial session was 15 min and five booster sessions lasted 7 min. GIM was delivered via a compact disc. Questionnaires for abdominal pain and disability at initiation, 1-week post-intervention and 3-month follow-up were collected. Guided imagery was associated with greater improvement in pain than RR. At 3 months, pain was still reduced from baseline in both GIM and RR group. No child was diagnosed with alternate disease in the 3-month follow-up. Investigators concluded that school nurse administered guided imagery for abdominal pain was feasible and that larger, prospective studies were needed to confirm these positive results.

Home-Based Interventions

Despite the good evidence in support of CBT for treating FAP in children, psychological services are often difficult for patients to access and may not be covered by insurance. It is also important to note that there is a paucity of therapists who are well trained in cognitive behavioral approaches with children. In addition, families may be resistant to a referral to a mental health professional when they are not well educated about the goals of treatment (learning to cope with pain and disability reduction) and rather see the referral as a sign the physician thinks the pain is "all in the child's head." As a consequence few patients with FAP are referred to mental health specialists unless they have additional psychiatric symptoms, with most children being treated exclusively by pediatricians or family physicians without integration with mental health care. Therefore, home-based interventions have been developed including delivery of CBT by phone, Internet, and CD which may increase access to this type of therapy.

CD Delivered CBT Components

Investigators have developed home-based, guided imagery treatment protocols, using audio and video recordings, which are inexpensive, easy for health-care professionals and patients to use, and may be applicable to a wide range of health-care settings [27]. In a pilot study, 34 children, 6–15 years of age, with a physician diagnosis of FAP were assigned randomly to receive 2 months of standard medical care with or without home-based, guided imagery treatment. Children who had received only standard medical care initially, received guided imagery treatment after 2 months. Patients were monitored for 6 months after completion of guided imagery treatment. All treatment materials were reported to be self-explanatory, enjoyable, and easy to understand and to use. The compliance rate was 98.5%. In an intention-to-treat analysis, 63.1% of children in the guided imagery treatment group were treatment responders, compared with 26.7% in the standard medical care-only group. When the children in the standard medical care group also received guided imagery treatment, 61.5% became treatment responders. Treatment effects were maintained for 6 months (62.5% responders). Investigators concluded that guided imagery treatment plus medical care was superior to standard medical care only for the treatment of abdominal pain, and treatment effects were sustained over a long period.

Internet Delivered CBT

Investigators from Sweden have investigated the treatment of adults with irritable bowel syndrome by CBT delivered via the World Wide Web [28, 29]. The aim of this study was to investigate if CBT based on exposure and mindfulness exercises delivered via the Internet would be effective. Eighty-six participants were included in the study and randomized to treatment or control condition (an online discussion forum). Participants in the treatment condition reported a 42% decrease and participants in the control group reported a 12% increase in primary IBS symptoms. Investigators concluded that CBT based on exposure and mindfulness delivered via the Internet can be effective in treating IBS patients, alleviating the total burden of symptoms and increasing quality of life.

Computerized CBT

These are cognitive behavioral therapy sessions in which the user interacts with computer software (either on a PC, or sometimes via a voice-activated phone service), instead of face to face with a therapist. For people who are feeling depressed and withdrawn, the prospect of having to speak to someone about their innermost problems can be off-putting. In this respect, computerized CBT can be a good option. Investigators from the Netherlands have piloted a feasibility and efficacy program utilizing PDA (personal digital assistants) or hand-held computers for the self-management of adults with irritable bowel syndrome [30]. The trial was conducted with 38 control group patients receiving standard care and 37 intervention group patients receiving standard care supplemented with a 4-week CBT intervention on PDAs. Between-group comparisons between baseline and follow-up showed improved quality of life improvement, and less catastrophizing thoughts as well as pain in the intervention group. Only improvement in catastrophizing thoughts persisted in the long term. Investigators concluded that CBT relying on pocket-type computers appears feasible and efficacious for improving IBS-related complaints and cognitions in the short term. Future studies should focus on unraveling the effective components of this innovative e-health intervention.

Proposed Mechanism of CBT: Physiological, Parent, Impaired Coping, or All Three?

Even though CBT has been found to be effective in FAP, it is still largely unknown by which mechanism these changes are driven. Identifying the active ingredients of treatment is of utmost importance given the variety of CBT approaches a therapist can choose from. Some approaches applied in CBT, such as guided imagery, have been shown to be effective by itself without addition of other techniques. This suggests that there may be active ingredients of therapy that are more important than other techniques in reducing symptoms. Cognitive behavioral intervention is based on the assumption that changes in active coping, cognitions, emotions, and care-giving strategies are responsible for improvement in FAP; however, these assumptions have not yet been widely validated as research on the mechanism of change is lacking from most treatment trials. Below we will discuss the evidence for various purposed mechanism of change.

Physiological Changes to the Brain and Gut?

Despite CBT's main focus on psychosocial variables, it has been suggested that it can be accompanied by physiological changes as well, especially in the central nervous system [31–33]. It has been speculated that CBT may affect symptoms through changes in the brain. Brain changes with CBT have been found with other disorders such as Obsessive Compulsive Disorder, Panic Disorder, Major Depressive Disorder, and phobias. In addition, there is some evidence that treatment of psychosocial symptoms in adults with IBS is associated with changes in the central nervous system. For example, Drossman and colleagues followed a young woman with a history of abuse, posttraumatic stress disorder, and functional GI complaints, before and after treatment. Treatment consisted of removing her from an abusive relation, treating posttraumatic distress, and weaning from narcotics. Clinical recovery was associated with reducing psychosocial distress and visceral hypersensitivity to normal levels. Functional Magnetic Resonance Imaging showed increases in area 40, 22 and the anterior insula as well as decreases in prefrontal area 6/44, midcingulate cortex, and the somatosensory cortex. A study on the placebo effect in adult irritable bowel syndrome patients showed a robust positive correlation between symptom amelioration and increases in regional cerebral blood flow as well as the ventrolateral prefrontal cortex, and this correlation was mediated by changes in the dorsal anterior cingulate (dACC), typically associated with pain unpleasantness [34].

Similar studies among children have not been performed but two trials show no effect of psychosocial treatments on pain thresholds. A randomized controlled trial of CBT among 32 children with FAP showed no decreases in somatic pain thresholds [35]. Similarly, a large study among 46 children with FAP receiving hypnosis did not show changes in rectal sensitivity to pain despite clinical recovery [36]. These studies suggest that at least in children no physiological changes in pain thresholds can be found with psychosocial treatments. Evidently more research is needed to study the physiological effects of CBT in FAP.

Changes in Parental Solicitousness

As described earlier in this chapter, Levy and colleagues tested the effect of CBT directed not only at the child but also at the cognitions, emotions, and behaviors of the parents. Specifically parents' responses to their child's pain were targeted as well as children's coping responses. The authors reported greater decreases in parental solicitous responses to their child's symptoms as well as decreases in parental perceived threat of their child's pain following CBT. In another study on family CBT, parental strategies such as reinforcing well-behavior, using distraction, ignoring pain, and avoiding modeling the sick role, were independent predictors of child pain behavior post-treatment [16]. These data suggest that changing parental behaviors and beliefs may be an active ingredient in reducing child's pain and disability.

Changes in Coping

Explanations of chronic pain increasingly highlight the role of coping in understanding FAP. The type of coping response used by the child has been shown to mediate the impact of pain. Active coping responses (efforts to function despite pain or to distract oneself from pain) are thought to increase the child's sense of control, whereas more passive reactions (depending on others for help and restricting activities) lead to withdrawal, decreased activity, and greater pain.

Children with severe and persistent FAP often have inadequate coping responses and perceive themselves as having little control over their symptoms. The potential usefulness of coping skills training for children with FAP has been suggested by uncontrolled clinical case reports. Relaxation training as a specific coping skill has been used in conjunction with other behavioral and dietary interventions. In addition, CBT has been found to improve active coping such as the use of distraction and pain minimization. No studies have examined whether a change in a child's coping strategies is the mechanism responsible for improvement in the child's pain.

It is not all in their Heads!

It is accepted that many FAP patients may suffer from a combination of subtle to overt comorbid psychological and related gastrointestinal dysfunctions often unfairly termed a FGIDs. The role of brain–gut physiology cannot be ignored, and the effects of longstanding symptoms that may indeed cause significant anxiety and depression in both child and caregiver need to be addressed. Given the effects of psychosocial factors on the expression and trajectory of FAP, it could be argued that the effects of CBT are mainly mediated through changes in psychological distress. Although studies in adults with irritable bowel syndrome have shown decreases in anxiety following CBT, there is no evidence that the therapeutic gains depend on changes in patient's level of psychological distress. In children, there is no evidence that psychological distress improves with CBT treatment. Sander and colleagues found that treatment of FAP decreases internalizing and externalizing behavior measured with the Child Behavior Checklist, but these effects were equal among children receiving CBT or standard medical care [12]. Levy and colleagues also found no effects of CBT on child reported anxiety and depression although parent report of child depression did improve [11]. A recent meta-analysis also observed that psychological therapies in children reduced abdominal pain but not emotional symptoms [23]. Thus, current data do not suggest that the effects of CBT occur through changes in psychological symptoms. CBT should therefore be equally effective in patients with and without psychological comorbidities. In fact, one study in adults found that CBT may be more effective in those without psychiatric comorbidity as CBT did not show benefit for IBS patients with comorbid depression.

Conclusions

In summary, CBT offers an opportunity to effectively treat children with abdominal pain related to FGIDs. Mechanism of action for the therapeutic benefit of CBT is yet to be fully elucidated but most likely reflects a targeted intervention at the root of these pain disorders; namely, a disturbed brain–gut access often leading to an amplification of pain in the setting of impaired coping environment. Thus, it is reasonable to accept that changing maladaptive cognitions is at the heart of CBT therapy and ultimately its success. As clinicians become increasing comfortable with the understanding of the role of the brain–gut axis in the etiology of these common disorders, it is expected that they ultimately will begin to offer CBT delivered in a variety of novel ways much earlier in the treatment paradigm rather than waiting for other comorbid conditions to develop such as anxiety, depression, and impaired function which may lead to a more refractory patient.

References

1. Szigethy E, Kenney E, Carpenter J, Hardy DM, Fairclough D, Bousvaros A, Keljo D, Weisz J, Beardslee WR, Noll R, DeMaso DR. Cognitive-behavioral therapy for adolescents with inflammatory bowel disease and subsyndromal depression. J Am Acad Child Adolesc Psychiatry. 2007;46:1290–8.
2. Patel A, Maissi E, Chang HC, Rodrigues I, Smith M, Thomas S, Chalder T, Schmidt U, Treasure J, Ismail K. Motivational enhancement therapy with and without cognitive behaviour therapy for Type 1 diabetes: economic evaluation from a randomized controlled trial. Diabet Med. 2011;28:470–9.
3. Gulliksson M, Burell G, Vessby B, Lundin L, Toss H, Svardsudd K. Randomized controlled trial of cognitive behavioral therapy vs standard treatment to prevent recurrent cardiovascular events in patients with coronary heart disease: Secondary Prevention in Uppsala Primary Health Care project (SUPRIM). Arch Intern Med. 2011;171:134–40.
4. van Dijk M, Benninga MA, Grootenhuis MA, Nieuwenhuizen AM, Last BF. Chronic childhood constipation: a review of the literature and the introduction of a protocolized behavioral intervention program. Patient Educ Couns. 2007;67:63–77.
5. Chitkara DK, Bredenoord AJ, Talley NJ, Whitehead WE. Aerophagia and rumination: recognition and therapy. Curr Treat Options Gastroenterol. 2006;9:305–13.
6. Chitkara DK, Van TM, Whitehead WE, Talley NJ. Teaching diaphragmatic breathing for rumination syndrome. Am J Gastroenterol. 2006;101:2449–52.
7. Barrett RP, McGonigle JJ, Ackles PK, Burkhart JE. Behavioral treatment of chronic aerophagia. Am J Ment Defic. 1987;91:620–5.
8. Holburn CS, Dougher MJ. Behavioral attempts to eliminate air-swallowing in two profoundly mentally retarded clients. Am J Ment Defic. 1985;89:524–36.
9. Slutsker B, Konichezky A, Gothelf D. Breaking the cycle: cognitive behavioral therapy and biofeedback

training in a case of cyclic vomiting syndrome. Psychol Health Med. 2010;15:625–31.
10. Huertas-Ceballos A, Logan S, Bennett C, MacArthur C. Psychosocial interventions for recurrent abdominal pain (RAP) and irritable bowel syndrome (IBS) in childhood. Cochrane Database Syst Rev. 2008; CD003014.
11. Levy RL, Langer SL, Walker LS, Romano JM, Christie DL, Youssef N, DuPen MM, Feld AD, Ballard SA, Welsh EM, Jeffery RW, Young M, Coffey MJ, Whitehead WE. Cognitive-behavioral therapy for children with functional abdominal pain and their parents decreases pain and other symptoms. Am J Gastroenterol. 2010;105:946–56.
12. Sanders MR, Shepherd RW, Cleghorn G, Woolford H. The treatment of recurrent abdominal pain in children: a controlled comparison of cognitive-behavioral family intervention and standard pediatric care. J Consult Clin Psychol. 1994;62:306–14.
13. Toner BB. Cognitive-behavioral treatment of irritable bowel syndrome. CNS Spectr. 2005;10:883–90.
14. Lackner JM, Jaccard J, Krasner SS, Katz LA, Gudleski GD, Blanchard EB. How does cognitive behavior therapy for irritable bowel syndrome work? A mediational analysis of a randomized clinical trial. Gastroenterology. 2007;133:433–44.
15. Drossman DA, Toner B, Whitehead WE, Diamant N, Dalton CB, Emmott S, Proffitt V, Akman D, Frusciante K, Meyer K, Blackman CJ, Hu Y, Jia H, Li Z, Morris C, Koch G, Bangdiwala S. A multi-center randomized trial of cognitive-behavioral treatment (CBT) vs education (EDU) in moderate to severe functional bowel disorder (FBD). Gastroenterology. 2003 Jul;125(1):19–31.
16. Walker LS, Williams SE, Smith CA, Garber J, Van Slyke DA, Lipani TA. Parent attention versus distraction: impact on symptom complaints by children with and without chronic functional abdominal pain. Pain. 2006;122(1–2):43–52.
17. Weinland SR, Morris CB, Dalton C, Hu Y, Whitehead WE, Toner BB, Diamant N, Leserman J, Bangdiwala SI, Drossman DA. cognitive factors affect treatment response to medical and psychological treatments in functional bowel disorders. Am J Gastroenterol. 2010;105(6):1397–406.
18. Humphreys PA, Gevirtz RN. Treatment of recurrent abdominal pain: components analysis of four treatment protocols. J Pediatr Gastroenterol Nutr. 2000; 31:47–51.
19. Walker LS, Baber KF, Garber J, Smith CA. A typology of pain coping strategies in pediatric patients with chronic abdominal pain. Pain. 2008;137:266–75.
20. Walker LS, Smith CA, Garber J, Claar RL. Testing a model of pain appraisal and coping in children with chronic abdominal pain. Health Psychol. 2005;24: 364–74.
21. Walker LS, Smith CA, Garber J, Claar RL. Appraisal and coping with daily stressors by pediatric patients with chronic abdominal pain. J Pediatr Psychol. 2007; 32:206–16.
22. Thomsen AH, Compas BE, Colletti RB, Stanger C, Boyer MC, Konik BS. Parent reports of coping and stress responses in children with recurrent abdominal pain. J Pediatr Psychol. 2002;27:215–26.
23. Palermo TM, Eccleston C, Lewandowski AS, Williams AC, Morley S. Randomized controlled trials of psychological therapies for management of chronic pain in children and adolescents: an updated meta-analytic review. Pain. 2010;148:387–97.
24. Claar RL, Baber KF, Simons LE, Logan DE, Walker LS. Pain coping profiles in adolescents with chronic pain. Pain. 2008;140:368–75.
25. Youssef NN, Murphy TG, Schuckalo S, Intile C, Rosh JR. School nurse knowledge and perceptions of recurrent abdominal pain: opportunity for therapeutic alliance? Clin Pediatr. 2007;46(4):340–4.
26. Youssef NN, van Tilburg MA, Langseder AL. School nurse administered guided imagery for functional abdominal pain: a pilot study. Gastroenterology. 2009;137(5):S1.
27. van Tilburg MA, Chitkara DK, Palsson OS, Turner M, Blois-Martin N, Ulshen M, Whitehead WE. Audio-recorded guided imagery treatment reduces functional abdominal pain in children: a pilot study. Pediatrics. 2009;124(5):e890–7.
28. Palermo TM, Wilson AC, Lewandowski A, et al. Randomized controlled trial of an Internet-delivered family cognitive-behavioral therapy intervention for children and adolescents with chronic pain. Pain. 2009;146:205–13.
29. Hicks CL, von Baeyer CL, McGrath PJ. Online psychological treatment for pediatric recurrent pain: a randomized evaluation. J Pediatr Psychol. 2006;31: 724–36.
30. Oerlemans S, van CO, Herremans PJ, Spreeuwenberg P, van DS. Intervening on cognitions and behavior in irritable bowel syndrome: A feasibility trial using PDAs. J Psychosom Res. 2011;70:267–77.
31. Siegel LJ, Smith KE. Children's strategies for coping with pain. Pediatrician. 1989;16:110–8.
32. Frewen PA, Dozois DJ, Lanius RA. Neuroimaging studies of psychological interventions for mood and anxiety disorders: empirical and methodological review. Clin Psychol Rev. 2008;28:228–46.
33. Drossman DA, Ringel Y, Vogt BA, Leserman J, Lin W, Smith JK, Whitehead W. Alterations of brain activity associated with resolution of emotional distress and pain in a case of severe irritable bowel syndrome. Gastroenterology. 2003;124:754–61.
34. Lieberman MD, Jarcho JM, Berman S, Naliboff BD, Suyenobu BY, Mandelkern M, Mayer EA. The neural correlates of placebo effects: a disruption account. Neuroimage. 2004;22:447–55.
35. Duarte MA, Penna FJ, Andrade EM, Cancela CS, Neto JC, Barbosa TF. Treatment of nonorganic recurrent abdominal pain: cognitive-behavioral family intervention. J Pediatr Gastroenterol Nutr. 2006;43:59–64.
36. Vlieger AM, van den Berg MM, Menko-Frankenhuis C, Bongers ME, Tromp E, Benninga MA. No change in rectal sensitivity after gut-directed hypnotherapy in children with functional abdominal pain or irritable bowel syndrome. Am J Gastroenterol. 2010;105: 213–8.

44 Complementary and Alternative Treatments for Motility and Sensory Disorders

Arine M. Vlieger and Marc A. Benninga

Introduction

Complementary and alternative medicine (CAM) is "diagnosis, treatment, and/or prevention which complements mainstream medicine by contributing to a common whole, by satisfying a demand not met by orthodoxy or by diversifying the conceptual frameworks of medicine" [1] a definition adopted by the Cochrane Collaboration. CAM incorporates many different approaches and methodologies ranging from ancient techniques like acupuncture and Ayurvedic medicine to chiropractics, homeopathy, spiritual healing, and body–mind medicine. CAM has a significant popularity with pediatric gastroenterology patients with a 1-year prevalence of CAM use of 36–41% [2–4]. Because of this high prevalence and the fact that some complementary therapies are not without adverse effects and may interfere with allopathic medications, it is important for pediatricians and gastroenterologists to become familiar with these therapies. CAM is especially used by children who have low perceived effect of conventional treatment and/ or experience significant school absenteeism [4]. Both situations occur frequently in motility and sensory disorders. For example, 30–50% of the children with functional constipation continue to have severe complaints despite intensive treatment with laxatives [5, 6]. Many patients are therefore dissatisfied with conventional treatment options. Also for pain-related disorders like functional abdominal pain, irritable bowel syndrome, and infantile colic, treatment options have limited efficacy, resulting in dissatisfied patients and parents. Moreover, Youssef et al. showed that adolescents with daily abdominal pain suffer from significant school absenteeism [7]. With the current increasing popularity of CAM in mind, it therefore seems just a matter of time before patients with chronic abdominal pain will consider an alternative route.

Another reason for parents to use CAM is a fear of side effects of allopathic medication, especially in young children. Many CAM therapies are considered "natural" by the general public and thus safer and gentler in some way than the armamentarium of modern medicine. This may explain the high use of CAM in young infants, for example infants with regurgitation and reflux [4].

In this chapter we will discuss the CAM treatment options for pediatric motility and sensory disorders in which CAM is used fairly often: infantile colic, gastro-esophageal reflux, chronic abdominal pain due to functional abdominal pain

A.M. Vlieger, M.D., Ph.D.
Department of Pediatrics, St. Antonius Hospital, Nieuwegein, The Netherlands

M.A. Benninga, M.D., Ph.D. (✉)
Department of Pediatrics, Emma Children's Hospital/ MAC, H7-248, Meibergdreef 9, 1105 AZ, Amsterdam, The Netherlands
e-mail: m.a.benninga@amc.nl

C. Faure et al. (eds.), *Pediatric Neurogastroenterology: Gastrointestinal Motility and Functional Disorders in Children*, Clinical Gastroenterology,
DOI 10.1007/978-1-60761-709-9_44, © Springer Science+Business Media New York 2013

and irritable bowel syndrome, and constipation. Since CAM treatments may vary widely and research on safety and efficacy of these treatments in children with these disorders is very limited, we will focus on those treatments that have been studied best and/or are being used most, including herbs, acupuncture, homeopathy, hypnotherapy, and manual-based therapies like chiropractics. The use of probiotics is not discussed in this chapter, because this has become mainstream medicine in the last decade.

General Remarks on Safety of CAM Therapies

Many CAM users consider CAM therapies "natural" and equate this with safety. They are often unaware of the fact that many of these therapies have the potential to be directly or indirectly harmful. There are several reports of severe adverse events in children, mostly due to contamination, drug interactions or direct toxic effects of herbs, and dietary supplements (reviewed by Cuzzolin et al. [8]). The problems of toxicity and drug interactions can be extra relevant in young children and infants whose metabolism and organ function is immature and less tolerant of even subtle changes in comparison to the adult. To date, only scant data on the frequency of adverse effects of CAM therapies in children are available. A recent review on safety and efficacy of acupuncture in children found a risk of adverse events of 1.55 in 100 treatments [9]. The authors concluded that acupuncture seems to be a safe CAM modality for pediatric patients, although the risk for an individual patient may be hard to determine because certain patients, such as immunosuppressed patients or infants, can be predisposed to an increased risk, and because acupuncturists may differ with respect to their qualifications, skills, and knowledge. Another study determined the frequency of concurrent use of conventional medications and natural health products and their potential interactions in 1,800 children [10]. Concurrent use of allopathic drugs and natural products was documented in 20% of patients with potential interactions in one quarter of them. The authors did not investigate whether these were true interactions resulting in clinical symptoms, but the significant number of children who used both drugs and natural products stresses the importance of studies investigating the safety of natural health products. A meta-analysis on adverse events associated with pediatric spinal manipulation identified 14 cases of direct adverse events involving neurologic or musculoskeletal events [11]. Incidence rates, however, could not be inferred from these observational data. Finally, some words on homeopathy, which is one of the most commonly used CAM treatments in children [12]. Over-the-counter homeopathic remedies are especially popular and used often for common self-limiting conditions. There is little published data on the safety of homeopathy. The few studies, which have been performed on this subject, show that adverse events to homeopathic drugs exist, but are rare and not severe. CAM therapies can also have indirect harmful effects due to missed diagnoses, delaying more effective treatments, and discontinuation of prescribed drugs [13]. These indirect effects are probably not a reason for concern in most motility and sensory disorders, for which conventional treatment options are often limited.

Infantile Colic

Infantile colic is a widespread clinical condition observed in 10–30% of infants [14]. It occurs mostly in healthy infants and is characterized by paroxysms of excessive, inconsolable crying, frequently accompanied by flushing of the face, drawing-up the legs, meteorism, and flatulence. These crying episodes tend to increase at the age of 6 weeks and usually resolve spontaneously at the end of 3 months. The etiology is not clear and its limited treatment options frustrate both parents and physicians. It is therefore not surprising that many parents turn towards CAM treatments for their infant.

Acupuncture

Acupuncture has long been used for infantile colic, especially in China, but the published literature is largely restricted to case studies. In 2008, Reinthal et al. investigated the effect of acupuncture in infantile colic in a randomized trial [15]. Forty children with excessive crying unresponsive to conventional therapies were quasi-randomized to control or light needling treatment. Parents were unaware of which group their child was assigned to. Children were given light needling acupuncture on one acupoint (LI4) on both hands for approximately 20 s on four occasions, or received the same care except needling. Acupuncture resulted in a significant reduction in the rated crying intensity, and also pain-related behavior, like facial expression, was significantly less pronounced in the light needling group. The results of this study are interesting, but need to be confirmed in larger, double-blind controlled trials.

Homeopathy

Homeopathic treatments, especially over-the-counter remedies, are very often used in infants with colic [12, 16], but data on its efficacy are lacking. One observational cohort study in 204 children compared the effect of a standard homeopathic preparation with a conventional drug (scopolamine) in the treatment of abdominal cramps. The analysis showed comparative improvements with both treatments in spasms, pain, sleeping disturbances, and crying. However, no double-blind RCT has been performed with this homeopathic preparation to confirm these findings, so the effect of this homeopathic product in the treatment of infantile colic is still unknown [17].

Manual-Based Treatments

One of the most frequently used treatments for infantile colic is spinal manipulation, given by chiropractors, manual therapists, osteopaths, or craniosacral therapists. It is often claimed by therapists that spinal manipulation is an effective treatment for colic. However, a systematic review in 2009 of three randomized clinical trials showed that the methodological quality of these trials was low with very low sample sizes and insufficient control of placebo effects [18]. It was concluded that to date there is no good evidence showing that spinal manipulation is effective for infantile colic. Moreover, the recent reported fatal adverse reaction on a 3-month-old baby upon craniosacral therapy demonstrates that spinal manipulation is not without risks and therefore should not be recommended for infantile colic [19].

Gastro-esophageal Reflux

Gastro-esophageal reflux (GER) is defined as the passive flow of gastric contents into the esophagus. It is important to recognize that GER is a normal physiologic phenomenon and therefore occurs to some extent in all infants and children. Symptoms, especially regurgitation, are very common in infancy and are reported by parents to occur at least regularly in 70% of 4-month-old babies [20].

Regurgitation and vomiting are the most typical symptoms related to GER [21]. However, most of the infants experiencing those symptoms are not considered to have GER disease. A combination of regurgitation and/or vomiting with excessive crying and feed-related irritability is most suggestive of GER disease in infants. Other symptoms such as hematemesis and failure to thrive are indicative of severe disease. Of the many extraesophageal symptoms such as apparent life-threatening events, laryngitis, hoarseness and asthma, only dental erosions, and Sandifer's syndrome are convincingly shown to be GER related [22].

Parental education, guidance, and support are usually sufficient to manage healthy, thriving infants with symptoms likely to be secondary to physiologic GER. If symptoms persist despite these conservative measures, it can be helpful to eliminate cow milk from the infant's diet (or in case of breastfeeding, from the mother's diet). Therefore, formula-fed infants with recurrent vomiting may benefit from a 2- to 4-week trial of an extensively hydrolyzed protein formula [23]. Thickening feeds has been shown to decrease the frequency of regurgitation, but not other symptoms and does not decrease acid exposure [24]. Many studies have been performed looking at the effect of posture in the postprandial position. Although some studies suggest a beneficial effect of lifting the head of the cot, there is not enough evidence to support this in clinical practice [24]. Compared to supine position, prone position significantly reduces the number of acid GER episodes, but increases the risk for sudden infant death syndrome (SIDS) [25, 26]. The major pharmacologic agents currently used for treating GERD in children are gastric acid-buffering agents, mucosal surface barriers, and gastric antisecretory agents.

Although many of the simple therapeutic interventions are helpful in infants and children with GER, 40% of the parents still seek help in the complementary medicine circuit. Despite this high percentage no well-designed trials exist which evaluate the efficacy of the complementary treatments that are used by parents for this disorder, such as osteopathy or naturopathy. Therefore, this review will only focus on acupuncture with respect to GERD.

Acupuncture

Transient lower esophageal sphincter relaxations (TLESR) have been shown to underlie most GER episodes in healthy volunteers and healthy premature infants as well as in adult and pediatric patients with GER disease [27]. Current data indicate that transient LES relaxations are mediated via a vago-vagal pathway initiated by tension receptors located in the proximal stomach musculature [28].

The mechanism by which acupuncture improves GERD-related symptoms remains to be elucidated. It has been shown that electric acupuncture at zusanli (ST-36) can increase the basal LES pressure, whereas transcutaneous electric nerve stimulation (TENS) at Hukou acupoint increases the degree of LES relaxation in volunteers (Fig. 44.1) [29]. Others have suggested that TENS at neiguan may inhibit the rate of TLESRs triggered by gastric distention and reduce the perception to gastric distention in human beings [30, 31]. A recent study in 12 healthy cats showed that electric acupoint stimulation at Neiguan significantly inhibits the frequency of TLESR

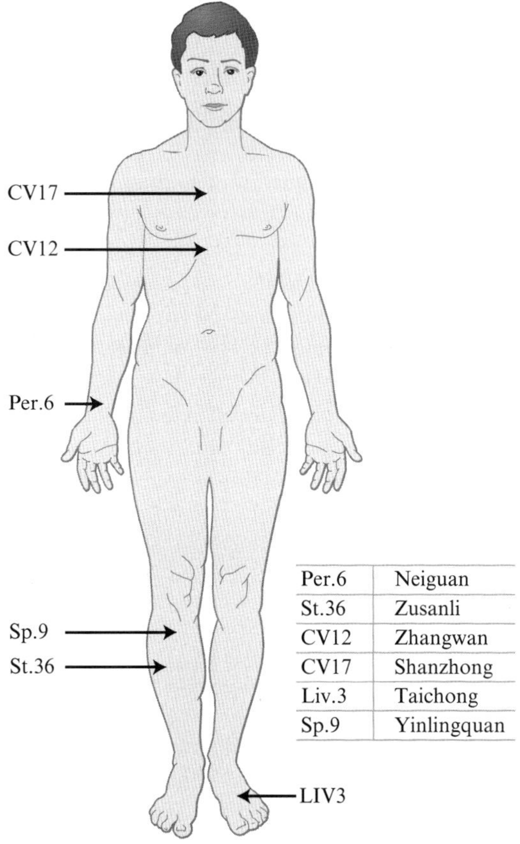

Fig. 44.1 Traditional Chinese Medicine acupuncture points used in the clinical trial: acupuncture versus doubling the proton pomp inhibitor dose in adults with gastro-oesophageal-related symptoms [32]

[32]. This effect appears to act on the brain stem, and may be mediated through nitric oxide, CCK-A receptor, and mu-opioid receptors.

A randomized parallel-group trial studied 30 adult patients (age > 18 years) with a 3-month history of GERD-related symptoms at least 2 days per week while taking standard-dose omeprazole 20 mg once daily [33]. The acupuncture protocol consisted of five acupuncture points according to the traditional Chinese medicine pattern diagnosis (Fig. 44.1). Treatment consisted of ten acupuncture sessions (25 min each) over 4 weeks. Acupuncture resulted in a significant improvement in daytime heartburn, night-time heartburn, and acid regurgitation when compared with doubling the PPI dose. A limitation of the study was the small sample size and the lack of a sham acupuncture arm. The authors point out, however, that increasing recognition in the acupuncture literature exists that superficial (needling of the skin), sham (needling of non-acupuncture points), and placebo (needling with blunt tip that does not penetrate the skin) acupuncture also provide an active therapeutic effect [34]. No such studies have been performed in either infants or children with gastro-esophageal reflux disease.

Functional Abdominal Pain and Irritable Bowel Syndrome

Irritable bowel syndrome (IBS) and functional abdominal pain (FAP) in childhood are pediatric functional gastrointestinal disorders, which are characterized by chronic or recurrent abdominal pain, and no evidence of an underlying organic disorder. By definition, altered bowel movements and/or relief of pain after defecation are seen in IBS, while defecation pattern is normal in patients with FAP [35]. IBS and FAP are among the most common pain complaints in childhood with reported prevalence's between 0.3 and 19% [36]. Quality of life scores of IBS and FAP children are significantly reduced and many children also suffer from anxiety and/or depression, highlighting the clinical significance [7, 37]. Standard medical treatment is symptomatic and consists of dietary advice, education, and/or pain medication. Sometimes patients are referred to a child psychologist for behavioral therapy. All these interventions may result in reduction of symptoms, but many children continue to experience symptoms for years, even into adulthood. It is therefore not surprising that a significant number of patients consider alternative treatments. Given the high placebo response shown in IBS studies, it is expected that many patients will experience at least a short-term benefit of any of these treatments.

Acupuncture

A 2006 Cochrane Database article reviewed six randomized trials using acupuncture in IBS [38]. It was concluded that the trials were generally of poor quality, included relatively small numbers of patients, and differed significantly in the acupuncture method utilized. The review found inconclusive evidence as to whether acupuncture is superior to sham acupuncture in IBS. Subsequently, two studies with in total 273 patients were published comparing real acupuncture to sham acupuncture or a waiting list. In both studies no significant difference was found between the response rates in patients receiving acupuncture and sham acupuncture on global improvement of IBS, although patients in both groups improved significantly compared to baseline [39, 40]. These results suggest that acupuncture has a potential role in the treatment of IBS, but its effect might be non-specific. However, Schneider et al. recently showed that real acupuncture in comparison to sham acupuncture had more specific physiological effects with a more pronounced decrease in salivary cortisol and an increased parasympathetic tone [41]. They concluded that different mechanisms seem to be involved in sham and real-acupuncture driven improvements, but the specific mode of action of acupuncture in IBS remains unclear and deserves further evaluation. Whether acupuncture is also effective in the treatment of children with IBS or FAP is unknown, since trials in this patient group are lacking. Awaiting such trials, physicians might already consider acupuncture as a potential treatment option in children with refractory IBS or FAP, since acupuncture is considered a safe CAM modality for pediatric patients [9].

Herbs

Herbals and botanicals have been used for hundreds of years for abdominal complaints in both adults and children, but good scientific evidence of their effectiveness is sparse. Two of three randomized-controlled trials (RCTs) demonstrated that (Chinese) herbal medicine may offer improvement in some adults with irritable bowel syndrome (IBS), and a superior post-treatment effect was found with individualized formulations in comparison to standardized preparations [42–44]. No studies have been performed in children. Peppermint, which is commonly found in over-the-counter preparations for IBS, has also been found effective [45]. The mechanism of action is thought to be from the menthol component of peppermint that relaxes gastrointestinal smooth muscle by blocking calcium channels [46]. In children with IBS the use of peppermint oil seems to be both safe and beneficial: in a small randomized, double-blind controlled 2-week trial, 76% of the patients receiving enteric-coated peppermint oil capsules reported a decrease in symptom severity versus only 19% in the placebo group [47]. Another popular herb in IBS is ginger (*Zingiber officinale*), especially used by patients with nausea and dyspepsia as one of the main complaints [48]. It has a prokinetic action probably mediated by spasmolytic constituents of the calcium antagonist type [49]. Ginger has been proven effective for reducing postoperative nausea and vomiting [50] and nausea in early pregnancy [51]. It seems to be relatively safe, although abdominal discomfort has been noted in some patients. NO RCT's have been performed in children with IBS, FAP, or functional dyspepsia.

Hypnotherapy

Brain–gut interactions are increasingly recognized in the pathogenesis of IBS and FAP, making body–mind medicine an appealing therapeutic approach. A body–mind technique that seems to be very useful in the treatment of children with FAP and IBS is gut-directed hypnotherapy. In this therapy a hypnotic trance is induced in which patients are given suggestions, directed towards control and normalization of gut function in addition to relevant ego-strengthening interventions. There is fairly strong evidence supporting the use of this CAM modality. A Cochrane review in 2006 found four RCT's in adults. The therapeutic effect of hypnotherapy was found to be superior to that of a waiting list control or usual medical management for abdominal pain and composite primary IBS symptoms [52]. Data were not pooled for meta-analysis due to differences in outcome measures and study design. One subsequent trial in children with FAP and IBS showed that developmentally appropriate gut-directed hypnotherapy was highly superior compared to standard medical care with complete remission of symptoms in 85% of children at 1-year follow-up versus 25% in the control group [53]. In an intriguing recent study, hypnotherapy based on self-exercises at home with the help of recorded scripts on CDs was used in a group of children with functional abdominal pain [54]. The CDs contained similar exercises as used in individual hypnotherapy. About two thirds responded favorably to this therapy compared to only 27% in the control group. Audio-recorded self-hypnosis can become an attractive first line therapy for children with FAP or IBS because of its low costs and direct availability, but further studies are needed to compare its effectiveness with individual hypnotherapy given by a therapist.

Manual-Based Therapies

Not many studies have been performed with manual-based therapies in patients with FAP or IBS. In adults with IBS a small single-blind trial did not show any benefit of reflexology foot massage on abdominal pain, defecation frequency, and abdominal distension [55]. A pilot study with 39 adult IBS patients investigated the effect of osteopathy, a manual treatment which relies on mobilizing and manipulating procedures in order to relieve complaints [56]. Compared to standard medical treatment, osteopathy resulted in a significantly lower disease severity index scores and a higher percentage of patients with definite overall improvement. It was concluded that osteopathic therapy might be a promising alternative in the treatment of patients with IBS. However, more studies are needed to confirm these findings before osteopathy can be advocated as a treatment option for IBS/FAP.

Constipation

The diagnosis functional constipation in infants and children is based on a complex of symptoms in the absence of an underlying organic cause. These children often have infrequent, painful, large, and hard bowel movements in combination with fecal incontinence. Furthermore, many of these children tend to show withholding behavior [35]. A recent systematic review reported that the worldwide prevalence of childhood constipation in the general population ranges from 0.7 to 29.6% [57]. As in children with functional abdominal pain chronic symptoms of functional constipation are associated with a lower quality of life, as measured with generic questionnaires [58]. Parents reported even lower quality of life than their children which was probably impacted by the duration of their child's symptoms and by family members having similar symptoms [58]. The backbone for treatment of functional constipation consists of education of the child and parents, behavioral modifications, and laxative therapy [59]. Once disimpaction is accomplished, maintenance therapy is essential to prevent re-accumulation of feces. Daily oral laxative therapy needs to be continued for 3 months or longer at a dose that produces a daily soft stool without side effects. In many children symptoms of constipation will resolve within this period. However, persistence of symptoms is reported in 30–52% of children in studies with at least 5 years of follow-up [60]. Not surprisingly Vlieger et al. showed that 36% of patients with constipation visiting a gastroenterology outpatient clinic used a least ≥CAM modality [4].

This review will discuss the effects of acupuncture, herbal therapies, reflexology, and body massage in the treatment of pediatric functional constipation. Since no well-designed studies could be identified on the effect of hypnotherapy, homeopathy, chiropractic and osteopathic manipulation, and energy therapies such as Reiki and healing touch these topics will not be discussed here.

Acupuncture

Little effort has been made to investigate the efficacy of acupuncture on constipation. A recently published review identified a total of 29 clinical studies evaluating the complementary effects of auriculotherapy as treatment option for constipation. However, generalization of these findings is limited because of two significant methodological flaws: (1) uncertainty in accurate acupoints identification and subjects' compliance to instructions resulted in varied doses of intervention received and (2) inconsistent intervention protocols and therapeutic outcome criteria make comparison among different studies difficult [61, 62].

Acupuncture can accelerate the release of opioid peptides in the central nervous system, but its effect on opioid activity and constipation is not known. Investigators in one study in children with chronic constipation looked at the effect of acupuncture on symptoms and on basal plasma panopioid levels—the ratio of plasma binding to opioid receptors in the brain [63]. The study regimen consisted of five weekly placebo acupuncture sessions followed by ten weekly true acupuncture sessions. A significant increase in frequency of bowel movements occurred in both boys and girls (1.5–4.4/week and 1.4–5.6/week, respectively, each $P<0.01$) after treatment. The panopioid activity was lower in the control children and increased only in the children who received the true acupuncture sessions. Out of 27 children who started, ten did not complete the study due to poor compliance. In contrast to the study in children, a study of acupuncture performed in adults with chronic constipation did not show any improvement in symptoms [64].

Herbs

Herbals and botanicals, and especially traditional Chinese medicine, have been used in many cultures over thousands of years for defecation disorders in both children and adults. Although there are many Chinese herbal medicine (CHM) interventions available, and some have been verified by clinical trials, their efficacy and safety are still questioned by both patients and health-care providers worldwide. A 2009 systematic review of the literature identified a total of 62 articles of which 35 were reviewed including a total of 3,571 patients (ranging in age from 1 month to 93 years) [65]. Although the authors conclude that the results of the different studies included, favored the tested CHM interventions in comparison with controls, the results of these trials should be interpreted with caution due to the generally low methodological quality of the included studies. First, all studies provided insufficient information on how the random allocation was generated and/or concealed, which is necessary to avoid selection bias. Second, none of the studies used any blinding method. Third, none of the included studies addressed incomplete outcome data, such as missing data due to attrition or exclusions. Fourth, none of studies had been registered and finally the majority of experimental CHM interventions were prepared by the investigators without detailed information describing underlying rationales on formulation, dosage, manufacturing process, etc.

A recent observational study investigated the use of a Japanese herbal medicine, Dai-Kenchu-To (DKT) composed of three herbs, zanthoxylum fruit, ginseng root, and dried ginger rhizomes, in ten children with non-defined severe constipation over a 3- to 12-month period [66]. In this small study the authors conclude that DKT had a favorable clinical effect on symptoms of constipation in children such as fecal incontinence. No data were, however, provided about the effect on defecation frequency, consistency of stools, and abdominal pain.

Historically, the botanical agents Rhamni purshiana and senna (Sannae folum) have been used as stimulant laxatives and are approved by the Food and Drug Administration for the treatment of constipation in children over 2 years of age. (NICE guideline), however studies evaluating safety and efficacy of these stimulants are lacking.

Reflexology

Reflexology is based on the notion that different areas on the hands and feet correspond to glands, organs, and other parts of the body and that pressure on those specific areas can have therapeutic effect. The mechanism underlying this treatment is unknown, but many believe that the effect is caused by an improvement of blood flow that encourages relaxation and the healing response [67]. The effect of reflexology has also been studied in 50 children, ages 3–14 years, with constipation and fecal incontinence [68]. After six weekly reflexology sessions of 30 min, results supported an increase in frequency of bowel movements and a decrease in fecal incontinence episodes with only 2% instead of 36% of the study children having fewer than one bowel movement a week during treatment. No side effects were reported, but double-blind studies with longer follow-up are needed to exclude placebo effect and determine the long-term outcome of this treatment.

Massage

Abdominal massage for the relief of constipation was a commonly practiced therapy in India, China, Arabia, Egypt, and Greece, but its use declined over time. As for other complementary therapies, there is now a resurgence of interest in the role that abdominal massage may play in relieving constipation, although preliminary studies have been disappointing although many patients perceived the therapy as agreeable [69].

Conclusion

Some CAM therapies and especially acupuncture and hypnotherapy show considerable promise in the treatment of children with motility and sensory disorders. Since so many patients are using CAM and because some of these modalities are not always devoid of risks, it is important for pediatricians and pediatric gastroenterologists to be familiar with these therapies. Moreover, given the ongoing interest in CAM by pediatric patients, it is in the public interest to establish more rigorous evidence on efficacy and safety of these therapies. Only this way, we can head towards integration of evidence-based CAM modalities into pediatric motility and sensory disorders. Until then, one should try to recognize both possibilities and limitations of CAM therapies in discussing these treatment options with parents and patients.

References

1. Ernst E, Resch K, Mills S, Hill R, Mitchell A, et al. Complementary medicine—a definition. Br J Gen Pract. 1995;45:506.
2. Day AS. Use of complementary and alternative therapies and probiotic agents by children attending gastroenterology outpatient clinics. J Paediatr Child Health. 2002;38:343–6.
3. Heuschkel R, Afzal N, Wuerth A, Zurakowski D, Leichtner A, et al. Complementary medicine use in children and young adults with inflammatory bowel disease. Am J Gastroenterol. 2002;97:382–8.
4. Vlieger AM, Blink M, Tromp E, Benninga MA. Use of complementary and alternative medicine by pediatric patients with functional and organic gastrointestinal diseases: results from a multicenter survey. Pediatrics. 2008;122:e446–51.
5. Staiano A, Andreotti MR, Greco L, Basile P, Auricchio S. Long-term follow-up of children with chronic idiopathic constipation. Dig Dis Sci. 1994;39:561–4.
6. van Ginkel R, Reitsma JB, Büller HA, van Wijk MP, Taminiau JA, Benninga MA. Childhood constipation: longitudinal follow-up beyond puberty. Gastroenterology. 2003;125:357–63.
7. Youssef NN, Murphy TG, Langseder AL, Rosh JR. Quality of life for children with functional abdominal pain: a comparison study of patients' and parents' perceptions. Pediatrics. 2006;117:54–9.
8. Cuzzolin L, Zaffani S, Murgia V, Gangemi M, Meneghelli G, et al. Patterns and perceptions of complementary/alternative medicine among paediatricians and patients' mothers: a review of the literature. Eur J Pediatr. 2003;162:820–7.
9. Jindal V, Ge A, Mansky PJ. Safety and efficacy of acupuncture in children: a review of the evidence. J Pediatr Hematol Oncol. 2008;30:431–42.
10. Johnston B, Vohra S. Which medications used in paediatric practice have demonstrated natural health product-drug interactions? Part A: Evidence-based answer and summary. Paediatr Child Health. 2006; 11:671–2.
11. Vohra S, Johnston BC, Cramer K, Humphreys K. Adverse events associated with pediatric spinal manipulation: a systematic review. Pediatrics. 2007; 119:e275–83.
12. Thompson EA, Bishop JL, Northstone K. The use of homeopathic products in childhood: data generated over 8.5 years from the Avon Longitudinal Study of Parents and Children (ALSPAC). J Altern Complement Med. 2010;16:69–79.
13. Ernst E. Risks associated with complementary therapies. In: Dukes MNG, editor. Meyler's side effects of drugs. 13th ed. Amsterdam: Elsevier Science; 2002. p. 1427–54.
14. Lucassen PL, Assendelft WJ, van Eijk JT, Gubbels JW, Douwes AC, van Geldrop WJ. Systematic review of the occurrence of infantile colic in the community. Arch Dis Child. 2001;84:398–403.
15. Reinthal M, Andersson S, Gustafsson M, Plos K, Lund I, et al. Effects of minimal acupuncture in children with infantile colic—a prospective, quasi-randomised single blind controlled trial. Acupunct Med. 2008;26:171–82.
16. Vlieger AM, van de Putte EM, Hoeksma H. The use of complementary and alternative medicine in children at a general paediatric clinic and parental reasons for use. Ned Tijdschr Geneeskd. 2006;150:625–30.
17. Muller-Krampe B, Oberbaum M, Klein P, Weiser M. Effects of Spascupreel versus hyoscine butylbromide for gastrointestinal cramps in children. Pediatr Int. 2007;49:328–34.
18. Ernst E. Chiropractic spinal manipulation for infant colic: a systematic review of randomised clinical trials. Int J Clin Pract. 2009;63:1351–3.
19. Holla M, Ijland MM, van d V, Edwards M, Verlaat CW. Diseased infant after craniosacral manipulation of the neck and spine. Ned Tijdschr Geneeskd. 2009;153:828–31.
20. Nelson SP, Chen EH, Syniar GM, Christoffel KK. Prevalence of symptoms of gastroesophageal reflux during infancy. A pediatric practice-based survey. Pediatric Practice Research Group. Arch Pediatr Adolesc Med. 1997;151:569–72.
21. Vandenplas Y, Rudolph CD, Di Lorenzo C, Hassall E, Liptak G, Mazur L, et al. Pediatric gastroesophageal reflux clinical practice guidelines: joint recommendations of the North American Society for Pediatric Gastroenterology, Hepatology, and Nutrition (NASPGHAN) and the European Society for Pediatric Gastroenterology, Hepatology, and Nutrition (ESPGHAN). J Pediatr Gastroenterol Nutr. 2009;49:498–547.
22. Pace F, Pallotta S, Tonini M, Vakil N, Bianchi Porro G. Systematic review: gastro-oesophageal reflux disease and dental lesions. Aliment Pharmacol Ther. 2008;27:1179–86.
23. Hill DJ, Heine RG, Cameron DJ, Catto-Smith AG, Chow CW, Francis DE, Hosking CS. Role of food protein intolerance in infants with persistent distress attributed to reflux esophagitis. J Pediatr. 2000; 136(5):641–7.
24. Craig WR, Hanlon-Dearman A, Sinclair C, Taback S, Moffatt M. Metoclopramide, thickened feedings, and positioning for gastro-oesophageal reflux in children under two years. Cochrane Database Syst Rev 2004;CD003502.
25. Orenstein SR, Whitington PF. Positioning for prevention of infant gastroesophageal reflux. J Pediatr. 1983;103:534–7.
26. Dwyer T, Ponsonby AL. Sudden infant death syndrome and prone sleeping position. Ann Epidemiol. 2009;19:245–9.
27. Dent J, Holloway RH, Toouli J, Dodds WJ. Mechanisms of lower oesophageal sphincter incompetence in patients with symptomatic gastrooesophageal reflux. Gut. 1988;29:1020–8.
28. Ireland AC, Dent J, Holloway RH. Preservation of postural control of transient lower oesophageal

sphincter relaxations in patients with reflux oesophagitis. Gut. 1999;44:313–6.
29. Chang FY, Chey WY, Ouyang A. Effect of transcutaneous nerve stimulation on esophageal function in normal subjects—evidence for a somatovisceral reflex. Am J Chin Med. 1996;24:185–92.
30. Zou D, Chen WH, Iwakiri K, Rigda R, Tippett M, Holloway RH. Inhibition of transient lower esophageal sphincter relaxations by electrical acupoint stimulation. Am J Physiol Gastrointest Liver Physiol. 2005;289:G197–201.
31. Coffin B, Azpiroz F, Malagelada JR. Somatic stimulation reduces perception of gut distention in humans. Gastroenterology. 1994;107:1636–42.
32. Wang C, Zhou DF, Shuai XW, Liu JX, Xie PY. Effects and mechanisms of electroacupuncture at PC6 on frequency of transient lower esophageal sphincter relaxation in cats. World J Gastroenterol. 2007;13:4873–80.
33. Dickman R, Schiff E, Holland A, Wright C, Sarela SR, et al. Clinical trial: acupuncture vs. doubling the proton pump inhibitor dose in refractory heartburn. Aliment Pharmacol Ther. 2007;26:1333–44.
34. Lund I, Lundeberg T. Are minimal, superficial or sham acupuncture procedures acceptable as inert placebo controls? Acupunct Med. 2006;24:13–5.
35. Rasquin A, Di LC, Forbes D, Guiraldes E, Hyams JS, Staiano A, et al. Childhood functional gastrointestinal disorders: child/adolescent. Gastroenterology. 2006; 130:1527–37.
36. Chitkara DK, Rawat DJ, Talley NJ. The epidemiology of childhood recurrent abdominal pain in Western countries: a systematic review. Am J Gastroenterol. 2005;100:1868–75.
37. Youssef NN, Atienza K, Langseder AL, Strauss RS. Chronic abdominal pain and depressive symptoms: analysis of the national longitudinal study of adolescent health. Clin Gastroenterol Hepatol. 2008; 6:329–32.
38. Lim B, Manheimer E, Lao L, Ziea E, Wisniewski J, Liu J, et al. Acupuncture for treatment of irritable bowel syndrome. Cochrane Database Syst Rev 2006;(4):CD005111.
39. Schneider A, Enck P, Streitberger K, Weiland C, Bagheri S, Witte S, et al. Acupuncture treatment in irritable bowel syndrome. Gut. 2006;55:649–54.
40. Lembo AJ, Conboy L, Kelley JM, Schnyer RS, McManus CA, et al. A treatment trial of acupuncture in IBS patients. Am J Gastroenterol. 2009;104:1489–97.
41. Schneider A, Weiland C, Enck P, Joos S, Streitberger K, Maser-Gluth C, et al. Neuroendocrinological effects of acupuncture treatment in patients with irritable bowel syndrome. Complement Ther Med. 2007;15:255–63.
42. Bensoussan A, Talley NJ, Hing M, Menzies R, Guo A, Ngu M. Treatment of irritable bowel syndrome with Chinese herbal medicine: a randomized controlled trial. JAMA. 1998;280:1585–9.
43. Madisch A, Holtmann G, Plein K, Hotz J. Treatment of irritable bowel syndrome with herbal preparations: results of a double-blind, randomized, placebo-controlled, multi-centre trial. Aliment Pharmacol Ther. 2004;19:271–9.
44. Leung WK, Wu JC, Liang SM, Chan LS, Chan FK, et al. Treatment of diarrhea-predominant irritable bowel syndrome with traditional Chinese herbal medicine: a randomized placebo-controlled trial. Am J Gastroenterol. 2006;101:1574–80.
45. Pittler MH, Ernst E. Peppermint oil for irritable bowel syndrome: a critical review and metaanalysis. Am J Gastroenterol. 1998;93:1131–5.
46. Hills JM, Aaronson PI. The mechanism of action of peppermint oil on gastrointestinal smooth muscle. An analysis using patch clamp electrophysiology and isolated tissue pharmacology in rabbit and guinea pig. Gastroenterology. 1991;101:55–65.
47. Kline RM, Kline JJ, Di PJ, Barbero GJ. Enteric-coated, pH-dependent peppermint oil capsules for the treatment of irritable bowel syndrome in children. J Pediatr. 2001;138:125–8.
48. van Tilburg MA, Palsson OS, Levy RL, Feld AD, Turner MJ, et al. Complementary and alternative medicine use and cost in functional bowel disorders: a six month prospective study in a large HMO. BMC Complement Altern Med. 2008;8:46.
49. Ghayur MN, Gilani AH. Pharmacological basis for the medicinal use of ginger in gastrointestinal disorders. Dig Dis Sci. 2005;50:1889–97.
50. Chaiyakunapruk N, Kitikannakorn N, Nathisuwan S, Leeprakobboon K, Leelasettagool C. The efficacy of ginger for the prevention of postoperative nausea and vomiting: a meta-analysis. Am J Obstet Gynecol. 2006;194:95–9.
51. Borrelli F, Capasso R, Aviello G, Pittler MH, Izzo AA. Effectiveness and safety of ginger in the treatment of pregnancy-induced nausea and vomiting. Obstet Gynecol. 2005;105:849–56.
52. Webb AN, Kukuruzovic RH, Catto-Smith AG, Sawyer SM. Hypnotherapy for treatment of irritable bowel syndrome. Cochrane Database Syst Rev 2007; (4):CD005110.
53. Vlieger AM, Menko-Frankenhuis C, Wolfkamp SC, Tromp E, Benninga MA. Hypnotherapy for children with functional abdominal pain or irritable bowel syndrome: a randomized controlled trial. Gastroenterology. 2007;133:1430–6.
54. van Tilburg MA, Chitkara DK, Palsson OS, Turner M, Blois-Martin N, et al. Audio-recorded guided imagery treatment reduces functional abdominal pain in children: a pilot study. Pediatrics. 2009;124:e890–7.
55. Tovey P. A single-blind trial of reflexology for irritable bowel syndrome. Br J Gen Pract. 2002;52:19–23.
56. Hundscheid HW, Pepels MJ, Engels LG, Loffeld RJ. Treatment of irritable bowel syndrome with osteopathy: results of a randomized controlled pilot study. J Gastroenterol Hepatol. 2007;22:1394–8.
57. van den Berg MM, Benninga MA, Di Lorenzo C. Epidemiology of childhood constipation: a systematic review. Am J Gastroenterol. 2006;101:2401–9.
58. Youssef NN, Langseder AL, Verga BJ, Mones RL, Rosh JR. Chronic childhood constipation is associ-

ated with impaired quality of life: a case-controlled study. J Pediatr Gastroenterol Nutr. 2005;41:56–60.
59. Bardisa-Ezcurra L, Ullman R, Gordon J, Guideline Development Group. Diagnosis and management of idiopathic childhood constipation: summary of NICE guidance. BMJ. 2010;340:c2585. doi:10.1136/bmj.c2585.
60. Bongers ME, van Wijk MP, Reitsma JB, Benninga MA. Long-term prognosis for childhood constipation: clinical outcomes in adulthood. Pediatrics. 2010;126:e156–62.
61. Li MK, Lee TF, Suen KP. A review on the complementary effects of auriculotherapy in managing constipation. J Altern Complement Med. 2010;16:435–47.
62. Ouyang H, Chen JD. Review article: therapeutic roles of acupuncture in functional gastrointestinal disorders. Aliment Pharmacol Ther. 2004;20:831–41.
63. Broide E, Pintov S, Portnoy S, et al. Effectiveness of acupuncture for treatment of childhood constipation. Dig Dis Sci. 2001;46:1270–5.
64. Klauser AG, Rubach A, Bertsche O, et al. Body acupuncture: effect on colonic function in chronic constipation. Z Gastroenterol. 1993;31:605–8.
65. Cheng CW, Bian ZX, Wu TX. Systematic review of Chinese herbal medicine for functional constipation. World J Gastroenterol. 2009;15:4886–95.
66. Iwai N, Kume Y, Kimura O, Ono S, Aoi S, Tsuda T. Effects of herbal medicine Dai-Kenchu-to on anorectal function in children with severe constipation. Eur J Pediatr Surg. 2007;17:115–8.
67. Hall N. Reflexology. London: Thorsons; 1996.
68. Bishop E, McKinnon E, Weir E, et al. Reflexology in the management of encopresis and chronic constipation. Paediatr Nurs. 2003;15:20–1.
69. Ernst E. abdominal massage for chronic constipation: a systematic review of controlled clinical trails. Forsch Komplementarmed. 1999;6:149–51.

Cellular-Based Therapies for Pediatric GI Motility Disorders

45

Ryo Hotta, Dipa Natarajan, Alan J. Burns, and Nikhil Thapar

Introduction

Currently, as has been discussed in other chapters, the therapeutic options for many gastrointestinal motility conditions remain inadequate. For the most severe, treatments are limited to palliative interventions such as surgery and the provision of artificial nutrition. This highlights the fact that current treatments aim to prevent the mortality and limit morbidity associated with the most significant complications of the diseases but are not designed to be curative.

Although it is clear that both surgery and parenteral nutrition (PN) have revolutionized management and overall survival of children suffering from severe intestinal motility disorders, most of whom would otherwise not have survived beyond the neonatal period [1–3], the conditions continue to be associated with high levels of morbidity and mortality. Mortality rates still remain in the order of 8–20%, and mostly relate to iatrogenic complications of central venous catheter-related sepsis and PN-related liver failure [1–6].

The poor outcome of gut motility disorders is perhaps best exemplified by Hirschsprung's disease (HSCR) where despite substantial surgical expertise and relatively rare use of PN, the post-operative morbidity data is compelling [7–11]. A long-term follow-up study of 48 HSCR patients with total colonic aganglionosis (TCA) by Tsuji et al. showed that 94% survived. Of the survivors, fecal incontinence was present in 82% of patients at 5 years, 57% at 10 years, and 33% at 15-year follow-up. On anthropometric follow-up, 63% of patients with TCA were failing to thrive at 15 years [7]. More recent studies suggest that such problems occur irrespective of the extent of aganglionosis [8] and persist in more than 50% of HSCR patients into early adulthood [9].

Such data highlights the need for improved, more curative, therapies for gut motility disorders, including those designed to definitively restore missing components or rescue dysfunctional ones. With particular attention to enteric neuropathies, this chapter summarizes the progress that has been made and the challenges that

R. Hotta, M.D., Ph.D.
Department of Anatomy and Neuroscience, The University of Melbourne, Melbourne, Australia

Department of Pediatric Surgery, Keio University School of Medicine, Tokyo, Japan

D. Natarajan, M.Sc., M.Phil., Ph.D. • A.J. Burns, Ph.D.
Neural Development Unit, UCL, Institute of Child Health, London, UK

N. Thapar, B.Sc.(hon), B.M.(hon), M.R.C.P., M.R.C.P.C.H., Ph.D. (✉)
Gastroenterology Unit, University College London, Institute of Child Health, Division of Neurogastroenterology and Motility, London, UK

Department of Paediatric Gastroenterology, Great Ormond Street Hospital for Children, London, UK
e-mail: n.thapar@ucl.ac.uk

C. Faure et al. (eds.), *Pediatric Neurogastroenterology: Gastrointestinal Motility and Functional Disorders in Children*, Clinical Gastroenterology,
DOI 10.1007/978-1-60761-709-9_45, © Springer Science+Business Media New York 2013

remain in the development of new curative cellular therapies for gut motility disorders.

Stem Cell Therapies for ENS Disorders: Background and Concepts

Recent advances in molecular biology and genetics have significantly enhanced our understanding of the development and function of the gut neuromusculature, especially its intrinsic innervation, the enteric nervous system (ENS). This has facilitated not only our appreciation of the pathogenesis of gut motility disorders but also the identification of novel tools and targets for therapy [12, 13]. Stem cells, defined by their unique ability to self-renew, proliferate extensively and differentiate into multiple lineages, provide one such tool. For the purposes of this review the term "stem cell" has been used to denote both progenitor cells, with limited self-renewal and differentiation capacities, as well as stem cells in the truest sense.

Successful stem cell therapy has already been performed for many years in the form of bone marrow transplants, and there is currently enormous interest in the potential of stem cell therapy to treat diseases of both the central nervous system (CNS) [14] and ENS [15–17]. Compared with other systems the use of stem cell therapy for treating diseases of the ENS has some potential advantages including accessibility to both source and deliver cells, as well as the possibility of autologous transplantation.

Sourcing Stem Cells for ENS Therapy

In the quest to develop cellular therapies for ENS disorders, a number of tissue sources have been explored to identify a cell type capable of generating ENS components upon transplantation. These are discussed below and summarized in Table 45.1.

Embryonic stem (ES) cells derived from the inner cell mass of the blastocyst are pluripotent and capable of giving rise to all the cell types in the body [18]. Their initial discovery [19, 20] and subsequent isolation from human embryos [21] led to significant interest for their use in regenerative medicine, especially given their potential to generate "unlimited" quantities of cells for replacement therapies. ES cells from both mouse (mES) and human (hES) are capable of producing a range of neural cell types [22–28], including enteric neurons [29, 30]. Kawaguchi et al. demonstrated that neural crest (NC) progenitors (Sox10 expressing) derived from mES cells can colonize, and give rise to neurons (Hu- and TuJ1-expressing) within explants of aneural hindgut of mouse embryos [30]. Neural progenitors derived from hES cells also appear capable of generating NC-like cells that migrate along normal NC migratory pathways in quail embryos in vivo and colonize explants of embryonic mouse gut in vitro where they give rise to neurons [29].

Apart from neurons, mES cells also appear capable of generating "gut-like" structures [31–36]. These structures are 0.2–1.5 mm in diameter, and contain an endodermal epithelium, intestinal epithelial stem cells, a layer of smooth muscle cells, and interstitial cells of Cajal (ICCs); they also exhibit spontaneous contractions [31–36]. Although they show some similarities to normal gut organogenesis [35] the requirement for brain-derived neurotrophic factor (BDNF) for neuron development differs from normal enteric neuron development, which does not require BDNF [37]. It is still unclear whether gut-like structures derived from ES cells will be useful for cell therapy or whether they are a curiosity of interest to basic ES cell researchers only.

CNS-derived stem cells: Although it had long been believed that the CNS in mammals is incapable of regenerating after birth, adult neurogenesis is now well established, including in humans [38–44]. This neurogenesis appears to be effected by a population of self-renewing, multipotent progenitors known as neural stem cells (NSCs) [45, 46]. CNS–NSCs were one of the first cell types tested for ENS therapy as several features were thought to make them suitable [16]. Transplanting CNS–NSCs into the pyloric wall of an animal model of gastroparesis (nNOS$^{-/-}$ mice) Micci et al. showed that these cells predominantly gave rise to neuronal nitric oxide synthase (nNOS) expressing neurons, which resulted in significant improvements in

Table 45.1 Possible sources of stem cells to generate a putative ENS

Source	Selection/propagation	Recipient or host tissue	Differentiation in host tissue	Function	Reference
ES					
Mouse ES cells	EB	Mouse renal capsule	N, M, ICC, and EP	Regular slow wave activity and spontaneous spike action potentials	[31, 34, 35, 101]
Mouse ES cells	Sox10	Aneural hindgut explant from mouse embryo in vitro	N	ND	[30]
CNS					
Embryonic mouse brain	NS	nNOS−/− mice stomach in vivo	N + G	Improved gastric function	[47, 88]
Embryonic rat brain	NS	Chemically denervated rat rectum in vivo	N + G	Restored rectoanal inhibitory reflex	[48]
Embryonic rat neural tube	NS	Chemically denervated rat colon in vivo	N + G	Improved colonic motility	[49]
Neural crest ENS					
Embryonic mouse gut	Sorted Ret + cells	Aganglionic gut explant from Ret−/− mouse embryo in vitro	N + G	ND	[60, 62]
Embryonic/postnatal mouse gut	NS	Aganglionic gut explant from Ret−/− mouse embryo in vitro	N + G	ND	[65]
Postnatal/adult rat gut	Sorted p75+/α4 integrin + cells	Aganglionic gut explant from Ednrb−/− mouse embryo grown on chorioallantoic membrane of chick embryos	N	ND	[57, 59, 64]
Embryonic rat gut	Sorted p75+/α4 integrin + cells	Ednrbsl/sl rat bowel in vivo, *i.p.*	N + G	ND	[100]
Embryonic/postnatal human gut	NS	Human gut explant in vitro	N	ND	[70]
HSCR patient gut	NS	Aneural hindgut explant from mouse embryo in vitro	N + G + ICC	Restored motility patterns to hindgut	[71, 72]
Postnatal human gut mucosa	NS	Explant from aganglionic region of HSCR patient in vitro	N	ND	[73]
ENS cell line from immortomice	Sorted p75+ cells	Piebald or nNOS−/− mice colon in vivo	N	Improved colonic motility	[102]

(continued)

Table 45.1 (continued)

Source	Selection/propagation	Recipient or host tissue	Differentiation in host tissue	Function	Reference
embryonic mouse gut	Sox2	Aneural hindgut explant from mouse embryo in vitro	N	ND	[103]
Other NCCs					
Embryonic mouse neural tube	Neural tube explant	Dom/+ mouse colon in vivo, *i.p.*	N+G	ND	[58]
Embryonic rat peripheral nerve	Sorted p75+/α4 integrin+cells	into migratory pathway of embryonic chickens in vivo	Gut; no, peripheral nerve; N+G	ND	[57, 59]

CNS central nervous system, *EB* embryoid body, *ENS* enteric nervous system, *EP* epithelium, *ES* embryonic stem (cells), *G* glial cells, *HSCR* Hirschsprung's disease, *ICC* interstitial cells of Cajal, *i.p.* intraperitoneally, *M* myofibroblasts, *N* neuron, *NCCs* neural crest cells, *ND* not determined, *NS* neurospheres gastric emptying and in electric field stimulation-induced relaxation [47]. Although the mechanisms underlying such improvement of gastric function were unclear, the study provided the first demonstration that NSCs transplanted into the bowel were able to ameliorate a motility disorder [15]. More recently, transplantation of fetal cerebral cortex-derived CNS–NSCs into the rectum of adult rats, where enteric neurons had been destroyed chemically, resulted in the generation of neurons and glial cells, an increase in both the expression of nNOS and choline acetyltransferase (ChAT), and restoration of the rectoanal inhibitory reflex [48].

Cells isolated from the mid-embryonic rat neural tube or "neuroepithelial stem cells" have also been shown to give rise to enteric neurons in vivo in similar experimental animals to that described above [49]. Transplantation of these cells appeared to result in nNOS and ChAT expressing neurons and improvements in colonic motility in recipient colons in which the ENS had been chemically destroyed [49].

Neural crest stem cells: Perhaps the most attractive tools for ENS therapy are derivatives of those NC cells that initially gave rise to the ENS itself. This is described in detail in earlier chapters. Briefly, during embryogenesis NC cells emigrate from the NC, a transient structure that forms at the dorsolateral surface of the developing neural tube, and migrate along defined pathways to give rise to diverse structures including the ENS [50, 51]. Vagal (hindbrain) NC cells arising adjacent to somites 1–7 [52, 53] enter the foregut and migrate along the developing gastrointestinal tract to give rise to the majority of the ENS [54–56]. The capacity to rescue the ENS appears to be limited to NC cells fated to give rise to the ENS itself [57] and although there is some data to suggest that vagal NC have some therapeutic potential [58], the most promising avenue appears to be the use of NC derivatives isolated from the gut.

Enteric Neural Crest Stem Cells (ENS Stem Cells)

Nonhuman studies: Several studies have demonstrated that multipotent cells, with the ability to form the ENS when transplanted to uncolonized, or aganglionic gut, are present within the gastrointestinal tract during development and into postnatal life [59–64], including from the ganglionic portion of the gut from a HSCR mouse model (miRet51) [65–67]. The methodology used to isolate such cells is the culture of dissociated gut to give rise to neurospheres or neurosphere-like bodies (NLBs), akin to stem cell-containing CNS neurospheres. In addition to differentiated neurons and glia, NLBs also contain proliferating undifferentiated cells that not only express putative stem cell markers (e.g., Sox10), but are also capable of self-renewal and giving rise to both enteric neurons and glia. Grafting of postnatal NLBs into aganglionic embryonic mouse gut revealed that donor cells were able to colonize the gut and differentiate into appropriate enteric phenotypes, at the appropriate locations [65].

Recent in vivo studies have shown that ENS stem or progenitor cells have the potential to migrate, proliferate, and differentiate into appropriate phenotypes when transplanted into the colon of postnatal mice [68]. Such cells isolated from the embryonic (E14.5) mice gut survived for at least 16 weeks, and formed enteric ganglion-like clusters containing neurons and glia. Graft-derived neurons expressed some enteric neuron subtype markers, including NOS, ChAT, calbindin, and calretinin [69]. Importantly, intracellular electrophysiological recordings from graft-derived neurons showed that they fired action potentials and received fast excitatory postsynaptic potentials (fEPSPs) demonstrating that the graft-derived neurons had incorporated into the enteric circuitry [69].

Human studies: A number of groups including ours have reported the harvesting of ENS stem cells from postnatal human gut [70–73]. Although initial studies suggested that this required full thickness tissue, our most recent work has shown that gut mucosal biopsies obtained by routine endoscopic procedures can be used as a source of stem cells [73]. Neurospheres were generated in cultures of mucosal tissue from endoscopic biopsies obtained from children from the neonatal period up to 16 years, including HSCR patients (Fig. 45.1). The neurospheres were equivalent to

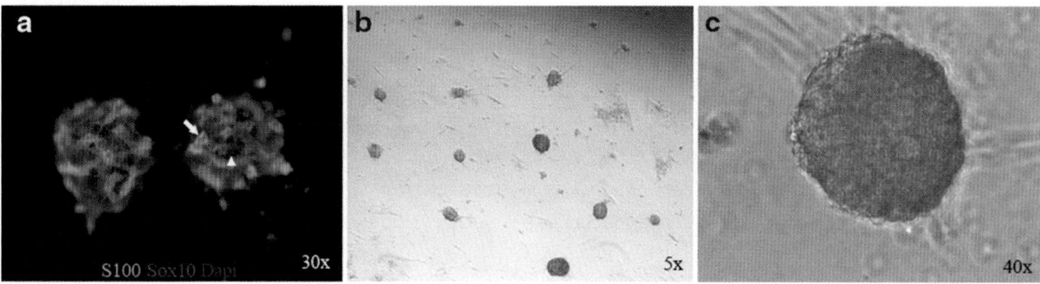

Fig. 45.1 Enteric neural stem cell-containing neurospheres can be harvested from postnatal gut. (**a**) Fluorescent immunostaining of day 14 cell cultures generated from postnatal mouse gut showing the presence of spherical multicellular aggregates of cells, termed neurospheres. These contain cells positive for Sox10 (red) and for S100 (green). Positivity for both markers (arrow) suggests the presence of glial cells, whereas the presence of cells positive for Sox10 only (arrowheads) suggests neural crest derived undifferentiated progenitors or stem cells. (**b** and **c**) Low power (**b**) and high-power (**c**) bright field images of cell cultures (day 21) generated from dissociated human colonic mucosal biopsies obtained from a 6 year old patient by conventional endoscopy. The cultures show numerous characteristic neurospheres, which have been shown to contain enteric neural stem cells and can be transplanted into recipient gut

those generated from human embryonic and full thickness postnatal gut tissue and contained putative ENS stem cells. When transplanted into segments of aganglionic gut, including human HSCR maintained in vitro, the neurosphere-derived cells colonized the recipient gut and generated neuronal phenotypes. These studies highlight a significant advance by identifying a regenerating source of tissue to generate ENS stem cells and confirming the feasibility of autologous transplantation. Although there is data that suggests that transplanted human cells are capable of influencing mouse embryonic gut function [72], current studies are more robustly assessing functional rescue of recipient postnatal gut following ENS stem cell transplantation in vivo.

Most recently, the development of newer endoscopic techniques that allow the acquisition of full thickness gut wall biopsies may enable harvesting of stem cells from all the layers of ENS plexuses overcoming potential limitations of sourcing cells from any one [74].

Practical Challenges in Developing Cell Therapies

Although there has been much progress in the sourcing of cells with potential for therapy for gut motility disorders, some key challenges still need addressing before effective clinical application.

What is the ideal target disease? HSCR has provided the archetypal disease for ENS stem cell therapy. The ENS deficiency (distal intestinal aganglionosis), however, is absolute and extensive, and it is unclear whether replenisment of the complex ENS circuitry is truly achievable. In view of this, perhaps disorders with a less severe anatomical or functional phenotype may be more amenable to therapy.

In esophageal achalasia, in the early stages of disease, functional and presumably neuronal loss appear more restricted to the lower esophagal sphincter presenting a smaller therapeutic target. The underlying immunologically mediated pathogenic processes [75], however, may need to be controlled prior to transplantation to prevent destruction of a neo-ENS. In intestinal pseudoobstruction and slow transit constipation the overall ENS "scaffold" appears intact but is clearly dysfunctional possibly due to deficiencies of particular elements of the neuromuscular circuitry [76–78]. These elements, once identified, may be easier to replenish than the entire ENS. Generalized involvement of the long gastrointestinal tract may, however, limit success, as would potential limitations in migration of transplanted cells [79, 80]. It is clear that all these potential disease targets need more detailed characterization of their specific defects and etiology prior to the development of any tailored replensihment strategies. Recent international initiatives to address these hold promise [81].

It should be noted that complete ENS restitution may not be necessary. Studies of the ageing gut, where despite substantial neuronal loss, a scanty surviving ENS functions in the absence of any overt functional obstruction, suggest that partial ENS reconstitution may be sufficient to restore some balance between inhibitory and excitatory influences within the neuropathic gut [82, 83]. This suggests that delivery of smaller number of appropriate cells may be an acceptable therapeutic goal.

What is the ideal cell type? It is likely that the therapeutic requirement for individual disorders will determine which cell source is most suitable, e.g., whether to use multipotent stem cells (e.g., from hES, iPS) or more committed neuronal precursors (e.g., "adult stem cells" or precursors sourced from gut). Limitations exist for each source ranging from uncontrolled proliferation and tumor formation (ES cells) to restricted harvesting and differentiation potential (adult stem cells).

The production of unlimited quantities of enteric neurons by direct induction of ES cells remains an exciting possibility, but there remains concern about their potential to form tumors [21, 84] and unwanted cell types. Strategies have been proposed to prevent this including partially differentiating ES cells, enriching for appropriate cell types and then screening for undifferentiated cells [84–86]. Certainly it would be advantageous to differentiate them into specific neuronal subtypes before transplantation. Protocols for such specific differentiation from each stem cell type have yet to be established although some progress has been made. Stem cells from fetal brain (CNS–NSCs) also have the ability to divide, form neurospheres and differentiate into neurons, and non-neuronal cells [45, 87]. Micci et al. have reported that CNS–NSCs preferentially differentiate into nNOS neurons [47, 88], which may be promising for conditions such as esophageal achalasia. For many patients, clinical practitioners and the general public at large, however, there are ethical problems associated with the use of hES cells and CNS–NSCs from fertilized human eggs and aborted fetal brain tissues, respectively.

Much focus has therefore shifted onto "adult" stem cells, especially given their presumed role in maintaining and repairing the tissue in which they are found and restricted potential to generate only those cell types (e.g., neurons and glia) of the required tissue (e.g., ENS), which limits the need for cell programming and reducing the risk of generating "ectopic" cell types and malignancy. Such cells, however, are present within much smaller number and appear to have a reduced potential to proliferate. Kruger et al. reported that NC stem cells comprise only <0.2% of cells within the gut wall of postnatal day 22 rats [64] and human studies have suggested that the generation of ENS stem cell-containing neurospheres declines with increasing postnatal age [73]. Although it is possible to enrich and expand neural stem cells obtained from the ENS [65, 70–73], it is not known whether the therapeutic potential is compromised with prolonged in vitro propagation. The paucity of specific markers for stem cells presents a further potential obstacle for the field. ENS stem cell harvesting has largely been restricted to their isolation within neurospheres, structures composed of a heterogenous mix of cells consisting of, in addition to the stem cells, differentiated cells including neurons, glia, and smooth muscle cells [65, 73]. Although it may be argued that pure isolation of stem cells is perhaps not necessary as neurospheres exist as potential readymade stem cells niches and complete therapeutic packages capable of colonizing aganglionic gut [65, 71, 73], unless specific isolation is possible the manipulation within, and generation of targeted cell types from, this heterogenous pool is likely to be a major problem.

One of the most exciting developments in stem cell science has been the generation of induced pluripotent stem (iPS) cells by the reprogramming of mouse embryonic or adult fibroblasts back to a pluripotent state by introducing four transcriptional factors—Oct4, Sox2, Klf4, and c-Myc [89]. Successful reprogramming of differentiated human somatic cells into a pluripotent state raised the possibility of creating patient-derived stem cells [90], which would bypass both immunological problems and bioethical issues associated with hES cells or those obtained from fetal brains. In terms of the gastrointestinal tract, iPS cells can produce intestinal tissue and gut-like structures in vitro. Three-dimensional intestinal organoids were derived from human iPS cells using activin A treatment to induce endoderm formation, followed by FGF4 and WNT3A manipulations to develop hindgut and intestinal specification [91]. Gut-like structures can also be derived from mouse iPS cells that contain a lumen with three distinct layers (epithelium, connective tissue, and muscle layer), neuronal networks, and ICCs, which exhibited spontaneous contractions [92]. It is unknown whether iPS cell-derived gut-like structures or neurons will have any therapeutic relevance for the treatment of enteric neuropathies. Studies will be required to elucidate the mechanisms of reprogramming of somatic cells into enteric neurons using exogeneously delivered transcription factors, and to establish a method of purifying desired cells with 100% frequency in vitro.

Is cell manipulation prior to transplantation likley to be necessary? The finding that stem cells can be generated from innervated or ganglionic portions of diseased gut makes it likely that in some cases, especially with autologous transplantation, that genetic modification of the cells may be necessary and possible before transplantation. Stem cells derived from the normo-ganglionic part of HSCR gut are likely to have defective biological function, underlining the inability of their predecessors to form a complete or functional ENS [93]. Indeed, enteric progenitors isolated from the monoisoformic Ret51 (miRet51) HSCR mouse model show delayed differentiation compared to controls [66]. These defective cells appear to be rescued by genetic manipulation, given that re-introducing the Ret^9 isoform within the $miRet^{51}$ ENS progenitor cells reverses the differentiation deficits (Natarajan and Pachnis, personal communication).

Injection of stem cells supplied with some missing neurotrophic factors might also be needed for their survival, migration, and differentiation [17]. Recent data suggests this may be possible. Endothelin 3, for example, inhibits reversibly the commitment and differentiation of ENS progenitor cells along the neurogenic and gliogenic lineages, suggesting a role for this factor in the maintenance of multilineage ENS progenitors [94]. Glial cell line-derived neurotrophic factor (GDNF) acting in the presence or absence of Endothelin 3 significantly increased the proliferation of ENS progenitors as well as increasing neurite outgrowth [65, 95]. Such findings and studies have enormous implications for pre-transplantation priming of ENS stem cells as well as the creation of receptive environments within recipient aganglionic gut.

Is the gut environment suitable for cell replenishment? In HSCR the average aganglionic segment measures almost 10 cm. Yet data from several groups including ours suggest that longitudinal migration of transplanted cells within recipient embryonic gut maintained in organ culture may be limited to a few millimeters at best [73]. Limited migratory ability of grafted stem cells appears special important in adolescent or older patients, where the mesenchyme is already well differentiated [47, 79, 80]. It is possible that the local gut environment of patients with congenital gut motility disorders might be defective and/or not be permissive for the grafts to survive or differentiate into appropriate cell types. For example, there are reports of decreased expression of GDNF in the aganglionic region of patients even with no mutation of GDNF [96]. GDNF has consistently been implicated in the process of directed migration of NC-derived ENS progenitors to facilitate colonization of the developing gut during embryogenesis [97, 98]. Therefore, similar to donor cells, the recipient gut may also require pre-treatment to optimize transplant success. More work needs to be done to confirm that pre-treatment of cells, the recipient gut or patients themselves does not have any adverse effects in other aspects of the health of patients.

Finally, immunological rejection of transplanted cells within the gut is also likely to be a problem [99] (Hotta, personal communication). This may well be overcome with improving protocols of immunosupression already in use with solid organ and cellular transplatation and use of autologous transplantation.

What is the most effective route to deliver cell therapy to the gut? The gut is easier to access compared to the brain or spinal cord and cells have been introduced into the gut wall of animals through the serosa via laparotomy [47–49, 58].

Stems cells have also been injected intraperitoneally into animals to replace enteric neurons, but further work is needed to identify all the sites colonized by using this method [58, 100]. A recent study has revealed the potential of NC stem cells to give rise to a small number of neurons and glial cells when injected into the peritoneal cavity of *Ednrb*$^{sl/sl}$ rat, but none of the injected cells were found in the aganglionic colon [100]. Injecting cells intravenously can allow cells to be delivered to a broader area which would be an advantage over mulitple injections. However, the vasculature has not yet been explored extensively as a delivery route for cells to gut.

Endoscopy is routinely practised to deliver drugs into the gut wall. This may be a better way for not only harvesting cells but also for their delivery into recipient guts especially when combined with imaging techniques for better precision (e.g., ultrasound, confocal). Disadvantages include the need to intubate entire segments of diseased gastrointestinal tract, some of which, e.g., mid-small intestine remain relatively inaccessible, and would require more complicated enteroscopy techniques.

What is the best measure of the success of cell therapy? The main aim of replacement cell therapy is to restore some function to the diseased gut. Grafted human ENS stem cells have been reported to differentiate into glia and neuronal subtypes reminiscent of a functional ENS within explants of aneural hindgut from chick and mouse embryos [72, 73]. Lindley et al. further reported that the newly generated neurons formed synapses and were able to regulate the rate of contraction of the recipient guts [72].

Although it is clear that further studies are required to determine whether introduced stem cells integrate into the circuitry of a preexisting ENS when introduced into a ganglionic region, or form an ENS with the appropriate circuitry to produce functional recovery when introduced into aganglionic regions, it is likely that functional data will only truly be understood within the context of in vivo studies, studying parameters ranging from simple gut transit to definitive measurements of peristaltic activity and sphincter function.

Summary and Future Directions

Cell therapy for gastrointestinal motility disorders is an exciting and promising prospect. The ENS has many potential advantages that favor the success of transplantation therapies. These include accessibility to both source and deliver cells, as well as the possibility of minimizing immunological rejection by expanding neural stem cells, obtained from unaffected regions of the intestine, for autologous transplantation.

The evidence to date suggests that cells with the potential of generating components of the ENS can be harvested from a range of allogeneic and autologous sources, have their biological properties manipulated, and ultimately be transplanted into diseased or dysmotile gut to replenish components of the ENS and rescue function. Although a number of significant hurdles remain, which will all need to be addressed, all is perhaps not so bleak. Aging-related neuronal loss is not associated with functional failure giving hope that restitution of a full normal ENS is perhaps not needed. Gene therapy is already established in clinical therapies and rescue of defective ENS stem cells derived from murine models of HSCR possible. Tissue transplantation and management of immunological aspects is well studied and potentially overcome with use of autologous transplantation. Recent work has shown that minimally invasive procedures such as endoscopy can be used to isolate ENS stem cells from a regenerating source of intestinal tissue and ultimately to deliver them back into gut. Transplantation of such cells into models of aganglionic gut suggests they are capable of colonization, generating components of the ENS, and effecting functional change. Although pleasing progress has been seen with enteric neuropathies, other motility disorders such as myopathies and mesenchymopathies will need to see similar initiatives in terms of understanding disease pathogenesis, pathology and ultimately cellular therapies.

There is no doubt that children and adults with gut motility disorders represent a significant challenge in management. Significant strides have been made in teasing away at the processes that underlie the complex workings of the gut neuromusculature, especially the ENS, and have given us tremendous insight into pathogenesis and the identification of putative treatments. Cellular therapies should now be considered alongside these and perhaps herald a shift towards definitive cures for gut motility disorders.

References

1. Duran B. The effects of long-term total parenteral nutrition on gut mucosal immunity in children with short bowel syndrome: a systematic review. BMC Nurs. 2005;4:2.
2. Guglielmi FW, Boggio-Bertinct D, Federico A, et al. Total parenteral nutrition-related gastroenterological complications. Dig Liver Dis. 2006;38:623–42.
3. Heneyke S, Smith VV, Spitz L, Milla PJ. Chronic intestinal pseudo-obstruction: treatment and long term follow up of 44 patients. Arch Dis Child. 1999;81:21–7.
4. Mousa H, Hyman PE, Cocjin J, Flores AF, Di Lorenzo C. Long-term outcome of congenital intestinal pseudoobstruction. Dig Dis Sci. 2002;47:2298–305.
5. Kelly DA. Intestinal failure-associated liver disease: what do we know today? Gastroenterology. 2006;130:S70–7.
6. Revel-Vilk S. Central venous line-related thrombosis in children. Acta Haematol. 2006;115:201–6.
7. Tsuji H, Spitz L, Kiely EM, Drake DP, Pierro A. Management and long-term follow-up of infants with total colonic aganglionosis. J Pediatr Surg. 1999;34:158–61. discussion 162.
8. Ludman L, Spitz L, Tsuji H, Pierro A. Hirschsprung's disease: functional and psychological follow up comparing total colonic and rectosigmoid aganglionosis. Arch Dis Child. 2002;86:348–51.
9. Conway SJ, Craigie RJ, Cooper LH, et al. Early adult outcome of the Duhamel procedure for left-sided Hirschsprung disease—a prospective serial assessment study. J Pediatr Surg. 2007;42:1429–32.
10. Catto-Smith AG, Trajanovska M, Taylor RG. Long-term continence after surgery for Hirschsprung's disease. J Gastroenterol Hepatol. 2007;22:2273–82.
11. Pini Prato A, Gentilino V, Giunta C, et al. Hirschsprung's disease: 13 years' experience in 112 patients from a single institution. Pediatric Surg Int. 2008;24:175–82.
12. Burns AJ, Pasricha PJ, Young HM. Enteric neural crest-derived cells and neural stem cells: biology and therapeutic potential. Neurogastroenterol Motil. 2004;16 Suppl 1:3–7.
13. Heanue TA, Pachnis V. Enteric nervous system development and Hirschsprung's disease: advances in genetic and stem cell studies. Nat Rev. 2007;8:466–79.
14. Lindvall O, Kokaia Z, Martinez-Serrano A. Stem cell therapy for human neurodegenerative disorders-how to make it work. Nat Med. 2004;10(Suppl):S42–50.
15. Young HM. Neural stem cell therapy and gastrointestinal biology. Gastroenterology. 2005;129:2092–5.
16. Micci MA, Pasricha PJ. Neural stem cells for the treatment of disorders of the enteric nervous system: strategies and challenges. Dev Dyn. 2007;236:33–43.
17. Schafer KH, Micci MA, Pasricha PJ. Neural stem cell transplantation in the enteric nervous system: roadmaps and roadblocks. Neurogastroenterol Motil. 2009;21:103–12.
18. Wobus AM, Boheler KR. Embryonic stem cells: prospects for developmental biology and cell therapy. Physiol Rev. 2005;85:635–78.
19. Evans MJ, Kaufman MH. Establishment in culture of pluripotential cells from mouse embryos. Nature. 1981;292:154–6.
20. Martin GR. Isolation of a pluripotent cell line from early mouse embryos cultured in medium conditioned by teratocarcinoma stem cells. Proc Natl Acad Sci USA. 1981;78:7634–8.
21. Thomson JA, Itskovitz-Eldor J, Shapiro SS, et al. Embryonic stem cell lines derived from human blastocysts. Science. 1998;282:1145–7.
22. Wichterle H, Lieberam I, Porter JA, Jessell TM. Directed differentiation of embryonic stem cells into motor neurons. Cell. 2002;110:385–97.
23. Li XJ, Du ZW, Zarnowska ED, et al. Specification of motoneurons from human embryonic stem cells. Nat Biotechnol. 2005;23:215–21.
24. Kawasaki H, Mizuseki K, Nishikawa S, et al. Induction of midbrain dopaminergic neurons from ES cells by stromal cell-derived inducing activity. Neuron. 2000;28:31–40.
25. Lee SH, Lumelsky N, Studer L, Auerbach JM, McKay RD. Efficient generation of midbrain and hindbrain neurons from mouse embryonic stem cells. Nat Biotechnol. 2000;18:675–9.
26. Zeng X, Cai J, Chen J, et al. Dopaminergic differentiation of human embryonic stem cells. Stem Cells. 2004;22:925–40.
27. Mizuseki K, Sakamoto T, Watanabe K, et al. Generation of neural crest-derived peripheral neurons and floor plate cells from mouse and primate embryonic stem cells. Proc Natl Acad Sci USA. 2003;100:5828–33.
28. Pomp O, Brokhman I, Ben-Dor I, Reubinoff B, Goldstein RS. Generation of peripheral sensory and sympathetic neurons and neural crest cells from human embryonic stem cells. Stem Cells. 2005;23:923–30.
29. Hotta R, Pepdjonovic L, Anderson RB, et al. Small-molecule induction of neural crest-like cells derived from human neural progenitors. Stem Cells. 2009;27:2896–905.
30. Kawaguchi J, Nichols J, Gierl MS, Faial T, Smith A. Isolation and propagation of enteric neural crest progenitor cells from mouse embryonic stem cells and embryos. Development. 2010;137:693–704.

31. Yamada T, Yoshikawa M, Takaki M, et al. In vitro functional gut-like organ formation from mouse embryonic stem cells. Stem Cells. 2002;20:41–9.
32. Kuwahara M, Ogaeri T, Matsuura R, Kogo H, Fujimoto T, Torihashi S. In vitro organogenesis of gut-like structures from mouse embryonic stem cells. Neurogastroenterol Motil. 2004;16 Suppl 1:14–8.
33. Matsuura R, Kogo H, Ogaeri T, et al. Crucial transcription factors in endoderm and embryonic gut development are expressed in gut-like structures from mouse ES cells. Stem Cells. 2006;24:624–30.
34. Takaki M, Nakayama S, Misawa H, Nakagawa T, Kuniyasu H. In vitro formation of enteric neural network structure in a gut-like organ differentiated from mouse embryonic stem cells. Stem Cells. 2006;24:1414–22.
35. Torihashi S, Kuwahara M, Ogaeri T, Zhu P, Kurahashi M, Fujimoto T. Gut-like structures from mouse embryonic stem cells as an in vitro model for gut organogenesis preserving developmental potential after transplantation. Stem Cells. 2006;24:2618–26.
36. Konuma N, Wakabayashi K, Matsumoto T, et al. Mouse embryonic stem cells give rise to gut-like morphogenesis, including intestinal stem cells, in the embryoid body model. Stem Cells Dev. 2008;18(1):113–26.
37. Young HM, Newgreen DF, Burns AJ. Development of the enteric nervous system in relation to Hirschsprung's disease. In: Ferretti P, Copp A, Tickle C, Moore G, editors. Embryos, genes and birth defects. Chichester: John Wiley and Sons Ltd; 2006. p. 263–300.
38. Rousselot P, Lois C, Alvarez-Buylla A. Embryonic (PSA) N-CAM reveals chains of migrating neuroblasts between the lateral ventricle and the olfactory bulb of adult mice. J Comp Neurol. 1995;351:51–61.
39. Kempermann G, Kuhn HG, Gage FH. More hippocampal neurons in adult mice living in an enriched environment. Nature. 1997;386:493–5.
40. Doetsch F, Caille I, Lim DA, Garcia-Verdugo JM, Alvarez-Buylla A. Subventricular zone astrocytes are neural stem cells in the adult mammalian brain. Cell. 1999;97:703–16.
41. Cameron HA, Woolley CS, McEwen BS, Gould E. Differentiation of newly born neurons and glia in the dentate gyrus of the adult rat. Neuroscience. 1993;56:337–44.
42. Gould E, Reeves AJ, Graziano MS, Gross CG. Neurogenesis in the neocortex of adult primates. Science. 1999;286:548–52.
43. Gould E, Reeves AJ, Fallah M, Tanapat P, Gross CG, Fuchs E. Hippocampal neurogenesis in adult Old World primates. Proc Natl Acad Sci USA. 1999;96:5263–7.
44. Eriksson PS, Perfilieva E, Bjork-Eriksson T, et al. Neurogenesis in the adult human hippocampus. Nat Med. 1998;4:1313–7.
45. Morrison SJ. Neuronal potential and lineage determination by neural stem cells. Curr Opin Cell Biol. 2001;13:666–72.
46. Temple S, Alvarez-Buylla A. Stem cells in the adult mammalian central nervous system. Curr Opin Neurobiol. 1999;9:135–41.
47. Micci MA, Kahrig KM, Simmons RS, Sarna SK, Espejo-Navarro MR, Pasricha PJ. Neural stem cell transplantation in the stomach rescues gastric function in neuronal nitric oxide synthase-deficient mice. Gastroenterology. 2005;129:1817–24.
48. Dong YL, Liu W, Gao YM, et al. Neural stem cell transplantation rescues rectum function in the aganglionic rat. Transplant Proc. 2008;40:3646–52.
49. Liu W, Wu RD, Dong YL, Gao YM. Neuroepithelial stem cells differentiate into neuronal phenotypes and improve intestinal motility recovery after transplantation in the aganglionic colon of the rat. Neurogastroenterol Motil. 2007;19:1001–9.
50. Farlie PG, McKeown SJ, Newgreen DF. The neural crest: Basic biology and clinical relationships in the craniofacial and enteric nervous systems. Birth Defects Res C Embryo Today. 2004;72:173–89.
51. Le Douarin NM, Kalcheim C. The neural crest. Cambridge: Cambridge University Press; 1999.
52. Le Douarin NM, Teillet MA. The migration of neural crest cells to the wall of the digestive tract in avian embryo. J Embryol Exp Morphol. 1973;30:31–48.
53. Le Douarin NM, Teillet MA. Experimental analysis of the migration and differentiation of neuroblasts of the autonomic nervous system and of neurectodermal mesenchymal derivatives, using a biological cell marking technique. Dev Biol. 1974;41:162–84.
54. Newgreen D, Young HM. Enteric nervous system: development and developmental disturbances–part 2. Pediatr Dev Pathol. 2002;5:329–49.
55. Newgreen D, Young HM. Enteric nervous system: development and developmental disturbances-part 1. Pediatr Dev Pathol. 2002;5:224–47.
56. Burns AJ, Thapar N. Advances in ontogeny of the enteric nervous system. Neurogastroenterol Motil. 2006;18:876–87.
57. Mosher JT, Yeager KJ, Kruger GM, et al. Intrinsic differences among spatially distinct neural crest stem cells in terms of migratory properties, fate determination, and ability to colonize the enteric nervous system. Dev Biol. 2007;303:1–15.
58. Martucciello G, Brizzolara A, Favre A, et al. Neural crest neuroblasts can colonise aganglionic and ganglionic gut in vivo. Eur J Pediatr Surg. 2007;17:34–40.
59. Bixby S, Kruger G, Mosher J, Joseph N, Morrison S. Cell-intrinsic differences between stem cells from different regions of the peripheral nervous system regulate the generation of neural diversity. Neuron. 2002;35:643–56.
60. Lo L, Anderson DJ. Postmigratory neural crest cells expressing c-RET display restricted developmental and proliferative capacities. Neuron. 1995;15:527–39.
61. Morrison SJ, White PM, Zock C, Anderson DJ. Prospective identification, isolation by flow cytometry, and in vivo self-renewal of multipotent mammalian neural crest stem cells. Cell. 1999;96:737–49.

62. Natarajan D, Grigoriou M, Marcos-Gutierrez CV, Atkins C, Pachnis V. Multipotential progenitors of the mammalian enteric nervous system capable of colonising aganglionic bowel in organ culture. Development. 1999;126:157–68.
63. Sidebotham EL, Kenny SE, Lloyd DA, Vaillant CR, Edgar DH. Location of stem cells for the enteric nervous system. Pediatr Surg Int. 2002;18:581–5.
64. Kruger G, Mosher J, Bixby S, Joseph N, Iwashita T, Morrison S. Neural crest stem cells persist in the adult gut but undergo changes in self-renewal, neuronal subtype potential, and factor responsiveness. Neuron. 2002;35:657–69.
65. Bondurand N, Natarajan D, Thapar N, Atkins C, Pachnis V. Neuron and glia generating progenitors of the mammalian enteric nervous system isolated from foetal and postnatal gut cultures. Development. 2003;130:6387–400.
66. Thapar N, Natarajan D, Caldwell C, Burns AJ, Pachnis V. Isolation of enteric nervous system progenitors from Hirschsprung's-like gut. Neurogastroenterol Motil. 2006;18:663–798.
67. De Graaff E, Srinivas S, Kilkenny C, et al. Differential activities of the RET tyrosine kinase receptor isoforms during mammalian embryogenesis. Genes Dev. 2001;15:2433–44.
68. Hotta R, Stamp L, Thacker M, et al. Migration and differentiation of enteric neural stem/progenitor cells transplanted into the post-natal bowel in vivo. Gastroenterology. 2010;138 Suppl 1:S-109.
69. Stamp LA, Hotta R, Thacker M, et al. Migration and differentiation of neural stem/progenitor cells from the embryonic gut after transplantation to the post-natal mouse colon. Neurogastroenterol Motil. 2010;22(Suppl s1):6.
70. Rauch U, Hansgen A, Hagl C, Holland-Cunz S, Schafer KH. Isolation and cultivation of neuronal precursor cells from the developing human enteric nervous system as a tool for cell therapy in dysganglionosis. Int J Colorectal Dis. 2006;21:554–9.
71. Almond S, Lindley RM, Kenny SE, Connell MG, Edgar DH. Characterisation and transplantation of enteric nervous system progenitor cells. Gut. 2007;56:489–96.
72. Lindley RM, Hawcutt DB, Connell MG, et al. Human and mouse enteric nervous system neurosphere transplants regulate the function of aganglionic embryonic distal colon. Gastroenterology. 2008;135:205–16.
73. Metzger M, Caldwell C, Barlow AJ, Burns AJ, Thapar N. Enteric nervous system stem cells derived from human gut mucosa for the treatment of aganglionic gut disorders. Gastroenterology. 2009;136:2214–25.
74. Rajan E, Gostout CJ, Lurken MS, et al. Evaluation of endoscopic approaches for deep gastric-muscle-wall biopsies: what works? Gastrointest Endosc. 2008;67:297–303.
75. Park W, Vaezi MF. Etiology and pathogenesis of achalasia: the current understanding. Am J Gastroenterol. 2005;100:1404–14.
76. Takahashi T. Pathophysiological significance of neuronal nitric oxide synthase in the gastrointestinal tract. J Gastroenterol. 2003;38:421–30.
77. Bassotti G, Villanacci V. Slow transit constipation: a functional disorder becomes an enteric neuropathy. World J Gastroenterol. 2006;12:4609–13.
78. De Giorgio R, Guerrini S, Barbara G, Cremon C, Stanghellini V, Corinaldesi R. New insights into human enteric neuropathies. Neurogastroenterol Motil. 2004;16 Suppl 1:143–7.
79. Druckenbrod NR, Epstein ML. Age-dependent changes in the gut environment restrict the invasion of the hindgut by enteric neural progenitors. Development. 2009;136:3195–203.
80. Hotta R, Anderson RB, Kobayashi K, Newgreen DF, Young HM. Effects of tissue age, presence of neurones and endothelin-3 on the ability of enteric neurone precursors to colonize recipient gut: implications for cell-based therapies. Neurogastroenterol Motil. 2010;22:331–86.
81. Knowles CH, De Giorgio R, Kapur RP, et al. The London Classification of gastrointestinal neuromuscular pathology: report on behalf of the Gastro 2009 International Working Group. Gut. 2010;59:882–7.
82. Thrasivoulou C, Soubeyre V, Ridha H, et al. Reactive oxygen species, dietary restriction and neurotrophic factors in age-related loss of myenteric neurons. Aging Cell. 2006;5:247–57.
83. Wade PR, Hornby PJ. Age-related neurodegenerative changes and how they affect the gut. Sci Aging Knowledge Environ. 2005;2005:pe8.
84. Murry CE, Keller G. Differentiation of embryonic stem cells to clinically relevant populations: lessons from embryonic development. Cell. 2008;132:661–80.
85. Laflamme MA, Chen KY, Naumova AV, et al. Cardiomyocytes derived from human embryonic stem cells in pro-survival factors enhance function of infarcted rat hearts. Nat Biotechnol. 2007;25:1015–24.
86. Mountford JC. Human embryonic stem cells: origins, characteristics and potential for regenerative therapy. Transfus Med. 2008;18:1–12.
87. Suhonen JO, Peterson DA, Ray J, Gage FH. Differentiation of adult hippocampus-derived progenitors into olfactory neurons in vivo. Nature. 1996;383:624–7.
88. Micci MA, Learish RD, Li H, Abraham BP, Pasricha PJ. Neural stem cells express RET, produce nitric oxide, and survive transplantation in the gastrointestinal tract. Gastroenterology. 2001;121:757–66.
89. Takahashi K, Yamanaka S. Induction of pluripotent stem cells from mouse embryonic and adult fibroblast cultures by defined factors. Cell. 2006;126:663–76.
90. Takahashi K, Tanabe K, Ohnuki M, et al. Induction of pluripotent stem cells from adult human fibroblasts by defined factors. Cell. 2007;131:861–72.
91. Spence JR, Mayhew CN, Rankin SA, et al. Directed differentiation of human pluripotent stem cells into intestinal tissue in vitro. Nature. 2011;470:105–9.

92. Ueda T, Yamada T, Hokuto D, et al. Generation of functional gut-like organ from mouse induced pluripotent stem cells. Biochem Biophys Res Commun. 2010;391:38–42.
93. Iwashita T, Kruger GM, Pardal R, Kiel MJ, Morrison SJ. Hirschsprung disease is linked to defects in neural crest stem cell function. Science. 2003;301:972–6.
94. Bondurand N, Natarajan D, Barlow A, Thapar N, Pachnis V. Maintenance of mammalian enteric nervous system progenitors by SOX10 and endothelin 3 signalling. Development. 2006;133:2075–86.
95. Barlow A, de Graaff E, Pachnis V. Enteric nervous system progenitors are coordinately controlled by the G protein-coupled receptor EDNRB and the receptor tyrosine kinase RET. Neuron. 2003;40:905–16.
96. Martucciello G, Thompson H, Mazzola C, et al. GDNF deficit in Hirschsprung's disease. J Pediatr Surg. 1998;33:99–102.
97. Natarajan D, Marcos-Gutierrez C, Pachnis V, de Graaff E. Requirement of signalling by receptor tyrosine kinase RET for the directed migration of enteric nervous system progenitor cells during mammalian embryogenesis. Development. 2002;129:5151–60.
98. Young HM, Hearn CJ, Farlie PG, Canty AJ, Thomas PQ, Newgreen DF. GDNF is a chemoattractant for enteric neural cells. Dev Biol. 2001;229:503–16.
99. Micci MA, Pattillo MT, Kahrig KM, Pasricha PJ. Caspase inhibition increases survival of neural stem cells in the gastrointestinal tract. Neurogastroenterol Motil. 2005;17:557–64.
100. Tsai YH, Murakami N, Gariepy CE. Postnatal intestinal engraftment of prospectively selected enteric neural crest stem cells in a rat model of Hirschsprung disease. Neurogastroenterol Motil. 2011;23:362–9.
101. Ishikawa T, Nakayama S, Nakagawa T, et al. Characterization of in vitro gutlike organ formed from mouse embryonic stem cells. Am J Physiol Cell Physiol. 2004;286:C1344–52.
102. Anitha M, Joseph I, Ding X, et al. Characterization of fetal and postnatal enteric neuronal cell lines with improvement in intestinal neural function. Gastroenterology. 2008;134:1424–35.
103. Heanue TA, Pachnis V. Prospective identification and isolation of enteric nervous system progenitors using SOX2. Stem Cells. 2011;29:128–40.

46 Chronic Intestinal Pseudo-obstruction Syndrome: Surgical Approach and Intestinal Transplantation

Olivier Goulet and Sabine Irtan

Chronic intestinal pseudo-obstruction syndrome (CIPO) is a severe, often unrecognized cause of neonatal or post-natal progressive intestinal failure (IF). This rare syndrome represents one of the main causes of IF and is characterized by impairment of physical growth and development as well as by a high rate of morbidity and mortality.

The diagnosis of CIPO is based on typical clinical manifestations, radiological evidence of distended bowel loops with air-fluid levels, and the exclusion of any organic obstruction of the gut lumen [1–5]. CIPO is often unrecognized, and the diagnosis, therefore, delayed by several years with useless and potentially dangerous surgeries.

CIPO can occur in patients with underlying diseases associated with gastrointestinal manifestations (scleroderma, amyloidosis, hypothyroidism, etc.) or be secondary to water-electrolyte disorders (e.g., hypokalemia), and toxic, viral, and parasitic causes. Most cases are idiopathic and sporadic, even though familial forms with either dominant or recessive autosomal inheritance have been described. Based on histological features intestinal pseudo-obstruction is classified into three main groups: neuropathies, and myopathies or "mesenchymopathies," according to the predominant involvement of enteric neurones, smooth muscle cells, and interstitial cells of Cajal, respectively [6–14]. Mitochondrial disorders have been reported [15, 16]. Regardless of the histologic type, CIPO always involves alterations of smooth muscle contractile function, leading to abnormal intestinal tract peristalsis and nutritional disorders. Manometry can play a supportive role in defining the diagnosis, as well as by showing differences in the manometric pattern of CIPO [17]. Accompanying uropathies must be sought in patients with CIPO [6, 18]. The clinical impact of these uropathies may be important and require specific management by using daily drainage and, sometimes, vesicostomy.

Longitudinal surveys have been published, including a large multicenter French pediatric study [19–23]. Long-term outcomes are generally poor despite surgical and medical therapies and characterized by disabling and potentially life-threatening complications. Treatment of CIPO involves nutritional, pharmacological, and surgical therapies but is often frustrating and does not change the natural course in the majority of cases [24–27]. Nutritional management is of crucial importance in the pediatric age group and involves enteral delivery of special formulae, by nasogastric tube, percutaneous gastrostomy, or

O. Goulet, M.D., Ph.D. (✉)
Department of Pediatric, Gastroenterology Hepatology and Nutrition, National Reference Center for Rare Digestive Diseases, Hospital Necker-Enfants Malades, University of Paris Descartes,
149 rue de Sèvres 75015, Paris, France
e-mail: olivier.goulet@nck.aphp.fr

S. Irtan, M.D.
Pediatric Surgery, Hôpital Necker-Enfants Malades, University of Paris, Paris, France

C. Faure et al. (eds.), *Pediatric Neurogastroenterology: Gastrointestinal Motility and Functional Disorders in Children*, Clinical Gastroenterology,
DOI 10.1007/978-1-60761-709-9_46, © Springer Science+Business Media New York 2013

jejunostomy [26]. In the most severe cases, parenteral nutrition becomes mandatory in order to satisfy nutritional requirements and appropriately manage obstructive episodes.

Surgery is one of the mainstays of CIPO therapeutic management. Surgery is performed in a variety of situations in pediatric patients but surgical options must be evaluated carefully. There is no consensus regarding indications and procedures. This short chapter aims to review the main situations in which surgery may be required.

Surgery for Diagnosis

Variable clinical presentation and lack of other specific diagnostic tests often leads to surgery being required for diagnosis. Nevertheless, unnecessary laparotomy could be avoided since diagnosis is mostly based on clinical and radiological symptoms of intestinal obstruction. It is not unusual, however, for some patients, especially children and adolescents with an acute presentation, to undergo an exploratory laparotomy. In the absence of organic obstruction observed at this laparotomy, we suggest that a medico-surgical discussion be undertaken to consider:

- Performing intestinal full-thickness biopsies at different levels for histopathologic analysis
- Performing an enterostomy according to the level of intestinal distension

In reality, in most cases, the acute presentation and subsequent surgical procedure do not occur at a specialized center, and these suggested interventions are not done. Such issues are controversial but we do propose that if the diagnosis of CIPO is strongly suggested from the surgical exploration, careful biopsies should be performed. Regarding enterostomy, our experience tends to suggest that if it is not performed at first laparotomy, it will need to be done later but with subsequent increased risk of peritoneal adhesions.

In summary, patients with evidence of CIPO from clinical and radiological presentation should not be operated on to make the diagnosis. Patients who undergo laparotomy for enterostomy because of permanent or recurrent intestinal obstruction should have intestinal full-thickness biopsies for specific diagnosis. This should be done regardless of the patient's age.

Gastrostomy Tubing

Bowel decompression by a gastrostomy and/or jejunostomy is often required. Repeated acute episodes of bowel obstruction as well as chronic intestinal distension require bowel decompression by using nasogastric suction. The placement of a venting gastrostomy is of great benefit in avoiding the recurrent placement of nasogastric tubes. When surgery is required, a gastrostomy may be performed during the same surgical procedure. If a gastrostomy is not surgically placed, percutaneous endoscopic gastrostomy tube (GT) placement is easily achieved in these children. Since enteral feeding should always be preferred to using parenteral nutrition (PN), intragastric administration of feeding may be achieved by the GT as continuous or bolus enteral tube feeding.

Enterostomy

In neonates and young infants, intestinal obstruction may last several weeks requiring total parenteral nutrition (TPN) with subsequent complications including catheter-related sepsis and liver disease [4]. Enterostomy may offer the chance to restart intestinal transit allowing feeding and reducing the need for PN.

In some patients, attacks of intestinal obstruction are frequent and/or life threatening. Chronic bowel dilatation impairs intestinal motility creating a vicious circle which increases intraluminal bacterial overgrowth with the subsequent risk of intestinal translocation, enterotoxin release, and liver disease [28, 29]. Enterostomy should be performed to bypass the functional obstruction and obtain digestive decompression.

The location of the enterostomy is a matter of debate. In cases of obvious megacystis microcolon syndrome, a terminal ileostomy is certainly required. Otherwise, we do recommend performing a terminal ileostomy and avoiding a colostomy whatever the clinical presentation or histopathologic pattern. It is important to consider the so-called ileo-caecal brake as the segment that should be short-circuited. In our experience, all patients who first underwent a colostomy went on to have formation of a terminal ileostomy or jejunostomy.

The outcome after ileostomy or jejunostomy varies according to the location of the enterostomy and to the disease itself. The literature does not provide any evidence of a histopathology-related prognosis even if the survey reported by Henyeke et al. suggested worse prognosis of myopathies and that they all need ileostomies [22]. However, much fewer than 50% of patients improve after ileostomy by being weaned from PN. In our opinion, enterostomy, as distal as possible is the most logical approach. Terminal ileostomy usually enables transit to resume and leads to a major long-term reduction in obstructive episodes. We currently perform an ileostomy to obtain durable intestinal autonomy and PN weaning, with the future plan to do a total or subtotal colectomy with ileorectal or ileosigmoid pull-through [23].

Irtan et al. have reported stomal prolapse in children with chronic intestinal pseudo-obstruction as a frequent complication [30]. Twenty-two out of 34 (65%) CIPO children referred to their center between 1988 and 2008 had a stoma and were compared with 22 other children referred for another pathology necessitating a stoma. The incidence of stomal prolapse in CIPO children was 45% vs. 9% in non-CIPO children ($p=0.01$). Prolapse occurred between the first postoperative day and the tenth postoperative month, with a median of 2 months. Surgical management was required in 60%, with an intestinal necrosis rate of 20% leading to intestinal resection. The authors did not identify particular risk factors favoring stomal prolapse.

Percutaneous endoscopic cecostomy or colostomy (PEC) is increasingly proposed as an alternative to surgery to treat CIPO and relapsing sigmoid volvulus [31–34]. Cecostomies or even sigmoidostomies have been used to administer antegrade enemas when intractable constipation appears to be the prominent symptom. A few reports are available both in children and adults describing the indications, complications, and outcomes. A retrospective, single-center study involving eight adults was reported by Lynch et al. [33]. Six patients had CIPO and two had chronic constipation. Use in seven of eight cases resulted in clinical improvement with reduction of intestinal obstruction episodes and improved feed tolerance. One patient suffering chronic constipation required surgical removal of the percutaneous endoscopic cecostomy tube at 4 days for fecal spillage resulting in peritonitis despite successful tube placement. Removal of the cecostomy tube occurred in three of six cases of pseudo-obstruction (the other three remain in place). In the other patient with chronic constipation, clinical improvement occurred, but the patient died of underlying illness 21 days after placement. A case of acute stercoral peritonitis was reported [34]. At laparotomy, the colostomy flange was embedded in the abdominal wall but no pressure necrosis was found at the level of the colonic wall. This complication was likely related to inadvertent traction of the colostomy tube. Percutaneous endoscopic cecostomy is considered by some authors as a viable alternative to surgically or fluoroscopically placed cecostomy in a select group of patients with recurrent colonic pseudo-obstruction or chronic intractable constipation.

Closure of the Stoma

In children whom a decompression ileostomy has produced relief, but there is diffuse disease, the urge to re-establish connection with the defunctioned limb of the bowel should be resisted as this will only result in further episodes of obstruction. In other words, performing an ileostomy and closing it because of clinical improvement results in the patient undergoing two surgical procedures without resolution of the primary issues. This should be avoided. Conversely, in patients in which clear improvement from ileostomy is observed, with PN weaning and at least 2 years follow up on enteral tube feeding or oral feeding without exacerbations, total colectomy and ileorectal anastomosis with the Duhamel procedure may be considered. In our experience, two-third of the patients who underwent this procedure remain off PN for a long period of time [23].

Recurrent Laparotomies and Enterectomy

In the past, many patients underwent multiple surgical procedures. Unnecessary abdominal surgery in children with CIPO should be avoided because they bear the risk of prolonged postoperative ileus and developing adhesions, creating a diagnostic problem each time there is a new obstructive episode. Mechanical obstruction should be considered in patients with an enterostomy who continue to present with exacerbations of bowel obstruction. In an earlier study involving only seven patients, surgery was performed as a treatment 21 times with a mean of three procedures per patient [20]. This is similar to other data reported. In one study, 67 surgical procedures were performed in 22 patients [8], and in another study involving 105 pediatric infants and children, 71 patients underwent surgery during their illness, with 217 surgical procedures [21]. An ostomy was the most performed procedure. Surgery may cause adhesions, so interpretations of postoperative obstructive episodes are difficult. Exploratory laparotomy for obstruction should be performed only when a clear mechanical obstruction has been demonstrated which remains very difficult to assess. Signs of peritonitis, extreme dilatation and pain in association with specific episodes of obstruction point more towards mechanical rather than functional obstruction, and a laparotomy may be required to relieve it.

Patients with CIPO or chronic intractable constipation (CIC) may develop anatomical obstruction such as colonic volvulus, with presenting symptoms mimicking those of underlying pseudo-obstruction. Patient records of 8 children with colonic volvulus were retrospectively reviewed [35]. The mean age at presentation with colonic volvulus was 13.2±5.05 years. All patients presented with worsening of abdominal distension and pain. The mean duration of symptoms of colonic volvulus before seeking medical help was 4.2 days (range 1–7 days). Water-soluble contrast enema was the single most useful investigation for confirming the diagnosis. All patients required surgery. There was no mortality associated with colonic volvulus. Clinicians should be vigilant and include volvulus in the differential diagnosis of the acute onset of abdominal distension and pain in patients with CIPO and CIC. Delay in diagnosis can result in bowel ischemia and perforation.

Some patients, in whom there is segmental bowel dilatation but no evidence of mechanical obstruction, have been reported to benefit from segmental resections or to have improved following placement of a jejunostomy tube within the dilated loop [36, 37]. In our experience, the use of this jejunostomy button device for daily intermittent bowel decompression can effectively improve bowel function allowing decreased PN intake. However, one should consider the quality of life (QOL) of a child with three tubes and, for most of the time, a central line.

Patients suffering from CIPO clearly benefit from home parenteral nutrition (HPN) to maintain adequate nutritional status and general health [38]. However, permanent and severe intestinal dysmotility can seriously disturb the QOL to the point of making it intolerable. Subtotal enterectomy [39, 40] or bilateral thoracoscopic splanchnicectomy have been proposed in severe CIPO [41]. A retrospective study of eight patients with end-stage CIPO maintained on HPN and suffering from chronic occlusive symptoms refractory to medical treatment underwent extensive small bowel resection preserving less than 70 cm of total small bowel and less than 20 cm of ileum [40]. The jejunum was anastomosed either to the ileum or to the colon. Six patients were completely relieved from obstructive symptoms. Two patients needed a second operation to remove the residual ileum because of recurrent symptoms. Both were significantly improved and there was no postoperative death. All patients experienced a significant improvement in their QOL. Near total small bowel resection appears to be a safe and effective procedure in end-stage CIPO patients, refractory to optimal medical treatment.

The implantation of gastric or intestinal pacemakers aimed at improving motility constitutes a promising investigational approach in patients with severe motility disorders. The use of gastric electrical stimulation has been shown to significantly improve nausea and vomiting not only in patients with diabetic gastroparesis, but more recently also in three adult patients with familial and one with postsurgical CIPO with disabling nausea and vomiting [42]. The weekly vomiting frequency decreased from 24 before implantation of the gastric pacemaker to 6.9 after 12 months. The clinical response was unrelated to the presence of, or improvement in, delayed gastric emptying in these patients. Although placements of the electrodes along the anterolateral surface of the stomach was successful in most patients by laparoscopic implantation, the procedure was not without risk since the electrodes caused ileus necessitating explantation and short intestinal resection [42].

Intestinal Transplantation

Intestinal transplantation (ITx) has become a lifesaving procedure for patients with irreversible intestinal failure (IF) [43–45]. Indications for ITx include not only extreme short bowel syndromes but also all situations in which the small intestine is unable to achieve nutritional requirements; these include inborn errors of intestinal mucosa development (intestinal epithelial dysplasia, microvillus inclusion disease) or severe motility disorders such as CIPO [46–50]. Approved indications for ITx include liver dysfunction, loss of major venous access, frequent central line-related sepsis, and recurrent episodes of severe dehydration despite intravenous fluid management. Surgical options include transplantation of the isolated intestine, combined liver–intestine transplantation, or multivisceral transplantation of the stomach, duodenum, pancreas, and small bowel (with or without the liver). Immunosuppression for ITx is based on tacrolimus therapy, often with induction immunosuppression using antilymphocyte antibodies (e.g., antithymocyte antibody and alemtuzumab). Experience at centers of excellence demonstrate 1- and 5-year patient survival rates of 95% and 77%, respectively, with ongoing investigations focusing on lowering long-term causes of graft loss such as chronic rejection [45].

In many cases of CIPO, outcome is poor, with a constant risk of sepsis from intestinal bacterial overgrowth, and water-electrolytic disorders related to intraluminal fluid retention. ITx is the only definitive curative treatment especially when many medical and surgical attempts have failed. ITx with or without liver transplantation is required in patients with primary neuro-muscular disease and PN-related complications such as progressive or end-stage liver disease or for those whose intravenous access has become unreliable and precarious because of repeated sepsis and extensive thrombosis. Transplant procedures vary according to indication for liver transplant and based on the experience of the transplant surgical team [47–49]. Combined small bowel–liver transplantations or multivisceral transplantations including the stomach have been performed in refractory forms of CIPO associated with end-stage liver disease [47–49]. Multivisceral transplantation (MVTx) was reported in 16 children with a median age of 4 years [47]. Indications for MVTx were liver failure ($n=10$), loss of venous access ($n=3$), or sepsis ($n=3$). Modified MVTx without the liver was performed in six patients. Reported actuarial patient survival for 1 year/2 years were 57.1% to 88.9%/42.9% to 77.8% according to immunosuppressive regimens. Currently, none of the long-term survivors are on PN and all tolerate enteral feeding. Gastric emptying was substantially affected in one case. Bladder function did not improve in those with urinary retention problems. MVTx for CIPO offers a lifesaving option with excellent function of the transplanted pancreas and stomach among survivors.

ITx may represent the only definitive cure for patients with permanent intestinal failure due to CIPO. However, graft rejection, and immunosuppression-related lymphoproliferative disorders are more common than other organ transplants. It is not yet established whether the results of ITx achieved in CIPO patients are equivalent to those experienced with other causes of IF such as short gut syndrome, total aganglionosis, microvillous inclusion disease, or epithelial dysplasia [51]. Complications seem to be more common due to multiple previous abdominal surgeries, dysmotility of the stomach and esophagus, and extra-intestinal manifestations including associated anomalies of the urological, immune, and neurological systems. An extensive workup including a search for mitochondrial disorders should be performed before any discussion of ITx and careful consideration is required before transplantation is undertaken. Determining the extent of the disease process (which may involve any part of the gastrointestinal tract) and the type of organ transplantation required is mandatory. Early referral is essential on initial presentation of these patients to enable optimal medical care and ensure that transplantation remains an option [43, 52].

Ethical dilemmas may arise with children who will never be able to tolerate full enteral feeding. Some patients with severe CIPO may be disabled because of chronic, massive GI dilatation refractory to stomal decompression or partial enterectomy. The poor QOL might serve as an indication for ITx, and not the usual criteria, which include progressive liver disease, loss of vascular access, and repeated life-threatening sepsis. In any case, parents must be extensively informed about the risks of the procedure and about the outcomes of all decisions.

Conclusion

Primary CIPO is a rare condition with a variable clinical expression. Medical management remains difficult and prognosis poor. Histological studies are essential to classify the syndrome, even if manometric data are able to differentiate between myopathic and neuropathic forms, and although histological type does not appear to influence management and long-term outcome. A trained multidisciplinary team, including surgeons, gastroenterologists, nutritionists, and a home PN coordinator, should assume the management of these patients which may involve a PN program and transplant surgery. For many reasons (nutrition, prevention of infectious complications, etc.), an enterostomy (preferably an ileostomy) is often performed as one of the first therapeutic measures. The "permanent" surgical reconstruction, designed to be minimally obstructive, is only envisaged after a long period of stability and if possible when the child is weaned from long-term PN. Intestinal transplantation may be the last therapeutic option when all medical and surgical approaches have failed.

References

1. Byrne WJ, Cipel L, Euler AR, et al. Chronic idiopathic intestinal pseudo-obstruction syndrome in children clinical characteristics and prognosis. J Pediatr. 1977;90:585–9.
2. Rudolph CD, Hyman PE, Altschuler SM, et al. Diagnosis and treatment of chronic intestinal pseudo-obstruction in children: report of consensus workshop. J Pediatr Gastroenterol Nutr. 1997;24:102–12.
3. Krishnamurthy S, Schuffler MD. Pathology of neuromuscular disorders of the small intestine and colon. Gastroenterology. 1987;93:610–39.
4. Goulet O, Ruemmele F. Causes and management of intestinal failure in children. Gastroenterology. 2006;130(2 Suppl 1):S16–28.
5. Connor FL, Di Lorenzo C. Chronic intestinal pseudo-obstruction: assessment and management. Gastroenterology. 2006;130(2 Suppl 1):S29–36.
6. Kern IB, Leece A, Bohane T. Congenital short gut, malrotation, and dysmotility of the small bowel. J Pediatr Gastroenterol Nutr. 1990;11:411–5.
7. Schuffler MD, Pagon RA, Schwartz R, Bill AH. Visceral myopathy of the gastrointestinal and genitourinary tracts in infants. Gastroenterology. 1988;94:892–8.
8. Krishnamurthy S, Heng S, Schuffler M. Chronic intestinal pseudo-obstruction in infants and children caused by diverse abnormalities of myenteric plexus. Gastroenterology. 1993;104:1398–408.
9. Ciftci AO, Cook RCM, Van Velzen D. Megacystic microcolon intestinal hypoperistalsis syndrome: evidence of a primary myocellular defect of contractile fiber synthesis. J Pediatr Surg. 1996;31:1706–11.
10. Feldstein AE, Miller SM, El-Youssef M, et al. Chronic intestinal pseudoobstruction associated with altered interstitial cells of cajal networks. J Pediatr Gastroenterol Nutr. 2003;36:492–7.
11. Kohler M, Pease PW, Upadhyay V. Megacystis-microcolon-intestinal hypoperistalsis syndrome (MMIHS) in siblings: case report and review of the literature. Eur J Pediatr Surg. 2004;14:362–7.

12. De Giorgio R, Sarnelli G, Corinaldesi R, Stanghellini V. Advances in our understanding of the pathology of chronic intestinal pseudo-obstruction. Gut. 2004;53:1549–52.
13. Gilbert J, Ibdah JA. Intestinal pseudo-obstruction as a manifestation of impaired mitochondrial fatty acid oxidation. Med Hypotheses. 2005;64:586–9.
14. Stanghellini V, Cogliandro RF, De Giorgio R, Barbara G, Cremon C, Antonucci A, Fronzoni L, Cogliandro L, Naponelli V, Serra M, Corinaldesi R. Natural history of intestinal failure induced by chronic idiopathic intestinal pseudo-obstruction. Transplant Proc. 2010; 42:15–8.
15. Wedel T, Tafazzoli K, Sollner S, Krammer HJ, Aring C, Holschneider AM. Mitochondrial myopathy (complex I deficiency) associated with chronic intestinal pseudo-obstruction. Eur J Pediatr Surg. 2003; 13:201–5.
16. Galmiche L, Jaubert F, Sauvat F, Sarnacki S, Goulet O, Assouline Z, Vedrenne V, Lebre AS, Boddaert N, Brousse N, Chrétien D, Munnich A, Rötig A. Normal oxidative phosphorylation in intestinal smooth muscle of childhood chronic intestinal pseudo-obstruction. Neurogastroenterol Motil. 2010;23(1):24–9.
17. Di Lorenzo C, Youssef NN. Diagnosis and management of intestinal motility disorders. Semin Pediatr Surg. 2010;19:50–8.
18. Lapointe SP, Rivet C, Goulet O, Fekete CN, Lortat-Jacob S. Urological manifestations associated with chronic intestinal pseudo-obstructions in children. J Urol. 2002;168:1768–70.
19. Vargas J, Sachs P, Ament ME. Chronic intestinal pseudo-obstruction syndrome in pediatrics. Results of a national survey by members of the NASPGN. J Pediatr Gastroenterol Nutr. 1988;7:323–32.
20. Nonaka M, Goulet O, Arhan P, et al. Primary intestinal myopathy, a cause of chronic intestinal pseudo-obstruction syndrome. Pediatr Pathol. 1989;9:409–24.
21. Faure C, Goulet O, Ategbo S, et al. Chronic intestinal pseudoobstruction syndrome. Clinical analysis, outcome, and prognosis in 105 children. Dig Dis Sci. 1999;44:953–9.
22. Heneyke S, Smith VV, Spitz L, Milla PJ. Chronic intestinal pseudo-obstruction: treatment and long term follow up of 44 patients. Arch Dis Child. 1999;81:21–7.
23. Goulet O, Jobert-Giraud A, Michel J-L, et al. Chronic intestinal pseudo-obstruction syndrome in pediatric patients. Eur J Pediatr Surg. 1999;9:83–90.
24. Stanghellini V, Cogliandro RF, de Giorgio R, Barbara G, Salvioli B, Corinaldesi R. Chronic intestinal pseudo-obstruction: manifestations, natural history and management. Neurogastroenterol Motil. 2007;19:440–52.
25. Cogliandro RF, De Giorgio R, Barbara G, Cogliandro L, Concordia A, Corinaldesi R, Stanghellini V. Chronic intestinal pseudo-obstruction. Best Pract Res Clin Gastroenterol. 2007;21:657–69.
26. Cucchiara S, Borrelli O. Nutritional challenge in pseudo-obstruction: the bridge between motility and nutrition. J Pediatr Gastroenterol Nutr. 2009;48 Suppl 2:S83–5.
27. Gariepy CE, Mousa H. Clinical management of motility disorders in children. Semin Pediatr Surg. 2009;18:224–38.
28. Kaufman SS, Loseke CA, Lupo JV, et al. Influence of bacterial overgrowth and intestinal inflammation on duration of PN in children with short bowel syndrome. J Pediatr. 1997;131:356–61.
29. Forchielli ML, Walker WA. Nutritional factors contributing to the development of cholestasis during total parenteral nutrition. Dev Pediatr. 2003;50:245–67.
30. Irtan S, Bellaïche M, Brasher C, ElGhoneimi A, Cézard JP, Bonnard A. Stomal prolapse in children with chronic intestinal pseudoobstruction: a frequent complication? J Pediatr Surg. 2010;45:2234–7.
31. Nitsche H, Pirker ME, Montedonico S, Hoellwarth ME. Creation of enteral shortcuts as a therapeutic option in children with chronic idiopathic intestinal pseudoobstruction. J Pediatr Gastroenterol Nutr. 2007;44:643–5.
32. Einwächter H, Hellerhoff P, Neu B, Prinz C, Schmid R, Meining A. Percutaneous endoscopic colostomy in a patient with chronic intestinal pseudo-obstruction and massive dilation of the colon. Endoscopy. 2006;38:547.
33. Lynch CR, Jones RG, Hilden K, Wills JC, Fang JC. Percutaneous endoscopic cecostomy in adults: a case series. Gastrointest Endosc. 2006;64:279–82.
34. Bertolini D, De Saussure P, Chilcott M, Girardin M, Dumonceau JM. Severe delayed complication after percutaneous endoscopic colostomy for chronic intestinal pseudo-obstruction: a case report and review of the literature. World J Gastroenterol. 2007; 13:2255–7.
35. Altaf MA, Werlin SL, Sato TT, Rudolph CD, Sood MR. Colonic volvulus in children with intestinal motility disorders. J Pediatr Gastroenterol Nutr. 2009;49:59–62.
36. Nayci A, Avlan D, Polat A, Aksoyek S. Treatment of intestinal pseudo obstruction by segmental resection. Pediatr Surg Int. 2003;19:44–6.
37. Shibata C, Naito H, Funayama Y, et al. Surgical treatment of chronic intestinal pseudo-obstruction: report of three cases. Surg Today. 2003;33:58–61.
38. Colomb V, Dabbas-Tyan M, Taupin P, Talbotec C, Révillon Y, Jan D, De Potter S, Gorski-Colin AM, Lamor M, Herreman K, Corriol O, Landais P, Ricour C, Goulet O. Long-term outcome of children receiving home parenteral nutrition: a 20-year single-center experience in 302 patients. J Pediatr Gastroenterol Nutr. 2007;44:347–53.
39. Mughal MM, Irving MH. Treatment of end stage chronic intestinal pseudo-obstruction by subtotal enterectomy and home parenteral nutrition. Gut. 1988;29:1613–7.

40. Lapointe R. Chronic idiopathic intestinal pseudo-obstruction treated by near total small bowel resection: a 20-year experience. J Gastrointest Surg. 2010;14(12):1937–42.
41. Khelif K, Scaillon M, Govaerts MJ, Vanderwinden JM, De Laet MH. Bilateral thoracoscopic splanchnicectomy in chronic intestinal pseudo-obstruction: report of two paediatric cases. Gut. 2006;55:293–4.
42. Andersson S, Lonroth H, Simren M, et al. Gastric electrical stimulation for intractable vomiting in patients with chronic intestinal pseudoobstruction. Neurogastroenterol Motil. 2006;18:823–30.
43. Goulet O, Lacaille F, Jan D, Ricour C. Intestinal transplantation: indications, results and strategy. Curr Opin Clin Nutr Metab Care. 2000;3:329–38.
44. Grant D, Abu-Elmagd K, Reyes J, Tzakis A, Langnas A, Fishbein T, Goulet O, Farmer D, On behalf of the Intestine Transplant Registry. 2003 report of the intestine transplant registry: a new era has dawned. Ann Surg. 2005;241:607–13.
45. Mazariegos GV, Squires RH, Sindhi RK. Current perspectives on pediatric intestinal transplantation. Curr Gastroenterol Rep. 2009;11:226–33.
46. Gambarara M, Knafelz D, Diamanti A, Ferretti F, Papadatou B, Sabbi T, Castro M. Indication for small bowel transplant in patients affected by chronic intestinal pseudo-obstruction. Transplant Proc. 2002;34:866–7.
47. Loinaz C, Mittal N, Kato T, Miller B, Rodriguez M, Tzakis A. Multivisceral transplantation for pediatric intestinal pseudo-obstruction: single center's experience of 16 cases. Transplant Proc. 2004;36:312–3.
48. Masetti M, Di Benedetto F, Cautero N, et al. Intestinal transplantation for chronic intestinal pseudo-obstruction in adult patients. Am J Transplant. 2004;4:826–9.
49. Bond GJ, Reyes JD. Intestinal transplantation for total/near-total aganglionosis and intestinal pseudo-obstruction. Semin Pediatr Surg. 2004;13:286–92.
50. Colledan M, Stroppa P, Bravi M, Casotti V, Lucianetti A, Pinelli D, Zambelli M, Guizzetti M, Corno V, Aluffi A, Sonzogni V, Sonzogni A, D'Antiga L, Codazzi D. Intestinal transplantation in children: the first successful Italian series. Transplant Proc. 2010;42:1251–2.
51. Goulet O, Ruemmele F, Lacaille F, Colomb V. Irreversible intestinal failure. J Pediatr Gastroenterol Nutr. 2004;38:250–69.
52. Silk DB. Chronic idiopathic intestinal pseudo-obstruction: the need for a multidisciplinary approach to management. Proc Nutr Soc. 2004;63:473–80.

Index

C. Faure et al. (eds.), *Pediatric Neurogastroenterology: Gastrointestinal Motility and Functional Disorders in Children*, Clinical Gastroenterology,
DOI 10.1007/978-1-60761-709-9, © Springer Science+Business Media New York 2013

B

C

D

E

H

I

K

L

M

Q

R

Printed by Printforce, the Netherlands